BRITISH COLUMBIA CANCER AGENCY
LIBRARY
600 WEST 10th AVE.

D0554000

BRITISH COLUMBIA CANCER AGENCY
LIBRARY
600 WEST 10th AVE.
VANCOUVER, B.C.   CANADA
V5Z 4E6

BONE MARROW AND STEM CELL PROCESSING:
A Manual of Current Techniques

BONE MARROW AND STEM CELL PROCESSING:
A Manual of Current Techniques

ELLEN M. AREMAN, S.B.B.(ASCP)
Bone Marrow Processing Laboratory
Division of Transfusion Medicine
Georgetown University Hospital
Washington, D.C.

H. JOACHIM DEEG, M.D.
Fred Hutchinson Cancer Research Center
Bone Marrow Transplantation Program
University of Washington
Seattle, Washington

RONALD A. SACHER, MB, BCH, DTM&H, FRCP(C)
Professor of Medicine and Pathology
Director, Transfusion Medicine
Georgetown University Hospital
Washington, D.C.

 F. A. Davis Company • Philadelphia

Copyright © 1992 by F. A. Davis Company

All rights reserved. This book is protected by copyright. No part of it may be reproduced, stored in a retrieval system, or transmitted in any form or by any means, electronic, mechanical, photocopying, recording, or otherwise, without written permission from the publisher.

Printed in the United States of America

Last digit indicates print number: 10 9 8 7 6 5 4 3 2 1

acquisitions editor: Robert G. Martone
production editor: Rose Gabbay
cover design by: Donald B. Freggens, Jr.

As new scientific information becomes available through basic and clinical research, recommended treatments and drug therapies undergo changes. The author(s) and publisher have done everything possible to make this book accurate, up to date, and in accord with accepted standards at the time of publication. The authors, editors, and publisher are not responsible for errors or omissions or for consequences from application of the book, and make no warranty, expressed or implied, in regard to the contents of the book. Any practice described in this book should be applied by the reader in accordance with professional standards of care used in regard to the unique circumstances that may apply in each situation. The reader is advised always to check product information (package inserts) for changes and new information regarding dose and contraindications before administering any drug. Caution is especially urged when using new or infrequently ordered drugs.

Library of Congress Cataloging-in-Publication Data

Bone marrow and stem cell processing : a manual of current techniques
  [edited by] Ellen M. Areman, H. Joachim Deeg, Ronald A. Sacher.
     p. cm.
   Includes bibliographical references and index.
   ISBN 0-8036-0266-9 (hardbound : alk. paper)
    1. Bone marrow—Transplantation.   2. Hematopoietic stem cells—
Transplantation. I. Areman, Ellen M., 1943- . II. Deeg, H. J. (Hans Joachim),
1945- . III. Sacher, Ronald A.
    [DNLM: 1. Bone Marrow—cytology. 2. Bone Marrow Transplantation—
methods. 3. Stem Cells—cytology. 4. Stem Cells—transplantation.
WH 380 B7085]
RD123.5.B647 1992
617.4′4—dc20
DNLM/DLC
for Library of Congress   92-4730
                                                          CIP

Authorization to photocopy items for internal or personal use, or the internal or personal use of specific clients, is granted by F.A. Davis Company for users registered with the Copyright Clearance Center (CCC) Transactional Reporting Service, provided that the fee of $.10 per copy is paid directly to CCC, 27 Congress St., Salem, MA 01970. For those organizations that have been granted a photocopy license by CCC, a separate system of payment has been arranged. The fee code for users of the Transactional Reporting Service is: 8036-0266/92 0 + $.10.

Foreword

More than four decades ago Jacobson and colleagues showed that mice exposed to otherwise lethal doses of total body irradiation would survive if the spleen were shielded. It was first thought that a humoral factor, released from the spleen, stimulated recovery of hemopoiesis. Subsequent experiments showed, however, that mice also survived if normal spleen or marrow cells were infused and that lympho-hemopoietic reconstitution was accomplished by donor-derived cells. At the same time, it was noted that mice receiving transplants from genetically different (allogeneic) but not from genetically identical (syngeneic) donors developed a syndrome which is now known as graft-versus-host disease (GVHD), i.e., the clinical manifestations of a reaction of donor-derived lymphoid cells, in particular T lymphocytes, against antigens on recipient cells that were not present in the donor. Soon a similar syndrome was also observed in patients receiving transplants from an allogeneic donor.

Studies in animal models demonstrated that GVHD could be completely prevented even with transplants across major histocompatibility barriers if T lymphocytes were removed in vitro before marrow infusion. Therefore, similar approaches were taken in clinical marrow transplantation, using polyclonal or monoclonal antibodies, immunotoxins, chemical compounds with predominant anti-T-cell reactivity, and physical separation procedures. In vitro elimination of T lymphocytes from human marrow, although successful in preventing GVHD, resulted in an unacceptably high incidence of graft failure as well as an increased incidence of leukemic relapse. Apparently, some T lymphocytes or certain subpopulations of cells that were eliminated during marrow treatment in vitro were necessary to ensure engraftment. In fact, several investigators have since undertaken studies in which the marrow was aggressively depleted of T lymphocytes and subsequently graded numbers of lymphocytes were added back to facilitate engraftment. Unfortunately, problems with engraftment were encountered, particularly in those patients who needed GVHD prophylaxis most, that is, in those given transplants from donors not completely HLA-matched with the recipient.

Because of complications associated with allogeneic transplants and because a suitable donor cannot be found for every patient, attempts have been made to utilize the patients' own (autologous) bone marrow. It was thought that in certain diseases in which hemopoietic stem cells were not directly affected, such as in patients with lymphoma or acute leukemia, it should be possible to eliminate malignant cells and retain hemopoietic stem cells which would be capable of reconstituting hemopoiesis in the patient after marrow ablative cytotoxic therapy. It is clear now that autologous marrow can be used successfully in certain patients. However, frequently hemopoietic reconstitution has been incomplete, suggesting that functionally impaired or insufficient numbers of stem cells have been transplanted. In others, the underlying malignant disease recurred early after transplantation, suggesting the possibility of infusion of malignant cells with the autologous marrow.

To improve the cell yield and the probability of successful autologous transplantation, investigators are now using peripheral blood stem cells. Animal models had shown earlier that precursor cells with the potential of repopulating marrow were circulating in peripheral blood. We now know that this is true for humans as well. The frequency of these cells in blood can be increased by treating the patient with moderate doses of cytotoxic agents such as cyclophosphamide, and more recent studies show that these "peripheral" stem cells can be used as the only source of stem cells for transplantation.

Finally, modern approaches to marrow transplantation have reawakened an interest in Jacobson's early speculation that a humoral factor released from the spleen may play a role in hemopoietic reconstitution. A series of cytokines and hemopoietic growth factors originally isolated from spleen cells and other lympho-hemopoietic tissues are now available as a result of recombinant molecular biological research, and many are currently undergoing clinical investigation. Studies have clearly shown that the administration of factors such as G-CSF or GM-CSF after transplantation can accelerate hemopoietic reconstitution in both the allogeneic and the autologous setting. Also, administration of these factors to patients before peripheral blood stem cell harvest increases the yield and the repopulating ability of these cells in autologous transplantation.

This manual summarizes in vivo and in vitro techniques of marrow and peripheral blood stem cell harvesting, enrichment, cryopreservation, and transplantation. Immense progress has been made over only a few decades. The techniques described in this manual represent the current state of the art and should be useful for all who work in this field.

E. Donnall Thomas, M.D.
Seattle, WA

Preface

Thirty years ago, when bone marrow transplantation was in its infancy, bone marrow was processed minimally, if at all. The researchers involved in these experimental procedures used materials available to them in the tissue culture laboratory to dilute and anticoagulate the marrow. When Drs. Thomas and Storb published their procedure for collecting, filtering, and transplanting marrow grafts in 1970, the literature of bone marrow processing had its beginning. Since those early days, which in actual fact were relatively recent, the discipline of in vitro manipulation of marrow and peripheral blood stem cells has been rapidly expanding.

As the numbers and types of transplants increased, some of these "experimental procedures" started to become more or less "routine" within the institution and found their way into clinical applications. Such techniques as red blood cell and plasma removal for ABO-mismatched transplants and cryopreservation of autologous bone marrow could be performed more expeditiously by a trained technical staff than by the workers in the research laboratory. However, as immune aberrations and hemopoietic reconstitution have become better understood in both transplantation and tumor biology, more elaborate methods of purifying, enriching, and purging the marrow have been and continue to be developed. As the research laboratory explores and develops these new techniques, the processing laboratory must be a partner in translating the experimental studies into working clinical protocols.

For those of us involved in these research/clinical partnerships, the work can be exciting, challenging, and, on occasion, intimidating. Often the translation of a procedure from the test tube to the marrow bag can be a difficult one involving many hours of developmental work. The processing laboratory often finds itself in an identity crisis, fitting comfortably in neither the clinical service area nor in the research and development sphere. Yet it is probably this unique combination and variety of tasks involved in marrow and peripheral stem cell processing, purging, and cryopreservation that makes the cell processing laboratory an exciting place to work.

Many of us have visited other centers in order to observe, and occasionally to perform, some of the processing and purging techniques being used. All of us have telephoned other processing laboratories, sometimes in desperation, for help in performing a particular procedure or for advice on how to proceed when a problem has arisen. It is to these people, both the helpers and the helped, that this book is dedicated. A book can never take the place of individual instruction or personal discussion, but our hope is that it will have a useful place, near at hand in the laboratory.

We are grateful to all of the laboratory personnel who were so generous in sharing their techniques with us. Some are quite similar to others, differing primarily in the instrumentation or the materials used. However, because some items may not be easily accessible internationally, we wanted to include as broad a variety as possible in the hope that our counterparts around the world could also benefit from this work. The techniques described in this volume are assumed to be accurate. Those individuals who have shared them with us are cited in the text should the need arise to contact them.

Although we have attempted to include as many of the different techniques currently in use as possible, not all the marrow and stem cell processing and purging procedures available are included in this book. Because the field is expanding so rapidly, with new methods appearing almost daily, this manual would never have been published had we attempted to incorporate every new technique. It is our hope, however, that the methods presented will encompass most situations where there is a need to further process or purge marrow or other hematopoietic stem cells intended for transplantation.

The editors would like to acknowledge Janice M. Davis, M.T. (ASCP), S.B.B., Cell Processing Laboratory, The Johns Hopkins Oncology Center, Baltimore, Maryland and Thomas R. Spitzer, M.D., Bone Marrow Transplant Program, Georgetown University Hospital, Washington, D.C., who also served as contributing editors.

Ellen M. Areman
H. Joachim Deeg
Ronald A. Sacher

Contributors

Tauseef Ahmed, M.D.
Bone Marrow Transplantation
Services
New York Medical College
Valhalla, New York

Ellen M. Areman,
S.B.B.(ASCP)
Bone Marrow Processing
Laboratory
Division of Transfusion Medicine
Georgetown University Hospital
Washington, D.C.

Kelvin Bailey, B.S.
Department of Medicine
University of Kentucky Medical
Center
Lexington, Kentucky

Edward D. Ball, M.D.
University of Pittsburgh
Pittsburgh Cancer Institute
Pittsburgh, Pennsylvania

Susan Barker, C.T.
University of Chicago Medical
Center
Chicago, Illinois

Bonny Bass, B.S.
Life Technologies, Inc.
Gaithersburg, Maryland

Eric X. Beck, B.S.
Ohio State University
Pediatric Bone Marrow
Transplantation Program
Columbus, Ohio

Suzanne Beckner, Ph.D.
Life Technologies, Inc.
Gaithersburg, Maryland

Barbara E. Bierer, M.D.
Hematology-Oncology Division
Brigham and Women's Hospital
Division of Pediatric Oncology
Dana-Farber Cancer Institute
Boston, Massachusetts

Sharon A. Bleau, M.S.
Memorial Sloan-Kettering Cancer
Center
New York, New York

Ridha Bouzgarou, M.D.
Centre Régional de Transfusion
Sanguine de Bordeaux
Bordeaux, France

Hal E. Broxmeyer, Ph.D.
Walther Oncology Center
Indiana University School of
Medicine
Indianapolis, Indiana

Regina Bryan
Hahnemann University
Philadelphia, Pennsylvania

Stephen Bulova, M.D.
Hahnemann University
Philadelphia, Pennsylvania

ix

Anne Canty, R.N.
Apheresis Unit
Institute of Medical and Veterinary
Science
Adelaide, South Australia

Carmelo Carlo-Stella
Department of Hematology
Bone Marrow Transplantation
Unit
University of Parma
Parma, Italy

Charles S. Carter
Special Services Laboratory
Department of Transfusion
Medicine
National Institutes of Health
Bethesda, Maryland

Richard Champlin, M.D.
The University of Texas M.D.
Anderson Cancer Center
Houston, Texas

K. W. Chan, M.B., B.S., FRCP(C)
Bone Marrow Transplant Program
British Columbia Children's
Hospital
Vancouver, British Columbia
Canada

Niculae Ciobanu, M.D.
Montefiore Medical Center
Bronx, New York

Nancy H. Collins, Ph.D.
Memorial Sloan-Kettering Cancer
Center
New York, New York

Scott Cooper, B.S.
Walther Oncology Center
Indiana University School of
Medicine
Indianapolis, Indiana

Michele Cottler-Fox, M.D.
National Institutes of Health
Department of Transfusion
Medicine
Bethesda, Maryland

Gérald Cristol, M.D.
Centre Régional de Transfusion
Sanguine de Bordeaux
Bordeaux, France

Herbert Cullis, B.S.
Fenwal Division
Baxter Healthcare
Deerfield, Illinois

Janice M. Davis, M.T.(ASCP), S.B.B.
Cell Processing Laboratory
The Johns Hopkins Oncology
Center
Baltimore, Maryland

H. Joachim Deeg, M.D.
Fred Hutchinson Cancer Research
Center
Bone Marrow Transplantation
Program
University of Washington
Seattle, Washington

Larry G. Dickson, M.D.
Clinical Laboratory
University of Kentucky Medical
Center
Lexington, Kentucky

Sarah F. Donnelly, M.T.(ASCP),
S.B.B.
University of Virginia Health
Sciences Center
Blood Bank and Transfusion
Services
Charlottesville, Virginia

Albert D. Donnenberg, Ph.D.
The Johns Hopkins Oncology
Center
Baltimore, Maryland

Gordon Douglas, M.D.
Department of Obstetrics and
Gynecology
New York University Medical
Center
New York, New York

Rory D. Duncan, SSG, U.S. Army
Brooke Army Medical Center
Department of Clinical
Investigation
Fort Sam Houston, Texas

Pamela G. Dyson, B.Sc. (Hons)
Leukaemia Research Unit
Institute of Medical and Veterinary
Science
Adelaide, South Australia

Denis English, Ph.D.
Bone Marrow Transplant
Laboratory
Methodist Hospital of Indiana
Indianapolis, Indiana

Mary Jane Farmelo, B.A., C.L.Sp.
(CG)
Bone Marrow Processing and
Evaluation Laboratory
H. Lee Moffitt Cancer Center and
Research Institute
University of South Florida
Tampa, Florida

Linda S. Fox, M.T.(ASCP)
Bone Marrow Transplant Program
University Hospital
Denver, Colorado

Naohisa Fujita, M.D.
Second Department of Medicine
Kyoto Prefectural University of
Medicine
Kyoto, Japan

Adrian P. Gee, Ph.D.
Department of Pediatrics
University of Florida
Gainesville, Florida

and

Baxter Healthcare Corporation
Santa Ana, California

Holly Goetzman, M.T.(ASCP)
Special Services Laboratory
Department of Transfusion
Medicine
National Institutes of Health
Bethesda, Maryland

N.C. Gorin, M.D.
Bone Marrow Transplantation
Unit
Centre National de Transfusion
Sanguine
Hôpital Sainte-Antoine
Paris, France

Vicki L. Graves, M.T.(ASCP)
Indiana University Hospital
Indianapolis, Indiana

Mary Ann Gross, M.T.(ASCP)
Shands Hospital
University of Florida
Gainesville, Florida

Samuel Gross, M.D.
Pediatric Hematology/Oncology
Bone Marrow Transplant Unit
University of Florida
Gainesville, Florida

Françoise Hau, M.D.
Centre Régional de Transfusion
Sanguine de Bordeaux
Bordeaux, France

David N. Haylock, B.App.Sc.
Leukaemia Research Unit
Department of Haematology
Institute of Medical and Veterinary
Science
Adelaide, South Australia

P. Jean Henslee-Downey, M.D.
Department of Medicine
University of Kentucky Medical
Center
Lexington, Kentucky

Sharon Herd, A.R.T.
British Columbia Children's
Hospital
Vancouver, British Columbia
Canada

G. P. Herzig, M.D.
Washington University School of
Medicine
St. Louis, Missouri

Roger H. Herzig, M.D.
James Graham Brown Cancer
Center
University of Louisville
Louisville, Kentucky

Marita G. Hill, M.T.(ASCP), S.B.B.
University of Kentucky Medical
Center
Lexington, Kentucky

Kristi Hollingsworth, M.A.
University of Chicago Medical
Center
Chicago, Illinois

Alix L. Howell, Ph.D.
Dartmouth-Hitchcock Medical
Center
Hanover, New Hampshire

Charles E. Hutcheson, M.T.(ASCP)
Shands Hospital
University of Florida
Gainesville, Florida

Tohru Inaba, M.D.
Second Department of Medicine
Kyoto Prefectural University of
Medicine
Kyoto, Japan

Jan Jansen, M.D.
Methodist Hospital
Indianapolis, Indiana

William E. Janssen, Ph.D.
Bone Marrow Processing and
Evaluation Laboratory
Bone Marrow Transplant Program
H. Lee Moffitt Cancer Center and
Research Institute
University of South Florida
Tampa, Florida

Elaine K. Jeter, M.D.
Medical University of South
Carolina
Charleston, South Carolina

Robert Jiang, M.T.(ACSP)
Mount Sinai Medical Center
New York, New York

Nancy L. Johnson, M.T.(ASCP),
S.B.B.
Memorial Blood Center of
Minneapolis
Minneapolis, Minnesota

Charles S. Johnston, M.T.(AMT)
Bone Marrow Transplant Program
University Hospital
Denver, Colorado

Christopher A. Juttner, M.B.,
B.Med.Sc., FRACP
Division of Haematology
Institute of Medical and Veterinary
Science
Adelaide, South Australia

and
Royal Adelaide Hospital
Adelaide, South Australia

Neena Kapoor, M.D.
Ohio State University
Pediatric Bone Marrow
Transplantation Program
Columbus, Ohio

Nancy A. Kernan, M.D.
Memorial Sloan-Kettering Cancer
Center
New York, New York

Anne Kessinger, M.D.
University of Nebraska
Medical Center
Omaha, Nebraska

Arnalda Lanfranchi, Ph.D.
Ohio State University
Pediatric Bone Marrow
Transplantation Program
Columbus, Ohio

Larry C. Lasky, M.D.
Memorial Blood Center of
Minneapolis
Minneapolis, Minnesota

Miriam F. Leach, M.T. (ASCP), S.B.B.
Dartmouth-Hitchcock Medical
Center
Hanover, New Hampshire

Jane Lebkowski, Ph.D.
Applied Immune Sciences Inc.
Menlo Park, California

Carlos E. Lee, M.T.
Bone Marrow Processing and
Evaluation Laboratory
Bone Marrow Transplant Program
H. Lee Moffitt Cancer Center and
Research Institute
University of South Florida
Tampa, Florida

Kyoung Lee, M.T.
University of California, Los
Angeles Center
for Health Sciences
Los Angeles, California

Lina Mangoni
Department of Hematology
Bone Marrow Transplantation
Unit
University of Parma
Parma, Italy

Ewa Marciniak, M.D.
Department of Medicine
University of Kentucky Medical
Center
Lexington, Kentucky

Leo J. McCarthy, M.D.
Indiana University Hospital
Indianapolis, Indiana

Ann McMican, M.S., M.T.(ASCP),
S.B.B.
University of Rochester School of
Medicine and Dentistry
Rochester, New York

Richard C. Meagher, Ph.D.
James Graham Brown Cancer
Center
University of Louisville
Louisville, Kentucky

Satoshi Murakami, M.D.
Second Department of Medicine
Kyoto Prefectural University of
Medicine
Kyoto, Japan

Masao Nakagawa, M.D.
Second Department of Medicine
Kyoto Prefectural University of
Medicine
Kyoto, Japan

Robert Negrin, M.D.
Hematology Department
Stanford University Hospital
Stanford, California

Doris Neurath, A.R.T.
Transfusion Medicine
Foothills Hospital
Calgary, Alberta
Canada

Stephen J. Noga, M.D., Ph.D.
The Johns Hopkins Oncology
Center
Baltimore, Maryland

Thomas Okarma, Ph.D., M.D.
Applied Immune Sciences, Inc.
Menlo Park, California

David H. Oldenburg
Section of Hematology/Oncology
Loyola University Medical Center
Maywood, Illinois

Richard J. O'Reilly, M.D.
Memorial Sloan-Kettering Cancer
Center
New York, New York

Gerda Pirsch, M.S.
University of Virginia Health
Sciences Center
Charlottesville, Virginia

John Graham Pole, M.D.
Pediatric Hematology/Oncology
Bone Marrow Transplant Unit
University of Florida
Gainesville, Florida

Robert Preti, Ph.D.
Hudson Valley Blood Services
Valhalla, New York

Elizabeth J. Read, M.D.
Department of Pathology
University of Utah Medical Center
Salt Lake City, Utah

Barbara A. Reeb, M.T.(ASCP)
Brooke Army Medical Center
Department of Clinical
Investigation
Fort Sam Houston, Texas

Josy Reiffers, M.D.
Bone Marrow Transplant Unit
Centre Hospitalier Régional
Bordeaux, France

Vittorio Rizzoli, M.D.
Department of Hematology
Bone Marrow Transplantation Unit
University of Parma
Parma, Italy

Vickie M. Robertson, M.T.(ASCP),
S.B.B.
University of Kentucky Medical
Center
Lexington, Kentucky

Oksana Rosina, M.T.(ASCP)
Mount Sinai Medical Center
New York, New York

Ruth E. Ross, M.H.S., M.T.(ASCP),
S.B.B.
Medical University of South
Carolina
Charleston, South Carolina

Scott D. Rowley, M.D., FACP
Fred Hutchinson Cancer Research
Center
Seattle, Washington

Ronald A. Sacher, MB, BcH, DTM&H,
FRCP(C)
Division of Transfusion Medicine
Georgetown University Hospital
Washington, D.C.

Lamia M. Schwarz, B.S.
Dartmouth-Hitchcock Medical
Center
Hanover, New Hampshire

Eileen Scigliano, M.D.
Mount Sinai Medical Center
New York, New York

Chichiro Shimazaki, M.D.
Second Department of Medicine
Kyoto Prefectural University of
Medicine
Kyoto, Japan

Elizabeth J. Shpall, M.D.
Bone Marrow Transplant Program
University Hospital
Denver, Colorado

Mark Singer
Biomedicon
Moorestown, New Jersey

Lorraine Y. Soken, M.T.(ASCP)
St. Francis Medical Center
Department of Pathology
Tissue Bank
Honolulu, Hawaii

Thomas R. Spitzer, M.D.
Bone Marrow Transplant Program
Georgetown University Hospital
Washington, D.C.

Carol Stanley, A.R.T.
British Columbia Children's
Hospital
Vancouver, British Columbia
Canada

Patrick J. Stiff, M.D.
Section of Hematology/Oncology
Loyola University Medical Center
Maywood, Illinois

Robert K. Stuart, M.D.
Medical University of South
Carolina
Charleston, South Carolina

Donna Tabrizi, M.D.
Mount Sinai Medical Center
New York, New York

Christopher J. Thoburn, B.S.
The Johns Hopkins Oncology
Center
Baltimore, Maryland

John S. Thompson, M.D.
Department of Medicine
University of Kentucky Medical
Center
Lexington, Kentucky

Lynda Thoreen, R.N.
American Red Cross
Midwest Region
Omaha, Nebraska

Dawn Thorp, R.N.
Apheresis Unit
Institute of Medical and Veterinary
Science
Adelaide, South Australia

Luen Bik To, M.D., M.B.B.S.
Leukemia Research Unit
Division of Haematology
Institute of Medical and Veterinary
Science
Adelaide, South Australia

and
Royal Adelaide Hospital
Adelaide, South Australia

Gérard Vezon, M.D.
Centre Régional de Transfusion
Sanguine de Bordeaux
Bordeaux, France

L. D. Wadsworth, M.B., FRCP(C),
FRCPath
Hematopathology/
Immunohematology
British Columbia Children's
Hospital
Vancouver, British Columbia
Canada

Roy S. Weiner, M.D.
University of Florida
Gainesville, Florida

Robert G. Whiddon, Ph.D.
Brooke Army Medical Center
Department of Clinical
Investigation
Fort Sam Houston, Texas

Stephanie F. Williams, M.D.
University of Chicago Medical
Center
Chicago, Illinois

Mitsi Wood, B.S.
University of Virginia Health
Sciences Center
Charlottesville, Virginia

David Wuest, M.D.
Hudson Valley Blood Services
Valhalla, New York

Jean T. Yao, M.S., S.B.B.(ASCP)
Blood Bank
Methodist Medical Center
Peoria, Illinois

Shengly Zhou, M.D.
Mount Sinai Medical Center
New York, New York

Contents

Chapter 11 QUALITY ASSURANCE IN MARROW PROCESSING 386

BONE MARROW PROCESSING FOR TRANSPLANTATION

1

Commentary by RONALD A. SACHER and ELLEN M. AREMAN

Although early transplants were generally ineffective, work in the late 1960s elucidating the human histocompatibility antigens opened the door to successful bone marrow transplantation between HLA-identical siblings.[1,2] Recently, indications for bone marrow transplantation have increased, and the number of transplants carried out annually has grown. Of the 9500 transplants performed between 1955 and 1984, 50 percent were performed in 1983 and 1984 alone.[3] The total number of bone marrow transplants that have been performed has now risen to more than 20,000 throughout the world.[4] Today allogeneic bone marrow transplantation is performed for acute and chronic leukemias,[3,5,6] Hodgkin's and non-Hodgkin's lymphomas,[6] myelofibrosis,[4] congenital immunodeficiencies,[7] and severe aplastic anemia.[3,6,8] Some successful results have also been reported with allogeneic transplantation for thalassemia, thrombasthenia, osteopetrosis, and other inherited metabolic abnormalities.[7]

Autologous transplantation can play an important role to rescue patients from intensive chemoradiotherapy for certain acute leukemias,[9] Hodgkin's and non-Hodgkin's lymphomas,[10,11] multiple myeloma,[11] and selected solid tumors.[12,13] Transplantation of autologous peripheral blood stem cells has recently become an option for those patients for whom allogeneic and conventional autologous bone marrow transplantation are not possible.[14–16] Promising experimental work is currently being done in the areas of transplantion of cultured autologous bone marrow for chronic myelogenous leukemia,[17–19] transplantation of purified hematopoietic stem cells,[20] transplantation of umbilical cord blood,[21] and gene replacement therapy using genetically engineered hematopoietic stem cells.[22,23] All of these uses for bone marrow transplantation bring with them the requirement for specific treatment of the marrow before it can be infused into the recipient. This section summarizes the categories of bone marrow processing that are covered in detail in later chapters.

BONE MARROW COLLECTION

Bone marrow is usually harvested, using specially designed stainless steel needles, from the posterior iliac crest, although the anterior crest and sternum are occasionally used if the yield from the primary site is likely to be insufficient. Marrow is collected into glass or plastic luer-lock syringes in aliquots of 2 to 10 mL and placed in a sterile container (usually a stainless steel beaker)[1]

1

containing tissue culture medium with heparin to prevent coagulation.[13] These media, originally developed for in vitro culturing of mammalian cells, contain combinations of electrolytes, buffers, amino acids, and vitamins or minerals or both. It is probable that many of these ingredients are unnecessary for storage of aspirated marrow for the short period of time between harvest and infusion or processing. Work in the area of blood component collection and storage has demonstrated the superiority of other anticoagulants such as acid-citrate-dextrose (ACD), citrate-phosphate-dextrose (CPD), and CPD-adenine (CPDA-1) over heparin for preservation of red blood cells, platelets, granulocytes, and lymphocytes.[24]

Immediately following the harvest, usually in the operating room, the collected marrow is filtered through a number of stainless steel mesh screens (usually 300- and 200-μm mesh size) to remove small clots, bone fragments, fat, and fibrin and is transferred to a sterile container (usually a blood bag) that is sealed and labeled.

Following the initial processing, the bone marrow may need to undergo a number of additional manipulations before it is suitable for infusion into an allogeneic or autologous recipient. Indeed, the only time that a bone marrow graft may be infused without any further processing is when the donor and recipient are ABO identical. Even in these cases many centers choose to reduce the volume of the infused marrow, as discussed in Chapters 6 and 7.

PERIPHERAL BLOOD STEM CELL COLLECTION

Even under normal conditions, pluripotent cells capable of hematopoietic differentiation constitutively circulate in the vascular compartment, albeit in low concentration. These cells, however, may be increased 25-fold under conditions of stress or recovery from myelosuppressive therapy, as may occur following chemotherapy.[25,26] It is possible to harvest these cells by modified leukapheresis techniques[14,15,27] and adoptively to transfer them to reconstitute hematopoietic elements. Timing of collection seems to be critically important, and these procedures are discussed in Chapters 5 and 9.

Leukapheresis may be performed during the rebound phase following pretreatment with a chemotherapeutic agent such as cyclophosphamide, or apheresis can be performed during the steady state of hematopoiesis, in certain circumstances.[25,28] Assays for the presence of cells positive for the CD34 antigen may also be performed as an indication of the marrow repopulating ability of the cells collected[26] (see Chapters 9 and 11). Although progenitor cell cultures can provide useful information on the colony-forming unit ability of the peripheral blood stem cells (PBSCs) collected, this information can be used only for retrospective analysis because of the 2 weeks required for culture growth.

The use of colony-stimulating factors (CSFs) as a means of mobilizing stem cells in the peripheral blood is also being explored.[26,28]

BONE MARROW COMPONENT PROCESSING

Harvested bone marrow can be thought of as equivalent in composition to a unit or number of units of whole blood: both of these contain a variety of cellular and noncellular components in an anticoagulant medium. Both marrow and whole blood can be separated into different fractions for specific purposes.

Plasma Removal

The marrow can be centrifuged to separate the plasma from the cellular elements. This procedure is useful for volume reduction when transplanting a small recipient, as discussed in Chapters 6 and 10. Plasma removal is also necessary when there is a minor ABO or other red blood cell incompatibility between the recipient and donor in which the donor plasma contains antibodies to certain of the recipient's red blood cell antigens. Although a small amount of donor plasma remains in the marrow product, this is rarely sufficient to cause frank hemolysis of the recipient's erythrocytes and can be diluted, if desired, by addition of saline or compatible donor plasma.[29] If the donor's isohemagglutinin titer is high, the marrow can be washed manually or in a cell washer to remove the plasma antibodies. Of course, this treatment does not remove the capacity of the immunocompetent donor lymphocytes to produce antibodies to the host's circulating red blood cells. The red cells, with a life span of approximately 120 days, can continue to survive for at least 3 months after transplantation, enough time for donor antibody production to occur and to induce immune hemolysis.[30]

Buffy Coat Preparation

One technique for fractionating the bone marrow is to prepare a concentrated *buffy coat* (white cell–rich product) by removal of the plasma and the bulk of the red blood cells (see Chapter 6, Buffy Coat Concentration/Buffy Coat Preparation). The buffy coat product is convenient for cryopreservation, as a marrow harvest of 1000 to 2000 mL can be concentrated to approximately 10 percent of the original volume.

Buffy coat can also be prepared for transplantation in case of major ABO incompatibility in which the recipient has antibodies to the donor red blood cells. It is important in this type of incompatibility, however, to assess the hemolytic potential of the graft based on the number of red blood cells remaining in the buffy coat and the isohemagglutinin titer of the recipient. Other methods of purification that remove a greater quantity of red blood cells might be preferable in high-risk situations (see Chapter 6, Mononuclear Cell Preparation). However, even with red blood cell depletion, just as the minor ABO incompatibility poses a risk for immediate and delayed hemolysis, so does the major ABO incompatibility. Although one can prevent the immediate event by removing the red blood cells in the graft, it is possible for host antibody to continue to be produced by lymphocytes that have escaped the preparative regimen. This antibody can then attach to donor-type red blood cells being produced in the marrow and cause their destruction. It is not unusual for recipients of this type of transplant to experience delayed erythroid reconstitution and to be dependent on red blood cell transfusion for a longer period than in an ABO-matched transplant.[30]

Although automated techniques are usually used to concentrate the buffy coat, manual techniques, which are generally more time consuming and labor intensive, may be necessary in the event that the volumes harvested are less than the minimum amounts that the automated instruments can process.

Mononuclear Cell Purification

Experimentation and experience have shown that the cells responsible for lymphohematopoietic reconstitution are found within the mononuclear cell population of the bone marrow.[31,32] Red blood cells, platelets, and mature granulocytes can be thought of as contaminants in the marrow graft, although some of them may eventually have value as blood components. Some of these cells can be detrimental to the recipient and can interfere with further processing and purging.

RED BLOOD CELLS

In addition to erythrocyte incompatibility mentioned earlier, a number of cases of acute renal failure have been reported following autologous transplantation with grafts containing large numbers of red blood cells.[33] This may occur because the erythrocytes do not freeze and thaw well in the cryopreservation process used for bone marrow and can hemolyze, exposing the recipient to large amounts of free hemoglobin and red cell stroma. In addition, red blood cell enzymes can interfere with some purging procedures[34,35] (see Chapter 8).

GRANULOCYTES AND PLATELETS

Because the marrow is not filtered during infusion, contaminating aggregates of granulocytes and platelets can be infused and may be trapped in the lungs of the recipient, causing ventilation-perfusion difficulties and hypoxemia. Leukoagglutinins produced by the recipient to neutrophil antigens can induce febrile reactions. Mature granulocytes do not survive standard bone marrow freezing and thawing techniques and can cause clumping of the thawed marrow product when DNA and lysosomal products are released. Furthermore, these cells can neutralize or diminish the effectiveness of monoclonal antibodies in some tumor cell purging procedures, requiring larger quantities of scarce and expensive reagents.

Finally, platelets in the suspension can become activated during any stage of processing, causing the marrow to clump.

Numerous techniques have been developed for mononuclear cell purification. Most of these require initial preparation of a buffy coat, which is then layered over a density gradient and subsequently centrifuged. The less dense mononuclear cells remain above the density gradient, whereas the heavier granulocytes and red blood cells fall below. The mononuclear cells are harvested and washed several times. This procedure can be performed manually or by using any of several semiautomated cell separation devices (see Chapter 6). Methods of mononuclear cell purification without a density gradient have also been developed.

Following preparation of a mononuclear cell product, the marrow is ready for infusion, cryopreservation, or further processing.

BONE MARROW PURGING

Purging of Allografts: T-Lymphocyte Depletion (Table 1–1)

Allogeneic transplantation involves the transfer of cells capable of reestablishing the donor hematopoietic and immune systems in the recipient. A severe complication of this engraftment may occur called graft-versus-host (GVH) disease. In this condition immunocompetent donor cells mount an immune attack against the immunoincompetent recipient (host). The recipient's skin, liver, and gastrointestinal tract bear the brunt of this immunologic response. This reaction can occur as an acute or chronic syndrome and, if allowed to progress, can result in irreversible damage to the involved tissues.[36] Immunosuppressive drugs such as cyclosporine have made GVH disease in matched allogeneic transplantation somewhat easier to prevent or manage, but it is still frequently a serious complication.[36]

The option of applying allogeneic transplantation as treatment for hematologic and immunologic diseases has been increasing, due in part to an expansion in the pool of available donors. Marrow from mismatched related and phenotypically matched unrelated donors has been transplanted successfully and is now being used as an alternative for patients who lack HLA-matched related donors.[4] The formation of registries of HLA-typed unrelated volunteers such as the National Marrow Donor Program in the United States, the Anthony Nolan Registry in Great Britain, and others throughout the world has made it possible for many patients without an HLA-matched sibling to locate an HLA-phenotypically matched volunteer donor. In the mismatched or unrelated setting, however, GVH disease still presents a significant barrier to an uncomplicated and successful transplant. The use of in vitro T-lymphocyte depletion has been found to abrogate GVH disease in many cases,[38–40] although the incidence of graft failure and disease relapse appears to be increased in patients receiving transplants with T-lymphocyte–depleted marrow.[41–44] To counteract this problem, some institutions are adding a measured number of the depleted lymphocytes back to the marrow inoculum.[45] There is also some evidence that a subpopulation of T lymphocytes contributes to a graft-versus-leukemia effect.[37,46,47] Many workers are attempting to determine whether there are separate and specific T-lymphocyte subsets that facilitate engraftment, are

Table 1–1 T-LYMPHOCYTE DEPLETION

Nonimmunologic
Soybean lectin with E rosetting
Counterflow centrifugation
Pharmacologic agents
    L-leucyl-L-leucine methyl ester
    Methylprednisolone/vincristine

Immunologic
Monoclonal antibodies with complement
Monoclonal antibodies with toxins
Monoclonal antibodies with magnetic polymer microspheres

instrumental in GVH disease, and participate in the graft-versus-leukemia effect. If such subpopulations do indeed exist and can be identified and isolated, it may someday be possible to remove specifically only the GVH cells (see Chapter 2).

T-LYMPHOCYTE DEPLETION BY NONIMMUNOLOGIC METHODS

Early attempts at T-lymphocyte depletion made use of the phenomenon by which T lymphocytes form rosettes around sheep erythrocytes (see Chapter 7, Cell Depletion of Bone Marrow by Treatment with Soybean Agglutinin and Sheep Red Blood Cell Rosetting). These rosettes can then be removed by density gradient centrifugation.

A physical technique for lymphocyte depletion uses elutriation to fractionate bone marrow by means of counterflow centrifugation.[47,48] Following a mononuclear purification procedure, the cells are suspended in an elutriation medium and are separated and harvested according to size (see Chapter 7, Counterflow Centrifugation).

Methods aimed at pharmacologically depleting the cytotoxic or alloreactive T-lymphocyte subpopulations involved in GVH disease, while sparing those cells that may be involved in the engraftment process and in the graft-versus-leukemia effect, have also been developed. The marrow is incubated with pharmacologic agents, such as methylprednisolone/vincristine, which preferentially remove the CD4-positive T-cell subset and modulate the alloreactive response (see Chapter 7, Methylprednisolone and Vincristine Treatment of Bone Marrow in HLA-Mismatched Bone Marrow Transplants).

IMMUNOLOGIC T-LYMPHOCYTE DEPLETION (TABLE 1-2)

One means of selecting specific populations of T lymphocytes for removal is to incubate the marrow with monoclonal antibodies directed against specific T-cell antigenic determinants. These antibodies can be used in conjunction with complement for lysis of the sensitized antigen-positive T cells[36,43,49,50] or immunotoxins such as the ricin A chain[51,52] (see Chapter 7, Immunologic). A recently developed technique involves binding of the anti–T-cell monoclonal

Table 1-2 MONOCLONAL ANTIBODIES USED FOR T-LYMPHOCYTE DEPLETION

Campath-1
CT-2
OKT3
Anti-CD3
Anti-CD2 + CD5 + CD7
Anti-CD5
Anti–Leu-2 (CD8)
Anti-CD6 (in mouse)
Anti-CD2 + anti-TCR/CD3

---

antibody to magnetic polymer microspheres, incubating the marrow with the microspheres, and exposing the container with the cell suspension to a strong magnet. The microsphere-cell complexes are held to the wall of the vessel, allowing the unbound cells to be removed[53-55] (see Chapter 8, Immunomagnetic Purging of Neuroblastoma Cells from Autologous Bone Marrow).

The percentage of T lymphocytes in the marrow should be determined before and after treatment to ensure sufficient depletion. This assessment can be made by staining a sample of the cell suspension with fluorescein-conjugated monoclonal antibodies to T-cell antigens and assaying with a fluorescence-activated cell sorter or with a fluorescence microscope (as outlined in Chapter 11). A more sensitive method of determining residual T-cell contamination after purging is by means of limiting dilution analysis.[56,57] This assay is based on the ability of T lymphocytes to proliferate in media that contain phytohemagglutinin (PHA) and interleukin-2 (IL-2) and, therefore, is capable of differentiating between viable T cells and those damaged by the depletion treatment but still bearing identifiable T-cell markers (see Chapter 11, Evaluation of T-Cell Depletion). However, because the assay takes 2 to 3 weeks to complete, its usefulness is limited to retrospective analysis of the T-cell depletion technique.

Purging of Autografts: Tumor Cell Depletion

Autologous marrow transplantation has not been universally embraced as treatment for hematologic malignancies. Even when patients are in complete clinical remission, some workers have been able to culture clonogenic tumor cells from the marrow.[58]

If relapse is, in some cases, induced by the contaminating tumor cells reinfused with the marrow, it is logical to attempt to remove these cells prior to marrow infusion. This must be done, of course, without injuring the hematopoietic progenitor cells. Many techniques have been developed for in vitro purging of occult clonogenic tumor cells from harvested autologous bone marrow, and these are outlined in Chapter 8 and are listed in Table 1–3. They can be broadly categorized as immunologic and nonimmunologic procedures.

TUMOR CELL DEPLETION BY NONIMMUNOLOGIC METHODS

Cytotoxic agents have been used as a means of eradicating clonogenic leukemic cells while sparing uncommitted hematopoietic progenitor cells. Derivatives of cyclophosphamide such as 4-hydroperoxycyclophosphamide, ASTA-Z (mafosfamide), as well as other chemotherapeutic drugs, have been widely used.[59-64] Purging is performed by incubating the marrow, generally a purified mononuclear cell suspension, with the drug for the appropriate time period, after which the marrow is washed and cryopreserved.

TUMOR CELL DEPLETION BY IMMUNOLOGIC METHODS

Surface markers have been identified that appear predominantly on certain tumor cells. Techniques identical to those described earlier for allogeneic marrow purging have been developed using combinations of monoclonal anti-

Table 1–3   AUTOGRAFT PURGING

Nonimmunologic
Pharmacologic
   4-hydroperoxycyclophosphamide
   ASTA-Z (mafosfamide)
   Etoposide (VP-16)
   Methylprednisolone
   Vincristine
   Alkyl-lysophospholipids (ALP)
Radioisotopes
Cytokines
   IL-3
   GM-CSF
   IL-2
Photoactivated dyes

Immunologic
Monoclonal antibodies with complement
Monoclonal antibodies with toxins
Monoclonal antibodies with magnetic polymer microspheres

Combination
Multiple cytotoxic drugs
Immunologic plus pharmacologic purging

bodies to these markers to remove or destroy contaminating tumor cells, while sparing the hematopoietic stem cells. One method uses monoclonal antibodies to sensitize the target cells, followed by incubation with complement to lyse the sensitized cells[65,66] (see Chapter 8, Manual Autologous Bone Marrow Purging with Monoclonal Antibodies and Complement).

Monoclonal antibodies bound to immunotoxins have also been used for cytotoxic purging of targeted tumor cells. Immunomagnetic beads incubated with monoclonal antibodies have been employed to deplete autologous marrow grafts of residual neuroblastoma cells[67,68] (see Chapter 8, Immunomagnetic Purging of Neuroblastoma Cells from Autologous Bone Marrow) and of B-lymphoma cells.[69]

In addition to purging with single agents, multiple drug procedures and combinations of immunologic and pharmacologic purging are being used in an attempt to remove heterogeneous populations of residual tumor cells.[70–76] As with in vivo antineoplastic therapy, the rationale for this type of treatment is to take advantage of the diverse mechanisms by which these agents act to disrupt the metabolism of the tumor cells.

Unique approaches to autologous marrow purging have been attempted, many of which mimic the therapeutic modalities used for in vivo cancer treatment. Radioisotopes have been bound to antibodies as a variation of the immunotoxin-antibody conjugate technique.[77] Many investigators are examining the effect of cytokines such as interleukin-3 (IL-3), granulocyte-macrophage colony-stimulating factor (GM-CSF), and IL-2 as agents that either enhance the killing ability of the purging chemicals or improve the hematopoietic potential of the cells remaining after purging.[78–81] Treatment of marrow with photoactivated dyes that preferentially localize in tumor cells is also being tried as an outgrowth of therapeutic photoradiation therapy.[82,83]

MARROW STORAGE

The concept of autologous marrow transplantation also requires a means of marrow preservation. The period between time of collection and time of reinfusion can range from a few days in institutions using a short preparative regimen to years for marrow stored in remission for use only in the event of relapse.

Most centers performing autologous transplantation cryopreserve the marrow in a solution containing dimethyl sulfoxide (DMSO) as the cryoprotectant.[13] This agent, although thought to be toxic to hematopoietic cells at temperatures above 4°C, is an excellent cryopreservative for cells stored at the extremely low temperature of liquid nitrogen.[84]

The marrow is reduced in volume and the red blood cells reduced or depleted by one of the separation techniques described in Chapter 6. The marrow cell suspension can then be adjusted to a specific concentration, although many centers do not find this adjustment necessary.[13] A freezing solution, usually containing 20 percent DMSO in tissue culture medium and autologous plasma, is prepared and added to an equal volume of concentrated marrow suspension in a plastic freezing bag, resulting in a final DMSO concentration of 10 percent.

The bags of marrow and cryopreservation solution are usually frozen in a programmable freezer at a constant rate and stored in either the liquid or the vapor phase of liquid nitrogen.[13] Freezing the marrow slowly (usually at 1°C per minute) beyond the phase change from liquid to solid seems to result in optimum colony-forming unit recovery.[85]

A technique has been developed for freezing and storing marrow in a mechanical freezer[86] (see Chapter 9, Mechanical Freezing). This method uses a cryopreservative consisting of hydroxyethyl starch (HES) with half as much 5 percent DMSO. Because the marrow is usually thawed and infused without removal of the DMSO, often producing unpleasant side effects in the recipient, it may be desirable to consider a freezing solution with a lower concentration of DMSO.

The cryopreserved marrow is thawed in a 37° to 40°C waterbath immediately prior to infusion and administered through a central venous catheter. It is possible to dilute and/or wash the marrow prior to infusion in order to remove the DMSO,[87] but this operation is rarely performed. Although the infusion of DMSO has been associated with toxicities including nausea, vomiting, flushing, dyspnea, changes in heart rate and blood pressure, and serum transaminase elevations,[88] most workers feel that manipulation of the thawed marrow may result in unacceptable cell losses.[35] The marrow may be either infused directly from the bag through an administration set or removed from the bag with a syringe and injected into the central line.[13]

Allogeneic marrow has also been successfully cryopreserved and transplanted.[89] With the increase in transplants from unrelated donors comes the increased danger that a donor may decline or be unable to donate after the preparative regimen has begun or that problems of transporting the marrow from distant collection sites may occur. If marrow were harvested from allogeneic donors and stored at the transplant center prior to the start of the conditioning regimen, there would be no risk of donor unavailability at the required time.

In addition to marrow storage in ultralow mechanical and liquid nitrogen freezers, there are also a number of published reports of marrow successfully transplanted after short-term storage at refrigerator temperatures.[90]

QUALITY ASSURANCE

Each of the steps in the processing of bone marrow for transplantation is also an opportunity to do harm to the precious product. Three areas of potential damage are as follows:

1. Loss of or injury to hematopoietic progenitor cells
2. Bacterial or fungal contamination
3. Failure of purging to adequately remove target cells

At every stage of processing, from collection to infusion, some type of test or assay should be available to ensure that the product of the specific procedure meets the established criteria. These criteria are generally determined by the individual institution, although the American Association of Blood Banks has recently published standards for bone marrow collection and processing.[91]

Number and Viability of Hematopoietic Progenitor Cells

Nucleated cell counts are usually performed using manual or automated techniques following each manipulation of the marrow. An automated cell counter is useful for this function because it is generally more accurate and faster than manual counting techniques (Chapter 4, Cell Counting and Calculations). It has been our experience, however, that a high fat content can falsely elevate the nucleated cell count of the marrow when an automated cell counter is used. A differential count to determine the percentage of mononuclear cells is also needed when a separation technique designed to isolate these cells is performed. Automated differential counters are not able to enumerate accurately the immature cell types in marrow suspensions.[96] A Wright- or Giemsa-stained smear is made and examined microscopically to determine the percentage of mononuclear cells in the marrow.

In addition to the requirement for rapid and accurate cell counts following each manipulation, the laboratory will also want a means of determining whether these cells are viable and whether they are capable of hematopoietic reconstitution. The traditional method for determining the viability of mononuclear cells is the dye exclusion technique (see Chapter 11, Dye Exclusion Test for Bone Marrow Viability). This technique depends on the ability of the viable cell membrane to exclude a dye such as trypan blue. This technique is rapid and simple but is not sensitive enough to distinguish cells that have been damaged but not yet killed.[92]

Although no culture system has yet been devised to assay predictably the number of pluripotent hematopoietic stem cells in a marrow aspirate, it is possible to analyze the marrow for committed hematopoietic progenitors (see Chapter 11, Bone Marrow Cell Culture). These progenitors, also known as colony-forming units, are cultured in a semisolid system for variable periods of time, after which colonies are enumerated. The medium can be either methylcellulose or agar, with various nutrients, proteins, and growth factors added. The resulting colonies in these cultures are erythroid (CFU-E and burst forming units—erythroid [BFU-E]), granulocyte-macrophage (CFU-GM) or granulocytic-erythroid-monocytic-megakaryocytic (CFU-GEMM). Although these colonies are probably not the immediate progeny of uncommitted progenitor cells, their growth in culture seems to be indicative of, although not necessarily proportional to, hematopoietic stem cells in the marrow suspension.[23]

Several workers have claimed to be able to use numbers of CFUs to predict engraftment in the autologous setting,[93-95] although others have not been able to confirm this. There have also been reports of some correlation between CFUs and engraftment in allogeneic transplantation[96] and peripheral blood stem cell transplantation.[97]

Another method of enumerating the number of early progenitor cells in the marrow is by means of immunofluorescence using a monoclonal antibody to the hematopoietic cell surface antigens, CD34 (see Chapter 11, Immunofluorescence). This antigen is present on less than 2 percent of low-density bone marrow mononuclear cells and does not appear on mature blood and bone marrow cells.[98] The CD34 marker does, however, appear on some acute as well as chronic myelogenous leukemia cells and on some tumors, so that one must be cautious when using this technique to quantify the cells capable of hematopoietic reconstitution in the marrow.

Bacterial or Fungal Contamination

Because the marrow is collected in an open environment and because many of the processing steps cannot be performed in a completely closed system, there are numerous opportunities for contamination with microorganisms. It is assumed that strict aseptic methods will be used in the operating room and in the processing laboratory. However, the danger of contamination rises in proportion to the number of manipulations the marrow must undergo. In one series, 17 percent of marrows were found to contain skin flora when cultured immediately after harvest.[99] Bacterial and fungal cultures should be performed at different stages of processing to determine whether any of the techniques and/or materials in use are compromising the purity of the marrow.

Adequacy of Purging

Numerous techniques have been devised to detect and quantify residual target cells following marrow purging (see Chapter 8). It is imperative that the laboratory be aware of the limitations of any of these assays when using them to measure the efficacy of any purging method, as there is great variability of sensitivity and specificity among the various assay systems. Even the same technique may yield inconsistent results owing to the differences in monoclonal antibodies, serum and complement lot, and other reagents and materials.

SUMMARY

As indications for bone marrow transplantation broaden, so do variations in bone marrow processing and manipulation techniques. Many centers have their own unique methods of mononuclear cell purification, concentration, and storage. This is particularly evident in the processing of marrow for autologous transplantation to allow dose intensification as salvage therapy for malignant disease. Unique procedures have also been developed in order to maximize yields, concentrate mononuclear cells necessary for engraftment, and reduce the likelihood of GVH disease in allogeneic transplants. Graft rejection and disease relapse still remain a problem in some of these manipulated marrows. Newer procedures may allow titration of the optimum numbers of immune reconstituting cells; however, at this time these techniques are not precise and the balance between preventing GVH disease at the expense of graft failure or relapse may still jeopardize disease-free survival. Innovative purging techniques that include pharmacologic and immunologic methods continue to evolve, necessitating that standards for bone marrow processing be flexible yet practical.

Quality control and viability assays are essential to verify the biologic proliferative potential of progenitor cells capable of marrow reconstitution. Although guidelines have now been established, these are quite broad and each transplant center should have internal criteria to monitor the quality of the processed marrow.

REFERENCES

1. Thomas, ED and Storb, R: Technique for human marrow grafting. Blood 36:507, 1970.
2. Santos, GW: History of bone marrow transplantation. Clin Haematol 12:611, 1983.
3. Bortin, MM and Gale, RP: Current status of allogeneic bone marrow transplantation: A report from the International Bone Marrow Transplant Registry. In Terasaki, P (ed): Clinical Transplants 1986. UCLA Tissue Typing Laboratory, Los Angeles, 1986, p 17.
4. Deeg, HJ: Bone marrow transplantation 1990. In Sacher, RA, McCarthy, LJ, and Smit Sibinga, CT (eds): Processing of Bone Marrow for Transplantation. American Association of Blood Banks, Arlington, VA, 1990, p 1.
5. Thomas, ED, et al: Marrow transplantation for the treatment of chronic myelogenous leukemia. Ann Intern Med 104:155, 1986.
6. Klingemann, H-G: When should marrow transplantation be considered? In Deeg, HJ, Klingemann, H-G, and Phillips, GL: A Guide to Bone Marrow Transplantation. Springer-Verlag, Berlin, 1988, p 18.
7. Deeg, HJ: How should marrow transplantation be approached? In Deeg, HJ, Klingemann, H-G, and Phillips, GL (eds): A Guide to Bone Marrow Transplantation. Springer-Verlag, Berlin, 1988, p 18.
8. Storb, R, et al: Allogeneic marrow transplants for treatment of severe aplastic anemia. In Gale, RP (ed): Recent Advances in Bone Marrow Transplantation. Alan R. Liss, New York, 1983, p 3.
9. Linch, DC and Goldstone, AH: Autologous bone marrow transplantation in acute leukemia. Bone Marrow Transplant 2:219, 1987.
10. Takvorian, T, et al: Prolonged disease-free survival after autologous bone marrow transplantation in patients with non-Hodgkin's lymphoma with a poor prognosis. N Engl J Med 316:1499, 1987.
11. Cheson, BD, et al: Autologous bone marrow transplantation: Current status and future directions. Ann Intern Med 110:51, 1989.
12. Advisory Committee for the International Autologous Bone Marrow Transplant Registry: Bone marrow autotransplantation in man: Report of an international cooperative study. Lancet 2:960, 1986.
13. Areman, EM, Sacher, RA, and Deeg, HJ: Processing and storage of human bone marrow: A survey of current practices in North America. Bone Marrow Transplant 6:203, 1990.
14. Reiffers, J, et al: Successful autologous transplantation with peripheral blood hemopoietic cells in a patient with acute leukemia. Exp Hematol 14:312, 1986.

15. Kessinger, A, et al: Reconstitution of human hematopoietic function with autologous cryopreserved circulating stem cells. Exp Hematol 14:192, 1986.
16. Kessinger, A, et al: Autologous peripheral hematopoietic stem cell transplantation restores hematopoietic function following marrow ablative therapy. Blood 71:723, 1988.
17. Coutinho, LH, et al: The use of cultured bone marrow cells in autologous transplantation. In Gross, SR, Gee, AP, and Worthington-White, DA (eds): Bone Marrow Purging and Processing. Alan R. Liss, New York, 1990, p 415.
18. Coulombel, L, et al: Long-term marrow culture reveals chromosomally normal hematopoietic progenitor cells in patients with Philadelphia chromosome-positive chronic myelogenous leukemia. N Engl J Med 308:1493, 1983.
19. Barnett, MJ, et al: Autografting in chronic myeloid leukemia (CML) after maintenance of marrow in culture (abstr). J Cell Biochem 14A:305, 1990.
20. Berenson, RJ, et al: Stem cell selection—clinical experience. In Gross, SR, Gee, AP, and Worthington-White, DA (eds): Bone Marrow Purging and Processing. Alan R. Liss, New York, 1990, p 403.
21. Gluckman, E, et al: Hematopoietic reconstitution in a patient with Fanconi's anemia by means of umbilical-cord blood from an LA-identical sibling. N Engl J Med 321:1174, 1989.
22. Hughes, PFD, et al: High-efficiency gene transfer to human hematopoietic cells maintained in long-term marrow culture. Blood 74:1915, 1989.
23. Lasky, LC and Bhatia, S: Future applications of marrow progenitor growth. In Sacher, RA, McCarthy, LJ, Smit Sibinga, CT (eds): Processing of Bone Marrow for Transplantation. American Association of Blood Banks, Arlington, VA, 1990, p 83.
24. Pegg, DE: Technical aspects of human bone marrow transplantation and storage. In Bone Marrow Transplantation. Lloyd-Luke, London, 1966, p 163.
25. To, LB, et al: High levels of circulating haemopoietic stem cells in very early remission from acute non-lymphoblastic leukaemia and their collection and cryopreservation. Br J Haematol 58:399, 1984.
26. Juttner, CA, et al: Peripheral blood stem cell selection, collection and auto-transplantation. In Gross, SR, Gee, AP, and Worthington-White, DA (eds): Bone Marrow Purging and Processing. Alan R. Liss, New York, 1990, p 447.
27. Williams, SF, et al: Peripheral blood-derived stem cell collections for use in autologous transplantation after high dose chemotherapy: An alternative approach. Bone Marrow Transplant 5:129, 1990.
28. Peters, WP, et al: GM-CSF primed peripheral blood progenitor cells (PBPC) coupled with autologous bone marrow transplantation (ABMT) will eliminate the absolute leukopenia following high dose chemotherapy (abstr). Blood 74:504, 1989.
29. Jansen, J: Processing of bone marrow for allogeneic transplantation. In Sacher, RA, McCarthy, LJ, and Smit Sibinga, CT (eds): Processing of Bone Marrow for Transplantation. American Association of Blood Banks, Arlington, VA, 1990, p 19.
30. Areman, EM: Bone marrow transplantation: Nuances of transfusion support implications for the blood bank. In Sacher, RA, McCarthy, LJ, and Smit Sibinga, CT (eds): Processing of Bone Marrow for Transplantation. American Association of Blood Banks, Arlington, VA, 1990, p 63.
31. Ekert, H, et al: Marrow function reconstitution by fraction 3 of percoll-density-gradient-separated cells. Transplantation 42:58, 1986.
32. Cottler-Fox, M, Bazar, LS, and Deeg, HJ: Isolation of hemopoietic precursor cells from human marrow by negative selection using monoclonal antibodies and immunomagnetic beads. In Gross, SR, Gee, AP, and Worthington-White, DA (eds): Bone Marrow Purging and Processing. Alan R. Liss, New York, 1990, p 277.
33. Smith, DM, et al: Acute renal failure associated with autologous bone marrow transplantation. Bone Marrow Transplant 2:196, 1987.
34. Jones, RJ, et al: Variability in 4-hydroperoxycyclophosphamide activity during clinical purging for autologous bone marrow transplantation. Blood 70:1490, 1987.
35. Davis, JM and Rowley, SD: Autologous bone marrow graft processing. In Sacher, RA, McCarthy, LJ, and Smit Sibinga, CT (eds): Processing of Bone Marrow for Transplantation. American Association of Blood Banks, Arlington, VA, 1990, p 41.
36. Champlin, R, et al: Selective depletion of CD8+ T lymphocytes for prevention of graft-versus-host disease after allogeneic bone marrow transplantation. Blood 76:418, 1990.
37. Deeg, HJ: Acute graft-versus-host disease. In Deeg, HJ, Klingemann, H-G, and Phillips, GL: A Guide to Bone Marrow Transplantation. Springer-Verlag, Berlin, 1988, p 86.

38. Racadot, E, et al: Prevention of graft-versus-host disease in HLA-matched bone marrow transplantation for malignant disease: A multicenter study using 3-pan-T monoclonal antibodies and rabbit complement. J Clin Oncol 5:426, 1987.

39. Maraninchi, D, et al: Impact of T-cell depletion on outcome of allogeneic bone marrow transplantation for standard risk leukaemias. Lancet 2:176, 1987.

40. Prentice, HG, et al: Depletion of T lymphocytes in donor marrow prevents significant graft-versus-host disease in matched allogeneic leukaemic marrow transplant recipients. Lancet 1:472, 1984.

41. Apperly, JF, et al: Bone marrow transplantation for patients with chronic myeloid leukaemia: T cell depletion with Campath-1 reduces the incidence of graft-versus-host disease but may increase the risk of leukaemic relapse. Bone Marrow Transplant 1:53, 1986.

42. Goldman, JM, et al: Bone marrow transplantation of chronic myelogenous leukemia in chronic phase. Increased risk of relapse associated with T-cell depletion. Ann Intern Med 108:806, 1988.

43. Mitsuyasu, RT, et al: Treatment of donor bone marrow with monoclonal anti-T cell antibody and complement for the prevention of graft-versus-host disease: A prospective, randomized, double-blind trial. Ann Intern Med 105:20, 1986.

44. Martin, PJ, et al: Graft failure in patients receiving T cell-depleted HLA-identical allogeneic marrow transplants. Bone Marrow Transplant 3:445, 1988.

45. Verdonck, LF, et al: A fixed low number of T cells in HLA-identical allogeneic bone marrow transplantation. Blood 75:776, 1990.

46. Gale, RP and Champlin, RE: How does bone marrow transplantation cure leukemia? Lancet 2:28, 1984.

47. DeWitte, T, Raymakers, R, and Plas, A: Bone marrow repopulation capacity after transplantation of lymphocyte-depleted allogeneic bone marrow using counterflow centrifugation. Transplantation 37:151, 1984.

48. Noga, SJ, et al: Rapid separation of whole human bone marrow aspirates by counterflow centrifugal elutriation. Transplantation 43:438, 1986.

49. Hale, G, et al: Removal of T cells from bone marrow for transplantation: A monoclonal antilymphocyte antibody that fixes human complement. Blood 62:873, 1983.

50. Waldmann, H, et al: Elimination of graft-versus-host disease by in vitro depletion of alloreactive lymphocytes with a monoclonal rat antihuman lymphocyte antibody (Campath-1). Lancet 2:483, 1984.

51. Antin, JH, et al: Depletion of bone marrow T-lymphocytes with an anti-CD5 monoclonal immunotoxin (ST-1 immunotoxin): Effective prophylaxis for graft-versus-host disease. In Gross, SR, Gee, AP, and Worthington-White, DA (eds): Bone Marrow Purging and Processing. Alan R. Liss, New York, 1990, p 207.

52. Martin, PJ, et al: Effects of treating marrow with a CD3-specific immunotoxin for prevention of acute graft-versus-host disease. Bone Marrow Transplant 3:437, 1988.

53. Egeland, T, et al: Immunomagnetic depletion of CD6+ cells from bone marrow and peripheral blood. Bone Marrow Transplant 5:193, 1990.

54. Knobloch, C, et al: T cell depletion from human bone marrow using magnetic beads. Bone Marrow Transplant 6:21, 1990.

55. Kogler, G, et al: High efficiency of a new immunological magnetic cell sorting method for T cell depletion of human bone marrow. Bone Marrow Transplant 6:163, 1990.

56. Taswell, C: Limiting dilution assay for the determination of immunocompetent cell frequencies. J Immunol 126:1614, 1981.

57. Kernan, NA, et al: Quantitation of T lymphocytes in human bone marrow by a limiting dilution assay. Transplantation 40:317, 1985.

58. Miller, CB, Zehnbauer, BA, and Jones, RJ: Detection of occult acute lymphocytic leukemia (ALL) by clonogenic assay (abstr). Exp Hematol 17:652, 1989.

59. Kaiser, H, et al: Autologous bone marrow transplantation in acute leukemia: A phase I study of in vitro treatment of marrow with 4-hydroperoxycyclophosphamide to purge tumor cells. Blood 65:1504, 1985.

60. Yeager, AM, et al: Autologous bone marrow transplantation in patients with acute nonlymphocytic leukemia, using ex vivo marrow treatment with 4-hydroperoxycyclophosphamide. N Engl J Med 315:141, 1986.

61. Gorin, NC, et al: Autologous bone marrow transplantation using marrow incubated with Asta Z 7557 in adult acute leukemia. Blood 67:1367, 1986.

62. Ciobanu, N, et al: Etoposide as an in vitro purging agent for the treatment of acute leukemias

and lymphomas in conjunction with autologous bone marrow transplantation. Exp Hematol 14:626, 1986.

63. Rizzoli, V, et al: Autologous bone marrow transplantation for acute leukemia: Optimal timing and mafosfamide treatment. In Dicke, KA, et al (eds): Autologous Bone Marrow Transplantation. Proceedings of the Fourth International Symposium. Houston, University of Texas M. D. Anderson Cancer Center, 1989, p 13.

64. Rizzoli, V, and Mangoni, L: Pharmacological-mediated purging with mafosfamide in acute and chronic myeloid leukemias. In Gross, SR, Gee, AP, and Worthington-White, DA (eds): Bone Marrow Purging and Processing. Alan R. Liss, New York, 1990, p 21.

65. Mitsuyasu, R, et al: Autologous bone marrow transplantation after *in vitro* marrow treatment with anti-Calla heteroantiserum and complement for adult acute lymphoblastic leukemia. In Gale, RP (ed): Recent Advances in Bone Marrow Transplantation. Alan R. Liss, New York, 1983, p 679.

66. Ramsay, N, et al: Autologous bone marrow transplantation for patients with acute lymphoblastic leukemia in second or subsequent remission: Results of bone marrow treated with monoclonal antibodies BA-1, BA-2, and BA-3 plus complement. Blood 66:508, 1985.

67. Seeger, RC, et al: Removal of neuroblastoma cells from bone marrow with monoclonal antibodies and magnetic immunobeads. In Transfusion Medicine: Recent Technological Advances. Alan R. Liss, New York, 1986, p 285.

68. Gee, AP, et al: Immunomagnetic purging and autologous transplantation in Stage D neuroblastoma. Bone Marrow Transplant 2(Suppl 2):89, 1987.

69. Kvalheim, G, et al: Immunomagnetic removal of B-lymphoma cells from human bone marrow: A procedure for clinical use. Bone Marrow Transplant 3:31, 1988.

70. Shimazaki, C, et al: Elimination of myeloma cells from bone marrow using monoclonal antibodies and magnetic immunobeads. Blood 72:1248, 1988.

71. Shimazaki, C, et al: Purging of myeloma cells from bone marrow using monoclonal antibodies and magnetic immunobeads in combination with 4-hydroperoxycyclophosphamide. In Gross, SR, Gee, AP, and Worthington-White, DA (eds): Bone Marrow Purging and Processing. Alan R. Liss, New York, 1990, p 311.

72. Shpall, EJ, et al: Immunopharmacologic purging of breast cancer from bone marrow for autologous bone marrow transplantation. In Gross, SR, Gee, AP, and Worthington-White, DA (eds): Bone Marrow Purging and Processing. Alan R. Liss, New York, 1990, p 321.

73. Cairo, MS, et al: Combination chemotherapy and verapamil to purge drug resistant leukemia cells from human bone marrow. In Gross, SR, Gee, AP, and Worthington-White, DA (eds): Bone Marrow Purging and Processing. Alan R. Liss, New York, 1990, p 47.

74. Deconinck, E, Tamayo, E, and Herve, P: In vitro chemosensitivity of leukemic progenitor cells (AML-CFU) to a combination of mafosfamide lysine (ASTA-Z 7654) and etoposide (VP16-213). Bone Marrow Transplant 5:13, 1989.

75. Jones, RJ, et al: In vitro evaluation of combination drug purging for autologous bone marrow transplantation. Bone Marrow Transplant 5:301, 1990.

76. Montgomery, RB, et al: Elimination of malignant clonogenic T cells from human bone marrow using chemoimmunoseparation with 2'-deoxycoformycin, deoxyadenosine and an immunotoxin. Bone Marrow Transplant 5:395, 1990.

77. Macklis, RM: Radioisotope-mediated purging in bone marrow transplantation. In Gross, SR, Gee, AP, and Worthington-White, DA (eds): Bone Marrow Purging and Processing. Alan R. Liss, New York, 1990, p 109.

78. Cramer, DV and Long, GS: Lymphokine-activated killer (LAK) cell purging of bone marrow. In Gross, SR, Gee, AP, and Worthington-White, DA (eds): Bone Marrow Purging and Processing. Alan R. Liss, New York, 1990, p 125.

79. Long, GS, et al: Lymphokine-activated (LAK) cell purging of leukemic bone marrow: Range of activity against different hematopoietic neoplasms. Bone Marrow Transplant 6:169, 1990.

80. Charak, BS, et al: A novel approach to purging of leukemia by activation of bone marrow with interleukin 2. Bone Marrow Transplant 6:193, 1990.

81. Slavin, S, et al: The use of recombinant cytokines for enhancing immunohematopoietic reconstitution following bone marrow transplantation. Effects of *in vitro* culturing with IL-3 and GM-CSF on human and mouse bone marrow cells purged with mafosfamide (ASTA-Z). Bone Marrow Transplant 4:459, 1989.

82. Sieber, F, et al: Dye-mediated photolysis of normal and neoplastic hematopoietic cells. Leuk Res 11:43, 1987.

83. Gulati, S, et al: Photoradiation methods for purging autologous bone marrow grafts. In Gross,

SR, Gee, AP, and Worthington-White, DA (eds): Bone Marrow Purging and Processing. Alan R. Liss, New York, 1990, p 87.

84. Gorin, NC: Collection, manipulation and freezing of haemopoietic stem cells. Clin Haematol 15:19, 1986.

85. Gorin, N, et al: Delayed kinetics of recovery of haemopoiesis following autologous bone marrow transplantation. The role of excessively rapid marrow freezing rates after the release of fusion heat. Eur J Cancer Clin Onc 19:485, 1983.

86. Stiff, PJ, et al: Autologous bone marrow transplantation using fractionated cells cryopreserved in dimethylsulfoxide and hydroxyethyl starch without controlled rate freezing. Blood 70:974, 1987.

87. Weiner, RS, Tobias, JS, and Yankee, RA: The processing of human bone marrow for cryopreservation and infusion. Biomedicine 24:226, 1976.

88. Davis, JM, et al: Clinical toxicity of cryopreserved bone marrow graft infusion. Blood 75:781, 1990.

89. Lasky, LC, et al: Successful allogeneic cryopreserved marrow transplantation. Transfusion 29:182, 1989.

90. Lasky, LC, McCullough, J, and Zanzani, ED: Liquid storage of unseparated human bone marrow: Evaluation of hematopoietic progenitors by clonal assay. Transfusion 26:331, 1986.

91. Rowley, SD and Davis, J: Standards of bone marrow processing laboratories. Transfusion 30:571, 1990.

92. Wilson, AP: Cytotoxicity and viability assays. In Freshney, RI (ed): Animal Cell Culture: A Practical Approach. IRL Press, Washington, DC, 1986, p 183.

93. Spitzer, G, et al: The myeloid progenitor cell—its value in predicting hematologic recovery after autologous bone marrow transplant. Blood 55:317, 1980.

94. Douay, L, et al: Recovery of CFU-GM from cryopreserved marrow and in vivo evaluation after autologous bone marrow transplantation are predictive of engraftment. Exp Hematol 14:358, 1986.

95. Rowley, SD, et al: CFU-GM content of bone marrow graft correlates with time to hematologic reconstitution following autologous bone marrow transplantation with 4-hydroperoxycyclophosphamide-purged bone marrow. Blood 70:271, 1987.

96. Jansen, J, et al: The impact of the composition of the bone marrow on engraftment and graft-versus-host disease. Exp Hematol 11:967, 1983.

97. To, LB, Dyson, PG, and Juttner, CA: Cell dose effect in circulating stem-cell autografting (letter). Lancet 2:404, 1986.

98. Civin, CI, et al: Positive stem cell selection—basic science. In Gross, SR, Gee, AP, and Worthington-White, DA (eds): Bone Marrow Purging and Processing. Alan R. Liss, New York, 1990, p 387.

99. Rowley, SD, et al: Bacterial contamination of bone marrow grafts intended for autologous and allogeneic bone marrow transplantation. Transfusion 28:109, 1988.

BONE MARROW AND HEMATOPOIETIC STEM CELL TRANSPLANTATION: SORTING THE CHAFF FROM THE GRAIN*

Commentary by H. JOACHIM DEEG

The first attempt at bone marrow transplantation was made approximately a century ago. However, it was not until the events of Alamogordo, New Mexico, and the observations in atomic bomb victims of Hiroshima and Nagasaki in 1945, that systematic investigations into the field of marrow transplantation were undertaken.[1] Jacobsen and Lorenz and their colleagues[2,3] showed that mice irradiated with bone marrow-toxic doses of gamma irradiation would survive if the spleen, a hematopoietic organ in the mouse, was shielded, or if spleen or marrow cells were infused or implanted following irradiation. While relatively small numbers of cells were needed when taken from a syngeneic (genetically identical) donor, 10 to 100 times as many cells were required if they were obtained from an allogeneic (genetically different) donor. Furthermore, mice given genetically nonidentical marrow generally developed skin changes, hair loss, diarrhea, and liver abnormalities—a syndrome initially termed secondary disease and subsequently known as graft-versus-host (GVH) disease.[4] This syndrome was apparently mediated by small mononuclear cells, lymphocytes,[5] which were contained in bone marrow and derived from hematopoietic stem cells.[6]

Bone marrow failure can be acquired, following an identifiable insult to the marrow (e.g., irradiation or chemotherapy, colloidal gold therapy), or can develop spontaneously, as with idiopathic severe aplastic anemia. Alternatively, marrow failure can result from congenital predisposition (as with Fanconi's anemia, Wiskott-Aldrich syndrome).[7] Accordingly, bone marrow transplantation represents either rescue or replacement therapy. Both indications were tested in the 1950s and early 1960s, but results were generally disappointing except in patients who happened to have an identical twin (syngeneic) donor.[8,9] Following the recognition and characterization of the major histocompatibility complex (MHC), termed HLA in humans,[10] transplant efforts were renewed in the late 1960s and early 1970s.[11] Concurrently, attempts were made to use the patient's own (autologous) marrow. Over the ensuing two decades, the field has developed rapidly, and currently at least 300 institutions worldwide are involved in bone marrow transplantation, carrying out approximately 4000 allogeneic and 3000 autologous transplants a year.

---

*Supported in part by grants CA 18221, CA 18029, CA 15704, and CA 47748 from the National Cancer Institute and HL 36444 from the National Heart, Lung and Blood Institute, NIH, DHHS.

TYPE OF TRANSPLANT

Among patients who have siblings, about 30 to 40 percent have at least one HLA-identical sister or brother suitable to serve as marrow donor.[12] Although transplants from related donors who differ from the recipient for only one HLA antigen result in long-term survival comparable to that with HLA-identical donors, transplants from donors who differ for two or more HLA antigens often result in severe GVH disease and a low probability of survival.[13] As an alternative approach, the feasibility of transplantation of bone marrow obtained from HLA–phenotypically matched unrelated volunteer donors has been explored over the past decade.[14] Results are encouraging; however, because of GVH disease and infectious complications even in good risk patients (e.g., with chronic myelogenous leukemia in chronic phase), long-term survival may be only 30 to 35 percent.[15] Furthermore, depending on the frequency of the patient's HLA haplotype, large numbers of unrelated individuals (at least 50 to 100×10^3) must be HLA typed before a suitable donor can be identified.[16] Thus, donor availability and GVH disease remain limiting factors for allogeneic marrow transplantation.

Therefore, investigators also explored the possibility of using the patient's own bone marrow for "trans"-plantation. Although, with conventional approaches, this was unlikely to hold any promise for congenital disorders or patients with marrow aplasia, concepts were developed that provided a rationale for using the patient's own marrow cells in chronic or acute leukemias and lymphomas. Autologous transplant recipients were usually not at risk of developing GVH disease; however, it appeared that they were at high risk of recurrent disease, not only because of residual malignant cells surviving aggressive chemoradiotherapy in the patient (which applies to allogeneic transplantation as well), but also because of reinfusion of clonogenic malignant cells with the patient's marrow.

Thus, for both allogeneic and autologous marrow transplantation, there has been great interest in eliminating those cells that are potentially detrimen-

Table 2–1 DIAGNOSIS AND SOURCE OF HEMATOPOIETIC STEM CELLS

Bone Marrow (BM)

Syngeneic	Acquired malignant or nonmalignant diseases with or without hematopoietic stem cell involvement
Allogeneic	Acquired diseases with or without hematopoietic stem cell involvement; congenital disorders
Autologous	Acquired, usually malignant disorders, generally without hematopoietic stem cell involvement

Peripheral Blood (PBSC)

Syngeneic	Experimental
Allogeneic	Experimental
Autologous	Acquired, usually malignant disorders with or without marrow involvement

Umbilical Cord Blood

Allogeneic	Experimental (Fanconi's anemia)

Fetal Liver

Allogeneic	Immunodeficiencies, various disorders

tal (i.e., lymphocytes capable of initiating GVH disease, after allogeneic transplantation, and malignant cells resulting in recurrent disease, after autologous marrow infusion) and in characterizing and positively selecting cells that are required for hematopoietic reconstitution (i.e., hematopoietic stem cells). As illustrated in Table 2–1, the option of using a certain source of hematopoietic stem cells depends on availability and the patient's diagnosis.

Syngeneic Transplants

Conditions should be ideal with a healthy syngeneic donor: transplanted cells are genotypically identical to those of the recipient (comparable to autologous cells); that is, there should be no risk for GVH disease, and, because cells were obtained from a healthy individual, there would be no contamination by tumor cells. Unfortunately only a few patients will have a syngeneic donor. Also, it has recently been shown that a syndrome similar to GVH disease can develop after syngeneic transplants[17] and that in patients with leukemia the probability of disease recurrence is higher with syngeneic transplants than with allogeneic transplants, presumably because of the absence of a graft-versus-leukemia (GVL) effect.[18] Nevertheless, patients with an acquired disorder (e.g., leukemia, lymphoma, aplastic anemia, and possibly some solid tumors) who have a healthy identical twin sibling may benefit from a syngeneic transplant. By definition the option of employing a syngeneic transplant would not exist in patients who suffer from a genetically determined disease because the identical twin would have inherited the same genes as the patient.

Allogeneic Transplants

Extensive work in experimental models and clinical studies has shown convincingly that donor T lymphocytes are responsible for the initiation of GVH disease in the allogeneic transplant recipient. GVH disease occurs frequently even with donor-recipient identity for MHC (HLA) antigens because donor cells recognize so-called minor (non-MHC) antigens, apparently sufficient to trigger an alloaggressive response.[11,19]

In murine models, experiments using T-lymphocyte depletion have shown that CD8-positive cells preferentially initiate GVH disease across MHC class I and CD4-positive cells across class II differences. If both antigens differ between donor and recipient, either CD4- or CD8-positive cells can induce GVH disease. With non-MHC or minor histocompatibility differences, predominantly CD8-positive cells are involved, although CD4-positive cells can participate in certain donor-host combinations.[20] There is also evidence that cells other than classic T cells contribute to the organ manifestations of GVH disease. Large granular lymphocytes (LGLs) with natural killer (NK) activity are recruited following activation of T cells, and antigen-presenting cells may contribute as well.[21] In addition, cytokines including interleukin-2 (IL-2), interferon gamma, and tumor necrosis factor alpha also play a central role in the development of GVH disease.[22,23] Thus, elimination of T cells or possibly LGLs, or neutralization of the cytokines they release, should interfere with and ideally prevent the development of GVH disease.

Table 2–2   IN VITRO T-CELL DEPLETION FROM
ALLOGENEIC MARROW

Monoclonal antibodies and complement
Monoclonal antibodies coupled to:
  Magnetic beads
  Immunotoxins
Agglutination (soybean lectin plus SRBCs*)
Counterflow elutriation
Chemoseparation

*Sheep red blood cells.

In agreement with animal experiment data, extensive clinical studies using various techniques (Table 2–2) have shown that T-cell depletion is effective in preventing GVH disease.[24,25] However, the clinical situation proved to be more complex, and several problems have emerged. First, elimination of T lymphocytes from the donor marrow frequently resulted in failure of sustained engraftment not only with HLA-nonidentical but even with HLA–genotypically identical transplants (as high as 60 percent and 30 percent, respectively, compared with approximately 5 to 10 percent and 1 to 2 percent, respectively, without T-cell depletion).[26] Second, there was an increased probability of recurrence of the underlying malignant disease, especially in patients with chronic myelocytic leukemia and possibly other diagnoses.[27,28] Because experimental and clinical studies have shown that the development of either acute or chronic GVH disease (or both) reduces the risk of leukemic recurrence, particularly in patients receiving transplants during an advanced stage of their disease,[29,30] a role of T lymphocytes in this GVL effect is likely. Whereas it has been possible in animal models to separate a GVL effect from GVH disease, clinical studies have not succeeded in doing so. In fact, one study showed a GVL effect to be manifest only in patients with clinically apparent GVH disease but not in patients with subclinical disease.[29] Nevertheless, studies have been undertaken aimed at selectively depleting different lymphocyte subsets from the bone marrow in an attempt to eliminate GVH disease while maintaining the graft facilitating function and possibly a GVL effect of lymphocytes contained in the donor marrow.[31,32]

Positive selection of hematopoietic precursor cells applied extensively with autologous transplantation (see further on) has so far not been applied to allogeneic transplantation. Because stem cell purification represents a quasi-mirror image of T-cell depletion, it is expected that with currently used conditioning regimens, the probability of graft failure and possibly disease recurrence would be even higher than with T-cell depletion.

Autologous Transplants

Somewhat surprisingly, an occasional patient given an autologous marrow graft will develop a GVH disease–like syndrome similar to that observed after allogeneic transplantation.[17] However, this complication is infrequent and usually self-limited. The problems that threaten the success of autologous transplantation are of a different nature.

For an autologous transplant to be successful, three prerequisites must be met[33]: First, it must be possible to obtain sufficiently large numbers of viable hematopoietic stem cells capable of self-replication and differentiation. Second, the cell preparation should be free of tumor stem cells, which might lead to disease recurrence. Third, the patient's malignancy must be responsive to chemoradiotherapy administered in preparation for marrow transplantation. This requirement applies, of course, to allogeneic transplantation as well; however, it may be even more important with autologous transplants, as no allogeneic or GVL effects can be expected with this procedure.

Stem cells obtained from the patient's bone marrow (or from peripheral blood; see further on) have usually been exposed to chemotherapy, irradiation, or both, given during initial treatment of the patient's disease. Thus, it is conceivable that these stem cells have been damaged (DNA breaks, enzyme defects, and the like) and that their ability to reconstitute hematopoietic and immunologic functions after transplantation may be impaired. Furthermore, cells with chromosomal damage may survive, expand clonally, and give rise to a new malignancy.

There is experimental and clinical evidence that the yield (and possibly the quality) of stem cells depends on when they are harvested (relative to chemoradiotherapy administration). Depending on the agents used and the time of harvest, the number of cells with in vitro colony-forming capacity varies.[34] Although these colony-forming cells are not thought to measure stem cell content (but rather later stages of hematopoietic precursors),[35] experimental and clinical data indicate that the rate of hematopoietic recovery in the autologous setting reflects the number of colony-forming units (CFUs). If the number of CFUs is low, recovery is slow, and the time period of pancytopenia and transfusion dependence is prolonged[36]; this in turn carries an increased risk of infections and transfusion-related problems.

To obtain the largest possible number of hematopoietic cells is even more important for both autologous and allogeneic transplants when in vitro manipulation is planned; already a single-step density gradient separation may result in a loss of 50 percent of all nucleated cells. With unmanipulated marrow the goal usually is to infuse at least 1 to 2×10^8 cells per kilogram for autologous and 2 to 4×10^8 cells per kilogram for allogeneic recipients.

Some techniques used for autologous marrow purging are similar to those described for T-cell depletion of allogeneic marrow, whereas others differ (Table 2-3). As outlined earlier, the emphasis is not on the prevention of GVH disease but on the removal of tumor cells. Hence, monoclonal antibodies employed here are directed at antigens expressed on tumor cells (and only in patients with T-cell leukemia or lymphoma will this include T cells). Pharmacologic methods require compounds that are active in vitro (i.e., not necessitating metabolic activation).[37,38] Most methods have evolved empirically, and it is not always clear why the compounds used preferentially destroy malignant cells.

In vitro culture methods are based on the intriguing concept that, under defined culture conditions, normal hematopoietic precursor cells can be provided with all nutrients necessary for proliferation and differentiation, whereas leukemia cells lack an essential factor and consequently do not replicate, which leads to marrow purging in culture.[39] Several patients with acute and chronic myelocytic leukemia have received transplants with culture-purged marrow,

Table 2–3   IN VITRO PURGING OF AUTOLOGOUS MARROW

Antibody (MAb)-Mediated
MAb + Complement
MAb + Magnetic beads
MAb + Immunotoxin

Pharmacologic
4-Hydroperoxycyclophosphamide
Mafosfamide (Asta Z)
Etoposide
Ether lipids
Combinations of agents

In Vitro Culture

Photoinactivation
Merocyanine 540
Phthalocyanine
Others

---

and some are surviving in remission.[40,41] Additional experience is necessary before the validity of this approach can be assessed. It should be pointed out that even simple cryopreservation may exert some purging effect—for example, on multiple myeloma cells.[42]

Another modality involves photoinactivation. Most experience has been accrued with merocyanine 540, a dye activated by fluorescent light.[43] This approach apparently results in a preferential uptake and cytocidal effect in leukemia cells, while sparing normal hematopoietic precursors. Lymphocytes can be inactivated as well.[44] Experience with other dyes such as phthalocyanine is more limited.[45]

Finally, bone marrow or peripheral blood stem cells harvested for autologous transplantation usually need to be cryopreserved in liquid nitrogen until later use. Several cryopreservation protocols are described elsewhere in this volume (see Chapter 9). Most investigators use a cryoprotectant such as dimethyl sulfoxide (DMSO) and subject cells to controlled-rate freezing, a gradual lowering of temperature (usually 1°C per minute) along with compensation for temperature fluctuations. It has now been shown that marrow cryopreserved for as long as 5 to 10 years can be used successfully for autologous reconstitution after marrow ablative therapy.[46] However, occasionally there have been patients with incomplete reconstitution of hematopoiesis. Often these patients die of hemorrhage or infection. Most transplant teams have, therefore, established the policy of storing a second (backup) marrow that is maintained unmanipulated to serve as a rescue should the first transplant (with or without in vitro manipulation) be unsuccessful.[46]

SOURCES OF HEMATOPOIETIC STEM CELLS

Hematopoiesis evolves through three embryologic stages: mesodermal (yolk sac), hepatosplenic, and medullary.[47] The first lineage that can be identified is erythropoiesis, followed by myelopoiesis, thrombopoiesis, and finally lymphopoiesis. At the time of birth, the bone marrow has generally become the only site of hematopoiesis, although some blood-forming ability may still be detectable in the spleen. In contrast to other species such as mice, in whom splenic hematopoesis persists throughout life, in adult human beings extramedullary hematopoiesis occurs only under pathologic conditions (e.g., chronic myelogenous leukemia, myelofibrosis). Accordingly, hematopoietic stem cells can be obtained from fetal (but not adult) livers,[48] whereas an adult donor usually can donate stem cells only in the form of bone marrow[49] or from peripheral blood wherein some stem cells circulate.[50] The presence of circulating stem cells in blood had previously been proven in animal models by the fact that transplants with cells exclusively obtained from peripheral blood resulted in complete lymphohematopoietic reconstitution.[51,52] This finding was not necessarily surprising (but was reassuring nevertheless) because bone marrow cells are usually transplanted via transfusion into a vein, then cross the pulmonary vascular bed, and through bone arteries "home" to the marrow cavity.

Table 2-1 lists potential sources of hematopoietic stem cells. The availability (and usefulness) depends largely on the patient's disease and the histocompatibility barrier that has to be overcome at transplantation.

Bone Marrow

Currently, most hematopoietic transplants are carried out with bone marrow cells (see Table 2-1). Generally, marrow cells are aspirated (harvested) with syringes through large bore needles from the posterior iliac crests and pelvic rim and in some patients also from anterior iliac crests and sternum.[8,49] If any one of these areas was previously exposed to irradiation, as, for example, in patients with Hodgkin's disease, it may be difficult and at times impossible to obtain cell numbers sufficient for transplantation.

Every aspirate consists of a mixture of marrow cells and peripheral blood (owing to perfusion of the marrow space and damage inflicted by needle placement and aspiration). It appears that the larger the volume aspirated, the greater the relative contribution of blood, including T lymphocytes. This has led to the recommendation to remove, with a single aspirate, no more than 3 to 5 mL. Some investigators have suggested surgical removal of bone chips (or even ribs) to avoid blood contamination and obtain concentrated marrow.[53] This approach, however, has not been followed routinely in clinical transplantation.

Of course, if the plan is to process the aspirated marrow before infusion into the patient, peripheral blood contamination need not be a concern. Treatment of marrow with monoclonal antibodies and complement,[54] magnetic beads,[55] or other techniques[56] (Table 2-2)—that is, those aimed at removing marrow T lymphocytes—will also remove T lymphocytes contributed by blood. This leaves the problem of donor blood loss and the need for allogeneic transfusion. A recent study[57] has suggested minimizing this need by reinfusing blood separated from the marrow-blood mixture during the marrow harvest. The harvest volume is generally limited to 10 to 15 mL per kg donor weight, a consideration particularly important in small pediatric donors.[58] The cell yield

Table 2-4 MARROW CELL YIELD BY DONOR AGE[1]

Age (Years)	ALLOGENEIC			AUTOLOGOUS		
	Volume[2]	Cells[3]	Concentration[4]	Volume	Cells	Concentration
≤9	13.0	4.5	3.2	14.4	2.4	2.5
10–19	10.8	2.8	2.6	13.6	2.7	1.9
20–59	9.5	2.2	2.4	10.7	2.3	2.7
≥60	8.5	2.0	2.2	9.6	2.4	2.4

1. Adapted from Buckner, CD, et al[59] and Jin, NR, et al[60]; only first harvests are considered.
2. mL/kg donor weight (median).
3. Nucleated marrow cells $\times 10^8$/kg donor weight (median).
4. Nucleated marrow cells $\times 10^7$/mL marrow (median).

declines somewhat with donor age (Table 2-4) but does not appear to be significantly different in allogeneic (normal) and autologous marrow harvests.[59,60]

Peripheral Blood Stem Cells

It was first shown in animal models that stem cells capable of complete hematopoietic reconstitution circulate in peripheral blood.[51,52,61] In nonhuman primates,[51] in dogs,[61] and in other species,[52] these cells are capable not only of autologous but also of allogeneic hematopoietic reconstitution. Although the allogeneic approach has not been explored extensively in humans, many patients have received transplants with autologous cells obtained by leukapheresis from peripheral blood prior to conditioning for transplantation.[34,50,62] The concentration of these cells in healthy individuals and in patients is usually quite low. It was observed, however, that with a delay following chemotherapy, there was a rebound burst of precursor cells as determined by in vitro colony formation.[34,62] The interval between chemotherapy and the peak concentration of precursor cells depends on the agent used. One can take advantage of this phenomenon and administer a cytotoxic drug such as cyclophosphamide, and then carry out leukaphereses at predetermined times and store the cells for transplantation after full-dose conditioning.[34,50,62] Assuming that in vitro colony formation correlates with in vitro repopulating ability, many investigators feel that this approach is advantageous (compared with the use of marrow), particularly in patients with malignant marrow involvement, with myelodysplastic disorders, or with prior irradiation to marrow-bearing bones that represent the usual site for marrow harvesting.

The characteristics of stem cells from peripheral blood may differ from those obtained from bone marrow.[63] Nevertheless, hematopoietic reconstitution has been shown to be complete, although in some patients, especially those with acute myelogenous leukemia, substantial time lags in recovery or incomplete recovery can be seen. The combined use of autologous bone marrow and peripheral blood stem cells has been even more encouraging in that recovery of hematopoietic function was faster, thus shortening the duration of marrow aplasia and leukopenia and thereby reducing the risk of intervening infections.[64] This approach has been further exploited by the administration of growth factors such as granulocyte-macrophage colony-stimulating factor

(GM-CSF) or interleukin-3 (IL-3) before leukapheresis, and patients given stem cells obtained with this manipulation appear to recover even faster than control individuals.[65]

Fetal Liver

As outlined earlier, for several months during fetal development, the liver is physiologically part of the hematopoietic tissues. It is during this time (from the second to the seventh month of pregnancy)—and ideally before the onset of lymphopoiesis—that fetal liver cells (a mixture of hepatocytes and hematopoietic cells) can be used for transplantation.[66] Fetal liver cells have been studied extensively in experimental models and have been shown clinically to reconstitute successfully both hematopoietic and immunologic systems in children with congenital immunodeficiencies.[67]

Fetal liver cells can be obtained only from aborted fetuses, and, therefore, are not available routinely. Because of ethical concerns and the development of alternative approaches (HLA-nonidentical donors, T-cell depletion), fetal liver cells have recently been used only by a few investigators and for very selected indications.[67]

Umbilical Cord Blood

Barnes, Ford, and Loutit[68] reported 25 years ago that the blood of fetal mice contained large numbers of hematopoietic stem cells. As discussed earlier, during ontogeny of hematopoiesis the major site of blood formation shifts from the mesenchyme to the liver (and spleen) and eventually to the bone marrow. In this process, stem cells reach the blood and circulate.

Cord blood, representing an integral part of the placentofetal circulation, therefore, also contains circulating stem cells.[69] The advantage of cord blood is that it can be accessed at the time of birth without affecting the fetus (or the mother). Indeed, it has been shown that with refined techniques up to 200 mL of cord blood can be obtained, containing as many as 4×10^6 myeloid progenitors.[70] A recent report[71] shows that these cells may be used, even after cryopreservation, to carry out a successful transplant in an older sibling suffering from Fanconi's anemia. Some investigators have expressed concern that these cells may carry high GVH disease potential, owing either to competent fetal cells or to contaminating maternal cells.

Ethical concerns exist about the use of cord blood and the issue is problematic. Conceivably, the parents of a child with a congenital disorder that could be corrected by marrow transplantation could decide to have another child to serve as a donor. However, the second child (fetus) might have the same genetically determined disorder and, therefore, would not be a suitable donor but instead would also need treatment. Alternatively, the fetus might be healthy but might have inherited the two parental HLA haplotypes not present in the patient. On that basis the fetus would not be a suitable donor; moreover, if a transplant were carried out, there would be a high risk of severe GVH disease.

Could cord blood be stored for later autologous use? This issue was discussed in a recent editorial.[72] The answer is probably yes, but the logistics, implications, and economic aspects are difficult to oversee at present.

ENUMERATION OF STEM CELLS

The earliest murine studies of marrow transplantation revealed that the number of marrow cells required for allogeneic transplants was substantially higher than for syngeneic transplants. This was subsequently confirmed in other species and is probably also true (but difficult to test) in humans. The usual aim is to infuse 2 to 4×10^8 cells per kg for an allogeneic transplant,[73] although successful transplants with lower cell numbers have been carried out. However, regardless of what cell number is required, it would be desirable to have a test that would provide an in vitro measurement allowing for a correlation with in vivo outcome.

Recent studies indicate a correlation between the number of CD34-positive cells contained in the marrow and the number of CFUs observed in vitro.[74] So far, it has not been possible to purify hematopoietic stem cells to the same degree in humans as has recently been achieved in mice, where the injection of a few cells was sufficient for complete reconstitution.[75] Nevertheless, CD34 appears to be a marker for very early hematopoietic precursor cells, and a correlation between CD34-positive cells and in vitro colony formation may thus give an approximation of the number of stem cells transplanted. As a rough guide for successful reconstitution, 1×10^5 CFU-GM per kg recipient weight have been suggested.[36] At doses of 5×10^4 CFU-GM or less recovery appeared to be slow. It is also important to note, however, that results vary considerably from study to study. For the time being, it seems prudent for every laboratory to establish its own standards. Ongoing studies using the supravital dye rhodamine 123 may offer further insight into which cells carry the capacity for long-term reconstitution versus short-term colony formation and in vitro function versus in vivo propagation.[76]

SUMMARY

Numerous methods of bone marrow transplantation are currently available. Regarding marrow purging, the "gold standard" will be the purification of the human stem cell[77] such that a limited number of cells can be transplanted without carrying the risk of contaminating tumor cells in the autologous setting or introducing immunocompetent lymphocytes, which would cause GVH disease after allogeneic transplantation. The impact of recombinant hematopoietic growth factors is only beginning to become apparent.[78] It is possible that their preharvest use will increase the yield of transplantable cells, and it is likely that their post-transplant effects will allow modification of the minimally required dose of stem cells to be transplanted. It is also conceivable that culture systems can be developed in which combinations of growth factors will allow in vitro expansion of stem cells harvested by a small marrow aspirate. Such an approach will also be important if gene transfer into defective cells is to be effective.[79] The individual chapters in this book address the various issues listed here and show how current applications and ongoing research strive to achieve those goals.

REFERENCES

1. Santos, GW: History of bone marrow transplantation. Clin Haematol 12:611, 1983.
2. Jacobson, LO, et al: Recovery from radiation injury. Science 113:510, 1951.
3. Lorenz, E, et al: Modification of irradiation injury in mice and guinea pigs by bone marrow injections. J Natl Cancer Inst 12:197, 1951.
4. van Bekkum, DW and de Vries, MJ: Radiation chimaeras. Radiobiological Institute of the Organization for Health Research TNO, Rijswijk ZH Netherlands. Academic Press, New York, 1967.
5. Gowans, JL: The fate of parental strain small lymphocytes in F1 hybrid rats. Ann NY Acad Sci 99:432, 1962.
6. McGregor, DD: Bone marrow origin of immunologically competent lymphocytes in the rat. J Exp Med 127:953, 1968.
7. Deeg, HJ, Klingemann, HG, and Phillips, GL: A guide to bone marrow transplantation. Springer-Verlag, New York, 1988.
8. Robins, MM and Noyes, WD: Aplastic anemia treated with bone-marrow transfusion from an identical twin. N Engl J Med 265:974, 1961.
9. Pillow, RP, et al: Treatment of bone-marrow failure by isogeneic marrow infusion. N Engl J Med 275:94, 1966.
10. Bach, FH and vanRood, JJ: The major histocompatibility complex—genetics and biology. N Engl J Med 295:806, 872, 927, 1976.
11. Thomas, ED, et al: Bone-marrow transplantation. N Engl J Med 292:832, 895, 1975.
12. Gale, RP: Potential utilization of a national HLA-typed donor pool for bone marrow transplantation. Transplantation 42:54, 1986.
13. Beatty, PG, et al: Marrow transplantation from relatives other than HLA-identical siblings. In Gale, RP and Champlin, R (eds): Bone Marrow Transplantation: Current Controversies. Alan R. Liss, New York, 1989, p 619.
14. Hansen, JA, et al: Transplantation of marrow from an unrelated donor to a patient with acute leukemia. N Engl J Med 303:565, 1980.
15. McGlave, PB, et al: Therapy for chronic myelogenous leukemia with unrelated donor bone marrow transplantation: Results in 102 cases. Blood 75:1728, 1990.
16. Beatty, PG, et al: Probability of finding HLA-matched unrelated marrow donors. Transplantation 45:714, 1988.
17. Hood, AF, et al: Acute graft-vs-host disease. Arch Dermatol 123:745, 1987.
18. Weiden, PL, et al: Antileukemic effect of chronic graft-versus-host disease—contribution to improved survival after allogeneic marrow transplantation. N Engl J Med 304:1529, 1981.
19. Perreault, C, et al: Minor histocompatibility antigens. Blood 76:1269, 1990.
20. Korngold, R and Sprent, J: T cell subsets in graft-vs.-host disease. In Burakoff, SJ, et al (eds): Graft-vs.-Host Disease: Immunology, Pathophysiology, and Treatment. Marcel Dekker, New York, 1990, p 31.
21. Ghayur, T, Seemayer, T, and Lapp, WS: Histologic correlates of immune functional deficits in graft-vs-host disease. In Burakoff, SJ, et al (eds): Graft-vs.-Host Disease: Immunology, Pathophysiology, and Treatment. Marcel Dekker, New York, 1990, p 109.
22. Piguet, PF: Tumor necrosis factor and graft-vs.-host disease. In Burakoff, SJ, et al (eds): Graft-vs.-Host Disease: Immunology, Pathophysiology, and Treatment. Marcel Dekker, New York, 1990, p 225.
23. Deeg, HJ and Cottler-Fox, M: Clinical spectrum and pathophysiology of acute graft-vs.-host disease. In Burakoff, SJ, et al (eds): Graft Versus Host Disease: Immunology, Pathophysiology and Treatment. Marcel Dekker, New York, 1990, p 311.
24. Prentice, HG, et al: Use of anti-T-cell monoclonal antibody OKT3 to prevent acute graft-versus-host disease in allogeneic bone-marrow transplantation for acute leukaemia. Lancet 1:700, 1982.
25. deWitte, T, et al: Depletion of donor lymphocytes by counterflow centrifugation successfully prevents acute graft-versus-host disease in matched allogeneic marrow transplantation. Blood 67:1302, 1986.

26. Martin, PJ, et al: Effects of treating marrow with a CD3-specific immunotoxin for prevention of acute graft-versus-host disease. Bone Marrow Transplant 3:437, 1988.

27. Mitsuyasu, RT, et al: Treatment of donor bone marrow with monoclonal anti-T-cell antibody and complement for the prevention of graft-versus-host disease. Ann Intern Med 105:20, 1986.

28. Hale, G, Cobbold, S, and Waldmann, H: T cell depletion with Campath-1 in allogeneic bone marrow transplantation. Transplantation 45:753, 1988.

29. Sullivan, KM, et al: Graft-versus-host disease as adoptive immunotherapy in patients with advanced hematologic neoplasms. N Engl J Med 320:828, 1989.

30. Horowitz, MM, et al: Graft-versus-leukemia reactions after bone marrow transplantation. Blood 75:555, 1990.

31. Champlin, R, et al: Selective depletion of CD8 positive T-lymphocytes for prevention of graft-versus-host disease following allogeneic bone marrow transplantation. Transplant Proc 21:2947, 1989.

32. Maraninchi, D, et al: Selective depletion of marrow-T cytotoxic lymphocytes (CD8) in the prevention of graft-versus-host disease after allogeneic bone-marrow transplantation. Transplant Int 1:91, 1988.

33. Körbling, M, Hunstein, W, and Fliedner, TM: Die autologe Knochenmarktransplantation. Dtsch Med Wochenschr 109:265, 271, 1984.

34. Juttner, CA, et al: Circulating autologous stem cells collected in very early remission from acute non-lymphoblastic leukaemia produce prompt but incomplete haemopoietic reconstitution after high dose melphalan or supralethal chemoradiotherapy. Br J Haematol 61:739, 1985.

35. Jones, RJ, et al: Separation of pluripotent haematopoietic stem cells from spleen colony-forming cells. Nature 347:188, 1990.

36. Rowley, SD, et al: CFU-GM content of bone marrow graft correlates with time to hematopoietic reconstitution following autologous bone marrow transplantation with 4-hydroperoxycyclophosphamide. Blood 70:271, 1987.

37. Kaizer, H, et al: Autologous bone marrow transplantation in acute leukemia: A phase I study of in vitro treatment of marrow with 4-hydroperoxycyclophosphamide to purge tumor cells. Blood 65:1504, 1985.

38. Gorin, NC, et al: Autologous bone marrow transplantation using marrow incubated with asta Z 7557 in adult acute leukemia. Blood 67:1367, 1986.

39. Coulombel, L, et al: Long term marrow culture of cells from patients with acute myelogenous leukemia (AML): Selection in favour of normal phenotypes in some but not all cases. J Clin Invest 75:961, 1985.

40. Chang, J, et al: The use of bone marrow cells grown in long-term culture for autologous bone marrow transplantation in acute myeloid leukaemia: An update. Bone Marrow Transplant 4:5, 1989.

41. Barnett, MJ, et al: Successful autografting in chronic myeloid leukaemia after maintenance of marrow in culture. Bone Marrow Transplant 4:345, 1989.

42. Barlogie, B, et al: High-dose chemoradiotherapy and autologous bone marrow transplantation for resistant multiple myeloma. Blood 70:869, 1987.

43. Sieber, F, et al: Dye-mediated photolysis of human neuroblastoma cells: Implications for autologous bone marrow transplantation. Blood 68:32, 1986.

44. Lum, LG, et al: Merocyanine 540-sensitized photoirradiation inhibits T and B cell functions. Exp Hematol 18:540, 1990.

45. Singer, CRJ, et al: Differential phthalocyanine photosensitization of acute myeloblastic leukemia progenitor cells: A potential purging technique for autologous bone marrow transplantation. Br J Haematol 68:417, 1988.

46. Areman, EM, Sacher, RA, and Deeg, HJ: Processing and storage of human bone marrow: A survey of current practices in North America. Bone Marrow Transplant 6:203, 1990.

47. Clara, M: Entwicklungsgeschichte Des Menschen, ed 6. Leipzig, 1966.

48. Lucarelli, G, et al: Fetal liver transplantation in aplastic anemia and acute leukemia. In Gale, RP (ed): Recent Advances in Bone Marrow Transplantation. Alan R. Liss, New York, 1983, p 865.

49. Thomas, ED and Storb, R: Technique for human marrow grafting. Blood 36:507, 1970.

50. Reiffers, J, et al: Successful autologous transplantation with peripheral blood hemopoietic cells in a patient with acute leukemia. Exp Hematol 14:312, 1986.

51. Storb, R, et al: Demonstration of hemopoietic stem cells in the peripheral blood of baboons by cross circulation. Blood 50:537, 1977.

52. Micklem, HS, Anderson, N, and Ross, E: Limited potential of circulating haemopoietic stem cells. Nature 256:41, 1975.
53. Herrmann, RP and Davis, RE: Technique for human bone marrow harvest. Acta Haematol 68:309, 1982.
54. Hale, G, et al: Removal of T cells from bone marrow for transplantation: A monoclonal anti-lymphocyte antibody that fixes human complement. Blood 62:873, 1983.
55. Vartdal, F, et al: Depletion of T lymphocytes from human bone marrow. Transplantation 43:366, 1987.
56. Autran, B, et al: T-cell depletion of bone marrow transplants: Assessment of standard immunological methods of quantification. Exp Hematol 15:1121, 1987.
57. Rosenfeld, CS, et al: Transfusion of bone marrow red cells during bone marrow harvests. Exp Hematol 16:702, 1988.
58. Sanders, J, et al: Experience with marrow harvesting from donors less than two years of age. Bone Marrow Transplant 2:45, 1987.
59. Buckner, CD, et al: Marrow harvesting from normal donors. Blood 64:630, 1984.
60. Jin, NR, et al: Marrow harvesting for autologous marrow transplantation. Exp Hematol 13:879, 1985.
61. Storb, R, Epstein, RB, and Thomas, ED: Marrow repopulating ability of peripheral blood cells compared to thoracic duct cells. Blood 32:662, 1968.
62. Körbling, M, et al: Successful engraftment of blood-derived normal hemopoietic stem cells in chronic myelogenous leukemia. Exp Hematol 9:684, 1981.
63. Gianni, AM, et al: Granulocyte-macrophage colony-stimulating factor to harvest circulating haemopoietic stem cells for autotransplantation. Lancet 2:580, 1989.
64. Gianni, AM, et al: Rapid and complete hemopoietic reconstitution following combined transplantation of autologous blood and bone marrow cells: A changing role for high dose chemo-radiotherapy? Hematol Oncol 7:139, 1989.
65. Blazar, BR, et al: Augmentation of donor bone marrow engraftment in histoincompatible murine recipients by granulocyte/macrophage colony-stimulating factor. Blood 71:320, 1988.
66. O'Reilly, RJ, et al: Fetal liver transplantation in man and animals. In Gale, RP (ed): Recent Advances in Bone Marrow Transplantation. Alan R. Liss, New York, 1983, p 799.
67. Touraine, JL: Transplantation of both fetal liver and thymus in severe combined immunodeficiencies: Interaction between donor's and recipient's cells. In Lucarelli, G, Fliedner, TM, and Gale, RP (eds): Fetal Liver Transplantation. Excerpta Medica, Amsterdam, 1980, p 276.
68. Barnes, DWH, Ford, CE, and Loutit, JF: Haemopoietic stem cells. Lancet 1:1395, 1964.
69. Linch, DC, et al: Studies of circulating hemopoietic progenitor cells in human fetal blood. Blood 59:976, 1982.
70. Broxmeyer, HE, et al: Human umbilical cord blood as a potential source of transplantable hematopoietic stem/progenitor cells. Proc Natl Acad Sci USA 86:3828, 1989.
71. Gluckman, E, et al: Hematopoietic reconstitution in a patient with Fanconi's anemia by means of umbilical-cord blood from an HLA-identical sibling. N Engl J Med 321:1174, 1989.
72. Linch, DC and Brent, L: Can cord blood be used? Nature 340:676, 1989.
73. Storb, R, Prentice, RL, and Thomas, ED: Marrow transplantation for treatment of aplastic anemia: An analysis of factors associated with graft rejection. N Engl J Med 296:61, 1977.
74. Siena, S, et al: Circulation of CD34+ hematopoietic stem cells in the peripheral blood of high-dose cyclophosphamide-treated patients: Enhancement by intravenous recombinant human granulocyte-macrophage colony-stimulating factor. Blood 74:1905, 1989.
75. Spangrude, GJ, Heimfeld, S, and Weissman, IL: Purification and characterization of mouse hematopoietic stem cells. Science 241:58, 1988.
76. Darzynkiewicz, Z, et al: Interactions of rhodamine 123 with living cells studied by flow cytometry. Cancer Res 42:799, 1982.
77. Berenson, RJ, et al: Antigen CD34+ marrow cells engraft lethally irradiated baboons. J Clin Invest 81:951, 1988.
78. Appelbaum, FR: The clinical use of hematopoietic growth factors. Semin Hematol 26:7, 1989.
79. Kaleko, M, et al: Expression of human adenosine deaminase in mice after transplantation of genetically-modified bone marrow. Blood 75:1733, 1990.

3 | ESTABLISHING A MARROW PROCESSING LABORATORY*

Commentary by ANN McMICAN

This chapter discusses the factors that require consideration in the establishment of a new laboratory for processing of bone marrow for transplantation. The main focus is for support of an autologous transplantation program, but some references are made to additional requirements for support of allogeneic and peripheral blood stem cell processing as well. Planning, space, and staffing considerations as well as equipment, training, and safety concerns are discussed. Also included are a list of materials and reagents commonly used in bone marrow processing, information on licensing issues, and quality assurance.

PLANNING CONSIDERATIONS

Several key issues need to be addressed in the planning of a bone marrow transplantation processing laboratory.

Which Procedures Will Be Performed?

The decision as to which types of procedures will be performed is first. Current possibilities include autologous transplantation, allogeneic or syngeneic transplants, or both, and peripheral or other types of stem cell harvests for transplantation. Start-up planning should be done in consideration of all procedures likely to be performed now or in the future to ensure flexibility and easy transition from one procedure to another.

Where Should the Processing Be Performed?

Current sites for bone marrow processing include hospital blood banks, HLA or tissue culture laboratories, research laboratories, specialized separate laboratories, and blood collection facilities.

---

*Thanks to the staff of the Blood Bank of the University of Rochester–Strong Memorial Hospital; especially to Kate Finke, Sue Frauenhofer, and Katie McNeice for their enthusiasm and support in the development of the Bone Marrow Processing Service.

Hospital blood banks are a good choice for a number of reasons. They are often located near the place where the actual bone marrow collection will be performed, which is helpful in avoiding long transportation times or other delays in collection or processing. Blood banks have well-trained technologists on staff who are usually already familiar with meticulous blood product manipulation under aseptic conditions. Also, preexisting equipment or other support technologies may be readily at hand (cell sorters, cell counters, blood cell separators, and the like). Finally, blood bank staff members are also heavily involved in the transfusion support of these patients and are committed to the highest quality of care. They are usually scheduled around the clock and can therefore more easily handle the procedures that may go across standard shift times because of their length or complexity. On the other hand, the hospital blood bank may not have sufficient existing free space, or the staffing or time to accomplish these additional highly specialized procedures in addition to a busy clinical service.

HLA or tissue culture laboratories are also well suited to bone marrow processing. The staff members in these areas are familiar with methods of mononuclear cell separation and cell culture techniques. They have often performed the transplantation-related histocompatibility testing and can easily assimilate continued support of the treatment process. Although these laboratories are often not staffed around the clock, an on-call system is usually in place to provide support for renal, liver, or cardiac transplantation. More flexibility is often available in staffing for the following day, compared with the blood bank, which must carry on its routine functions regardless of the special procedures performed. As in the blood bank, space may be a limitation here. Also, the small total staff size limits flexibility, and extra on-call responsibilities may be a burden.

Research laboratories have the advantage of procedure development experience and flexibility—both requirements for bone marrow processing. Often, procedures are modified slightly on the day of use to fit specific patient circumstances. It is sometimes difficult for the clinical technologist to feel confident about change that has not been well worked out before hand. Yet the personalized processing that is called for in bone marrow work is critical to the success of the patients and program. Research technologists are expected to have a more flexible approach to standard experimentation, which many of the procedures require, and can more easily handle subtle changes from day to day. However, these individuals' backgrounds may be too limited to enable them to make good decisions when troubleshooting unexpected occurrences. Often, one would be starting from the ground up in training and equipment acquisition in the research laboratory.

Specialized bone marrow processing laboratories are another possible place for these activities. They have the advantage of a single focus and mission. The disadvantages include those of any isolated work space—small budgets, less flexibility in staffing, and starting from the ground up in hiring staff who will be creative in their approaches yet meticulous in the technical aspects of the processing. Hiring staff with experience in either blood bank or histocompatibility testing or immunology could lessen the impact in this area.

Blood collection centers are considered good processing sites, for a number of reasons. First, they have many of the same advantages as the hospital blood bank. In addition, they may be able to serve several institutions in their blood collection region, resulting in better use of staff, consistency of patient care, and economic efficiency. These centers most certainly participate in apheresis procedures and can easily make the switch to peripheral stem cell harvests with little additional time and funding. Transportation of bone marrow and materials to the admitting facility may present special challenges because accidents such as losing precious marrow to a bag broken in transport must be avoided.

Each of the laboratories detailed here can make suitable processing sites. Institutions should review each of the possibilities before choosing one site over another.

What Parts of the Procedure Require Laboratory Involvement?

Autologous marrow and peripheral stem cell procedures are the most labor-intensive for the laboratory, consisting of at least five distinct components: collection, processing, storage, reinfusion, and quality assurance. The laboratory may be responsible for all or part of these functions. Collections are usually performed in the operating room (or donor room in peripheral stem cell harvest). It is often helpful to perform cell counts at intervals during the marrow collection process to ensure that adequate numbers of cells are being collected for subsequent reinfusion and engraftment. Counts can be done at the collection site or in the processing laboratory if transportation and turnaround time can be kept short. Processing (stem cell concentration or isolation) and freezing are the next major steps. These can be done in one laboratory or several—again, if transportation is not a problem. Storage mainly requires freezer space and an inventory and monitoring system. Large amounts of freezer space are needed if many marrows will be collected for use in the distant future. Many programs channel patients directly from the collection procedure to transplant. For reinfusion, laboratories are usually asked to provide only the frozen marrow and a waterbath. Transplant nurses or other medical personnel are more often directly responsible for the reinfusion itself. Finally, a variety of people and laboratories may need to be involved in the complex program of quality assurance recommended for marrow processing. Microbiologists provide sterility culture information, and flow cytometry studies or cell culture techniques monitor the efficiency and effectiveness of the processing techniques.

Which Methods Will Be Used?

Many different methods for bone marrow and stem cell processing are now in use. Several are described in detail elsewhere in this book. Most of them begin with a concentration step in which the fraction of material containing stem cells is concentrated into a small volume (50 to 150 mL) from the large volume (500 to 2500 mL) of marrow collected. This may be done manually, using aseptic technique and many conical centrifuge tubes, or in an automated fashion, using any one of a number of automated blood cell processors. Most technologists opt for the efficiency of an automated procedure, one that guarantees good stem cell recovery, low contamination rates, and less technologist time; an automated procedure can cut the processing time in half. On the other hand, a manual backup method should also be in place to enable continuation in times of instrument failure.

Density gradient separations add 30 to 90 minutes to the processing time. These are useful in decreasing red blood cell, platelet, and mature granulocyte contamination and are often used to ready the concentrate for purging techniques. Density gradient purification may decrease the frequency or severity of patient reactions to reinfusion[1] but may also lower overall stem cell recovery.

There are two main stem cell cryopreservation techniques.[2,3] Dimethyl sulfoxide (DMSO) is the common cryoprotectant used in both methods, although at different concentrations in the final suspension to be frozen. The first method uses controlled-rate freezing in liquid nitrogen. The concentrates may be stored either in liquid nitrogen itself or in the vapor phase. The second method does not require controlled-rate freezing, adds hydroxyethyl starch (HES) to the freezing media, and makes use of a standard mechanical freezer for both freezing and storage. Although freezing and storing in liquid nitrogen is significantly more costly, some investigators feel that it may contribute to better postprocedure stem cell function and viability. Both procedures have been proven to enable stem cell preservation and engraftment in patients undergoing bone marrow transplantation.

Bone marrow and stem cell concentrates may be manipulated prior to freezing in an attempt to further eradicate tumor cells (in autologous transplants) or deplete T lymphocytes and lessen the severity of graft-versus-host (GVH) disease (in allogeneic transplants). These manipulations are referred to as purging techniques. To date, a variety of chemicals, monoclonal antibodies, and drugs have been used to purge grafts. As mentioned previously, many of these techniques require the use of better stem cell purification. They may also result in a significant reduction in stem cell recovery. The major implications for the laboratory are increased processing time, the purchase of purging reagents, and the technical ability to wash or otherwise remove excess reagent from the marrow before freezing. Some of the reagents have special storage requirements resulting in additional expense.

The final key in the planning process is to determine the number of procedures that will be performed. All programs will begin with a modest proposal for the first year or two, but most programs escalate rapidly once success is obtained. It is always advisable to plan for a larger number of procedures than is actually expected; if that number is not actually reached, the plans allow for additional practice runs, which may be necessary.

SPACE CONSIDERATIONS

The amount of space required depends on the answers to the previous questions, and is particularly sensitive to the parts of the procedure that require laboratory involvement and the methods to be used. Space is somewhat less sensitive to the number of procedures to be performed: 300 to 400 square feet is adequate to perform cell counts, automatically process (including density separation and purging), and freeze and store marrow. Additional space may be needed if either stem cell culturing or flow cytometry services need to be included. The space may need to be increased if the service becomes particularly large (more than 200 procedures performed each year) but should not be reduced significantly even if the number is small owing to the absolute size required for capital equipment, work space, liquid nitrogen tanks, and other equipment.

One should assess whether two or more staff members will be working in the area at the same time. The general scheme of marrow processing lends itself to a person working sequentially through the steps independently, but if two or more procedures are performed at the same time, space may have to be increased. Thought should be given to backup freezer space in the event of instrument failure. If alternate emergency storage is not available somewhere within the facility or nearby, then additional space should be planned within the laboratory. This should usually be in the form of a duplicate freezer or liquid nitrogen–holding tank, both requiring significant additional floor space. Storage space for materials and reagents is included in the previous estimate, however. Thawing and reinfusion usually take place at the patient's bedside, so the only space required to support this part of the process is room for a waterbath or a transport container or both to be stored.

EQUIPMENT

A list of both capital and minor equipment needed for bone marrow processing is in Table 3-1. Many facilities will have some of these instruments already in place, used for other applications. Several items that are specific to bone marrow procedures may not be commonly available. A general list of materials and reagents is in Table 3-2. Many of the reagents currently used in bone marrow processing are not licensed for in vivo use, including the tissue culture media, reagents such as DNAse, density gradients, and most of the purging materials. However, most of these reagents have been in general use for this application without significant untoward reactions in the recipients. There may be specific state or federal regulations that should be taken into

---

Table 3–1   EQUIPMENT

Processing
Freezer space, including canisters and racking system
    a. Liquid nitrogen
    b. Mechanical freezer
Sterile work space, certified
Automated blood cell processor/separator
Controlled-rate freezer
Peristaltic pump
Heat sealer, storage bag dependent
Automated cell counter

Cell Culturing
CO_2 incubator
Inverted phase microscope

Reinfusion
Waterbath
Transport container

Table 3–2   MATERIALS AND REAGENTS

Precision pipettes and tips	DMSO
Pipettes: 1, 5, 10 mL	Hank's balanced salt solution
Test tubes	Ficoll-Hypaque
Freezing bags	DNAse
Freezing vials	Heparin
Culture plates	Trypan blue
Transfer packs: 300 mL to 2 L	HES
Needles: 16 to 18 gauge, and spinal	RPMI/^{199}Tc
Syringes: tuberculin to 60 mL	Liquid nitrogen
Alcohol wipes	CO_2 gas
Sampling site couplers	Ethyl alcohol
Conical centrifuge tubes: 15 to 50 mL	Growth stimulators
Plasma transfer sets	Purging materials
Clamps and crimper	McCoy's 5A Medium
Processing software	Fetal bovine serum
Hemostats	Penicillin-strep solution
Wrench	L-glutamine
Gloves: latex and cold protective	Agar
Thermometers	Sterile dH_2O
Plastic bags	
Unopettes/diluter	
Hemocytometer	
Microscope	
Autoclave	
Stirrer	
Refrigerator	
Centrifuge	

account when using such materials, and all personnel involved in the development and practice of these techniques should be made aware of this.

STAFFING

At least two staff members should be able to perform bone marrow processing in each facility, so that the procedures can be performed even if one person is unavailable. Often collections cannot wait for a person to return from vacation or absence due to illness; even if the total number of procedures performed is small, it is in the patients' best interest to have at least two people available.

The processing staff should report to a laboratory director or supervisor. The management of this type of program takes from 0.1 to 1 FTE, depending on the level and type of involvement of the manager and where the laboratory is in the implementation of the program. For example, once in operation, a laboratory that performs only processing and storage for a moderate number of procedures would require far less management time (perhaps 0.1 FTE) than would a laboratory in the development stage expecting to perform significant research and a large and varied number of procedures to carry primary responsibility for collection of peripheral blood stem cells (perhaps 1 FTE). The types of people qualified for managerial work depend on the same factors.

The length and complexity of bone marrow processing and support procedures often necessitate long hours or, alternatively, involvement of staff on more than one shift. This is a feature that makes the clinical laboratory, with its 24-hour staffing schedule, a desirable place to initiate such a program. Although most collections take place during daylight hours, the processing and stem cell culturing that must be performed sequentially often run into the evening and night hours. Using multiple staff members on other shifts to perform these different functions allows for ready availability and flexibility in the provision of services. One staff member is not overwhelmed, and several others may get the opportunity to participate in the program. In contrast, in a dedicated bone marrow laboratory, staff members may be either exhausted after 12 hours of work or may sit idle if a scheduled procedure is canceled. Many of the ancillary support services such as stem cell culturing may be delegated to other laboratories to avoid overly lengthy workdays.

OTHER ISSUES

In addition to planning, space, equipment, and staffing concerns are several issues that are important to laboratory development. These include training, developing a procedure manual, and personnel safety.

Bone marrow processing is a specialized and complex activity, and staff members should be extensively trained. If at all possible, money should be earmarked for adequate supplies for practice procedures and travel for off-site training. Each facility should plan to support multiple practice runs of processing and freezing, including all quality assurance procedures, so that techniques can become solidly established before material from the first actual patient is handled. Because significant volumes of bone marrow to work with are difficult to obtain, provision should be made to obtain pooled buffy coats (not very satisfactory) or apheresis products, or perhaps to work with local surgeons to collect marrow as a part of surgical procedures (e.g., from sternums opened during open heart procedures). The last option requires surgeon cooperation and patient consent.

No good substitute is available for direct observation of procedures performed in an established laboratory. Most facilities are willing to share their expertise as time permits. The budget for this should be sufficient to support travel to at least two different sites in the first year. Additional funds should continue to be allocated to ensure continuing proficiency, updating of procedures, and acquisition of new skills.

Procedures should be documented in writing as soon as possible, a practice that helps to ensure consistency of the work performed as well as ease of training of additional technologists. Many established laboratories are willing to share some of their written procedures; many procedures are also found in this book. Records should be kept of all work performed. It would be good practice to follow standard blood bank procedures with regard to record keeping.[4,5] State, local, and other regulatory agencies may also have specific guidelines or requirements.

Laboratory personnel should follow standard safety guidelines for handling potentially infectious materials, sharp instruments, and carcinogenic agents, as well as for the appropriate disposal of all of these materials. Aseptic technique should be used in all phases of the program. All patient materials should be considered potentially infectious. The use of sharp instruments or needles should be discouraged and suitable alternatives instituted whenever possible. Disposal of used materials and carcinogenic agents should be as directed by the facility health and safety policies. All biohazardous materials should be either autoclaved or incinerated. Staff should wear protective attire as appropriate. As always, good handwashing is essential.

SUMMARY

Several important questions need to be addressed in the planning of a laboratory for bone marrow processing in support of a transplantation service. These include what types of procedures will be performed, where it should be done, what phases require laboratory involvement, what methods will be used, and how many procedures are likely to be performed. The space, equipment, and staffing requirements depend largely on the answers to these questions. Finally, adequate training, written procedures, and safety guidelines that are carefully followed are necessary for the successful development of a laboratory for bone marrow processing for transplantation.

REFERENCES

1. Davis, JM, et al: Clinical toxicity of cryopreserved bone marrow graft infusion. Blood 75:781, 1990.
2. English, D, et al: Semiautomated processing of bone marrow grafts for transplantation. Transfusion 29:12, 1989.
3. Stiff, PJ, et al: Autologous bone marrow transplantation using unfractionated cells cryopreserved in dimethyl sulfoxide and hydroxyethyl starch without controlled-rate freezing. Blood 70:974, 1987.
4. Widmann, F (ed): Standards for blood banks and transfusion services. American Association of Blood Banks, Arlington, VA, 1989.
5. Walker, RH (ed): Technical manual. American Association of Blood Banks, Arlington, VA, 1990.

4 | BONE MARROW COLLECTION TECHNIQUES

Commentary by MICHELE COTTLER-FOX

BONE MARROW HARVEST AND
  FILTRATION
Bone Marrow Harvest: Traditional Method
Bone Marrow Harvest: Disposable Collection
  Kit
Rapid Method for Filling a Transfer Bag in
  the Operating Room
Bone Marrow Filtration

CELL COUNTING AND CALCULATIONS
Counting Nucleated Cells with a
  Hemacytometer
Automated and Manual Cell Counting of
  Bone Marrow Suspensions
Automated Cell Counting during
  Hydroxyethyl Starch Sedimentation of
  Incompatible Red Blood Cells from Bone
  Marrow

The important parameters in marrow procurement for transplantation were clearly identified prior to the first reports of successful marrow transplantation in humans in the 1960s.[1-5] These parameters, as reviewed by Wilson in 1959,[6] include type of anesthesia, sites of aspiration, technique of and equipment for aspiration, type of suspension fluids used including anticoagulants, preparation of marrow suspension for infusion or storage, and number of cells needed. In 1970 Thomas and Storb[7] described their technique for marrow harvest, addressing each of these questions and noting their own successful solutions. Their methods have undergone few major changes, and are still the basis for marrow harvesting today. However, with almost 200 marrow transplant centers now active in the United States alone, variations on the original Seattle method have developed. This overview is meant as a guide to marrow collection in general, pointing out areas where changes have been made and questions that remain to be answered.

WHEN TO HARVEST

Marrow from an identical twin (syngeneic) or other related donor (allogeneic) is generally harvested at the recipient's transplant center on the day of transplant. However, if marrow is harvested from an unrelated donor at a center far from the recipient, marrow may sometimes be collected a day earlier in order to accommodate time requirements for transportation. Freezing autologous marrows remains the standard practice at present; however, marrow cells permit hematologic reconstitution after liquid storage for 34 to 48 hours at 4°C,[8] potentially eliminating the need to freeze an autologous marrow for a short conditioning regimen or allowing cells to be exposed for some period of time to growth factors in vitro prior to freezing. Freezing allogeneic marrow has not usually been a consideration owing to fears that stem cell loss upon freezing and thawing would lead to failure of engraftment. Despite such concerns, at least two centers have performed successful marrow transplantation using a frozen allogeneic graft.[9,10]

The decision about when to harvest autologous marrow remains problematic. A marrow free of malignant cells is preferred, although centers that purge autologous marrow may accept low-level contamination with malignant cells. How long after cessation of chemotherapy an autologous marrow is best harvested remains unclear. Although the marrow needs to recover from toxic effects of chemotherapy, the minimum interval required to do so is unknown and probably varies with therapeutic regimen and individual patient. If the patient remains in remission and a second or third harvest is needed, the yield of the repeat harvest has been reported to be best if performed more than 7 weeks after the previous harvest.[11] A second collection may be performed if the total number of mononuclear cells is deemed inadequate or if the transplant team prefers to have a backup should the initial marrow fail to engraft, containing more cells than can be provided by dividing the initial harvest volume. The need for a second collection can be determined only after evaluation of the completed first harvest.

EVALUATING MARROW QUALITY

Parameters currently available for evaluating the quality of harvested marrow include mononuclear cell count, colony-forming assays of precursor cells, and fluorescence-activated cell sorting (FACS) using an anti-CD34 monoclonal antibody to identify the most primitive recognized hematopoietic stem cell population. All three methods give only a relative measure of marrow quality. Although a total nucleated cell count of 1 to 3×10^8 per kg recipient body weight is generally considered adequate for engraftment in the autologous setting, 2 to 4×10^8 per kg recipient body weight is suggested for an allogeneic transplant[12] owing to the phenomenon of genetic resistance or the host-versus-graft reaction. For a marrow containing large amounts of fat it may be advisable to perform a manual count, as fat may be read by an automated cell counter as mononuclear cells. Further, allowance should be made for the number of granulocytes and band forms present, as these cells are part of the automated total white cell count but do not contribute to lasting engraftment. Whereas most centers that carry out marrow harvests also correct the total nucleated cell count for the donor's peripheral white blood cell count, the need to do so may depend on the technique used for harvest—that is, the amount of peripheral blood contaminating the harvested marrow. In the case of an exceptionally overweight recipient it is not clear whether cell dose requirements should be based on ideal body weight or on real weight and the decision will have to be a pragmatic one.

Although a relationship has been demonstrated for time to engraftment relative to number of autologous colony-forming units—culture (CFU-C) or colony-forming units—granulocyte-macrophage (CFU-GM) infused,[13,14] these colony assays reflect committed progenitor cells whose relationship to pluripotent stem cells in a given graft remains to be determined. It is also unclear how few such colony-forming cells reliably lead to engraftment, as available data have been acquired retrospectively, from marrow harvested on the basis of 10 to 20 mL marrow per kg recipient body weight. Although no linear relationship has been noted for time to engraftment versus mL marrow per kg recipient body weight or the number of cells per kg recipient body weight, there are animal data that suggest a strong correlation between the number of cells versus time to engraftment. The minimum number of CD34-positive cells required for engraftment remains unknown, although autologous grafts of as few as 1 to 4.5×10^6 CD34-positive enriched cells per kg have been successful.[15] Recent work by Jones and colleagues[16] in a mouse model suggests, in fact, that early hematopoietic recovery after transplant depends on relatively committed progenitor cells (post harvest days 8 and 12 colony-forming units—spleen [CFU-S], CFU-GM), whereas long-term reconstitution depends on pluripotent stem cells. Thus, for successful early engraftment and long-term reconstitution a marrow harvested for transplantation may need an as yet undetermined ratio of committed progenitors and pluripotent stem cells.

ANESTHESIA AND RISKS OF MARROW HARVEST

Marrow harvests are most frequently performed with patients under general anesthesia, with epidural or spinal anesthesia as options available if the donor or anesthesiologist prefers. Autologous harvests have also been performed using sedation and local anesthesia alone, and repeat donors often prefer this method to general anesthesia despite an increased level of discomfort.[17] Anesthesia is usually induced by inhalation or intravenous agents (e.g., a neuroleptic combination such as fentanyl and droperidol), followed by maintenance with nitrous oxide and oxygen. Other supplementary inhalation agents have sometimes been used as well.[18] Effects of anesthetic agents on the marrow harvested have not been well studied. At least one early report notes an increased yield of cells after inhalation agents compared with local anesthesia.[6] However, a more recent report notes a decrease in CFU-GM in harvested marrow as a function of time under nitrous oxide anesthesia.[19] If this is confirmed, it may become more important to determine accurately how little marrow is needed because time under anesthesia is dependent primarily on the volume harvested. Offsetting this potential risk from nitrous oxide is its potential antileukemic effect in the autologous setting,[20] a result of methylcobalamin coenzyme inactivation and subsequent folate deficiency.

Marrow harvests have commonly been performed on an in-patient basis, with the donor being admitted to the hospital the night before or early on the morning of harvest and discharged the day after harvest. The desire to decrease hospital costs, however, has led to a recent study of autologous harvest carried out as a same-day surgery, out-patient procedure.[21] If the donor is prepared to be admitted to the hospital in the event of hypotension, excessive pain, or unexpected complication of harvest it would appear that the majority of autologous donors may be harvested in this way and discharged within 12 hours. A similar study of allogeneic donors remains to be done.

Major risks of marrow harvest are those associated with anesthesia. An initial analysis of 2027 allogeneic harvests reported to the International Bone Marrow Transplant Registry[22] and 1270 such harvests reported by the Seattle team[23] revealed an overall combined incidence of 0.27 percent major, life-threatening complications including nonfatal cardiac arrest, pulmonary embolus, aspiration pneumonitis, ventricular tachycardia, and cerebral infarction. One fatality in an older donor owing to cardiac arrest during induction of general anesthesia at an unidentified institution is quoted in one of these reports.[24] Other complications such as bacteremia, local infection at aspiration sites, transient pressure neuropathies due to hematomas at the aspiration sites, postoperative fever, broken harvest needle requiring surgical removal, fractured anterior iliac crests, and spinal headache have also been reported,[23] as have diffuse intravascular coagulopathy[24] and air embolism.[25] Indeed, a recent analysis from the Seattle transplant team of another 1245 harvests shows 27 percent of allogeneic donors have complicating events, of which 92 percent were considered minor.[26] Roughly half of the serious complications in this series were related to anesthesia, with no relationship to length of anesthesia noted. Care must also be taken with autologous donors to avoid anesthetic agents associated with liver toxicity, as hepatic veno-occlusive disease is a major cause of post-transplant morbidity and mortality, and its incidence is increased in the setting of abnormal liver functions at the time of transplant.[27] Thus, although the risks of marrow donation are small, they are real and require careful preoperative assessment and close postoperative follow-up of the donor.

MARROW COLLECTION TECHNIQUES

Marrow may be harvested from both posterior and anterior iliac crests, sternum, and, rarely, from the tibia in the case of a very young donor. Historically donors were harvested from both anterior iliac crests, sternum, and posterior iliac crests by the Seattle team in an effort to acquire the maximum number of marrow cells possible.[7] However, with time and increasing experience it became clear that in the majority of cases posterior iliac crest harvests from allogeneic donors were adequate.[11,23,28] With a large difference between donor (small) and recipient (large) size, however, it may still be necessary to harvest anterior iliac crests, sternum, or even the tibia (in a donor under 1 year of age). Thus, after anesthesia is induced the donor is placed in the prone position either on pillows placed across the operating table to support hips and lower rib cage such that the diaphragm is free to move, or on a spinal frame (e.g., Wilson convex adjustable frame) such as is used for laminectomy. Harvest in the lateral position, although not common, has been described[6] and may be of use with a pregnant donor. A sterile field is prepared and two members of the transplant team harvest simultaneously, one on either side of the donor, while a third member of the team is responsible for processing the marrow.

The manner in which marrow is aspirated varies from center to center and has changed somewhat with time. Older literature[7] suggests that the needle should be advanced with frequent rotation and aspiration continuously through the bone until a total of 20 mL (posterior iliac crest) or 5 mL (sternum) has been acquired. The needle and syringe are then removed and the syringe is emptied into a container with tissue culture medium and preservative-free heparin, rinsed in saline and then in preservative-free heparin; the needle, meanwhile, is freed of bone particles and reinserted to begin the process again. More recent data[29-31] suggest that no more than 3 to 5 mL should be collected with a single aspiration, as any volume larger than this will simply be due to contamination by peripheral blood, decreasing the yield of stem cells and increasing the number of lymphocytes (T cells) in the harvested marrow, which may increase the risk of graft-versus-host disease after allogeneic transplantation. Indeed, repetitive aspiration of larger volumes from both iliac crests simultaneously may lead to increased blood transfusion requirements as the anesthesiologist responds to decreased blood pressure resulting from hypovolemia. Thus, a harvest ideally becomes a rapid ballet of aspiration and reaspiration, with each needle insertion being at a different site, depth, or angle from the previous one, the skin being moved over the bone to minimize postoperative scarring. An average harvest (less than 1000 mL) may be done in this way with one to six skin puncture sites in each iliac crest. Some harvest teams use a scalpel incision in the skin to allow easier needle insertion, but this is not usually necessary.

Over time many different types of needles have been used for harvest, general requirements being a handle that is comfortable for prolonged use and a strong needle with beveled edge that will not bend on repeated use and of large enough diameter not to clog with marrow. Early reports of marrow harvest for transplant used the Sahli[32] or Waterfield marrow biopsy needle[33] or Bierman 16-gauge marrow aspiration needle.[6] Thomas and Storb[7] noted that a Westerman-Jensen aspiration needle could be used but that it plugged easily if advanced without the stylet in place, as was then the custom. They also noted that with the Bierman needle, which has a side opening that did not plug, the yield was often poor. They therefore designed a needle of their own, 6 to 8 cm, with a side opening and locking notch to prevent the stylet from being dislodged during placement (Thomas needle). Later, the Seattle group adopted a 16-gauge Rosenthal aspiration needle with a variably sized handle on the stylet for operator comfort.[11,23,28] This needle is available in lengths of 6.25 cm or more and remains the standard harvest needle at Seattle today. Another variant is the Steis needle, with a transverse handle designed to conform to the operator's palm. Although comfortable to use, the stylet protrudes beyond the needle necessitating a scalpel incision for placement and forcing aspiration through a pool of blood after the stylet is removed. Disposable harvest needles are now available, but the handles, while transverse, are short and less comfortable than the Seattle instrument.

The syringe used to aspirate marrow is usually 20 or 50 mL in volume, in order to obtain good suction, dislodge cells from the marrow sinuses, and, thus, speed the harvest. Many harvesters prefer glass syringes, which slide more quickly and easily. However, glass syringes may break with time and repeated harvests, leaving the harvest field or operator's hand filled with glass. For this reason some centers prefer plastic syringes. Although somewhat more difficult to pull back on, the marrow theoretically should be less likely to clot in plastic than in glass.

Early descriptions of marrow harvest depicted marrow as being aspirated into syringes already containing small amounts of heparinized tissue culture medium.[6,32] At present marrow is usually harvested into empty syringes that have been rinsed with heparinized culture medium. Whether the type of heparin used (i.e., beef or pork) is important has not been investigated, but the ethylenediaminetetraacetic acid (EDTA) preservative used for heparin has been shown to inhibit DNA synthesis in aspirated marrow.[34] Thus, preservative-free pork heparin is most frequently used. At least one marrow processing team, however, has their pharmacy specially prepare preservative-free beef heparin (Scott Rowley, Johns Hopkins University, personal communication, 1991), and another group[35] has used beef heparin with benzyl alcohol preservative. How much heparin is used varies among centers. In some cases the donor has also been given a bolus of intravenous heparin at the start of harvest to improve hemodynamic instability thought to be due to fatty microemboli from the marrow harvest.[18]

After harvest, citrate may also be added for further anticoagulation during automated processing. Citrate alone has been tested as an anticoagulant for marrow harvest with generally unsatisfactory results, possibly because the calcium in culture medium overwhelms the citrate. Traditionally, plain TC-199 has been used, although Hank's balanced salt solution, MEM, and RPMI 1640 (Gibco, Grand Island, NY) have also been used.[35] The role and value of tissue culture medium in the collection of marrow is unclear. The effect of the phenol red pH indicator in medium on marrow cells is unknown but potentially hazardous. Culture medium without phenol red is available and is being used successfully by at least one center (E. Areman, Georgetown University, personal communication, 1991).

After aspiration, marrow has traditionally been expelled into an open stainless steel beaker containing heparinized culture medium, held in a support stand to prevent tipping over.[7] It may also be collected into a covered glass flask with a magnetic mixing bar to help prevent clumping. When the harvest is completed, marrow is passed through stainless steel mesh screens of decreasing size (0.307 mm, 0.201 mm) to break up clumps that may cause pulmonary emboli in the recipient and to remove bone fragments.[7] Fat, however, is poorly removed by these screens.

More recently, a commercial marrow collection bag that hangs from a metal stand has become available (Fenwal Division, Baxter Healthcare, Deerfield, IL). This is a more protected system because there is a top that can be closed to cover the marrow during harvest and three sterile filters of graduated size are attached at the bottom of the bag. This collection system has the additional advantage of leaving most, if not all, fat behind in the collection bag after the heavier marrow cells have drained out through the bottom of the bag and the in-line filters. It is preferable to eliminate fat as early as possible in the processing as it interferes with automated cell counting and complicates automated marrow processing using apheresis machines as well as manual processing. There has been some concern that many nucleated cells are lost during the filtering process and that small cell clumps rather than single cell suspensions are produced. An alternative method for producing a single cell suspension without clumps using a Potter-Elvehjem homogenizer has been developed and tested successfully in human marrow transplant[32] but has not been widely adopted.

After filtration, marrow is placed in a standard blood collection bag and samples are taken for quality control (e.g., colony assays, microbiologic cultures to identify possible contamination). Any procedures necessary to prepare the marrow for the intended transplant are then performed. At this point it is possible to remove contaminating red cells and return them to the donor, decreasing the need for homologous blood transfusion. Allogeneic marrow may be purged of T cells, whereas autologous marrow may be purged of contaminating malignant cells. Autologous marrows are then usually cryopreserved because conditioning regimens most often last longer than the length of time marrow cells are likely to survive under other conditions, although a short-term liquid culture method has been tested.[8] Syngeneic and allogeneic marrows are usually infused immediately following aspiration, or as soon as in vitro processing has been completed.

HOW MUCH TO COLLECT

The volume of marrow to be harvested is based on the recipient's body weight (at least 2 to 4×10^8 nucleated cells per kg for allogeneic and 1 to 3×10^8 per kg for autologous transplant) and the amount of any extra marrow required for a purging protocol or as backup marrow. Some centers do not transfuse red blood cells until after the harvest to prevent marrow dilution and eliminate any risk that third-party lymphocytes in the transfusion product, although irradiated, might survive and cause graft-versus-host disease. In most centers, however, red blood cell transfusion is at the discretion of the anesthesiologist and depends on the volume of marrow harvested, hemodynamic status, and vital signs of the donor.

As blood transfusion is another area of potential risk to the donor, recent attention has been focused on the need for transfusion and the ability of marrow donors to provide autologous blood for transfusion. In an analysis of 192 evaluable autologous harvests a median of 10.6 mL per kg donor weight yielding a median of 2.23×10^8 nucleated cells per kg donor weight was obtained. Twenty-two percent required no red blood cell transfusions, 35 percent one unit, 41 percent two units, and 2 percent more than two units.[11] In a comparable study of allogeneic donors, 24 percent received no transfusions, 59 percent received one unit, 14 percent two units, and 3 percent more than two units.[23] These data led to a prospective study of red blood cell transfusion requirements in the autologous setting where specific criteria for transfusion included hemoglobin less than 110 g per L or harvest volume more than 1400 mL.[21] If donors fulfilled criteria for transfusion but were clinically stable postoperatively (minimal symptoms of anemia, hemodynamically stable) they were not given transfusions. In 59 harvests, 56 percent of donors required transfusion, and in all cases two units or less were needed. It is probable, therefore, that the majority of harvests can be performed using autologous preoperative blood donations.[36] Should a larger, nonstandard harvest be required, as in the case of centers preparing a purged and a backup marrow,[37] red blood cells collected during harvest may successfully be returned to the donor after marrow processing. In the future, erythropoietin therapy to stimulate hematopoiesis may make autologous donation possible even in these latter cases, where the time interval available for blood storage before marrow harvest would ordinarily not permit collection of more than two units.

AFTER THE HARVEST

After marrow is harvested the donor's aspiration sites are bandaged with a pressure dressing and analgesia is supplied as needed. Minor narcotic medications (acetaminophen with codeine or oxycodone) given per os usually provide adequate analgesia[38] and are rarely needed for more than a few days after harvest. Ice applied to the bandaged harvest site in the immediate postoperative and recovery room period may also be beneficial to reduce pain and swelling. Most donors will be able to eat, drink, and walk soon after return from the recovery room. Harvest sites should be checked for signs of local infection 24 to 48 hours postoperatively and donors cautioned to contact a physician should fever or signs of infection occur after discharge from the hospital.

ALTERNATIVE SOURCES OF MARROW

Surgically resected ribs are potential sources of marrow,[39-41] as are cadaveric vertebral bodies[39-42] and complete ilia.[40,43] Femora and scapulae have also been examined but yields of marrow are too small to make these bones a good source of marrow for transplant.[40] The general principle of harvest using surgically resected specimens is to open the bone to expose the marrow cavity and to remove marrow-rich matrix into a buffered salt solution containing DNAse but no heparin.[40] Gentle agitation permits release of the cells from their bone matrix, and the cell suspension may then be filtered, washed, and prepared for immediate use or freezing. Alternatively, marrow may be pressed out into a sterile fluid.[43]

Cadaveric vertebral marrow is obtained from the thoracic and lumbar vertebral column after kidney harvest,[40] or at autopsy if performed within 4[42] to 14 hours of death.[43] The vertebral column may be transected at disk spaces permitting removal of a block of vertebrae, which can be separated into individual vertebrae from which outer cortical bone is removed with an osteotome,[40] leaving a cell-rich matrix to be handled like a surgically resected bone marrow. Alternatively, the anterior of the vertebral column may be removed with a bone saw and chisel, after which a sterile bone scoop, chisel, and gauge are used to remove marrow in pieces 1 to 2 cm in diameter from exposed vertebral bodies (usually 100 to 200 cm of cancellous bone marrow can be obtained). These pieces of marrow are chopped using a stainless steel chopper in a balanced salt solution in suspension, and free cells are filtered through mesh screens to remove bone particles.[41]

Marrow cell yield is a function of the amount of bone removed and its cellularity. Marrow from older individuals tends to be fatty. In a series of 25 harvests of bone marrow from partial collections of ribs and vertebrae from adult cadavers ranging in age from 34 to 86 years, an average of 12×10^9 cells was obtained.[42] Cell yield from lumbar vertebrae is reported to be greater than that from thoracic vertebrae.[43] In a series of surgically resected specimens the mean yield was 3.2×10^8 nucleated cells per rib in a total of 35 specimens after separation on a Ficoll gradient, 1×10^8 cells per femur in a total of seven harvests, and 1.9×10^8 cells per ilium in three cases in which one quarter to one half of the entire bone was resected.[40] Among cadaver donors in this series the mean yield per ilium was 1.6×10^9 cells in five harvests and a mean yield per vertebral body of 3.1×10^9 cells in four harvests. Another report of marrow yields from vertebral body harvested without Ficoll separation gave a number of 5.9 $\times 10^9$ cells per vertebra.[43] A further report comparing yields pre- and post-Ficoll from cadaveric vertebral bodies gave a mean harvest of 4.4×10^9 cells per vertebral body pre-Ficoll and 3.4×10^9 cells per vertebral body post-Ficoll.[41]

With the cell requirement for an allogeneic human marrow transplant estimated at 3×10^8 cells per kg recipient weight from a graft harvested by aspiration from a living donor, it seems likely, based on numbers alone, that cadaveric marrow transplants could be carried out successfully. Indeed, there is at least one report of hematologic reconstitution by cadaveric marrow, in this case from a designated donor who suddenly died 48 hours before the scheduled harvest.[9] Furthermore, with estimated contamination by peripheral blood cells in aspirated marrow ranging from 15 to 20 percent[29,45] it is possible that surgically resected bone or cadaveric marrow may be a better source of hematopoietic stem or progenitor cells than cell counts alone would suggest. While acute graft-versus-host disease is an anticipated problem with cadaveric marrow transplantation, there are fewer T cells in cadaveric or surgically resected marrow[46] than in marrow aspirated from living donors,[41,44] and T-cell depletion techniques are now available to deal with this problem. Thus, cadaveric marrow is an option for marrow transplant that is not widely used owing to problems with HLA matching, storage costs, and the personnel problems inherent in its acquisition. Nevertheless, this approach may be of importance in the future either as a means of inducing tolerance for solid organ transplant[47] or possibly for gene transfer therapy.

REFERENCES

1. Mathé, G, et al: Successful allogeneic bone marrow transplantation in man: Chimerism, induced specific tolerance and possible antileukemic effects. Blood 25:179, 1965.
2. Gatti, RA, et al: Immunological reconstitution of sex-linked lymphopenic immunological deficiency. Lancet 2:1366, 1968.
3. Thomas, ED, et al: Aplastic anemia treated by marrow transplantation. Lancet 1:284, 1972.
4. Robins, MM and Noyes, WD: Aplastic anemia treated with bone marrow transfusion from an identical twin. N Engl J Med 265:974, 1961.
5. Buckner, CD, et al: Allogeneic marrow engraftment following whole body irradiation in a patient with leukemia. Blood 35:741, 1970.
6. Wilson, RE: Technics of human-bone-marrow procurement by aspiration from living donors. N Engl J Med 261:781, 1959.
7. Thomas, ED and Storb, R: Technique for human marrow grafting. Blood 36:507, 1970.
8. Burnett, A, et al: Haematological reconstitution following high dose and supralethal chemo-radiotherapy using stored, non-cryopreserved autologous bone marrow. Br J Haematol 54:309, 1983.
9. Lasky, LC, et al: Successful allogeneic cryopreserved marrow transplantation. Transfusion 29:182, 1989.
10. Gluckman, E, et al: Hematopoietic reconstitution in a patient with Fanconi's anemia by means of umbilical cord blood from an HLA identical sibling. N Engl J Med 321:1174, 1989.
11. Jin, NR, et al: Marrow harvesting for autologous marrow transplantation. Exp Hematol 13:879, 1985.
12. Deeg, HJ, Klingemann, HG, and Phillips, GL: A Guide to Bone Marrow Transplantation. Springer-Verlag, New York, 1988.
13. Rowley, SD, Piantadose, S, and Santos, GW: Correlation of hematologic recovery with CFU-

GM content of autologous bone marrow grafts treated with 4-hydroperoxycyclophosphamide culture for cryopreservation. Bone Marrow Transplant 4:553, 1989.

14. Spitzer, G, et al: The myeloid progenitor cell—its value in predicting hematopoietic recovery after autologous bone marrow transplantation. Blood 55:317, 1980.

15. Berenson, RJ, et al: Engraftment of autologous CD34+ marrow cells in patients with advanced cancer. Exp Hematol 18:672, 1990.

16. Jones, RJ, et al: Separation of pluripotent haematopoietic stem cells from spleen colony-forming cells. Nature 347:188, 1990.

17. deVries, EGE, et al: No narcosis for bone marrow harvest in autologous bone marrow transplantation. Blut 49:419, 1984.

18. Filshie, J, et al: The anaesthetic management of bone marrow harvest for transplantation. Anaesthesia 39:480, 1984.

19. Reman, O, et al: Quantitation of CFU(GM) of bone marrow harvested after general anesthesia. Influence of nitrous oxide. Bone Marrow Transplant 5:114 (Suppl 2), 1990.

20. Abels, J, et al: Anti-leukemic potential of methylcobalamin inactivation by nitrous oxide. Am J Hematol 34:128, 1990.

21. Brandwein, et al: An evaluation of out-patient bone marrow harvesting. J Clin Oncol 7:648, 1989.

22. Bortin, MM and Buckner, CD: Major complications of marrow harvesting for transplantation. Exp Hematol 11:916, 1983.

23. Buckner, CD, et al: Marrow harvesting from normal donors. Blood 64:630, 1984.

24. McCarthy, DM, et al: DIC after bone marrow harvesting in a patient with Hodgkin's disease in remission. Bone Marrow Transplant 5:443, 1990.

25. Mangan, KF, et al: Rapid detection of venous air embolism by mass spectrometry during bone marrow harvesting. Exp Hematol 13:639, 1985.

26. Petersen, FB, et al: Marrow harvesting from normal donors. Exp Hematol 18:676, 1990.

27. Gentet, JC, et al: Veno-occlusive disease in children after intensive chemo- and radiotherapy and repeated halothane anesthesias. Acta Oncol 27:5879, 1988.

28. Sanders, JE, et al: Experience with marrow harvesting from donors less than two years of age. Bone Marrow Transplant 2:45, 1987.

29. Batinic, D, et al: Relationship between differing volumes of bone marrow aspirates and their cellular composition. Bone Marrow Transplant 6:103, 1990.

30. Holdrinet, RSG, et al: A method for quantification of peripheral blood admixture in bone marrow aspirates. Exp Hematol 8:103, 1980.

31. Batinic, D, et al: Lymphocyte subsets in normal human bone marrow harvested for routine clinical transplantation. Bone Marrow Transplant 4:229, 1989.

32. Herrmann, RP and Davis, RE: Technique for human bone marrow harvest. Acta Haematol 68:309, 1982.

33. Pegg, DE and Kemp, NH: Collection, storage, and administration of autologous human bone marrow. Lancet 2:1426, 1960.

34. Lochte, HL, Ferrebee, JW, and Thomas, ED: The effect of heparin and EDTA on DNA synthesis by marrow in vitro. J Lab Clin Med 55:435, 1960.

35. Jansen, J: Processing of bone marrow for allogeneic transplantation. In Sacher, RA, McCarthy, LJ, and Smit Sibinga, CT (eds): Processing of Bone Marrow for Transplantation. American Association of Blood Banks, Arlington, VA, 1990.

36. Thompson, HW and McCullough, J: Use of blood components containing red cells by donors of allogeneic bone marrow. Transfusion 26:98, 1986.

37. Rosenfeld, CS, et al: Transfusion of bone marrow red cells during bone marrow harvests. Exp Hematol 16:702, 1988.

38. Hill, HF, et al: Assessment and management of donor pain following marrow harvest for allogeneic bone marrow transplantation. Bone Marrow Transplant 4:157, 1989.

39. Haurani, FI, Repplinger, E, and Tocantins, LM: Attempts at transplantation of human bone marrow in patients with acute leukemia and other marrow depletion disorders. Am J Med 28:794, 1960.

40. Sharp, TG, et al: Harvest of human bone marrow directly from bone. J Immunol Methods 69:187, 1984.

41. Lucas, PJ, et al: Alternative donor sources in HLA-mismatched marrow transplantation: T-cell depletion of surgically resected cadaveric marrow. Bone Marrow Transplant 3:211, 1988.

42. Ferrebee, JW, et al: The collection, storage and preparation of viable cadaver marrow for intravenous use. Blood 14:140, 1959.

43. Mugashimi, H, Terasaki, P, and Sueyoshi, A: Bone marrow from cadaver donors for transplantation. Blood 65:392, 1985.

44. Ray, RN, Cassell, M, and Chaplin, H: A new method for the preparation of human cadaver bone marrow for transfusion. Blood 17:97, 1964.

45. Fauci, AS: Human bone marrow lymphocytes. I. Distribution of lymphocyte subpopulations in the bone marrow of normal individuals. J Clin Invest 56:98, 1975.

46. Saunders, EF, et al: Graft vs host disease is reduced in allogeneic bone marrow transplantation using marrow obtained surgically. Blood 76(10 Suppl 1):563, 1990.

47. Barber, WH, et al: Use of cryopreserved donor bone marrow in cadaver kidney allograft recipients. Transplantation 47:66, 1989.

BONE MARROW HARVEST AND FILTRATION

BONE MARROW HARVEST: TRADITIONAL METHOD

DESCRIPTION	Bone marrow is aspirated from the iliac crests, mixed with heparinized media, and filtered to obtain a suspension suitable for buffy coat processing. Harvest procedures are performed in the sterile field of the operating room. The cells per kg harvested depend on the laboratory procedure to be performed. This can also serve as a backup procedure for the disposable harvest sets.
TIME FOR PROCEDURE	Approximately 1 to 2 hours (harvest time)

SUMMARY OF PROCEDURE

1. Bone marrow is aspirated from the posterior (and, in some cases, the anterior) iliac crests and dispensed into a flask containing medium and preservative-free heparin.
2. The total volume to be harvested is determined by the cells per kg obtained and the cells per kg needed for laboratory processing.
3. When harvesting is complete, the marrow is filtered to remove any bone spicules or small clots.
4. The filtered marrow is placed into a transfer bag and transported to the laboratory for processing.

EQUIPMENT

1. 2 Jamshidi biopsy needle sets: American Pharmaseal Laboratories No. BRC-4011A (4 inches × 11-gauge for adults) or No. BRC-3513A (3½ inches × 13-gauge for pediatrics)
2. 4 Becton Dickinson 10-gauge × 4 inches Westerman-Jensen needle sets, No. 1573; Lee disposable harvest needles for adults No. TP-114 (11-gauge × 4 inches), No. TP-133 pediatric needle (13-gauge × 3½ inches)
3. Gripping handle for Westerman-Jensen needle set BD No. 1459
4. 1 pair scissors
5. 1 hemostat
6. 2 University of Washington filtering syringe sets No. BFA; each includes a polycarbonate cutoff syringe (barrel, plunger, and screw-on end cap), one 300-μm coarse screen, one 200-μm fine screen with silicone gaskets fused to both sides of the screens.
7. 1 ring stand with clamp
8. 2 magnetic stir bars
9. 1 magnetic stirrer
10. 2 plastic collection flasks (adult 1000-mL, pediatric 600-mL)
11. 2 plastic filtering pitchers (adult 1000-mL, pediatric 600-mL)
12. One 500-mL plastic beaker to rinse syringes

SUPPLIES AND REAGENTS

1. 100 mL of Medium 199 with Earle's salts and L-glutamine with 10,000 USP units of preservative-free heparin added.
2. Six 60-mL luer-lock syringes

3. Two 20-mL luer-lock syringes

4. Three 18-gauge $\times$ 3 inches spinal needles

5. Two 5-mL luer-lock syringes

6. Two 2000-mL transfer packs for adults, or two 600-mL transfer packs for pediatric patients

7. 2 stopcocks (3-way)

8. 2 transfer lines

9. Fenwal hand sealer clips No. 4R4418

PROCEDURE

1. SURGICAL FIELD SETUP

   A. Perform standard surgical scrub as per operating room procedure. Glasses or goggles are worn to protect the eyes from the aerosols that may be produced.

   B. Assemble the appropriate harvest and biopsy needles.

   C. Place the ring stand on the Mayo tray and the magnetic stirrer on top of the ring stand base. When the procedure is ready to begin the stirrer is connected to an extension cord.

   D. If a transfer pack is to be used to transport the marrow to the laboratory, cut the coupler line and insert a stopcock. An extension tubing is attached to the stopcock.

   E. To the collection flask, add 10 mL of medium heparin solution for every 100 mL of marrow to be harvested. Add approximately 20 mL of medium heparin to the 500-mL beaker to be used to rinse the syringes.

   F. Assemble the filtering syringes by placing into the screw-on base a coarse filter that has silicone gaskets on each side. Attach the barrel to the base and insert the plunger into the barrel. The other filtering syringe is assembled using the fine screen.

   G. Rinse the harvest needles with medium heparin solution.

2. HARVESTING

   A. If biopsies are to be performed, hand the physician a Jamshidi needle. When the biopsy is obtained it is placed on gauze and, if adequate, placed into a sterile specimen container to which sterile saline has been added. The specimen container is handed to the circulating nurse, who labels it appropriately.

   B. If aspiration for tissue examination is to be performed, give the physician a 20-mL luer-slip syringe after the aspiration needle is positioned. Two to 3 mL from each side are withdrawn and given to the circulating nurse, who places it into EDTA tubes and labels them.

   C. Harvesting of the marrow now begins. Adjust the magnetic stirrer so the bone marrow is gently mixed. Give the physician a 60-mL luer-slip syringe. Five to 10 mL of marrow will be withdrawn each time and the syringe handed to the technologist. The marrow is gently dispensed down the side of the collection flask. The syringe is rinsed in the medium heparin solution and handed back to the physician.

   D. When half of the expected volume of marrow has been harvested, collect a 1-mL specimen for a nucleated cell count. For adults a count is performed at a volume of 500-mL, and for pediatric patients a cell count is performed when 10 to 20 mL of marrow per kg body weight have been harvested.

3. CALCULATIONS
   A. Cells per kg can be determined by the following calculation:

$$\frac{\text{Cells/mm}^3 \times 10^3 \times \text{volume}}{\text{kg weight}} = \text{Nucleated cells/kg}$$

   B. A table that displays cells per mm³ and weight can be made to determine the cells per kg. This number is expressed in cells $\times\ 10^8$. The adult table (shown here) is based on a volume of 500 mL, and the pediatric table on a volume of 250 mL.
   C. To estimate the cells per kg at 1000 mL, multiply the cells per kg at 500 mL by 2.

MARROW VOLUME 500

	WEIGHT, POUNDS (KILOGRAMS)										
Cells/mm³	100 (45)	110 (50)	120 (55)	130 (59)	140 (64)	150 (68)	160 (73)	170 (77)	180 (82)	190 (86)	200 (91)
12000	1.32	1.20	1.10	1.02	0.94	0.88	0.83	0.78	0.73	0.69	0.66
13000	1.43	1.30	1.19	1.10	1.02	0.95	0.89	0.84	0.79	0.75	0.72
14000	1.54	1.40	1.28	1.18	1.10	1.03	0.96	0.91	0.86	0.81	0.77
15000	1.65	1.50	1.38	1.27	1.18	1.10	1.03	0.97	0.92	0.87	0.83
16000	1.76	1.60	1.47	1.35	1.26	1.17	1.10	1.04	0.98	0.93	0.88
17000	1.87	1.70	1.56	1.44	1.34	1.25	1.17	1.10	1.04	0.98	0.94
18000	1.98	1.80	1.65	1.52	1.41	1.32	1.24	1.16	1.10	1.04	0.99
19000	2.09	1.90	1.74	1.61	1.49	1.39	1.31	1.23	1.16	1.10	1.05
20000	2.20	2.00	1.83	1.69	1.57	1.47	1.38	1.29	1.22	1.16	1.10
21000	2.31	2.10	1.93	1.78	1.65	1.54	1.44	1.36	1.28	1.22	1.16
22000	2.42	2.20	2.02	1.86	1.73	1.61	1.51	1.42	1.34	1.27	1.21
23000	2.53	2.30	2.11	1.95	1.81	1.69	1.58	1.49	1.41	1.33	1.27
24000	2.64	2.40	2.20	2.03	1.89	1.76	1.65	1.55	1.47	1.39	1.32
25000	2.75	2.50	2.29	2.12	1.96	1.83	1.72	1.62	1.53	1.45	1.38
26000	2.86	2.60	2.38	2.20	2.04	1.91	1.79	1.68	1.59	1.51	1.43
27000	2.97	2.70	2.48	2.28	2.12	1.98	1.86	1.75	1.65	1.56	1.49
28000	3.08	2.80	2.57	2.37	2.20	2.05	1.93	1.81	1.71	1.62	1.54
29000	3.19	2.90	2.66	2.45	2.28	2.13	1.99	1.88	1.77	1.68	1.60
30000	3.30	3.00	2.75	2.54	2.36	2.20	2.06	1.94	1.83	1.74	1.65
31000	3.41	3.10	2.84	2.62	2.44	2.27	2.13	2.01	1.89	1.79	1.71
32000	3.52	3.20	2.93	2.71	2.51	2.35	2.20	2.07	1.96	1.85	1.76
33000	3.63	3.30	3.03	2.79	2.59	2.42	2.27	2.14	2.02	1.91	1.82
34000	3.74	3.40	3.12	2.88	2.67	2.49	2.34	2.20	2.08	1.97	1.87
35000	3.85	3.50	3.21	2.96	2.75	2.57	2.41	2.26	2.14	2.03	1.93
36000	3.96	3.60	3.30	3.05	2.83	2.64	2.48	2.33	2.20	2.08	1.98
37000	4.07	3.70	3.39	3.13	2.91	2.71	2.54	2.39	2.26	2.14	2.04
38000	4.18	3.80	3.48	3.22	2.99	2.79	2.61	2.46	2.32	2.20	2.09
39000	4.29	3.90	3.58	3.30	3.06	2.86	2.68	2.52	2.38	2.26	2.15
40000	4.40	4.00	3.67	3.38	3.14	2.93	2.75	2.59	2.44	2.32	2.20
41000	4.51	4.10	3.76	3.47	3.22	3.01	2.82	2.65	2.51	2.37	2.26
42000	4.62	4.20	3.85	3.55	3.30	3.08	2.89	2.72	2.57	2.43	2.31
43000	4.73	4.30	3.94	3.64	3.38	3.15	2.96	2.78	2.63	2.49	2.37
44000	4.84	4.40	4.03	3.72	3.46	3.23	3.03	2.85	2.69	2.55	2.42
45000	4.95	4.50	4.13	3.81	3.54	3.30	3.09	2.91	2.75	2.61	2.48

4. FILTRATION
   A. When sufficient marrow has been collected, remove the flask from the magnetic stirrer. The marrow is poured through the coarse-screened

filtering syringe into the 1000-mL pitcher and then through the fine-screened filtering syringe into the other 1000-mL pitcher.

B. Place the filtered marrow into a transfer pack using the stopcock, syringe, and extension set. The pack is clamped using Fenwal clips and transported to the laboratory.

ANTICIPATED RESULTS	From 10 to 40 mL of marrow per kg of body weight are harvested to give the desired cells per kg needed for laboratory processing. Final marrow volumes collected range from 100 mL for pediatric patients to more than 2000 mL for adult patients.

NOTES

1. Disposable harvest sets are now available that are used for the collection and filtration of the aspirated marrow. These eliminate the risk of contamination posed by the open containers and replace many of the equipment items. This procedure is used as a backup for the disposable sets. Also available are disposable harvest needles in a variety of sizes and styles.

2. The marrow should be mixed gently to avoid hemolysis and aerosol production.

3. The filtering of the marrow should be done over a tray to contain the marrow if a spill should occur.

AUTHORS

Barbara A. Reeb, M.T.(ASCP)
Brooke Army Medical Center
Department of Clinical Investigation
Fort Sam Houston, TX 78234-6200

Robert G. Whiddon, Ph.D.
Brooke Army Medical Center
Department of Clinical Investigation
Fort Sam Houston, TX 78234-6200

REFERENCE

1. Thomas, E and Storb, R: Technique for human marrow grafting. Blood 36:507, 1970.

BONE MARROW HARVEST: DISPOSABLE COLLECTION KIT

DESCRIPTION	Collection of human iliac crest bone marrow stem cells using the Fenwal bone marrow collection kit to separate the marrow cells from bone spicules, fat, and cellular debris.
TIME FOR PROCEDURE	1 to 2 hours for harvest; 5 to 10 minutes for filtration
SUMMARY OF PROCEDURE	Collection of bone marrow stem cells is performed by repeated insertion of a large-bore (10- to 14-gauge) marrow aspirating needle into the iliac marrow cavity and aspiration of the marrow cells into a disposable 20-mL heparinized syringe. The marrow is transferred to the collection bag of the Fenwal bone marrow collection kit (Fig. 4–1), which contains 100 mL of heparinized balanced salt solution (e.g., TC-199 for RPMI-1640). Upon completion of the bone marrow harvest, the bone marrow cells are gravity-filtered through a series of successively smaller-diameter stainless steel mesh filters and collected in a sterile plastic transfer pack.

EQUIPMENT

1. Fenwal bone marrow collection kit: 2 sterile wraps, two 1.2-L collection containers, 2 each of 500-μm (red), 300-μm (yellow), and 200-μm (blue) stainless steel mesh filters in plastic housing, two 600-mL transfer packs, 2000-mL transfer pack, plastic pouch with three nonvented tip protectors
2. Bone marrow collection stand (4R2105)
3. 4 hemostats or Kelly clamps, rubber-shod

SUPPLIES AND REAGENTS

1. 2 marrow aspiration and 2 biopsy needles
2. 6 to 8 sterile disposable 20-mL syringes
3. 100-mL RPMI-1640 without phenol red, with L-glutamine
4. 40,000 units of sodium heparin

PROCEDURE

1. Assemble collection stand and collection kit according to manufacturer instructions within the sterile operating field (steps 1 through 6 of Fenwal instructions).
2. Close collection container clamp at the bottom of the collection container. For added precaution, a large rubber-shod hemostat or Kelly clamp is positioned along the outlet tubing below the container clamp.
3. Open collection container cap and add 90 to 95 mL of the sterile heparinized collection medium. Place remaining 5 to 10 mL in a small specimen cup (to be used as rinse media, to rinse and reheparinize syringes between aspirations).
4. Perform marrow aspiration and expel marrow into collection container. Gently knead bag to thoroughly mix marrow and collection media after each syringe transfer of marrow. The marrow should be gently expelled from the syringe. Pointing the syringe toward the rear of the collection container bag and allowing the marrow to run down the bag will prevent excessive foaming that may be experienced if the marrow is injected straight downward into the media.
5. Continue to aspirate marrow until desired amount is obtained. Add the 5 to 10 mL rinse medium to the marrow collection, and close and secure cap

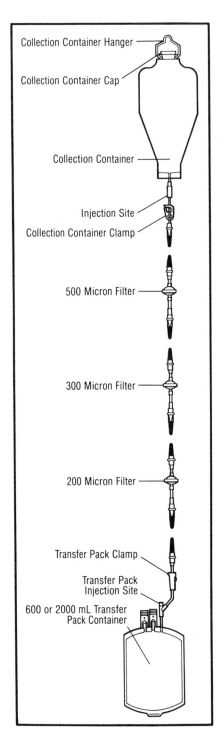

Collection Container Hanger

Collection Container Cap

Collection Container

Injection Site

Collection Container Clamp

500 Micron Filter

300 Micron Filter

200 Micron Filter

Transfer Pack Clamp

Transfer Pack Injection Site

600 or 2000 mL Transfer Pack Container

FIGURE 4–1 Components of disposable bone marrow collection kit.

on the collection container. Be sure cap is secured before attempting to move the marrow collection kit.

6. Remove the collection container from the collection stand and hang on an IV pole, using the hanger strap attached to the collection container.

7. If additional marrow is required or the collection container is full, use another collection kit setup. Repeat steps 1 through 6.

8. For filtration, connect one group of stainless steel mesh filters provided in the collection kit in descending order, as follows: 500- (red), 300- (yellow), 200- (blue) μm filters.

9. Twist each filter connection to ensure tight connections between filters.

10. Attach the series of filters to the collection container (red filter).

11. Attach the 2000-mL plastic transfer pack supplied in the collection kit to the blue filter. Other transfer packs (600-mL) may also be used, depending on the volume of marrow collected.

12. Thoroughly mix the bone marrow suspension in the collection container bag. Sampling of marrow before filtration may be obtained from the side-port injection site or from the top of the collection container.

13. Open the clamps on the collection container and the transfer pack. As the marrow suspension enters each filter unit, invert the filter unit temporarily and tap gently to expel air from the filters.

14. Allow marrow to flow by gravity through the filters into the transfer pack. Filtration pressure and flow rate may be adjusted by raising or lowering the collection container.

15. If a filter unit becomes clogged, change the filter using aseptic technique: (a) Close the clamps on the collection container and transfer pack, and (b) clamp tubing above and below the clogged filter using the rubber-shod clamps. Remove the clogged filter and replace with same size spare filter provided in the collection kit.

16. Continue to filter the bone marrow suspension by unclamping the tubing and opening the clamps on the collection container and transfer pack; then resume the marrow suspension flow through the series of filters.

17. Upon completion of marrow filtration, an additional aliquot of physiologic sterile saline may be passed through the filtration setup to rinse any residual cells through the filters.

18. After the filtration procedure is complete, clamp the transfer pack to seal and remove the transfer pack from the series of filters.

19. Discard collection container and filters after single use. Label filtered bone marrow cell suspension with patient name, date of collection, medical record number, and other relevant information. Take bone marrow suspension to the bone marrow transplant processing laboratory for further processing and cryopreservation, if necessary.

ANTICIPATED RESULTS	Volume markings on the collection container read 10 to 15 percent lower than actual volume collected (e.g., if bag reads 1000 mL, it actually contains 1100 mL).

AUTHORS	Roger H. Herzig, M.D.	Richard C. Meagher, Ph.D.
	James Graham Brown Cancer Center	James Graham Brown Cancer Center
	University of Louisville	University of Louisville
	Louisville, KY 40292	Louisville, KY 40292

REFERENCE   1. Linn, A, et al: Evaluation of a disposable bone marrow collection and filtration kit. Transfusion 27:526, 1987.

RAPID METHOD FOR FILLING A TRANSFER BAG IN THE OPERATING ROOM

DESCRIPTION	A modified beaker (Biomedicon) was constructed from a stainless steel straightedge beaker (Fisher). This beaker has a tapered drain spout in the center of the bottom and a 25-cm sidearm extension for attachment to an IV pole. This beaker allows the marrow to flow into the transfer bag by gravity at a rapid rate when compared with the slower method of using a transfer needle and syringe.
TIME FOR PROCEDURE	Approximately 10 to 15 minutes for 2 L of bone marrow
EQUIPMENT	1. Standard marrow filtering apparatus
	2. 1000-mL stainless steel beaker with drain spout and sidearm (beaker has a 1.8-cm long, 0.6-cm inside-diameter drainage spout welded to the bottom; a 25-cm long, 1.2-cm diameter rod is welded to the top to allow attachment to an IV pole by a clamp [Fig. 4–2])
	3. 2-L transfer bag with attached coupler on tubing
	4. IV pole
PROCEDURE	1. Collect and filter bone marrow in the usual manner.
	2. Attach the stainless steel beaker to the IV pole using a large clamp holder capable of holding heavy apparatus. The transfer bag is then firmly secured by friction into the tapered drain spout by the coupler attached to the tubing.
	3. Pour the bone marrow into the beaker and allow it to drain into the bag (Fig. 4–3). After all the bone marrow has drained into the transfer bag, the air is expressed out by forcing it through the tubing (Fig. 4–4). The bag is clamped and final volume is obtained by weight. Weight may be converted to volume by dividing by 1.058.
	4. Take the marrow to the laboratory for further processing or give it to the patient.

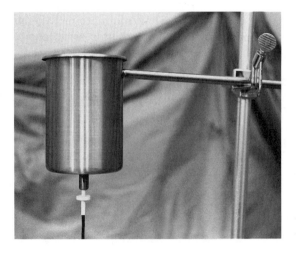

FIGURE 4–2 Showing stainless steel beaker with drain spout and side-arm used for transferring bone marrow to transfer bag.

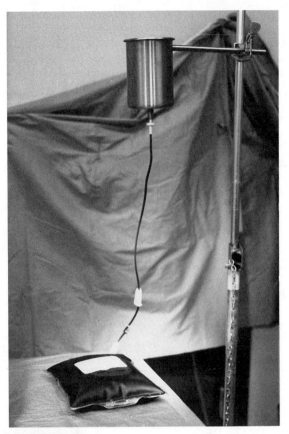

FIGURE 4–3 Showing marrow draining from stainless steel beaker into marrow transfer bag.

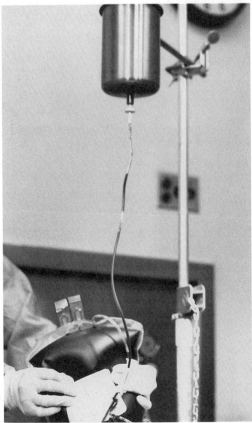

FIGURE 4–4 After all the marrow has drained into the transfer bag, the remaining air is expressed out by forcing it through the tubing.

AUTHORS   Regina Bryan   Stephen Bulova, M.D.
                    Hahnemann University   Hahnemann University
                    Philadelphia, PA 19102   Philadelphia, PA 19102

                    Mark Singer
                    Biomedicon
                    Moorestown, NJ 08057

BONE MARROW FILTRATION

DESCRIPTION	Bone marrow filtration using a Cutter bone marrow transfer bag with filter to remove particulate matter and to prevent clumping and occlusion of the infusion set.
TIME FOR PROCEDURE	Approximately 2 to 3 minutes to filter 300 mL
SUMMARY OF PROCEDURE	1. Harvested bone marrow is delivered to the recovery room in up to three 300-mL transfer packs. 2. Bone marrow is filtered by gravity using the transfer bag with filter. 3. Filtered bone marrow is labeled and stored at room temperature before infusion.
EQUIPMENT	1. Sebra tube sealer 2. IV stand
SUPPLIES AND REAGENTS	1. Three 300-mL transfer packs 2. 3 Cutter bone marrow transfer bags with filter, Code 890-77Y.
PROCEDURE	1. Enter the harvested bone marrow pack with the spike of the sterile transfer bag with filter. 2. Hang the bone marrow pack on the IV stand. 3. Open roller clamp on the filter set. 4. Filter bone marrow by gravity into the 600-mL transfer bag, occasionally applying gentle pressure to the marrow pack. 5. Gently squeeze drip chamber and filter to remove any trapped bone marrow. 6. Close roller clamp. 7. Seal and cut the tubing going into the transfer bag. 8. Discard the filter and the attached original bone marrow pack. 9. Label the filtered bone marrow bag and store at room temperature until infused.
ANTICIPATED RESULTS	The procedure should yield 98 percent of harvested bone marrow free of particulate matter.
NOTE	In the event of filter occlusion due to particle accumulation, filtration has to be interrupted and a new sterile transfer bag with filter used.
AUTHOR	Doris Neurath, A.R.T. Transfusion Medicine Foothills Hospital Calgary, Alberta T2N 4N2 Canada
REFERENCE	1. Neurath, D and Russell, JA: A simple disposable system for bone marrow filtration. Bone Marrow Transplant 3:522, 1988.

CELL COUNTING AND CALCULATIONS

COUNTING NUCLEATED CELLS WITH A HEMACYTOMETER

DESCRIPTION	Manual cell counts obtained with a hemacytometer have the following advantages: 1. Fast; no need to wait for a Coulter counter to be available 2. Simple; use existing laboratory equipment and aliquots of diluents at any preferred dilutions; can be prepared in advance 3. All nucleated cells counted; no cell size threshold limits
TIME FOR PROCEDURE	Approximately 6 minutes per cell count
SUMMARY OF PROCEDURE	Small aliquot of specimen is diluted with diluent which contains 5 percent acetic acid to lyse the red cells. Cell counts are obtained by counting with a microscope and calculating the dilution factor and volume factor.
EQUIPMENT	1. Light microscope 2. High light transmission counting chamber (e.g., improved Neubauer Plane Spotlight double)
SUPPLIES AND REAGENTS	1. Crystal violet stain (0.05 percent) with 5 percent acetic acid: • 0.1 g crystal violet • 10.0 mL glacial acetic acid • 190.0 mL distilled water 2. 1.5 mL microfuge tubes: • For 1:20 dilution, use 10-μL specimen in 190-μL aliquot of crystal violet stain solution. • For 1:100 dilution, use 8-μL specimen in 792-μL aliquot of crystal violet stain solution.
PROCEDURE	1. Wipe and clean the hemacytometer and cover glass with methanol, dry with Kim wipes. 2. Wet the ridges on both ends of the counting chamber with water to mount the cover glass. 3. Invert the specimen to mix well, pipette 10 μL of specimen and wipe the outside of the pipette tip with Kim wipe away from the tip without touching the tip. 4. Deliver the specimen into one of the prepared 190-μL aliquots of crystal violet stain solution in microfuge tubes. 5. Mix well; discharge carefully into the counting chamber to avoid overfill. 6. Let cells settle to the bottom of the chamber; count with low power (100$\times$) all 4 W areas. 7. The dilution factor is 20, and

$$\text{MNC/mL} = \frac{\text{Count/0.1 mm}^3 \times 20}{4}$$

$$= \frac{\text{Count} \times 10^4/\text{mL} \times 20}{4}$$

where: MNC = marrow nucleated cells

8. The dilution factor is 100 when 8-μL specimen is mixed with 792 μL crystal violet stain solution.

ANTICIPATED RESULTS

1. For peripheral blood specimens, use 1:20 dilution.
2. The results range from 1 to 20 $\times$ 10^6 per mL.
3. Use 1:100 dilution when the concentration is higher than 20 $\times$ 10^6 per mL.

NOTES

Prepared aliquots of diluent in airtight microfuge tubes may have condensation inside the tube after standing. They can be spun down in microfuge before use.

AUTHOR

Jean T. Yao, M.S., S.B.B.(ASCP)
Blood Bank
Methodist Medical Center
221 N.E. Glen Oak Ave.
Peoria, IL 61636

AUTOMATED AND MANUAL CELL COUNTING OF BONE MARROW SUSPENSIONS

DESCRIPTION	**PURPOSE OF CELL COUNTING**

Although methods for cell counting of peripheral blood have become standardized in most clinical laboratories, methods for counting cells in suspensions of harvested bone marrow have not. For the bone marrow processing laboratory, the two main reasons for developing accurate and consistent cell counting methods are:

1.   Animal and human data have suggested a relationship between the number of bone marrow cells infused and engraftment of the marrow in autologous and allogeneic transplantation. Although there is controversy over what the minimum criterion for cell counts in the infused marrow suspension should be, many transplant centers use such criteria. One example of a standard for minimum cell content is the National Marrow Donor Program standard for unrelated allogeneic bone marrow requiring a minimum of 2.0×10^8 marrow nucleated cells per kg recipient body weight. Even in centers where the decision to transplant is not based on the cell counts of the marrow, the cell counts are still considered an essential part of the database for clinical investigations aimed at identifying predictors of the marrow's potential for engraftment.

2.   Quantitation of cell loss is critical in the assessment of procedures for processing, purging, and cryopreservation. Intralaboratory and interlaboratory comparisons of new procedures are facilitated by accurate, consistent cell counting methods.

DEFINITIONS

The following definitions will be used in the subsequent discussion and procedure:

Non-nucleated cells include mature erythrocytes and platelets. The presence of such cells in harvested bone marrow results from the presence of admixed peripheral blood, which is unavoidable with current methods of marrow aspiration.

Nucleated cells in the harvested bone marrow include *marrow nucleated cells,* consisting of mature and immature cells of all lineages (erythroid, myeloid, lymphoid), and the admixed *peripheral blood nucleated cells,* consisting mainly of mature leukocytes of both the myeloid and lymphoid series. Many centers calculate a *corrected marrow nucleated cell count* by applying a formula that estimates the contribution of peripheral blood nucleated cells to the total nucleated cell count of the harvested marrow; two such formulas are provided in the procedure that follows.

Nucleated cells of the bone marrow or peripheral blood can be classified morphologically into *mononuclear cells* and *polymorphonuclear cells.* Mononuclear cells in the harvested bone marrow include cells of marrow or peripheral blood origin that contain a single (nonlobulated) nucleus and cannot be readily identified as a nucleated red blood cell (in the polychromatophilic erythroblast stage or beyond) or as a mature cell of the granulocytic series (a band or polymorphonuclear form). Mononuclear cells in harvested marrow will therefore include not only lymphocytes and monocytes from peripheral blood and marrow, but also many immature erythroid and myeloid forms from the marrow that would not normally contribute to the peripheral blood mononuclear cell count. Estimation of the mononuclear cell count requires a slide differential count of the marrow preparation.

Although the nucleated cell count has been the most widely used and reported measure of cellular content of marrow grafts, the mononuclear cell content and yield is now used by many marrow processing laboratories. Mononuclear cell content may be preferable for assessment of processing methods, because many common marrow separation methods result in the concentration of hematopoietic progenitor cells in the light density mononuclear cell fraction. In addition, the mononuclear cell count excludes nucleated red blood cells (RBCs) and more mature cells of the myeloid series that clearly do not contribute to hematologic reconstitution and, in fact, are undesirable because they may contribute to infusion toxicity in the recipient. It is important to understand that neither nucleated cell count nor mononuclear cell count can be used to predict precisely the progenitor cell content of the marrow or its potential for engraftment.

CELL COUNTING METHODS

Nucleated cell counts may be obtained by either manual or automated techniques. In general, automated counts are recommended over manual counts because they are more rapid, less labor intensive, and more precise. However, manual counts may in fact be more accurate for samples of unseparated marrow. This may be due in part to the fat content of bone marrow, which can cause an artifactual increase in the white blood cell (WBC) count (nucleated cell count) owing to fat particles being counted in the lower end (by size) of the leukocyte channel. Another possible factor contributing to inaccuracy of automated counts is that the programs for some automated counters are based on expectations for peripheral blood counts. Manual counts may also be useful as backup when the automated counter is not operational.

Several automated cell counters are capable of providing automated differential leukocyte counts based on analysis of the leukocyte size histograms and programmed expectations for size distribution of leukocytes in normal peripheral blood. Because bone marrow samples are more complex than peripheral blood in terms of cell content, such automated differentials cannot be directly applied to bone marrow samples. Accurate estimation of bone marrow mononuclear cell content requires microscopic examination of a Wright- or Giemsa-stained smear. Despite difficulties with automated differentials, several laboratories, including our own, are investigating the utility of the leukocyte size histograms (provided by some automated counters) in assessing loss of specific cell populations during processing.

Although the marrow nucleated cell count is of most interest in bone marrow transplantation, most processing laboratories will need to assess hematocrit (Hct) in order to estimate packed cell volume of the initial harvest (necessary for some automated procedures) or to quantitate and adjust the red cell content prior to use of purging techniques (e.g., 4-hydroperoxycyclophosphamide [4-HC] purging).

TIME FOR PROCEDURE	1.	Manual cell counting: 20 minutes per sample
	2.	Automated cell counting: 2 minutes per sample

3. Differential: 10 minutes slide preparation, 5 to 15 minutes reading time per slide

SUMMARY OF PROCEDURE	1. Samples are taken from the bone marrow suspension at selected time points during processing and cryopreservation. A total volume of 1.0 mL per sample should be adequate for all counting procedures, including automated and manual counting and the slide differential.
	2. Automated cell counting is carried out on all samples, including Hct and WBC (nucleated cell count). (Other cell counts available on most automated counters are not essential for most purposes.)
	3. Manual counting of nucleated cells is carried out on one or more samples obtained before and during processing, in order to make a comparison of manual and automated counts within the laboratory. This is advisable for all samples of harvested bone marrow prior to separation.
	4. A smear of the marrow sample is made on a glass slide, stained with Wright or Giemsa stain, and examined microscopically. A differential is done to categorize cells into nucleated RBCs, mononuclear cells, and non-mononuclear leukocytes (bands and polymorphonuclear leukocytes).
	5. Calculations are carried out to express the cell content of the marrow in terms of total nucleated cells, corrected marrow nucleated cells, and mononuclear cells in the total suspension and per kg body weight of the recipient.
EQUIPMENT	1. Automated cell counter (although we use the Coulter S-Plus 5, many other instruments are also excellent for basic cell counting)
	2. Light microscope, with 100× and 430× magnifications
	3. Scale and balance bags
SUPPLIES AND REAGENTS	1. For manual counting: hemacytometer, petri dish with moist filter paper on bottom, Unopette microcollection system (Becton Dickinson, Rutherford, NJ)
	2. For automated counting: tubes and diluents appropriate for specific counter
	3. For differential counts: glass slides, staining materials (Wright or Giemsa)
PROCEDURE	1. OBTAIN 1.0-ML SAMPLE FROM EACH SUSPENSION REQUIRING COUNTING: For each sample, record identification and volume of the suspension from which the sample was obtained. (Our convention is to consider volume equal to weight, rather than consider correcting the weights for various specific gravities of the suspensions.)
	2. AUTOMATED CELL COUNTING: Following directions for specific cell counter, perform Hct and total nucleated cell (WBC) count on an undiluted sample of bone marrow suspension. Do not add anticoagulant in addition to the anticoagulant already present in the harvested marrow, and do not count the samples more than a few hours after they are obtained. If the WBC count is greater than 50,000 per μL, dilute the sample 1:10 with saline or other isotonic solution and perform a count on diluted sample.
	3. MANUAL CELL COUNTING: Follow manufacturer's directions for carrying out leukocyte count by Unopette method. This method uses an ammonium

oxalate diluent to lyse red blood cells, a glass hemocytometer, and light microscope for counting cells. A secondary dilution should always be done for high leukocyte counts. After loading cell suspension into hemacytometer with coverslip on top of chamber, place hemacytometer in petri dish with moistened filter paper on bottom for at least 10 minutes before reading.

4. DIFFERENTIAL CELL COUNT: Make thin smear of bone marrow suspension on glass slide. Allow to dry, then stain with Wright or Giemsa polychrome stain using conventional methods. When examining slides under light microscope, perform a 200-cell differential, placing cells in one of the following three categories:
    A. Nucleated red blood cells—any nucleated erythroid form at the stage of polychromatophilic erythroblast or beyond
    B. Mature granulocytic cells—polymorphonuclear and band forms
    C. Mononuclear cells—all other cells with one nucleus

Each of these categories should be expressed as a percentage.

5. CALCULATIONS AND REPORTING
    A. To obtain the *nucleated cell content* of marrow suspension, multiply leukocyte count (nucleated cell count) by marrow volume. Note that the Coulter WBC count is reported as a count $\times 10^6$ per mL. After multiplying by volume (in mL), it is easy to move the decimal point over and express the total cell content as cells $\times 10^8$ or 10^9.
    B. To obtain a *corrected nucleated cell content* of the marrow suspension, use one of the following methods:
        (1) Seattle method: Calculate the contribution of peripheral blood leukocytes in the marrow as follows: Correct the volume of the marrow by subtracting the volume of the added anticoagulant. Multiply this corrected volume by the donor's peripheral leukocyte count. Subtract this figure from the total nucleated cell content of the harvested marrow. The resulting figure will be a corrected marrow nucleated cell content.
        (2) Holdrinet method: Calculate the fraction of marrow nucleated cells that came from the peripheral blood as follows:

$$\text{Fraction} = [\text{Hct (bm)}/\text{Hct (pb)}] \times [\text{NC (pb)}/\text{NC (bm)}] \times 100\%$$

        where: Hct = hematocrit
                 NC = nucleated cells
                 pb = peripheral blood
                 bm = bone marrow

        Subtract this fraction from 100 percent, and multiply the resulting percentage by the nucleated cell content of the marrow suspension to obtain the corrected marrow nucleated cell content.
    C. To obtain the *mononuclear cell content* of the marrow suspension, multiply the percentage of mononuclear cells from the slide differential by the nucleated cell content (uncorrected).
    D. All of the aforementioned cell content values may be expressed as cells per kg of recipient body weight by dividing the cell content by the kg

body weight of the recipient. (It is conventional to express the cell content as cell number $\times 10^8$ per kg recipient body weight.)

E. Calculation of the *cell yield* following a manipulation or series of manipulations is done by dividing the cell content after the manipulation(s) by the cell content before the manipulation(s), and expressing the resulting number as a percentage.

AUTHORS

Elizabeth J. Read, M.D.
Department of Pathology
University of Utah Medical Center
Salt Lake City, UT 84132

Charles S. Carter, B.S.
Special Services Laboratory
Department of Transfusion
  Medicine
National Institutes of Health
Bethesda, MD 20892

REFERENCES

1. Williams, WJ, Nelson, DA, and Morris, MW: Examination of the blood. In Williams, WJ, et al: Hematology, ed 4. McGraw-Hill, New York, 1990, p 9.
2. Tatsumi, J, Tatsumi, Y, and Tatsumi, N: Counting and differential of bone marrow cells by an electronic method. Am J Clin Pathol 86:50, 1986.
3. Williams, WJ: Polychrome staining. In Williams, WJ, et al: Hematology, ed 4. McGraw-Hill, New York, 1990, p 1699.
4. Shafer, JA: Preparation and interpretation of peripheral blood smears. In Hoffman, R, et al: Hematology. Basic principles and practice. Churchill Livingstone, New York, 1991, p 1790.
5. Holdrinet, RSG, et al: A method for quantification of peripheral blood admixture in bone marrow aspirates. Exp Hematol 8:103, 1980.

AUTOMATED CELL COUNTING DURING HYDROXYETHYL STARCH SEDIMENTATION OF INCOMPATIBLE RED BLOOD CELLS FROM BONE MARROW

DESCRIPTION	White blood cell counts and hematocrit measurements of marrow are taken before processing, after processing, and when the red cells are to be reprocessed. These values are used to calculate the amount of Hank's balanced salt solution and hydroxyethyl starch (HES) to add to the marrow and to calculate the numbers of white cells and red cells infused.
TIME FOR PROCEDURE	1 minute per sample
SUMMARY OF PROCEDURE	1. Samples for counts are removed from the marrow pack at the same time as samples for bacterial cultures, to minimize the possibility of contamination. 2. White cell counts and hematocrits are measured using an automated cell counter.
EQUIPMENT	1. Baker 8000 cell counter or other automated cell counter 2. Dilutor for Baker 8000 3. Clay-Adams Readacrit centrifuge, Becton Dickinson, or other hematocrit centrifuge
SUPPLIES AND REAGENTS	1. Diluvials 2. Haemline diluting solution 3. Haemrinse cleaning solution
PROCEDURE	1. Mix marrow pack. 2. Remove sample for testing as described in Chapter 11, "Sterility Checks during Bone Marrow Processing." 3. Follow manufacturer's instructions for cell counting.
ANTICIPATED RESULTS	Quickly obtained hematocrit and white blood cell (WBC) values for use in calculations.
NOTES	1. The number of WBCs in the processed product may exceed the limits of the machine. In such case, follow manufacturer's instructions for dilutions. 2. The hematocrit of the processed product will be too low for measurement by automated cell counter. A hematocrit centrifuge such as the Clay-Adams Readacrit centrifuge can be used.
AUTHOR	Sarah F. Donnelly, M.T. (ASCP), S.B.B. University of Virginia Health Sciences Center Blood Bank and Transfusion Services Charlottesville, VA 22908
REFERENCE	1. Baker System 8000 Cell Counter Operator's Manual. Manual No. DS007, January 1986, Baker Instruments, Allentown, PA.

5 | COLLECTION AND PROCESSING OF PERIPHERAL BLOOD STEM CELLS

Commentary by CHRISTOPHER A. JUTTNER and LUEN BIK TO

COLLECTION

Timing of Recovery-Phase Peripheral Blood Stem Cell Collection

Harvesting of Recovery-Phase Peripheral Blood Stem Cells Using the CS3000 Blood Cell Separator

Peripheral Stem Cell Harvests in the Steady and Nonsteady States

Collection of Peripheral Blood Stem Cells Using the Haemonetics V-50

PROCESSING

Processing of Blood Stem Cells

Processing of Peripheral Blood Mononuclear Cells (PBMCs)

Elevated levels of colony-forming units—granulocyte-macrophage (CFU-GM) during hematopoietic recovery (HR) following chemotherapy-induced myelosuppression were first described in 1976,[1] but HR capacity in humans was initially demonstrated only with chronic myeloid leukemia peripheral blood stem cells (PBSCs) collected in chronic phase.[2,3] Later reports of successful mobilization, collection, and autotransplantation used postchemotherapy recovery-phase PBSCs and produced rapid HR after transplantation, with safe neutrophil and platelet counts by the beginning of the third week from stem cell infusion.[4-9]

The neutrophil recovery is as fast as that produced by autologous or allogeneic bone marrow transplants stimulated by granulocyte or granulocyte-macrophage colony-stimulating factor (G-CSF, GM-CSF) given after the transplant,[10,11] but platelet reconstitution is much faster, allowing discharge from hospital 7 to 10 days earlier. More recently PBSCs have been used in combination with bone marrow (BM) stem cells and CSFs in order to gain the advantages of rapid HR without the incompletely resolved uncertainties of longer-term HR occasionally associated with the use of PBSCs alone.[5,12] However, incomplete long-term HR is rarely seen with adequate doses of PBSCs, as measured by a CFU-GM level greater than 3×10^4 per kg body weight.

Steady-phase PBSC collection is an alternative approach.[13,14] It is easier logistically because stem cell apheresis can be scheduled to the workload of the apheresis unit rather than the incompletely predictable recovery phenomenon. However, more aphereses are required and HR after transplantation is slower than with recovery-phase PBSCs.[14]

Studies of HR after autotransplantation using recovery-phase PBSCs have shown a significant correlation between CFU-GM dose but not mononuclear cell dose and short- and long-term HR and have suggested that there is a threshold dose of CFU-GM below which there is not satisfactory HR.[12,15,16] Initial engraftment probably results from relatively late stem cells, adequately measured by the CFU-GM assay, whereas the sustained HR suggests that the high levels of CFU-GM in recovery-phase PBSCs are indirect indications of high levels of pluripotent stem cells. The collection of large numbers of CFU-GM is thus important in achieving rapid and sustained HR following transplant.

The CFU-GM dose is, however, an imperfect indicator of HR capacity. There is no agreed upon standardization of the bioassay so that results from different laboratories are not necessarily comparable. Furthermore, the CFU-GM dose does not always predict satisfactory HR in individual patients, especially in patients with acute myeloid leukemia (AML) and the threshold dose seems to be lower in leukemias other than AML.[12,17]

Further refinements under development include the use of hematopoietic growth factors alone,[18,19] synergistic combinations of growth factors with myelosuppressive chemotherapy for mobilization,[20,21] and the development of better means of quantitating PBSCs to determine timing of harvest and HR capacity. They may lead to safer mobilizations and autotransplantation, reducing the need for hospitalization. Repeated high-dose therapy and rescue with PBSCs to increase dose intensity is fast becoming a feasible approach.

TIMING OF COLLECTION OF PBSCs

Collecting enough PBSCs is clearly important, especially in those protocols where PBSCs are used without the addition of bone marrow. For practical reasons apheresis for stem cell collection is usually started when the leukocyte count reaches 0.9 to 1.0×10^9 per L. The problems associated with using the CFU-GM assay to determine the optimum time to perform apheresis are delineated and alternative approaches applicable in real time reviewed by Haylock, To, and Juttner.[25] Timing techniques based on changes in blood counts are simple but indirect, and the use of assays for absolute levels of CD34-positive cells are more promising, particularly as bone marrow cells enriched for CD34-positive cells have been shown capable of HR in humans and in subhuman primates, and the CD34-depleted bone marrow failed to reconstitute.[22] Further refinements will include analysis of subsets of CD34-positive cells (CD34-positive/mature lineage-negative, CD34-positive/CD33-negative). In addition Siena and associates[23] have developed a rapid cytofluorimetry assay of CD34-positive cells using 50 μL of whole blood, which apparently shows promising results.

We observed poor platelet reconstitution in two AML patients who were given PBSCs containing a high CFU-GM dose collected only during the late recovery period.[17] This suggests that there may be distinct populations of hematopoietic progenitors in the peripheral blood at different times during recovery. Late in recovery there may be many committed progenitors but relatively few pluripotent stem cells compared with the early phase of recovery. Until more is understood about the kinetics of recovery phase hematopoiesis, it would be prudent to perform stem cell aphereses throughout the recovery phase.

Timing of collection is not important when steady-phase PBSCs are collected, and collection can be timed to fit in with the routine of the apheresis unit. Recovery-phase collection is generally preferred because of the HR advantages and the need for fewer aphereses, which means that a smaller volume of product will subsequently be reinfused into the patient, with a possible lower risk of toxicity.[14]

HARVESTING OF PBSCs

Initial experience with PBSC collection involved the use of intermittent flow cell separators, and some units continue to use these devices. Most groups now use continuous flow cell separators. The techniques used by the Chicago and Adelaide groups are presented in this manual. Both groups use the Fenwal CS3000 or CS3000 Plus and use only procedure 1 (platelet procedure) in Chicago or either procedure 1 or procedure 3 (lymphocyte procedure) in Adelaide. Note that there are minor and probably irrelevant differences in the modifications to procedure 1 shown in the manual by the two groups.

Procedure 1 has lower levels of red blood cell contamination but higher levels of platelets, and Dr. Williams recommends a secondary spin to reduce platelet numbers. There are several reasons why the platelet level in the PBSC collection is important. First, excessive platelet removal may lead to clinically important thrombocytopenia in the patient, although our extensive experience with early-recovery apheresis has not shown this to be so with either procedure. Second, high numbers of platelets in the cryopreserved material may lead to increased cell aggregation after thawing with the potential loss of some or all of the stem cells. Third, high platelet levels may lead to underestimation of CFU-GM numbers by causing inhibition in the bioassay system.

We prefer to use procedure 3 to reduce platelet contamination while accepting a slightly higher level of red cell contamination. Red cell depletion in the patient is not a problem because red cell transfusion is often required during and after chemotherapy, and our processing protocol removes most of these red cells before cryopreservation.

The most relevant question is whether there is any evidence to suggest that one technique or one machine yields either higher levels of PBSC from each apheresis, or discrete populations of stem cells that offer advantages in either hematopoietic reconstitution or malignant contamination. There is no clear evidence that either procedure has an absolute advantage, although the manufacturer recommends procedure 1. It is uncertain whether any of the groups who are actively involved in the field are investigating this issue, and there is probably no need for such a study.

Preliminary data in our laboratory show that the CS3000 has an extremely high instantaneous collection efficiency (95 percent) for both mononuclear cells and CFU-GM in procedure 1 or 3 and that the lower overall or average collection efficiencies generally seen result from false overestimation of the actual blood volume processed as a result of the dead space in the apheresis system and dilution by anticoagulant and from an approximately 20 percent fall in the white blood cell count during apheresis. The latter effect appears to occur only in recovery-phase stem cell collection. These considerations probably apply to all apheresis machines and most studies have reported overall collection efficiencies between 50 and 70 percent, irrespective of machine or procedure.

PROCESSING OF PBSCs

The major requirements in processing PBSCs are to reduce the volume to be frozen and to increase the purity of the frozen product. Kessinger and colleagues[14] have reported significant toxicity related to the volume of cryoprotectant and the processing technique. It would therefore seem desirable to reduce the final cell volume as much as possible. Furthermore, a smaller final volume will be desirable if cryopreservation uses vials rather than bags, and particularly if the controlled rate freezer has a small-volume freezing chamber, which may make vials mandatory.

We consider it theoretically desirable to reduce red blood cell contamination in order to reduce potential renal damage from free hemoglobin after thawing, and to reduce platelet and granulocyte contamination in order to reduce the chance of major clumping or congelation of the PBSCs during reinfusion. Our protocol thus uses a density gradient step to remove most mature granulocytes and red blood cells. This is not recommended by the Peoria or University of Chicago groups in their sections in the manual (see Chapter 9). These centers report satisfactory HR after autografting without such extensive cell processing, so the choice of processing protocol depends on local preference.

CRYOPRESERVATION AND STORAGE OF PBSCs

The contributors to this manual recommend controlled rate freezing with the final concentration of dimethyl sulfoxide (DMSO) at 10 percent. Stiff and associates[24] reported satisfactory viability and HR using 5 percent hydroxyethyl starch (HES), 5 percent DMSO, and uncontrolled rate freezing and storage at $-80°C$. There is uncertainty about the cell concentration for cryopreservation and storage and whether the frozen cells should be kept in the liquid or vapor phase of liquid nitrogen, although there is some evidence to suggest that the lesser temperatures are associated with lower viabilities, at least over storage periods of months or years.[25] Gorin[26] recommends storage at cell concentrations less than or equal to 2×10^7 per mL, whereas we store at concentrations up to 5×10^7 per mL. Some centers store at cell concentrations as high as 10×10^7 per mL, and it is uncertain if this leads to reduced viability.

QUANTITATION OF PBSCs

Dyson and Haylock (see Chapter 11) present the details of the CFU-GM assay techniques used for quantitating PBSCs. A well-optimized peripheral blood CFU-GM assay is a vital part of any PBSC transplant program, and it appears necessary to plate the mononuclear cells at several concentrations in order to overcome the confounding effects of monocytes in culture.[27] This may explain why we report higher CFU-GM levels than many other groups.

It is important to emphasize that single recombinant hematopoietic growth factors will usually stimulate lower numbers of CFU-GM colonies in culture than combinations, and they are not necessarily comparable to optimized conditioned media such as human placental conditioned medium (HPCM). Each laboratory should establish its reference range.

The post-thaw or viability assay provides an important quality control assessment of the cryopreservation and storage technique. The CFU-GM viability is generally more than 80 percent of the fresh specimen, and storage in the liquid phase of liquid nitrogen allows this viability to persist for up to 5 years. The use of leukocyte feeder layers in addition to HPCM is of major importance in assessing viability, confirming the initial report by Schlunk, Ruber, and Schleyer.[28] It is arguable whether post-thaw rather than prefreeze CFU-GM numbers should be quoted in reports of HR in PBSC transplantation because viability testing adds a further variable. Gorin[26] suggested that viability should be at least 50 percent, and such a semiquantitative approach is probably as valid.

REFERENCES

1. Richman, CM, Weiner, RS, and Yankee, RS: Increase in circulating stem cells following chemotherapy in man. Blood 47:1031, 1976.
2. Körbling, M, et al: Successful engraftment of blood-derived normal hemopoietic stem cells in chronic myelogenous leukemia. Exp Hematol 9:684, 1981.
3. Goldman, JM and Lu, DP: New approaches in chronic granulocytic leukemia—origin, prognosis and treatment. Semin Hematol 19:241, 1982.
4. To, LB, et al: High levels of circulating haemopoietic stem cells in very early remission from acute non-lymphoblastic leukaemia and their collection and cryopreservation. Br J Haematol 58:399, 1984.
5. Juttner, CA, et al: Circulating autologous stem cells collected in very early remission from acute non-lymphoblastic leukaemia produce prompt but incomplete haemopoietic reconstitution after high dose melphalan and supralethal chemoradiotherapy. Br J Haematol 61:739, 1985.
6. Körbling, M, et al: Autologous transplantation of blood-derived hemopoietic stem cells after myeloablative therapy in a patient with Burkitt's lymphoma. Blood 67:629, 1986.
7. Reiffers, J, et al: Successful autologous transplantation with peripheral blood haemopoietic cells in a patient with acute leukaemia. Exp Hematol 14:312, 1986.
8. Bell, AJ, et al: Peripheral blood stem cell autografting (letter). Lancet 1:1027, 1986.
9. Tilly, H, et al: Haemopoietic reconstitution after autologous peripheral blood stem cell transplantation in acute leukaemia (letter). Lancet 2:154, 1986.
10. Sheridan, WP, et al: Effects of granulocyte colony stimulating factor (G-CSF) following high dose chemotherapy and autologous bone marrow transplantation. Lancet 2:891, 1989.
11. Brandt, SJ, Peters, WP, and Atwater, SK: Effect of recombinant human granulocyte-macrophage colony-stimulating factor on hematopoietic reconstitution after high dose chemotherapy and autologous bone marrow transplantation. N Engl J Med 318:869, 1988.
12. To, LB, et al: An unusual pattern of hemopoietic reconstitution in patients with acute myeloid leukaemia transplanted with autologous recovery phase peripheral blood. Bone Marrow Transplant 6:109, 1990.
13. Kessinger, A, et al: Autologous peripheral hematopoietic stem cell transplantation restores hematopoietic function following marrow ablative therapy. Blood 71:723, 1988.
14. Kessinger, A, et al: High-dose therapy and autologous peripheral blood stem cell transplantation for patients with lymphoma. Blood 74:1260, 1989.
15. Reiffers, J, et al: Haematopoietic reconstitution after autologous blood stem cell transplanta-

tion. In Gale, RP and Champlin, RE (eds): Bone Marrow Transplantation, Current Controversies, Proceedings of Sandoz-UCLA Symposium. Alan R Liss, New York, 1988.

16. To, LB, Dyson, PG, and Juttner, CA: Cell-dose effect in circulating stem cell autografting (letter). Lancet 2:404, 1986.

17. Juttner, CA, et al: Granulocyte macrophage progenitor numbers in peripheral blood stem cell autotransplantation. In Smit Sibinga, C Th and Kater, L (eds): Advances in Haemapheresis. Proceedings of the Third International Congress of the World Apheresis Association. April 9–12, 1990. Amsterdam. Third International Congress of the World Apheresis Association.

18. Sheridan, WP, et al: Granulocyte colony-stimulating factor (G-CSF) in peripheral blood stem cell (PBSC) and bone marrow (BM) transplantation (abstr). Blood 76(Suppl 1):565, 1990.

19. Socinski, MA, et al: Granulocyte-macrophage colony stimulating factor expands the circulating haemopoietic progenitor cell compartment in man. Lancet 1:1194, 1988.

20. Gianni, AM, et al: Granulocyte-macrophage colony-stimulating factor to harvest circulating haematopoietic stem cells for autotransplantation. Lancet 2:580, 1989.

21. Gianni, AM, et al: Rapid and complete hemopoietic reconstitution following combined transplantation of autologous blood and bone marrow cells: a changing role for high dose chemoradiotherapy. Hematol Oncol 7:139, 1989.

22. Berenson, RJ, et al: Antigen CD34+ marrow cells engraft lethally irradiated baboons. J Clin Invest 81:951, 1988.

23. Siena, S, et al: Flow cytometry for clinical estimation of circulating hematopoietic progenitors for autologous transplantation in cancer patients. Blood 77:400, 1991.

24. Stiff, PJ, et al: Autologous bone marrow transplantation using unfractionated cells cryopreserved in dimethylsulfoxide and hydroxylethyl starch without controlled-rate freezing. Blood 70:974, 1987.

25. Haylock, DN, To, LB, and Juttner, CA: A simplified bone marrow cryopreservation method (letter). Blood 72:1102, 1988.

26. Gorin, NC: Collection, manipulation and freezing of haemopoietic stem cells. Clin Haematol 15:9, 1986.

27. To, LB, et al: The effect of monocytes in the peripheral blood CFU-C assay system. Blood 62:112, 1983.

28. Schlunk, T, Ruber, E, and Schleyer, M: Survival of human bone marrow progenitor cells after freezing: improved detection in the colony-formation assay. Cryobiology 18:111, 1981.

COLLECTION

TIMING OF RECOVERY-PHASE PERIPHERAL BLOOD STEM CELL COLLECTION

DESCRIPTION

This section addresses the timing of peripheral blood stem collection during the recovery phase following myelosuppressive chemotherapy. The aim is to harvest an adequate dose of stem cells for safe transplantation with a minimum of aphereses. Protocols are described for peripheral blood stem cell (PBSC) collection in patients with acute myeloid leukemia (AML) following induction or consolidation chemotherapy and in patients treated with high-dose cyclophosphamide.

PROBLEMS WITH DETERMINING THE TIME FOR COLLECTION

The variable recovery pattern observed with the various chemotherapy regimens poses a problem for determining when to perform stem cell collection because there is no one simple and quick index that is predictive of the collection of stem cells that produce both early rapid and sustained hematopoietic reconstitution (HR). The number of myeloid progenitor cells, or colony-forming units—granulocyte-macrophage (CFU-GM), collected appear to correlate with rapid and sustained HR,[1,2] but the assay takes 14 days to yield results that are influenced by the methodology used. However, it is an imperfect indicator of HR, particularly of long-term HR. The following protocols are thus based on retrospective analyses correlating changes in blood counts with CFU-GM levels.[3-5]

Acute Myeloid Leukemia

For AML patients following induction or consolidation chemotherapy, apheresis is commenced when the platelet count rises above 50×10^9 per L and when the leukocyte count approaches 1×10^9 per L. This usually occurs between 12 and 16 days from the completion of the chemotherapy. Daily apheresis is continued while the blood counts are rising rapidly. We require an increase of 20 to 30 percent in both the leukocyte and platelet counts before the next apheresis is performed. Apheresis will be performed until a total of more than 3×10^8 mononuclear cells per kg have been collected.

Usually three to four aphereses are performed until the leukocyte count reaches normal levels. Additional indicators of vigorous recovery and remission are monocytosis and a reverse ratio of lymphoid to myeloid cells, which may persist until the leukocyte count returns to normal levels. Large atypical lymphocytes or monocytes and the occasional myeloblast in the peripheral blood can also be present in the very early remission phase.

In those patients who achieve only partial remission, the rate of recovery following induction chemotherapy is slow and a rebound increase in PBSCs does not occur. Consequently, insufficient stem cells are collected. If there is doubt as to the attainment of remission, a bone marrow biopsy can be performed to aid with the decision to continue or abandon apheresis.

PBSC Collection in Non-AML Patients

In patients with non-Hodgkin's lymphoma, multiple myeloma, and ovarian and breast carcinoma a single high dose of cyclophosphamide (4 g/m^2) is an effective way of producing high levels of PBSCs, especially in those who have normal or minimally involved bone marrow and who have not had intensive recent therapy.[4] Following a period of cytopenia the blood counts start to recover 13 to 18 days after cyclophosphamide. Our current protocol is:

1. Start apheresis when the leukocyte count reaches 1.0×10^9 per L or when the platelet count shows a rapid rise. Continue apheresis if either the leukocyte or the platelet count shows a rise of 20 percent or more compared with the count the previous day. Once the leukocyte count reaches 2.0×10^9 per L, do two aphereses on consecutive days whether the counts continue to rise or not. This is because we have seen sustained high levels of CFU-GM when the leukocyte count was around 2.0 to 2.5×10^9 per L, even when the counts were not rising.

2. A minimum of four aphereses are performed until mononuclear cell yield reaches 3.0×10^8 per kg body weight (BW) and when the leukocyte count reaches 3.0×10^9 per L. In patients whose leukocyte count takes more than 5 days to rise from 1.0 to 3.0×10^9 per L, high levels of CFU-GM are unlikely and apheresis may be abandoned.

Alternative Methods for Timing of PBSC Collection

MONOCYTOSIS   Other groups have used monocytosis as a guide to start of recovery-phase apheresis.[6,7] Although monocytosis is undoubtedly part of the recovery process, particularly in AML patients, we have not found a significant correlation with CFU-GM incidence, and its value remains questionable.

CD34-POSITIVE CELLS   It is now evident that CD34 antigen-bearing hematopoietic cells play a key role in hematopoietic reconstitution (HR) following transplantation.[8-10] CD34-positive cells that do not express T and B–mature myeloid and monocyte markers are present in normal peripheral blood,[11] and they are markedly increased during recovery phase and their levels correlate with CFU-GM.[12,13] CD34-positive cells and their immunophenotypic subsets can be accurately measured by flow cytometry and possibly by immunocytochemical staining of cells on cytospin preparations.

With use of these methods the level of CD34-positive hematopoietic cells may provide a rapid and reliable measure of when to collect PBSCs as well as an index of their HR capacity. It is essential that laboratories carefully develop their methods and validate the correlation between CD34-positive cells and CFU-GM before using these new techniques to determine the timing of PBSC collection.

AUTHORS

David N. Haylock, B.App.Sc.
Leukaemia Research Unit
Department of Haematology
Institute of Medical and Veterinary Science
Adelaide, South Australia 5000

Pamela G. Dyson, B.Sc.(Hons)
Leukaemia Research Unit

Institute of Medical and Veterinary Science
Adelaide, South Australia 5000

Luen Bik To, M.D., M.B.B.S.
Leukaemia Research Unit
Institute of Medical and Veterinary Science
Adelaide, South Australia 5000

REFERENCES

1. Reiffers, J, et al: Haemopoietic reconstitution after autologous blood stem cell transplantation. In Gale, RP and Champlin, RE (eds): Bone Marrow Transplantation, Current Controversies, Proceedings of Sandoz-UCLA Symposium. Alan R Liss, New York, 1988.
2. To, LB, et al: An unusual pattern of haemopoietic reconstitution in patients with acute myeloid leukaemia transplanted with autologous recovery phase peripheral blood. Bone Marrow Transplant 6:109, 1990.
3. To, LB, et al: The optimisation of collection of peripheral blood stem cells for transplantation for autotransplantation in acute myeloid leukaemia. Bone Marrow Transplant 4:41, 1989.
4. To, LB, et al: Single high doses of cyclophosphamide enable the collection of high numbers of haemopoietic stem cells from the peripheral blood. Exp Hematol 18:442, 1990.
5. To, LB and Juttner, CA: Stem cell mobilisation by myelosuppressive chemotherapy. In Autologous Blood Stem Cell Autografts. Springer-Verlag, New York, 1990.
6. Tilly, H, et al: Haemopoietic reconstitution after autologous peripheral blood stem cell transplantation in acute leukaemia (letter). Lancet 2:154, 1986.
7. Stiff, PJ, Koester, AR, and Lanzotti, VJ: Autologous transplantation using peripheral blood stem cells (abstr). Exp Hematol 14:311, 1986.
8. Civin, CI, et al: Antigenic analysis of hematopoiesis. III. A hematopoietic progenitor cell surface antigen defined by a monoclonal antibody raised against KG-1a cells. J Immunol 133:157, 1984.
9. Andrews, RG, Singer, JW, and Bernstein, ID: Precursors of colony forming cells in humans can be distinguished from colony forming cells by expression of CD33 and CD34 antigens and light scatter properties. J Exp Med 169:1721, 1989.
10. Berenson, RJ, et al: Antigen CD34+ marrow cells engraft lethally irradiated baboons. J Clin Invest 81:951, 1988.
11. Bender, JG, et al: Identification and comparison of CD34 positive cells from normal peripheral blood and bone marrow using multicolor flow cytometry. Blood (in press).
12. Siena, S, et al: Circulation of CD34+ hematopoietic stem cells in the peripheral blood of high dose cyclophosphamide-treated patients: Enhancement by intravenous recombinant human granulocyte-macrophage colony stimulating factor. Blood 74:1905, 1989.
13. Juttner, CA, et al: Approaches to blood stem cell mobilisation: Initial Australian clinical results. Bone Marrow Transplant 5:22, 1990.

HARVESTING OF RECOVERY-PHASE PERIPHERAL BLOOD STEM CELLS USING THE CS3000 BLOOD CELL SEPARATOR

DESCRIPTION	Peripheral blood stem cells are harvested from the patient during the period of hematopoietic regeneration following cytoreductive therapy. Three to five procedures are required so that sufficient stem cells for safe autotransplantation can be collected.
TIME FOR PROCEDURE	Approximately 2½ hours to process 7000 mL, 3½ hours to process 10,000 mL patient blood, plus 30 minutes for setup and cleanup (both procedures 1 and 3 operate with a whole blood flow rate of 50 mL per minute)
SUMMARY OF PROCEDURE	1.　Set and prime CS3000 machine. 2.　Make program changes. 3.　Establish patient vascular access. 4.　Harvest stem cells by CS3000. 5.　Disconnect patient from the machine. 6.　Resuspend stem cells, separate collection bag, and collect specimen. 7.　Send stem cells to laboratory for processing.
EQUIPMENT	Fenwal CS3000 blood cell separator No. 4R4531 or Fenwal CS3000 Plus blood cell separator No. 4R4539 with granulo separation chamber (Fenwal Division, Baxter Healthcare)
SUPPLIES AND REAGENTS	1.　Fenwal open apheresis kit No. 4R2210 2.　1000 mL 0.9 percent sodium chloride for intravenous (IV) infusion 3.　500 mL anticoagulant citrate dextrose solution formula A (ACD-A), containing 24.5 g dextrose (monohydrate), 22.0 g sodium citrate (dihydrate), and 8.0 g citric acid (monohydrate) per 1000 mL 4.　600-mL transfer pack 5.　Two 16-gauge A-V fistula needles with backeye Terumo No. AV-E16 or similar 6.　Venipuncture equipment 7.　Donor couch, recliner chair, or bed
STANDARD PROCEDURE (Procedure 3)	1.　INSTALL APHERESIS KIT AND PRIME 　　A.　Install the apheresis kit following the procedure outlined in the operator's manual. 　　B.　Select procedure 3, with PRIME and RUN switches in auto. (Procedure 1 may be chosen, see alternative procedure in notes.) 　　C.　Initiate autoprime as per operator's manual (6.6–6.8). 2.　REPROGRAM AUTO-RUN 　　A.　Change interface detector offset to 0200. Press and hold ENTER-2; using END-POINT switches, increase interface detector offset from 0150 to 0200. Release ENTER-2; press RESUME.

B. If desiring to process 10,000 mL patient blood, change END-POINT to 9990, using END-POINT switches.

Or if using CS3000 Plus:

3. REPROGRAM AUTO-RUN CS3000 PLUS
   A. Change interface detector offset to 0200. Press DISPLAY/EDIT key; using up/down arrow keys (↑↓), scroll through changeable parameters until interface detector offset is displayed in LED readout. Press ENTER and change offset to 0200 by using ↑↓ keys. Press ENTER again to store information and exit by pressing DISPLAY/EDIT.
   B. If desiring to process 10,000 mL, press DISPLAY/EDIT, scroll through changeable parameters by using ↑↓ keys until END-POINT volume is displayed. Press ENTER, change END-POINT volume to 10,000 by using ↑↓ keys. Store information by pressing ENTER and exit by pressing DISPLAY/EDIT key.

ALTERNATIVE PROCEDURE (Procedure 1 Modified)

1. INSTALL APHERESIS KIT AND PRIME
   A. Install the apheresis kit following the procedure as per the operator's manual.
   B. Use granulo separation chamber, A-35 collection container.
   C. Select procedure 1, with PRIME and AUTO-RUN switches in auto.
   D. Press PRIME switch. Prime as per the operator's manual.

2. REPROGRAM AUTO-RUN
   A. Reprogram the computer. To modify standard computer program press and hold "C" in CS3000 (on operator panel) while pushing RUN.

   After the indicator light on the ENTER-2 switch is lighted, use the ENTER-1 (to increment by tens) and the ENTER-2 (to increment by ones) switches to select the stop locations (shown in status display) to be modified.

   The preprogrammed values for each step should be altered as listed below using the switches underneath END-POINT display while holding "C" in CS3000.

   Existing and modified values will be shown in END-POINT display. Upon completion of each step alteration, use ENTER-1 and ENTER-2 switches to select the next steps to be modified.

   B. The following locations are changed:

Step	Blood Flow 50 mL/min
L-60 from (0240)	to 1750
L-61 from (0010)	to 0000
L-62 from (0160)	to no change (0160)
L-64 from (0320)	to no change (0320)
L-68 from (0450)	to Hct of patient (see table below)
L-71 from (0400)	to 1000
L-78 from (0850)	to 0950

PATIENT HEMATOCRIT (Hct) TABLE

Patient Hct%	Change L-68 to	Patient Hct%	Change L-68 to
20	0750	38	0550
22	0730	40	0520
24	0710	42	0500
26	0680	44	0480
28	0660	46	0460
30	0640	48	0430
32	0620	50	0410
34	0590	52	0390
36	0570	54	0360

    C. After all program modifications have been completed, press RESUME to incorporate the desired modifications and exit reprogramming mode.

    D. If desiring to process 10,000 mL of patient's blood, change END-POINT to 9990, using END-POINT switches.

    E. Blood flow rate is programmed to be maintained at 50 mL per minute to allow adequate dwell time in the separation chambers.

Or if using CS3000 Plus:

2. REPROGRAM AUTO-RUN CS3000 PLUS

    A. Reprogram computer (to modify standard computer program). Using the table EDIT keys, change the component separation data stored in the computer's memory.

    B. Press EDIT key; then, using the location arrow keys, scroll to desired location. To change the value of that location use the content's arrow key, then press STORE to commit the new value to memory. Continue this process until all steps are completed; then exit reprogramming mode by pressing EDIT.

    C. If desiring to process 10,000 mL, press DISPLAY/EDIT, scroll through changeable parameters by using ↑↓ keys until END-POINT volume is displayed. Press ENTER, change END-POINT volume to 10,000 by using ↑↓ keys. Store information by pressing ENTER, and exit by pressing DISPLAY/EDIT key.

    D. Blood flow rate is programmed to be maintained at 50 mL per minute to allow adequate dwell time in the separation chambers.

3. ACHIEVE VASCULAR ACCESS

    A. Perform venipuncture, using aseptic technique.

    B. Connect the inlet and return lines to needle tubing. Tape securely to the patient's arm.

    C. Initiate a "keep vein open" drip by adjusting the roller clamp on the inlet and vent lines.

4. HARVEST STEM CELLS

    A. Initiate auto-run (procedure as per the operator's manual).

    B. Check the anticoagulant flow rate by monitoring the ACD drip rate. Ratio should be 1 mL ACD:11 mL whole blood.

    C. After first spillover (status code 80) is complete and status code 00 is displayed, reset interface detector baseline as follows:

        1. *For the CS3000*

          a. Press SET BLOOD FLOW RATE such that red indicator light is illuminated.

          b. Simultaneously press and hold ENTER-2 and any of the three END-POINT switches until the RESUME light blinks. Release switch.

          c. Press RESUME to enter new baseline value.

        2. *For CS3000 Plus*

          a. Press DISPLAY/EDIT key.

          b. Use ↑↓ arrows to display interface detector baseline in message center.

          c. Press ENTER kcy to set the value.

          d. Press DISPLAY/EDIT key to exit.

    D. When end-point is reached, press REINFUSE to return the red cells from the machine to the patient.

    E. When auto-reinfuse is completed, remove the inlet line and return line needles from the patient; refer to the operator's manual.

5. REMOVE COLLECTED STEM CELLS FROM CS3000

    A. Open the centrifuge compartment doors.

    B. Remove the upper hex from its restraining collar.

    C. Release the lower hex from its restraining collar.

    D. Make two seals on each of the two collection container tubings. Cut each between the seals.

    E. Open the collection container holder clamp and remove the collection bag containing the harvested cells.

    F. Resuspend the stem cells by vigorously shaking the collection bag for 2 to 3 minutes.

    G. Label stem cell collection bag with the patient's name, unit record number, and date of collection.

6. TRANSPORT STEM CELLS TO LABORATORY

ANTICIPATED RESULTS	Each procedure results in 200-mL product volume. The quantity of stem cells will vary considerably depending on the patient's starting white cell count and circulating stem cell fraction.

NOTES	1. Procedure 1 modified and procedure 3 give similar results. The number of stem cells collected and machine collection efficiency compare favorably. There are fewer red cells but more platelets collected using modified procedure 1.
	
	Our unit uses procedure 3 with slight modification (the interface detector offset is changed to 0200).
	
	2. VASCULAR ACCESS
	  A. Preferred device is 16 gauge × 1 in A-V fistula set (Terumo Corporation No. AV-E16).
	  B. Installing the needle for return line in radial, cephalic, or ulnar vein in the forearm will allow the patient freedom of movement in this arm (inlet line needle should be placed in the largest vessel available—usually in the ante-cubital fossa).

    C. Needle size—preferably 16 gauge for inlet—never smaller than 18 gauge. Return line devices may include 18-gauge IV catheter (Jelco, Johnson and Johnson). At machine startup a code No. 40 (return line negative pressure) may show if this device is used. The operator may override this code with caution.

    D. If peripheral access sites have been exhausted the use of a central venous catheter may be a viable alternative. A dual-lumen device (i.e., Vas-Cath Dual Lumen Kit DLK-4400, Vas-Cath, Inc., Mississauga, Ontario, Canada) is preferred because it gives the necessary dual access and is rigid. These catheters may remain in situ for up to 6 weeks with proper care. Insertion is done by experienced medical staff using strict aseptic technique. Catheter placement is checked by x-ray examination before use.

3. PATIENT COMFORT

    A. Good communication is essential. The patient who has a clear understanding of the procedure, the time each procedure takes, and the reasons for uncertainty of commencement day for the harvest will be much more comfortable with the procedure.

    B. Planning vascular access: The apheresis staff members visit the patient during their admission for high-dose chemotherapy. At this visit the apheresis procedure is explained in detail and the patient visits the apheresis room. Apheresis staff members inspect the patient's peripheral blood vessels. Vascular access for the procedure is planned and a note made in the patient's record folder. If a central venous catheter is to be used, this can be inserted the day before the first collection day.

    C. Blood banks are notified to supply only irradiated blood products for patients from day 1 of cytotoxic infusion. Patients often require transfusion, as their hemoglobin may be reduced from 0.5 g per dL to 0.8 g per dL per stem cell harvest, when using procedure 3.

    D. During harvest procedure comfort measures include using a comfortable chair or bed, and using diversional therapy—books, TV, radio, interaction with staff, food and drinks—as well as good general nursing care.

    E. Vital signs monitoring: Temperature, pulse, and blood pressure (BP) are observed at the commencement of the procedure and pulse and BP are monitored every 10 minutes throughout the procedure.

    F. Pediatric and small blood volume patients: Prime the kit in the usual manner; attach a waste bag to the return line; initiate auto-run using cross-matched, irradiated whole blood connected to the inlet line, until the first spill-over step occurs; initiate halt-irrigate; close both inlet and return saline drips. Disconnect the whole blood pack and waste bag and connect the patient, resume the procedure, adjusting the end-point to take account of the amount of cross-matched blood processed.

AUTHORS

Dawn Thorp, R.N.
Apheresis Unit
Institute of Medical and Veterinary
  Science
Adelaide, South Australia 5000

David N. Haylock, B. App. Sc.
Leukaemia Research Unit
Department of Haematology
Institute of Medical and Veterinary
  Science
Adelaide, South Australia 5000

Anne Canty, R.N.
Apheresis Unit
Institute of Medical and Veterinary
    Science
Adelaide, South Australia 5000

REFERENCES

1. Haylock, D, et al: Assessing the stem cell collection efficiency of the Fenwal CS3000. Apheresis: Proceedings of the Second International Congress of World Apheresis Association, New York, Alan R. Liss, 1990.
2. To, LB, et al: The optimisation of collection of peripheral blood stem cells for autotransplantation in acute myeloid leukaemia. Bone Marrow Transplant 4:41, 1989.
3. Cullis, H: Fenwal Division, Baxter Healthcare, Deerfield, IL. Personal communication.

PERIPHERAL STEM CELL HARVESTS IN THE STEADY AND NONSTEADY STATES

DESCRIPTION	High-dose chemotherapy with autologous stem cell rescue has become an increasingly useful therapeutic regimen in many patients with hematologic as well as solid tumors. Many patients who might benefit from this therapy have bone marrow involved with the malignancy or hypocellular bone marrows, making it impossible to collect and cryopreserve autologous bone marrow. Alternative sources of these marrow stem cells include collection of circulating hematopoietic cells from the peripheral blood. These peripheral stem cells can be collected in an unprimed or steady state or during the myeloid recovery phase from myeloablative chemotherapy to increase numbers of circulating hematopoietic stem cells (mobilized or nonsteady state). The collection method is essentially similar. The method involves the use of the Fenwal CS3000 cell separator employing a closed, sterile system to obtain a concentrated mononuclear cell product that is subsequently cryopreserved and stored in the liquid phase of nitrogen.
TIME FOR PROCEDURE	Approximately 3 to 4 hours to process 8 to 10 L of whole blood (in steady state eight separate procedures are performed); after chemotherapy mobilization during recovery from neutropenia (nonsteady state) three to five separate procedures are performed).
SUMMARY OF PROCEDURE	1. All patients have double-lumen subclavian catheters placed prior to beginning apheresis procedures.
	2. A standard Fenwal apheresis kit is installed on the CS3000 and primed with 0.9 percent saline.
	3. The CS3000 is programmed to collect mononuclear cells according to the chart.
	4. 10 L of whole blood are processed using the double-lumen central vein catheter (one lumen as draw line and second lumen as return).
	5. A secondary spin is performed to remove platelets from mononuclear product.
	6. The mononuclear product collected is then cryopreserved in dimethyl sulfoxide (DMSO) (10 percent final concentration) and frozen in a controlled rate liquid nitrogen freezer.
EQUIPMENT	1. Fenwal CS3000 Blood Cell Separator with A-35 collection chamber and granulo separation chamber, Fenwal Division, Baxter Healthcare
	2. Cryomed controlled-rate liquid nitrogen freezer
SUPPLIES AND REAGENTS	1. Quinton Permacath, double lumen for central venous access
	2. Fenwal closed system apheresis cell collection kit (4R2230), which includes: A. 1000 mL 0.9 percent sodium chloride processing solution B. 1000 mL anticoagulant citrate dextrose solution, formula A (ACD-A) C. Two 1000-mL transfer packs D. 600-mL transfer pack
	3. 1000 USP units per mL preservative-free heparin

PROCEDURE

1. PREPROCEDURE
   A. All patients have double-lumen central vein access placed under sterile conditions in the operating room.
   B. Patients undergoing non–steady state collections are treated with myeloablative chemotherapy (such as cyclophosphamide 4.0 g per m^2). Blood counts are followed and as patients recover from neutropenia leukapheresis is begun (WBC greater than or equal to 1000 per mm^3).

2. INSTALLATION OF APHERESIS KIT AND PRIME
   A. Install apheresis kit according to operator's manual.
   B. Select procedure 1 on the manual control panel.
   C. Prior to prime mode, put 1 mL of heparin (1000 USP units per mL) in the air trap.
   D. Press PRIME switch.
      (1) Modify basic computer program to facilitate mononuclear cell collection as follows:
         (a) Select anticipated whole blood flow rate and modify the following:

	BLOOD FLOW			
Step	60 mL/min	70 mL/min	80 mL/min	85 mL/min
L-60 from 0240	to 2100	to 0245	to 0240	to 0420
L-61 from 0010	to 0000	to 0000	to 0010	to 0010
L-62 from 0160	to 0190	to 0210	to 0250	to 0270
L-64 from 0320	to 0380	to 0420	to 0500	to 0540
L-68 from 0450	*	*	*	*

*See chart in step (b), which follows.

         (b) Determine patient hematocrit and select value for step L-68 from chart.

Hct CHART FOR CS3000
MONONUCLEAR CELL
COLLECTION USING MODIFIED
PROCEDURE 1

Change L-68 in Program from 0450 to			
If Patient Hct%	Change L-68 to	If Patient Hct%	Change L-68 to
20	0750	38	0550
22	0730	40	0520
24	0710	42	0500
26	0680	44	0480
28	0660	46	0460
30	0640	48	0430
32	0620	50	0410
34	0590	52	0390
36	0570	54	0360

(c) Press and hold "C" in CS3000 (on operator panel) while pushing RUN to enter reprogramming mode. Use ENTER-1 and ENTER-2 switches to select step modification and press END-POINT switches to alter reprogrammed values, as earlier.

3. LEUKAPHERESIS OF PATIENT

A. 10 L of whole blood are processed using the closed system apheresis kit.

B. Follow procedure in Fenwal CS3000 operator's manual for "Production of Lymphokine Activated Killer Cells" (revised 4/25/88).

(1) Double-lumen central venous access device is placed for ease of access and patient comfort. Tip of catheter must be 2 cm above right atrium as shown on chest x-ray examination.

(2) ACD-A runs continuously during leukapheresis in a ratio of 1:9 (ACD-A to peripheral blood), although this may depend on patient's reaction to ACD-A.

(3) Blood flow rates between 60 and 85 mL per minute may be used, as tolerated by patient. This is possible using central catheters such as Permacaths.

C. Follow standard reinfusion procedure to return maximum number of red blood cells.

4. SECONDARY SPIN TO REMOVE PLATELETS FROM MONONUCLEAR CELL PRODUCT

A. 200 mL 0.9 percent sodium chloride processing solution should be collected prior to the start of RUN to rinse platelets from the 600-mL transfer pack and return line after secondary spin. This is collected according to the operator's manual.

B. Follow procedure in Fenwal CS3000 operator's manual "Double Secondary Spin to Remove Platelets from Mononuclear Cell Product" (revised 4/25/88).

C. Resuspension and transfer of product is also performed according to aforementioned manual. At any point before transfer of stem cell product put 2 mL of preservative-free heparin (1000 USP units per mL) in 1000-mL transfer pack in which stem cells product will be transferred.

ANTICIPATED RESULTS	In steady state collections eight apheresis procedures should yield 5 to 7×10^8 mononuclear cells per kg. In chemotherapy, non–steady state collections three to five procedures should yield 3×10^8 mononuclear cells per kg. Non–steady state collections will have much higher CFU-GM activity than steady state collections.
NOTE	Most patients have symptoms of oral numbness or tingling in their hands or toes owing to ACD-A. If symptoms persist beyond 10 to 15 minutes, 5 to 10 mL of calcium carbonate suspension (equal to 500 to 1000 mg elemental calcium) is given prophylactically. This is repeated as necessary. Infrequently, calcium by intravenous riders is also used.
AUTHORS	Stephanie F. Williams, M.D. University of Chicago Medical Center Chicago, IL 60637 Susan Barker, C.T. University of Chicago Medical Center Chicago, IL 60637

Kristi Hollingsworth, M.A.
University of Chicago Medical
Center
Chicago, IL 60637

REFERENCES

1. Williams, SF, et al: Peripheral blood-derived stem cell collections for use in autologous transplantation after high dose chemotherapy: An alternative approach in bone marrow purging and processing. Gross, S, Gee, AP, and Worthington-White, D (eds): Proceedings of the Second International Symposium 1989. Wiley-Liss, New York, 1990, p 461.
2. Williams, SF, et al: Peripheral blood-derived stem cell collections for use in autologous transplantation after high dose chemotherapy: An alternative approach. Bone Marrow Transplant 5:129, 1990.

COLLECTION OF PERIPHERAL BLOOD STEM CELLS USING THE HAEMONETICS V-50

DESCRIPTION	Peripheral stem cells are used in autologous transplantation for patients who have malignancy in the bone marrow or who have received previous radiation to the traditional bone marrow harvest sites. The collections are performed on the Haemonetics V-50 using the lymphocyte time saver return protocol. At the end of each procedure a secondary spin is performed on the final product in the blood processor to reduce the volume of red blood cells (RBCs) and plasma, to concentrate the buffy coat, and to return the unwanted components to the patient.

TIME FOR PROCEDURE	4 hours

SUMMARY OF PROCEDURE

1. The blood processor is set up for a lymphocyte time saver protocol using a Haemonetics 603 TSPP disposable kit. ACD Formula B is used as the anticoagulant.
2. The Haemonetics V-50 is programmed for lymphocyte program—non-surge; RBC volume is set at 40.
3. Collection is performed for approximately 3¾ hours.
4. At the end of the collection time the draw line from the patient is clamped and saline flow is initiated to keep the venous access patent.
5. The lymphocyte protocol on the machine is reprogrammed for a 60-mL RBC volume. The product is reintroduced into the bowl and a buffy coat concentration is done. On this cycle all of the buffy coat and 60 mL of RBCs are collected.
6. The unwanted components are returned to the patient at the completion of the buffy coat pass.
7. The product is removed from the blood processor and a sample is taken for cell cultures and to determine cell counts.

EQUIPMENT	Haemonetics V-50 Plus apheresis system

SUPPLIES AND REAGENTS

1. Haemonetics 603 TSPP component collection set
2. 600-mL transfer pack
3. 150-mL transfer pack
4. Two 500-mL ACD formula B (ACD-B)
5. 2 Haemonetics 8933 plasma exchange couplers
6. 500-mL 0.9 percent sodium chloride
7. Straight reinfusion set
8. Sampling site couplers
9. Supplies for venipuncture

PROCEDURE

SETUP FOR THE STANDARD LYMPHOCYTE COLLECTION

1. Press POWER ON. After the machine powers up, it displays "HAEMO-NETICS V-50" for approximately 2 seconds, indicating that the machine

is ready to run. It then displays "CHECK AIR DETECTOR" for 2 seconds. The machine then displays "SELECT PROTOCOL." At this time the four protocol panel lights (PPP, PRP, PEX, and COMP) flash, awaiting your selection.

2. Press LOAD. This opens all the valves simultaneously. The three valve buttons (valve 1, valve 2, and valve 3) on the control panel light to indicate the valves are open.

3. Install the disposable set according to standard operating procedure (SOP) for a 1-arm procedure and for a lymphocyte collection.

   Connect one 600-mL transfer pack to the port on valve 2 (platelet port). *Write patient's name and hospital number on the label of the collection bag.* Insert a sampling site coupler into this transfer pack for research sampling. Use ACD-B as the anticoagulant. DO NOT USE STARCH! Insert one surge line into air/plasma bag, thread through valve 1, and insert other end into surge line pigtail behind the blood pump. Insert second surge line into the other port on the air/plasma bag, thread through valve 6B, and insert the other end into the time saver return (TSR) port. Prepare a saline drip using a straight recipient set. Prime the machine according to SOP. Press LOAD to close all the valves.

PROGRAM FOR THE STANDARD LYMPHOCYTE COLLECTION

1. The display reads "SELECT PROTOCOL." Press COMP to select a component collection. The machine assumes preset valves for parameters such as centrifuge speed (4800 RPMs) and pump speed (20 mL/min).

2. As the V-50 prompts the different protocols, press NO until "LYMPHOCY? Y/N" shows on the screen. Press YES.
   "Time Saver? Y/N"
   Press YES.
   "Is weigher set? Y/N" Verify weigher is set at 0100 and the digital display reads 000. Press YES.
   "Volume Proc 4000? Y/N" Press YES.

3. The machine responds by displaying:
   "READY TS/L 0 50 0"

4. To select the standard collection protocol, press MOD. The machine prompts:
   "AC/BLOOD RATIO 08"
   Press MOD.
   "AUTOSURGE—YES"
   Press NO. The V-50 will then display "READY TS/L 000 0"

5. To modify the RBC vol press MOD. The V-50 will display: "AC Ratio 8: Press MOD RBC Vol 000." Enter 40 on the numeric key pad, and press ENTER.

6. The machine will then display "READY LYMPH 040 0"
   This indicates that the machine is ready to begin the collection process and that the optical mode is operational.

7. To modify the number of passes press the MOD key until "Number of

passes 08" is displayed. Enter the desired number of cycles (usually 15) by pressing the appropriate buttons on the numeric key pad and then pressing ENTER. This number can be readjusted during the procedure if needed.

8. Note that during the first pass the surge line will be primed with 30 mL of plasma and the TSR line will be primed with 20 mL of plasma. If using a therapeutic pump assist (TPA) line, be sure to remove this line from the blood pump when the surge lines are priming.

ALTERNATIVE PROCEDURE

The collection process will continue according to SOP for a 4-hour period, processing as many passes as possible. With the LY-TSP the reinfusion speed of each pass can be 150 mL per minute, or as the patient is able to tolerate.

1. After returning the last standard collection pass, stop reinfusion as air starts exiting the bowl, leaving tubing and monitor pouch primed.

2. Clamp off the whole blood/ACD line with a hemostat and open the saline to flush the needle. Adjust the saline drip to a "keep open" rate.

3. Obtain and record the weight of the product bag. Mix the product gently. Put a hemostat on the product bag line, unspike this from the collection port, and respike it into the surge port behind the blood pump. Unclamp the hemostat on this line, and clamp the whole blood line under the surge port.

4. Insert the end of the 150-mL prelabeled transfer pack into the platelet port on valve 2.

5. Place a hemostat on the ACD line and open the ACD pump handle.

6. Reprogram the RBC volume on the LY-TSP for 60.

7. Press FILL and increase the pump speed to 60 mL per minute to load the product into the bowl. Press CUFF button to deflate cuff on donor's arm. If using a TPA line, do not have it in the blood pump.

8. When all of the product is loaded into the bowl, press PUMP STOP. Rethread the ACD line and remove the hemostat from this line. Remove the hemostat from the tubing below the blood pump and close the red slide clamp on the surge port tubing.

9. Rethread the TPA line if using a catheter, or reinflate cuff on donor's arm if using a peripheral vein. Clamp off the saline, remove hemostat from the blood line, and push PUMP STOP to resume blood flow from the patient to finish filling the bowl with blood.

10. Start the stopwatch when blood starts entering the bowl. This will be used to determine how much additional blood you will add from the donor. When the blood pump speed drops to 20 mL per minute quickly note the time on the stopwatch and then clear and restart the stopwatch again. You will continue timing at 20 mL per minute until the collection is completed.

11. Manually open valve 2 when the platelet band is starting to exit the effluent line. When this line is turning red, the counter on the machine's display should start counting to 60 mL. If this counting should start early owing to high density in the line from a thick platelet band, note what the count was when the effluent line turned red and add this to your 60 mL for RBC volume to collect. *Be sure you are collecting 60 mL from the time the*

effluent line turned red. Remove the empty 600-mL bag and reinsert surge line (valve 1) into surge port by blood pump.

12. When the collection is finished the machine will automatically advance to return. While the bowl is emptying strip the product bag tubing, verify that the labeling on the bag is correct, double hemoclip the product bag tubing leaving only a short segment, and remove the product from the machine.

13. When all the blood is returned to the patient, discontinue according to SOP.

14. Obtain and record the weight of the product bag. Label bag and all specimens from this bag as post-60. Also label each tube with patient's name, hospital number, date, time, and bag weight. Obtain the following samples:

    - 1.0 mL for bone marrow culture
    - 0.5 mL for tissue typing

ANTICIPATED RESULTS	Approximately 6.5 to 8×10^8 mononuclear cells per kg body weight are collected over a 9-day period prior to transplant.
NOTES	1. ACD-A was used as the anticoagulant if the patient has a high precollection platelet count or if the product appeared to contain clumps of cells.
	2. If peripheral veins were inadequate, a central venous catheter was inserted.
	3. The volume of blood processed during each 4-hour collection was approximately 7 L.
AUTHORS	Lynda Thoreen, R.N. Anne Kessinger, M.D. American Red Cross University of Nebraska Midwest Region Medical Center Omaha, NE 68105 Omaha, NE 68198
REFERENCE	1. Haemonetics V-50 Standard Operating Procedure Manual, Braintree, MA, 1991.

PROCESSING

PROCESSING OF BLOOD STEM CELLS

DESCRIPTION	Peripheral blood stem cells collected by apheresis are processed:

1. To reduce the volume of cells to be cryopreserved
2. To remove the majority of red cells, thus reducing the amount of free hemoglobin and red cell stroma in the post-thaw infusion product
3. To remove platelets and thus reduce the risk of clumping when the final product is thawed

TIME FOR PROCEDURE	Approximately 2 hours

SUMMARY OF PROCEDURE

1. Peripheral blood cells collected by apheresis are delivered to the laboratory.
2. The mononuclear cell fraction is isolated using density gradient centrifugation.
3. Plasma and mononuclear cells are collected.
4. Mononuclear cells are washed to reduce platelet contamination.

EQUIPMENT	Class II biologic safety cabinet (BH series, Gelman Sciences, MI)

SUPPLIES AND REAGENTS

1. 50-mL sterile, disposable, graduated conical centrifuge tubes (Becton Dickinson, NJ)
2. Hank's balanced salt solution (HBSS) supplied as powder (Flow Laboratories, Australia)
3. Lymphoprep (Nycomed, Norway)
4. Sterile, individually wrapped, mixing cannulae (Indoplas, Cat. No. 500.11.012, Australia)
5. Sterile disposable 30-mL syringes (Terumo, Japan)
6. 40-cm single-use link sets (Tuta, Cat. No. 76-026, Australia)
7. Sterile, individually wrapped, 1-mL transfer pipettes (Samco, USA)

PROCEDURE

1. Carry out all processing aseptically in a biologic safety cabinet.
2. Collect peripheral blood stem cells by apheresis, as described in "Apheresis for blood stem cell collection," then deliver to the laboratory in a 200-ml pack.
3. Add 15-mL HBSS to each of ten 50-mL sterile centrifuge tubes.
4. Using a link set and clamp, add 20 mL of the cell suspension from the pack to each of the 50-mL tubes, ensuring adequate mixing.
5. Underlay the diluted cell suspension with 15 mL of Lymphoprep.
6. Centrifuge at 400g for 30 minutes at room temperature without braking.
7. Collect 10 mL of diluted plasma from above the interface in each tube, for a final volume of 100 mL. Centrifuge plasma at 600g for 10 minutes to remove platelets. Keep plasma on ice until required.

8. Remove remaining supernatant to within 2 cm of interface in each tube.

9. Using a sterile plastic transfer pipette, collect mononuclear cells from each interface.

10. Pool into five 50-mL tubes and add HBSS to bring the volume of each to 50 mL. Centrifuge at $400g$ for 10 minutes without braking.

11. Remove 35 to 40 mL of supernatant and discard. Resuspend cells and add HBSS to bring volume to 50 mL. Centrifuge at $400g$ for 10 minutes without braking.

12. Repeat step 11. Remove 35 to 40 mL of supernatant and discard. Resuspend cells, and pool into a weighed 50-mL tube. Adjust volume to approximately 50 mL with HBSS, and weigh to measure the volume of the cell suspension.

13. Keep on ice for cryopreservation procedure.

ANTICIPATED RESULTS	1. The procedure should yield at least 90 to 95 percent of the starting mononuclear cells with at least an 80 percent reduction in platelet numbers. The cell product should comprise 20 to 80 $\times$ 10^8 cells, of which approximately 90 percent are mononuclear cells.
	2. Plasma collected by this procedure is effectively diluted 1:2 with HBSS and is platelet depleted.

NOTES	1. It is essential that all centrifugation procedures be performed without braking, to maximize platelet removal.
	2. The procedure may be shortened by omitting one washing step; however, in this case the washing volume should be increased.
	3. A buffy coat cell suspension prepared from the apheresis product may be cryopreserved. However, the storage volume is markedly increased, and the thawed product contains a large amount of free hemoglobin and red cell stroma.

AUTHORS

Pamela G. Dyson, B.Sc. (Hons)
Leukaemia Research Unit
Institute of Medical and Veterinary
  Science
Adelaide, South Australia 5000

David N. Haylock, B.App.Sc.
Leukaemia Research Unit
Department of Haematology
Institute of Medical and Veterinary
  Science
Adelaide, South Australia 5000

Luen Bik To, M.D., M.B.B.S.
Leukaemia Research Unit
Institute of Medical and Veterinary
  Science
Adelaide, South Australia 5000

REFERENCES

1. To, LB, et al: High levels of circulating haemopoietic stem cells in very early remission from acute non-lymphoblastic leukaemia and their collection and cryopreservation. Br J Haematol 58:399, 1984.

2. To, LB, et al: The optimisation of collection of peripheral blood stem cells for autotransplantation in acute myeloid leukaemia. Bone Marrow Transplant 4:41, 1989.

PROCESSING OF PERIPHERAL BLOOD MONONUCLEAR CELLS (PBMCs)

DESCRIPTION	Peripheral stem cell concentrate, after autologous apheresis procedure, is consolidated and cryopreserved in the laboratory.
TIME FOR PROCEDURE	Approximately 2 hours from receiving the product to storing it in the freezer
SUMMARY OF PROCEDURE	The PBMC product is spun down in blood bag cup and extra clear plasma is removed by a plasma extractor. The cell pellet is resuspended in autologous plasma and cryopreserved dimethyl sulfoxide (DMSO) at a final concentration of 10 percent.

EQUIPMENT

1. Blood bag centrifuge
2. Plasma extractor
3. 60-mL disposable sterile syringes
4. 14-gauge cannulas

SUPPLIES AND REAGENTS

1. Heparin sodium, preservative-free; 1000 units per mL, 5-mL bottle
2. Cryoserve DMSO, CRS-70, Research Industries
3. ^{199}Tc, GIBCO

PROCEDURE

1. Prepare ^{199}Tc/DMSO solution beforehand, and store on ice or in the refrigerator:
   A. For each 100-mL freezer bag, one 50-mL tube is prepared with the following:
      (1) 20.4 mL TC-199
      (2) 10.2 mL DMSO
   B. Use 30 mL of this mixture at the freezing step.

2. Mononuclear cell (MNC) concentrate should have had 5000 units of heparin added in the bag before collection. Mix the product and take a 0.1-mL specimen with a tuberculin syringe from the coupler. Do a cell count.

3. Fit the product into a blood bag cup, with the top seam parallel to the cup flats.

4. Balance the loaded cup with a dummy bag and cup.

5. Centrifuge at $400g$ for 15 minutes with no brake at room temperature.

6. Carefully remove the product from the cup, and hook the bag onto the plasma extractor.

7. Gently release the plasma extractor handle.

8. Swab the coupler site with povidine-iodine and connect a 600-mL transfer pack with a 16-gauge needle.

9. Plasma will start flowing into the transfer pack. With a pair of hemostats handy, stop the flow when approximately 50 mL is left.

10. Resuspend cells in remaining autologous plasma; examine any clumps by gently massaging the bag.

11. Under the sterile hood, aspirate the product with a 60-mL syringe and a cannula; transfer into a freezer bag.

12. Release the hemostat and drain plasma into the product bag to rinse out the residual cells; be conservative about the volume.

13. Measure with the syringe to make a total of 70-mL cell suspension in the freezer bag. Mix well, and take a 0.2-mL sample sterilely for cell count, percentage MNC, and viability test.

14. Leave the freezer bag on wet ice or in the refrigerator for 10 minutes.

15. Precool the freezing chamber to 4°C.

16. Add 30 mL TC-199/DMSO mixture to each bag with agitation. Reserve 0.5 mL for one reference vial for post-thaw CFU-GM culture.

17. Start freezing with no delay.

ANTICIPATED RESULTS

Each 100-mL freezer bag can safely cryopreserve 10×10^9 nucleated cells.

NOTE

Before adding TC-199/DMSO solution, make sure everything is ready to go to minimize time delay for freezing:

- A bag holder cassette should be properly labeled, prechilled in the refrigerator.
- One reference vial should be labeled and sitting on ice bath with cap open, under the sterile hood.
- When prefreezer specimen is heavily contaminated with mature granulocytes, 20 units of DNAse can be added before freezing.

AUTHOR

Jean T. Yao, M.S., S.B.B.(ASCP)
Blood Bank
Methodist Medical Center
221 N.E. Glen Oak Ave.
Peoria, IL 61636

BONE MARROW COMPONENT PROCESSING | 6

Commentary by THOMAS R. SPITZER

Critical to the success of bone marrow transplantation is the infusion of marrow containing adequate lymphohematopoietic progenitor cells to ensure engraftment and adequate immune reconstitution. Although understanding of stem cell biology has increased dramatically in recent years, collection of marrow for transplantation purposes and knowledge of components necessary to ensure engraftment remain relatively crude. Goals for autologous and allogeneic transplantation, moreover, are not identical. In autologous transplantation, avoidance of contamination with tumor cells and infusion of an adequate number of viable lymphohematopoietic stem cells remain the primary objectives. In the setting of allogeneic transplantation, engraftment and immune reconstitution also are primary goals, but infusion of tumor cells is not an issue. Avoidance of clinically significant graft-versus-host (GVH) disease (while preserving a graft-versus-tumor effect), however, is of paramount importance to the long-term success following transplantation.

95

With these goals in mind, preparation of marrow for infusion usually involves separation of the various components both for avoidance of toxic effects (e.g., due to ABO incompatibility) and for isolation of a relatively pure mononuclear cell fraction. Although the morphologic and immunologic characterization of the human pluripotential stem cell has not been fully defined, cells capable of restoring trilineage hematopoiesis are known to reside in the mononuclear cell fraction of the marrow.[1] This fraction is known to contain cells capable of giving rise to myeloid/monocyte/macrophage (CFU-GM), erythroid (CFU-E, BFU-E) and mixed erythroid, myeloid, and megakaryocytic (CFU-GEMM) colonies in culture, and to express very early hematopoietic surface antigens such as CD34 or CD33 or both.[1-3] Isolation of this fraction has obvious advantages: (1) volume reduction, which minimizes the quantities of costly reagents such as monoclonal antibodies or chemotherapeutic agents used for in vitro treatment of the marrow and reduces toxic complications of transplantation such as dimethyl sulfoxide (DMSO) toxicity and volume overload, and (2) removal of unwanted, potentially stem cell–toxic components such as neutrophils.[3]

What constitutes the minimal marrow components necessary to ensure lymphohematopoietic engraftment is yet to be defined. Extrapolation of data from animal models has suggested that a minimum of 1×10^8 nucleated marrow cells per kg is necessary to ensure engraftment following autologous transplantation.[4] In allogeneic transplantation 3×10^8 nucleated cells per kg are generally desired, based on a series from the Fred Hutchinson Cancer Center showing an enhanced risk of engraftment failure in patients with aplastic anemia transplanted with a lesser cell number.[5] Nonetheless, successful engraftment has commonly been observed with significantly smaller cell numbers as evidenced by the range of infused cell numbers reported in most major series. Moreover, more recent series using relatively pure mononuclear cell preparations have reported uniformly successful engraftment with infused cell numbers significantly less (0.2 to 1.2×10^8 cells per kg) than previously accepted minimum cell numbers.[6]

Use of in vitro colony growth data has also been advocated by some as a means to predict adequacy of (and time to) engraftment.[7-9] Correlation with engraftment data has not been substantiated in other series, however, and at present no specific in vitro culture data are universally accepted as predictors of engraftment.[10,11] Moreover, following in vitro purging of marrow with drugs such as 4-hydroperoxycyclophosphamide, adequate trilineage engraftment may still be established even when the marrow fails to grow viable myeloid colonies in culture.

Successful engraftment has also occurred following infusion of more purified populations of progenitor cells obtained by either positive or negative selection techniques. Recently, autologous transplants using relatively pure CD34-positive hematopoietic progenitor cells (obtained by positive-selection monoclonal antibody–purging methods) have been associated with adequate engraftment following myeloablative conditioning therapy and infusion of the CD34-positive progenitors.[12] T cells or B cells may also be removed from autologous marrow in cases of T- or B-cell lymphoproliferative malignancies with adequate myeloid engraftment in most cases (although protracted cell-mediated immune deficiencies have been observed, particularly in the case of T-depleted autografts).[13,14] Removal of T cells from allogeneic marrow in an attempt to prevent GVH disease, however, results in a significantly increased risk of engraftment failure.[15] It is unclear, however, if these engraftment difficulties result from loss of lymphohematopoietic stem cells during processing or whether T cells (via lymphokines or hematopoietic growth factors or both) are necessary for optimal allogeneic engraftment.

In this chapter, three sections are devoted to descriptions of the methods used to separate the various marrow components. Investigators from the University of British Columbia present a method of plasma removal from bone marrow in the first section. In addition to volume reduction, plasma removal is of importance in removing alloantibodies before allogeneic transplantation. This is a particular concern in situations of minor ABO incompatibility between donor and patient because infusion of large quantities of isoagglutinins might induce clinically significant hemolysis.[16]

In the next section, multiple methods of preparing a buffy coat fraction are described. Historically, preparation of a buffy coat fraction with minimal loss of white cells has constituted the primary objective of marrow processing. Removal of plasma was important for the aforementioned reasons, whereas reduction in the number of red blood cells was essential in the setting of a major ABO-incompatible allogeneic marrow transplant. Contained in the white cell fraction, moreover, is the pluripotential stem cell compartment (and perhaps other components such as T cells) necessary for lymphohematopoietic engraftment. Although effective, manual methods are, by nature of the increased manipulation and exposure to the environment, more likely to result in bacterial contamination of the marrow. Also problematic with the manual buffy coat preparation is the inclusion of unwanted components including neutrophils and platelets. Although less likely to become contaminated, buffy coat fractions prepared using automated methods still contain undesirably high quantities of neutrophils and platelets. As described, with either manual or automated methods, recovery of nucleated cells is expected to be in excess of 75 percent of preprocessed cell numbers.

Sedimentation techniques for red blood cell removal are also described and offer alternative methods of buffy coat preparation. Although sedimentation techniques are highly efficient methods of removing red cells, newer automated techniques have apparent advantages in terms of preparation of more pure populations of mononuclear cells without subsequently exposing patients to reagents like hydroxyethyl starch.

Finally, methods of isolating a relatively pure mononuclear cell fraction have recently become an important goal in marrow processing laboratories. Multiple separation methods using either manual or automated density gradient separation techniques or automated non–density gradient separation (via the Fenwal CS3000 cell separator) are currently available. Both manual and automated methods have produced marrow fractions with minimal red cell and plasma contamination while preserving a high percentage of preprocessed mononuclear cells. Manual and some automated techniques have used density gradient reagents such as Ficoll-Hypaque; although mononuclear cell yields have generally been in excess of 50 percent of original cell numbers, concern has been raised about potential cell injury from these reagents based on the demonstration of a significant reduction in tritiated thymidine incorporation and loss of lymphocyte viability when cultured with Ficoll-Hypaque.[17] These reagents, moreover, have not been approved, nor were they even originally intended for clinical use.

Preliminary data have demonstrated that recovery of mononuclear cells and CFU-GM following automated methods of mononuclear cell isolation have ranged from 60 to 100 percent and 56 to 105 percent, respectively, whereas efficiency of red blood cell depletion has exceeded 92 percent.[3,5,18–21] Use of the Fenwal CS3000 cell separator, as described by Ellen Areman, Georgetown University Hospital, has the potential advantage of avoidance of potentially cytotoxic density gradient reagents while preserving a closed, sterile system. Mean mononuclear cell recovery and red cell depletion efficiencies of 53 percent and 95 percent, respectively, are comparable to automated methods using density gradient methods. Of 26 patients transplanted with CS3000-prepared marrow (containing a mean of $0.7 \pm 0.5 \times 10^8$ cells per kg), all have shown stable trilineage engraftment.[6]

In summary, marrow component processing has made substantial progress over recent years, as newer techniques to isolate mononuclear cell fractions without exposure to potentially toxic chemical reagents have been developed. Furthermore, given the ability to separate components within the mononuclear fraction successfully and the preliminary evidence showing that certain progenitors (such as CD34 antigen–expressing cells) can be effective in obtaining autologous engraftment whereas others (CD8 antigen–bearing cells) can be removed from allogeneic marrow with apparent attenuation of GVH disease,[22] the ultimate goals in marrow processing include preparation of a pure population of progenitor cells either free of tumor (for autologous transplantation) or with retention of graft-versus-leukemia– but not GVH disease–producing effects (for allogeneic transplantation). Of course, such marrow refinement should be associated with a minimum degree of manipulation (in terms of both physical manipulation and exposure to potentially stem cell toxic chemicals) and ideally be as free of contaminating plasma and red cells as possible. Ultimately, preparation of a small-volume stem cell–pure product will eliminate most of the risks of marrow infusion and of contamination of the marrow, while still preserving adequate and early lymphohematopoietic engraftment.

REFERENCES

1. Ekert, H, et al: Marrow function reconstitution by fraction 3 of percoll-density-gradient-separated cells. Transplantation 42:58, 1986.
2. Gilmore, MJ, et al: A technique for rapid isolation of bone marrow mononuclear cells using Ficoll, Metrizoate and the IBM 2991 blood cell processor. Br J Haematol 50:619, 1982.
3. Faradji, A, et al: Separation of mononuclear bone marrow cells using the Cobe 2997 blood cell separator. Vox Sang 55:133, 1988.
4. Vriesendorp, HM and van Bekkum, DW: Role of total body irradiation in conditioning for bone marrow transplantation. In Thierfelder, S, Rodt, HV, and Kolb, HJ (eds): Immunobiology of Bone Marrow Transplantation. Springer-Verlag, Heidelberg/New York, 1980, p 348.
5. Storb, R, Prentice, RL, and Thomas, ED: An analysis of factors associated with graft rejection. N Engl J Med 296:61, 1977.
6. Areman, EM, et al: Automated processing of human bone marrow results in a purified population of mononuclear cells capable of achieving engraftment following transplantation. Transfusion (in press)1991.
7. Spitzer, G, et al: The myeloid progenitor cell—its value in predicting hematopoietic recovery after autologous bone marrow transplantation. Blood 55:317, 1980.
8. Rowley, SD, et al: CFU-GM content of bone marrow graft correlates with time to hematologic reconstitution following autologous bone marrow transplantation with 4-hydroperoxycyclophosphamide-purged bone marrow. Blood 70:271, 1987.
9. Arnold, R, et al: Hemopoietic reconstitution after bone marrow transplantation. Exp Hematol 14:271, 1986.

10. Atkinson, K, et al: Lack of correlation between nucleated cell dose, marrow CFU-GM dose or marrow CFU-E dose and the rate of HLA identical sibling marrow engraftment. Br J Haematol 60:245, 1985.

11. Torres, A, et al: No influence of number of donor CFU-GM on granulocyte recovery in bone marrow transplantation for acute leukemia. Blut 50:89, 1985.

12. Berenson, RJ, et al: Stem cell selection—clinical experience. In Gross, SR and Gee, A (eds): Bone Marrow Purging and Processing. Proceedings of the Second International Symposium on Bone Marrow Purging and Processing. Progress in Clinical and Biological Research. Wiley-Liss, New York, 1990, p 403.

13. Anderson, KC, et al: Hematologic engraftment and immune reconstitution post-transplant with anti-B1 purged autologous bone marrow. Blood 69:597, 1987.

14. Anderson, KC, et al: T-cell depleted autologous bone marrow transplantation therapy: analysis of immune deficiency and late complications. Blood 76:235, 1990.

15. Mitsuyasu, RT, et al: Treatment of donor bone marrow with monoclonal anti-T-cell antibody and complement for the prevention of graft-versus-host disease. Ann Intern Med 105:20, 1986.

16. Lasky, LC, et al: Hemotherapy in patients undergoing blood group incompatible bone marrow transplantation. Transfusion 23:277, 1983.

17. Kurnick, JT, et al: A rapid method for the separation of functional lymphoid cell populations of human and animal origin on PVP-silica (Percoll) density gradients. Scand J Immunol 10:563, 1979.

18. Humblet, Y, et al: Concentration of bone marrow progenitor cells by separation on a percoll gradient using the Haemonetics model 30. Bone Marrow Transplant 3:63, 1988.

19. English, D, et al: Semiautomated processing of bone marrow grafts for transplantation. Transfusion 29:12, 1989.

20. Gilmore, MJ, et al: A technique for rapid isolation of bone marrow mononuclear cells using Ficoll-Metrizoate and the IBM 2991 blood cell processor. Br J Haematol 50:619, 1982.

21. Jin, N, et al: Preparation of red-blood cell-depleted marrow for ABO-incompatible marrow transplantation by density-gradient separation using the IBM 2991 blood cell processor. Exp Hematol 15:93, 1987.

22. Champlin, R, et al: Selective depletion of CD8$^+$ T lymphocytes for prevention of graft-versus-host disease after allogeneic bone marrow transplantation. Blood 76:418, 1990.

PLASMA REMOVAL FROM BONE MARROW

DESCRIPTION	When a bone marrow transplant involves minor ABO incompatibility, ABO isoagglutinins will be present in the bone marrow supernatant. Because transfusion of a large volume of ABO-incompatible plasma can cause hemolysis of recipient erythrocytes, it may be desirable to remove the plasma from the bone marrow prior to transplantation. The method described here involves centrifuging the bone marrow and removing the plasma using a plasma extractor.
TIME FOR PROCEDURE	Approximately 20 minutes to process 500 mL bone marrow
SUMMARY OF PROCEDURE	1. Harvested bone marrow is delivered as soon as possible to the processing laboratory. 2. Marrow is centrifuged in an upright position for 10 minutes at 2000g at 22°C. 3. Plasma is removed into a transfer pack using a plasma extractor.
EQUIPMENT	1. Plasma extractor (Fenwal Division, Baxter Healthcare) 2. Laminar flow hood
SUPPLIES AND REAGENTS	Two transfer packs (300-mL or 600-mL, depending on the volume of the bone marrow)

PROCEDURE	1. CENTRIFUGATION OF MARROW
	  A. If necessary, transfer the marrow to an appropriately sized transfer pack to allow good separation of the red cells and plasma.
	  B. Centrifuge the marrow in an upright position for 10 minutes at 2000g at 22°C.
	2. REMOVAL OF PLASMA
	  A. Place the marrow bag on the plasma extractor in a laminar flow hood. Attach a transfer pack to one port of the marrow bag.
	  B. Express off all but 2 cm of plasma into the transfer pack.

ANTICIPATED RESULTS	This procedure should decrease the volume of ABO-incompatible plasma by 70 to 75 percent. The original marrow volume should be decreased by 55 percent. The loss of nucleated cells should be less than 5 percent.
NOTE	Sampling for nucleated cell counts, cell cultures, or sterilities will vary with each processing laboratory.

AUTHORS

Carol Stanley, A.R.T.
British Columbia Children's
  Hospital
Vancouver, B.C.
Canada

Sharon Herd, A.R.T.
British Columbia Children's
  Hospital
Vancouver, B.C.
Canada

L. D. Wadsworth, M.B., FRCP(C),
  FRCPath
British Columbia Children's
  Hospital
Vancouver, B.C.
Canada

BUFFY COAT CONCENTRATION/BUFFY COAT PREPARATION

Manual Techniques

MANUAL BUFFY COAT SEPARATION USING CENTRIFUGE TUBES

DESCRIPTION	This procedure describes the separation and concentration of the buffy coat from harvested bone marrow by a manual technique using test tubes and centrifugation. This technique is useful for the preparation of marrow for cryopreservation.
TIME FOR PROCEDURE	Approximately 3 to 5 hours to process 500 to 1500 mL
SUMMARY OF PROCEDURE	1. Harvested bone marrow is delivered to the bone marrow processing laboratory in one or more 600-mL transfer bags.
	2. The marrow is centrifuged in the transfer bags at $4333g$ for 10 minutes at 20 to 24°C.
	3. The centrifuged marrow is expressed from the transfer bags to conical tubes to be divided into four separate pools: fat, plasma, buffy coat, and red cells.
	4. The marrow is centrifuged in the conical tubes to further separate and concentrate the buffy coat.
EQUIPMENT	1. Laminar flow hood
	2. Centrifuge and tube holders for 50 mL conical tubes
	3. Pipet Aid, vacuum-pressure
SUPPLIES AND REAGENTS	1. Disposable serologic pipettes (sterile): 25 mL, 10 mL, 2 mL
	2. Sterile polypropylene conical tubes with caps: 250 mL, 50 mL
	3. Plasma transfer sets with coupler
	4. 600-mL transfer bags with coupler
PROCEDURE	1. PREPROCESSING TESTS AND CENTRIFUGATION OF MARROW

A. Using standard procedures, collect harvested bone marrow in the operating room, and place into 600-mL plastic transfer bags. The marrow bags, labeled with donor name and hospital number, are delivered to the bone marrow processing laboratory for separation and concentration of the marrow buffy coat.

(1) Remove samples of bone marrow for nucleated cell count and other appropriate tests.

(2) Seal each bag of bone marrow and weigh to determine marrow volume.

B. Centrifuge the 600-mL marrow bags, port side up, at $4333g$ for 10 minutes at 20 to 24°C.

2. **TRANSFER OF MARROW FROM BAGS TO TEST TUBES**
   A. Place centrifuged bag on a plasma expresser. Insert one coupler of a transfer set into one port of the marrow bag. Release plasma expresser. Slowly transfer fat layer to 50-mL tubes. Close roller clamp on transfer set. Keep coupler sterile for later use.
   B. Insert coupler from an empty transfer bag into the free port of the marrow bag. Transfer fat-free plasma into this transfer bag, leaving ⅛ inch plasma, without disturbing buffy coat. Temporarily clamp the tubing between the primary marrow bag and the plasma transfer bag.
   C. Using the transfer set tubing attached to the primary marrow bag (see step 2A), express concentrated buffy coat into a 250-mL sterile conical tube. Do not allow the red cell layer to be expressed into the buffy coat tube.
   D. Using the same transfer set tubing (see step 2C), express the red cell layer into 50-mL sterile tubes. Close roller clamp on transfer tubing. Keep coupler sterile for later use.
   E. To rinse primary marrow bag, return plasma from the transfer bag (see step 2B) to the primary marrow bag. Seal tubing between bags. Cut tubing and discard empty secondary transfer bag.
   F. Using the transfer set attached to the primary marrow bag, aliquot plasma (see step 2E) into 50-mL sterile conical tubes.

3. **CONCENTRATION OF BUFFY COAT IN CONICAL TUBES**
   A. Centrifuge red cell and plasma tubes at $900g$ for 15 minutes at 20 to 24°C.
   B. Pool plasma
      (1) With a 25-mL sterile pipette, remove extra plasma (leave ¼ inch plasma) from tubes without disturbing the buffy coat layer and pool into 250-mL sterile conical tubes labeled "pooled plasma."
      (2) Transfer 25 mL of pooled plasma to a 50-mL sterile conical tube. Use this plasma to rinse pipettes used in pooling the buffy coat.
   C. Pool buffy coat
      (1) Remove the buffy coat from each 50-mL tube using a sterile pipette and add to the buffy coat obtained directly from the primary marrow bag (step 2C). Rinse the pipette with the "rinse" plasma before discarding pipette.
      (2) Pool remaining red cells into 50-mL sterile conical tubes.
   D. Recentrifuge red cell tubes at $900g$ for 15 minutes at 20 to 24°C. Pipette and add remaining buffy coat to buffy coat tube (see step 2C). Rinse the pipette with the "rinse" plasma before discarding.
   E. Centrifuge the "rinse" plasma at $900g$ for 10 minutes at 20 to 24° C.
      (1) Add plasma to pooled plasma.
      (2) Transfer cell button to pooled buffy coat.
   F. Remove a sample from the pooled buffy coat for nucleated cell count and other appropriate tests.
   G. Calculate the yield of nucleated cells. The yield should be approximately 1 to 3×10^8 cells per kg body weight of recipient. If the yield is not sufficient, recentrifuge the marrow red cells and repeat steps 3D through 3G.
   H. The nucleated cell count should be less than 200×10^6 per mL for

freezing. If the nucleated cell count is greater than or equal to 200×10^6 per mL, dilute pooled buffy coat with pooled autologous plasma. The concentrated marrow buffy coat is now ready to be cryopreserved.

ANTICIPATED RESULTS	The procedure should yield at least 1 to 3×10^8 cells per kg body weight of recipient, or at least 75 percent of the initial total nucleated cell count.
NOTE	All work for the entire procedure is performed in a laminar flow hood using sterile technique to prepare marrow for cryopreservation.

AUTHORS

Marita G. Hill, M.T.(ASCP), S.B.B.
University of Kentucky Medical
   Center
Lexington, KY 40536

Vickie M. Robertson, M.T.(ASCP),
   S.B.B.
University of Kentucky Medical
   Center
Lexington, KY 40536

Larry G. Dickson, M.D.
Clinical Laboratory
University of Kentucky Medical
   Center
Lexington, KY 40536

REFERENCES

1. Thomas, E and Storb, R: Technique for human marrow grafting. Blood 36:507, 1970.
2. Appelbaum, F, et al: Successful engraftment of cryopreserved autologous bone marrow in patients with malignant lymphoma. Blood 52:85, 1978.

MANUAL BUFFY COAT SEPARATION USING TRANSFER BAGS

DESCRIPTION	A bone marrow harvest results in the collection of marrow and peripheral blood cells in a total volume of as much as 2000 mL. It is frequently desirable to concentrate the marrow, both in the autologous setting as a means of reducing the volume of marrow to be cryopreserved and in the allogeneic setting as a means of red blood cell depletion in instances of ABO incompatibility. The manual procedure is necessary (1) when no automated equipment is available or (2) when the marrow volume is too small for automated processing, or both.

TIME FOR PROCEDURE	From 60 to 90 minutes

SUMMARY OF PROCEDURE	1. Marrow is distributed into four bags of a quadruple transfer pack and centrifuged.
	2. Buffy coat is removed into 150-mL transfer bags.
	3. Marrow and plasma are pooled and recentrifuged.
	4. Buffy coat is again removed.
	5. Individual buffy coat collections are pooled.

EQUIPMENT	1. Centrifuge with blood bag cups
	2. Plasma expressor
	3. Electric heat sealer
	4. Tube stripper
	5. Hemostats
	6. Sterile Connecting Device (SCD) (SteriCell, Terumo Medical Corp., Elkton, MD 21921) (optional)

SUPPLIES AND REAGENTS	1. Quadruple transfer pack (Fenwal No. 4R2958)
	2. 150-mL transfer packs (Fenwal No. 4R2001)
	3. 600-mL transfer packs with coupler (Fenwal No. 4R2023)
	4. 600-mL transfer packs with needle adaptor (Fenwal No. 4R2024)
	5. Sampling site couplers
	6. Extension set—51 cm (Travenol No. 2C0065)
	7. 60-mL syringes
	8. 16-gauge needles
	9. Three-way sterile disposable stopcock
	10. Plasma transfer set with coupler and needle adapter
	11. Hand sealer clips

PROCEDURE	1. When the marrow arrives from the operating room: it is weighed and aliquots removed for cell count, hematocrit, and other tests as required.
	2. Divide the marrow as evenly as possible into the four bags of the quadruple transfer pack. Strip the tubing and heat seal each bag.
	3. Centrifuge the four bags at 3500g for 10 minutes at 20°C with the brake on.

4. After centrifugation: place one bag in the plasma expressor.
    - Attach a 150-mL transfer pack clamped with a hemostat to the center port of the marrow bag.
    - Attach a 600-mL transfer pack clamped with a hemostat to the second port.

5. Release the press while stretching the marrow bag, being careful not to disturb the cell layers.

6. Open the hemostat to the 600-mL transfer pack and remove the plasma to approximately 2 cm of the cell layer. Temporarily clamp the tubing.

7. Open the hemostat to the 150-mL transfer pack. Gently squeeze the marrow bag to express the buffy coat. When all of the buffy coat appears to have been collected, seal the tubing.

8. Allow the separated plasma to flow back into the marrow bag. Mix thoroughly and transfer the suspension back to the plasma transfer bag so that the marrow is in a bag with two unused ports.

9. Repeat steps 4 through 8 with the remaining marrow bags.

10. Repeat steps 3 through 7 with the residual cells.

11. Strip the tubing to the 150-mL buffy coat transfer packs and heat seal. Place a sampling site coupler in the port of each bag.

12. To the three ports of a three-way stopcock attach:
    - 60-mL syringe
    - Extension tubing with 16-gauge needle attached
    - Needle adapter end of plasma transfer set

13. Spike an empty 600-mL transfer pack with other end of transfer set. With lever of stopcock pointing toward empty transfer pack, draw one buffy coat into the syringe. Turn lever toward 150-mL bag and expel contents of syringe into 600-mL bag. Repeat until all buffy coats have been pooled.

14. Label product appropriately.

15. Mix well and remove samples for cell count, cultures, and other tests as required.

ALTERNATIVE PROCEDURE

1. Divide the marrow as evenly as possible into the four bags of the quadruple transfer pack. Strip the tubing and heat-seal 8 to 10 inches from bag.

2. Using the Sterile Connecting Device (SCD) attach a 600-mL and a 150-mL transfer bag to each 600-mL bag of marrow. Use two hand sealer clips to close off tubing to each transfer bag, but *do not* squeeze the clips.

3. Centrifuge the four bags at 3500g for 10 minutes at 20°C with the brake on.

4. After centrifugation, place one bag in the plasma expressor.

5. Release the press while stretching the marrow bag, being careful not to disturb the cell layers.

6. Remove the clips from the 600-mL transfer pack and remove the plasma to approximately 2 cm of the cell layer. Temporarily clamp the tubing.

7. Remove the clips to the 150-mL transfer pack. Gently squeeze the marrow bag to express the buffy coat. When all of the buffy coat appears to have been collected, seal the tubing 6 to 8 inches from bag.

8. Allow the separated plasma to flow back into the marrow bag. Use hand sealer clips to close off 600-mL transfer pack, but *do not* squeeze the clips.

9. Repeat steps 6 through 9 with the remaining marrow bags.

10. Repeat steps 5 and 6 with the residual cells.

11. Attach a 150-mL transfer pack (with tubing clamped by hemostat) to one port of the 600-mL marrow bag.

12. Release the press while stretching the marrow bag, being careful not to disturb the cell layers.

13. Remove the clips from the 600-mL transfer pack and remove the plasma to approximately 2 cm of the cell layer. Heat seal the tubing.

14. Open the hemostat to the 150-mL transfer pack. Gently squeeze the marrow bag to express the buffy coat. When all of the buffy coat appears to have been collected, seal the tubing 6 to 8 inches from bag.

15. Connect empty 600-mL transfer pack with needle adapter to three-way stopcock. Attach extension set to opposite port of stopcock. Seal off free end of extension set.

16. Using SCD, connect eight buffy coat bags to extension tubing.

17. Open stopcock to buffy coat bags and draw up about 50 mL of buffy coat. Open stopcock toward empty transfer pack and expel contents of syringe. Repeat until entire buffy coat has been transferred to transfer bag.

18. Label product appropriately.

19. Mix well and remove samples for cell count, cultures, and other tests as required.

ANTICIPATED RESULT	At least 70 percent of the original nucleated cells should be recovered.
AUTHOR	Ellen M. Areman, M.L.T., S.B.B.(ASCP) Bone Marrow Processing Laboratory Division of Transfusion Medicine Georgetown University Hospital Washington, D.C. 20007
REFERENCE	1. Davis, J: Cell Processing Laboratory, Johns Hopkins Oncology Center, Baltimore, MD. (Personal communication.)

Automated Techniques

PROCESSING OF ABO-INCOMPATIBLE BONE MARROW WITH THE COBE 2991

DESCRIPTION	Depletion of ABO-incompatible red cells from bone marrow must be done before infusion to avoid hemolytic transfusion reaction. This method accomplishes efficient and almost complete removal of incompatible red cells allowing a good recovery of progenitor cells necessary for engraftment.
TIME FOR PROCEDURE	Approximately 2.5 hours for 1500 mL of bone marrow.
SUMMARY OF PROCEDURE	1. Harvested bone marrow containing approximately 4 to 6 $\times$ 10^8 nucleated cells per kg is taken to the blood bank in a 2-L transfer bag.
	2. Marrow is centrifuged on a COBE 2991 Blood Cell Processor. The buffy coat portion and part of the red cells are removed, containing about 85 percent of the nucleated cells.
	3. A unit of washed irradiated group O red cells is added to the buffy coat.
	4. This marrow group O red cell mixture is reprocessed on the COBE 2991, again removing the buffy coat and some red cells containing 85 percent of the nucleated cells. The group O red cells dilute the donor's remaining red cells. Therefore, very few of the donor's group A or B red cells remain in the final product.
	5. The marrow is resuspended in 5 percent human serum albumin and transfused.
EQUIPMENT	1. COBE 2991 Blood Cell Processor, COBE Laboratories
	2. Automated Cell Counter
SUPPLIES AND REAGENTS	1. 4 COBE blood cell processing kits
	2. 1000-mL bag 0.9 percent sodium chloride
	3. Three 1000-mL transfer bags
	4. Three 600-mL transfer bags
	5. 4 sampling site couplers
PROCEDURE	1. Install blood cell processing kit on COBE 2991. Do not use valves. Attach a 600-mL bag to the BLUE line and a 1000-mL bag to the YELLOW line. The marrow is connected to the RED line.
	2. The cell processor is set in the manual mode. Speed is set at 3000 rpm, Superout rate 450 mL per minute to remove supernatant and 100 mL per minute to remove buffy coat.
	3. Clamp all five lines as close to the T as possible. Hang marrow using RED line.
	4. Push blood in, unclamp RED line allowing bone marrow to flow by gravity into processing set. When marrow stops running, press AIR OUT. As soon as the air reaches the marrow bag, push BLOOD IN.

5. Press STOP/RESET, clamp RED line, press START/SPIN, and time for 3 minutes.

6. Set Superout rate at 250 mL per minute. Clear line of marrow cells by pushing SUPEROUT and release clamp on RED line. When line is clear, push HOLD, clamp the RED line, and unclamp the YELLOW line. Push CONTINUE and adjust Superout rate to 450 mL per minute.

7. Stop collecting supernatant when cells approach the silver ring. Push HOLD, clamp YELLOW line. Push CONTINUE, AGITATE/WASH in, and release clamp on RED line. Time for 60 seconds.

8. Push START/SPIN and time for 10 minutes.

9. Set Superout rate at 100 mL per minute and clear the line of cells first. Then collect the supernatant at a rate of 450 mL per minute through the YELLOW line.

10. When the cells are against the silver ring, press HOLD, clamp the YELLOW line, open the BLUE line, push CONTINUE, and collect the marrow buffy coat for *exactly 45 seconds.*

11. Repeat until all marrow is concentrated.

12. Combine the buffy coat bags. Determine volume and obtain hematocrit and cell counts. The red cell volume is determined by multiplying the total volume by hematocrit. This is buffy coat 1.

13. One unit of group O red blood cells, which has been cross-matched with the serum of the bone marrow recipient, is washed and irradiated. The volume of cells is recorded.

14. The unit of red blood cells is mixed with buffy coat 1.

15. The processing procedure is repeated again, removing the buffy coat for only 45 seconds. Measure the volume and hematocrit and obtain cell counts. Determine the red cell volume. This is buffy coat 2.

16. The concentration of marrow cells is diluted to 4×10^7 cells per mL with 5 percent human serum albumin before transfusion.

17. Formula used to obtain the total volume of incompatible red cells:

$$B \times \frac{A}{(A + C)} = \text{Volume incompatible cells infused}$$

where: A = red cell volume buffy 1
            B = red cell volume buffy 2
            C = red cell volume of added irradiated cells

ANTICIPATED RESULTS

No evidence of a hemolytic transfusion reaction has been noted in 14 allogeneic bone marrow transplants. The median nucleated cell recovery is 75 percent. Median volume of incompatible red cells was 10 mL.

NOTE

10,000 units of heparin are given to the patient prior to the marrow infusion. It is advisable to obtain 4 to 6×10^8 cells per kg at the harvest. This will allow recovery of enough cells for rapid engraftment (usually at least 3×10^8 cells per kg.)

AUTHORS

Regina Bryan
Hahnemann University
Philadelphia, PA 19102

Stephen Bulova, M.D.
Hahnemann University
Philadelphia, PA 19102

REFERENCES

1. Rosenfeld, CS: A double buffy coat method for red cell removal from ABO incompatible marrow. Transfusion 29:415, 1989.
2. Bone Marrow Concentration and Processing Using the COBE 2991 Blood Cell Processor. Issues in Bone Marrow Processing, COBE Laboratories, Lakewood, CO, 1986.

SEMIAUTOMATED SEPARATION USING THE COBE 2991

DESCRIPTION	The harvested marrow is processed in the laboratory to concentrate the nucleated cell layer and reduce the volume to 10 to 15 percent of that harvested. The processing uses the manual mode of the instrument and is not controlled by the pinch valves.
TIME FOR PROCEDURE	Approximately 1 to 2 hours to process 650 to 1500 mL of harvested marrow.

SUMMARY OF PROCEDURE

1. The harvested marrow transfer pack is connected to the COBE processing set and the marrow is allowed to flow into the centrifuge.
2. Padded forceps are used instead of the pinch valves to control the flow of the marrow.
3. The marrow is centrifuged to concentrate the nucleated cell layer.
4. Autologous plasma is collected for use in the freezing medium.
5. The nucleated cell layer is collected, and the remaining harvested marrow concentrated.

EQUIPMENT

1. COBE 2991 Blood Cell Processor, Model I
2. Sebra dielectric sealer or COBE clips and pliers

SUPPLIES AND REAGENTS

1. COBE 2991 blood cell processing set No. 912-647-819
2. Hank's balanced salt solution (HBSS) ($1\times$) without magnesium or calcium salts
3. 1000-mL transfer pack
4. 600-mL transfer pack
5. 4 sampling site couplers

PROCEDURE

1. COBE 2991 SETUP
   A. Prime the COBE 2991 as per the manufacturer's instructions.
   B. Install the COBE 2991 processing set into the instrument according to the manufacturer's directions, with the following exceptions:
      (1) Place all tubing in front of the valves. Before connecting the lines to any transfer pack, clamp the lines with padded hemostats near the red blood cell detector.
      (2) Do not use the red blood cell detector.
      (3) Connect the BLUE line to a tared 600-mL transfer pack. This will be used for the buffy coat collection. Place the 600-mL transfer collection pack on a balance to weigh the volume collected. Clamp the coupler line. Insert a sampling site coupler into the bag. Weigh the bag, hemostat, and coupler after the bag is connected to the processing set.
      (4) Connect the YELLOW line to a 1000-mL transfer pack for collection of the autologous plasma.
      (5) Connect the GREEN line to the 600-mL transfer pack of HBSS.
   C. Procedure parameters
      (1) Centrifuge speed: 3000 rpm
      (2) SUPEROUT volume: 600 mL

(3) SUPEROUT rate: 450 mL per minute for concentration steps
                   100 mL per minute for buffy coat collection

(4) Process control setting: manual

2. LOADING BONE MARROW INTO THE PROCESSING SET
   A. After determining the marrow volume and removing specimens for cell counts and cultures, connect the PINK line to the marrow bag.
   B. Release the hemostats from the GREEN line and allow approximately 20 to 50 mL of HBSS to enter the centrifuge.
   C. Remove the hemostat from the PINK line and press BLOOD IN. The marrow will flow into the centrifuge.
   D. When the marrow has stopped flowing into the bag, press AIR OUT. Excess air will be removed from the centrifuge.
   E. When marrow begins to enter the harvest pack or no more air is seen coming from the centrifuge, press BLOOD IN and more marrow enters the processing set.
   F. When the marrow has stopped entering the processing set (it is full), place the hemostats on the PINK line and press STOP/RESET.

3. AUTOLOGOUS PLASMA AND BUFFY COAT COLLECTION
   A. Press START/SPIN and centrifuge the marrow for 7 *minutes* at 3000 rpm.
   B. Unclamp the YELLOW autologous plasma collection line and press SUPEROUT. Collect plasma until the buffy coat layer is 90 mm from the center of the seal weight. This achieves a centrifugal force of 900g.
   C. Press HOLD and reclamp the YELLOW line. Centrifuge another 7 minutes.
   D. While the marrow is spinning, remove autologous plasma from the transfer pack, place into conical tubes and freeze at −70°C. This will be used in the freezing medium.
   E. Change the SUPEROUT setting to 100 mL per minute.
   F. Unclamp the YELLOW plasma line and press SUPEROUT. Collect plasma until the nucleated cell layer comes to within ½ inch of the silver plate in the centrifuge.
   G. Push HOLD and clamp the YELLOW line.
   H. Unclamp the BLUE line, press CONTINUE, and collect the volume of buffy coat needed based on weight.
      (1) Recover a volume that is approximately 10 percent of the volume harvested. If a volume of 1200 mL was harvested, a nucleated cell volume of 120 mL would be recovered.
      (2) Based on the volume harvested, determine the number of times the centrifuge will be filled and buffy coat collected. If a volume of 1200 mL was collected, the centrifuge would be filled two times (the centrifuge has a capacity of 650 mL). Collect 60 mL at each collection.
      (3) Set the balance for the volume to be collected.
   I. When the collection is complete, press HOLD and clamp the BLUE line.
   J. Unclamp the PURPLE waste line and press CONTINUE. The red cells will be collected in the waste bag.
   K. Press STOP/RESET. Clamp the PURPLE line.

L. Process the remaining harvested marrow following Section 2 (Autologous Plasma and Buffy Coat Collection) through Section 3 (Loading Bone Marrow into the Processing Set).

M. When processing is completed, mix the buffy coat well and remove a specimen for a nucleated cell count. If adequate cells have been collected, the BLUE line is sealed and the pack removed.

ANTICIPATED RESULTS

The total nucleated cells recovered from the harvested marrow is approximately 75 to 90 percent with a volume reduction of 85 to 90 percent of that harvested. The desired cell dose is 2.0×10^8 cells per kg.

NOTES

1. The parameters of centrifugation speed and time for this procedure were based on the manual processing method already in use.

2. Bone marrow should not be allowed to remain in the hexagonal seal for prolonged times. HBSS should be used to rinse the lines and the seal so bone marrow does not dry in the lines and cause the seal to break.

3. The seal weight should be kept clean and lubricated so that it can move freely and not ruin the integrity of the bag.

4. If adequate cells were not recovered, the waste bag and autologous plasma bag can be placed into the centrifuge and reprocessed.

AUTHORS

Barbara A. Reeb, M.T.(ASCP)
Brooke Army Medical Center
Department of Clinical Investigation
Fort Sam Houston, TX 78234-6200

Rory D. Duncan, SSG, U.S. Army
Brooke Army Medical Center
Department of Clinical Investigation
Fort Sam Houston, TX 78234-6200

REFERENCE

1. Lopez, M, et al: Human bone marrow processing in view of further in vitro treatment and cryopreservation. Transfusion Immunohaematol 28:411, 1985.

BUFFY COAT PREPARATION USING THE HAEMONETICS MODEL 30

DESCRIPTION	Harvested bone marrow grafts contain a large volume of marrow and peripheral blood cells. Centrifugation separates the nucleated cell fraction (buffy coat concentrate, containing the majority of the hematopoietic progenitor cells) from red blood cells and plasma present in the original marrow graft. Red blood cell removal is required when there is an ABO-incompatible donor-recipient pair. Volume reduction is required before additional processing (e.g., elutriation).
TIME FOR PROCEDURE	The time will vary according to the volume of the harvested graft. Approximately 1 L of marrow can be concentrated per hour.
SUMMARY OF PROCEDURE	1. Bone marrow graft is harvested. 2. Product is loaded into the Haemonetics Model 30 at 40 mL per minute. 3. The buffy coat cells are collected. 4. The bowl is emptied and the process repeated until the entire volume has been processed.
EQUIPMENT	1. Haemonetics Model 30 2. Tubing stripper 3. Heat sealer 4. Clamps 5. IV pole
SUPPLIES AND REAGENTS	1. 225-mL bowl apheresis set (or 125-mL bowl for smaller volumes) (Haemonetics) 2. 2000-mL transfer bag (Fenwal 4R2041) 3. 1000-mL transfer bag (Fenwal 4R2032) 4. 600-mL transfer bag (Fenwal 4R2023) 5. Y blood component recipient set (Fenwal 4C2196) 6. 500 mL 0.9 percent sodium chloride (Hospital Supply) 7. Anticoagulant citrate dextrose solution, formula A (ACD-A), 500 mL (Fenwal 4B7898) 8. Plasma transfer set (AE-7) (Fenwal 4C2240) 9. Plasma transfer set (AE-2) (Fenwal 4C2243) 10. Y connector (Abbott 4064) 11. Sampling site couplers (Fenwal 4C2025)
PROCEDURE	1. SETUP (FIG. 6–1) A. Remove the bowl and harness from the package. The volume of red blood cells in the harvested marrow will determine which bowl (125-mL or 225-mL) should be used. This red cell volume can be calculated (hematocrit × volume). When less than 200 mL of red blood cells are in the harvested marrow, the 125-mL bowl is used. If less than 120 mL of red blood cells are in the product, the marrow should be mixed with

MARROWPHERESIS

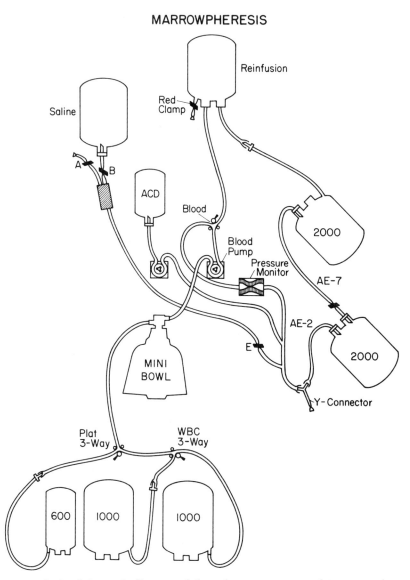

FIGURE 6-1 Schematic diagram of the software system used to process bone marrow grafts using the Haemonetics model 30.

a unit of red blood cells before processing. These red blood cells should be cross-match compatible with both the donor and recipient and *irradiated* before being added to the harvested marrow.

B. Check that the chuck screws are in the open position. Place the bowl in the chuck of the machine. With the highest port of the bowl pointing toward the back of the machine, insert the bowl by tilting it slightly as it enters the chuck ring and then exert firm pressure with the heels of your hands on the shoulders of the bowl. Hold the bowl with one hand and rotate the chuck to ensure proper insertion. Hold the bowl firmly in place while the chuck screws are tightened sequentially, first slightly and then firmly.

C. Secure the feed tube support arms, putting on the right one first, while raising the feed tube: make sure that the head of the bowl is straight, move the hook over and attach it to the locking cam. Tighten the cam by moving it 90 degrees clockwise.

D. The component collection set should be put through the three-way stopcock on the base of the machine with the color-coded labels matching.

E. Hang the reinfusion bag on the reinfusion bag pole.

F. Hold the Y tubing assembly upright so that tubing attached to the bowl is not twisted. Insert the collar on the tubing under the guide below the blood pump. Lay the tubing against the pump rollers and close the pump platen. Insert the line connected to the reinfusion bag into the right side of the three-way stopcock. Insert the other piece of the tubing into the left side of the three-way stopcock.

CAUTION: *It is essential to insert this tubing without any kinks or twists. The rapid emptying of blood through twisted tubing in this three-way stopcock can cause hemolysis.*

G. Insert the spike of anticoagulant line into a 500-mL ACD-A bag and hang the bag in the cradle above the pump, feed the tubing through the pump, and hook the tubing stopper spot under the tubing guide. Then close the platen handle.

NOTE: *Be careful not to let any solution drip into the pump. This will cause the rollers to stick.*

H. Place the pressure monitor on the right side of the machine; thread the tubing at each end into the tubing guides.

 I. Insert the spike of a Y recipient set into a 500-mL bag of 0.9 percent sodium chloride and hang the bag on left IV pole. Place the tubing in the guides below the bag to secure the filter.

J. Insert the end of the long tubing of the Y recipient set into the "keep open connection" of the harness.

K. Insert the harness into one of the female arms of a Y connector and an AE-2 plasma transfer set into the other female arm. Heat seal the tubing extending off the male port.

L. Put the coupler of a 600-mL bag into the platelet (green) port of component collection set. This bag will be used to collect the buffy coat cells.

M. Put the coupler of a 1000-mL bag into the WBC (blue) port of component collection set. This bag will be used to collect plasma.

N. Put the coupler of a 2000-mL bag into the medium-length tubing coming from the reinfusion bag and clamp the tubing.

O. Close the red clamp on the short line of the tubing on the reinfusion bag.

P. Attach one end of an AE-7 plasma transfer set to the 2000-mL bag. Close the roller clamp on the transfer set.

2. PRIME

A. Refer to Figure 6–1 for priming. Close clamp E and open clamps A and B. Fill the filter and half fill the drip chamber of the Y recipient set. Close clamp A. Open clamp E, turn on the power with the pump speed set at 0. Press the FILL button (this causes the centrifuge to spin).

B. Turn the pump speed to 40 mL and check the following:
   (1) Be sure the saline and anticoagulant are dripping.
   (2) Be sure air is being displaced from the bowl into the bag on the yellow line.
   (3) Tilt the pressure monitor pouch to allow air to run into the bowl.
C. When 150 mL of saline has been pumped, close clamp E. When the pressure monitor has collapsed, turn the pump speed to 0 and depress the STOP button.
D. When the bowl has stopped spinning, push the EMPTY button, turn the pump speed to 80 to 100 mL per minute and empty the bowl, allowing air to run to just above the blood three-way stopcock.
E. Turn the pump speed to 0, open the blood pump platen, and allow just enough solution to run back into the bowl to refill the tubing. Close the pump platen and depress the STOP button.
F. Turn the power off. The marrow should be processed within 4 hours of priming.

3. SEPARATION
   A. Weigh the harvested marrow and record the weight. Calculate the volume harvested by first subtracting the tare weight of the bag then dividing by 1.058 (specific gravity of whole blood).
   B. Sample the graft for appropriate specimens based on the type of marrow processing.
   C. Transfer the marrow to another 2000-mL transfer bag. Insert the AE-2 plasma transfer set that is attached to the harness into the marrow bag. Insert the AE-7 plasma transfer set (attached to the 2000-mL bag from step 1P) to the remaining port.
   D. Open the roller clamp on the AE-2 plasma transfer set and start to fill the bowl at 40 mL per minute.
   E. When the buffy coat line is approximately ¼ inch from the center of the bowl, turn the pump speed to 0.
   F. Collect the buffy coat cells by depressing the PLATELET button and setting the pump speed to 20 mL per minute. When processing an ABO-incompatible marrow, collect the buffy coat cells into the 600-mL bag until red blood cells are seen at the entrance port of the transfer bag, then continue to collect for 40 seconds. When working with a marrow that will be further processed (e.g., elutriated), collect the buffy coat cells into the 600-mL bag until red cells are seen at the entrance port of the transfer bag, then continue to collect for 60 seconds.
   G. Depress the STOP button after the buffy coat cells are collected.
   H. Empty the bowl at 80 mL per minute. Drain the reinfusion bag into the attached 2000-mL bag.
   I. Refill the bowl again following the same procedure.
   J. Run the next marrow aliquot through. When the marrow bag is almost empty (approximately 5 mL remaining), open the roller clamp on the AE-7 plasma transfer set from the 2000-mL bag (attached to the reinfusion line) to the original marrow product bag. Use these cells to fill the bowl; then collect the buffy coat cells as in step F.
   K. Plasma should be collected during the second pass into the 1000-mL bag by depressing the WBC button.

L. Label all bags with identifying number and contents before removal from the machine. Weigh and sample as necessary.

M. Chart the information on the appropriate processing forms.

ANTICIPATED RESULTS

Thirty marrows (15 ABO-incompatible, 15 pre-elutriation) processed using this procedure had the following recoveries:

1. Marrow processed to remove red blood cells contained 40 ± 12 percent of the nucleated cells harvested with an average of 4.3 ± 1.0 mL of red blood cells.

2. Marrow processed in preparation for further treatment contained 45 ± 9 percent of the nucleated cells harvested with an average of 6.7 ± 3.8 mL of red blood cells.

AUTHORS

Janice M. Davis, M.T.(ASCP), S.B.B.
Cell Processing Laboratory
The Johns Hopkins Oncology Center
Baltimore, MD 21205

Scott D. Rowley, M.D., FACP
Fred Hutchinson Cancer Center
Seattle, WA 98104

REFERENCE

1. Braine, HG, et al: Bone marrow transplantation with major ABO blood group incompatibility using erythrocyte depletion of marrow prior to infusion. Blood 60:420, 1982.

BUFFY COAT SEPARATION USING TERUMO STERICELL PROCESSOR

DESCRIPTION	Cells are centrifuged in a bell-shaped latham bowl. Erythrocytes, which are denser than nucleated cells, will not rise through the bowl, while a buffy coat consisting mostly of nucleated white cells will rise to the top of the bowl from where they may be collected.
TIME FOR PROCEDURE	Approximately 2 hours from receipt of marrow to end of buffy coat collection
EQUIPMENT	1. SteriCell processor (Terumo Medical Corp. Elkton, MD 21921) 2. SteriCell Sterile Connecting Device (SCD) sterile tubing welder 3. Tube sealer 4. Hemacytometer (Neubauer ruled) 5. Timer with sweep second hand 6. Hemostats (at least 6)
SUPPLIES AND REAGENTS	1. SteriCell gradient/wash set (Terumo Cat. No. NCC-902) and/or SteriCell pediatric gradient/wash set (Terumo Cat. No. NCC-903) 2. Fenwal 2000-mL transfer packs (Fenwal No. 4R-2041) 3. 2 SteriCell Y adaptors (Terumo Cat. No. NCC-951) 4. 2 SteriCell nonvented spike adaptors (Terumo Cat. No. NCC-953) 5. 3 percent glacial acetic acid—100 mL distilled water + 3.0 mL glacial acetic acid—or Unopette for counting white blood cells (WBCs) 6. Unopette for counting red blood cells (RBCs) 7. Microbiologic assay vials 8. Syringes: 1-mL and 3-mL 9. Fenwal 1000-mL transfer packs (Fenwal No. 4R-2032) 10. PlasmaPlex (PPF) 11. Medium 199 (Gibco formula 79-0415PJ) in 10-L pack aliquoted into ten 1-L transfer packs

PROCEDURE	1. PREPARATIVE STEPS TO PERFORM IN ADVANCE OF SPECIMEN ARRIVAL IN LABORATORY
	  A. Thoroughly clean biologic safety cabinet with disinfecting agent. Cleaning should include ceiling of cabinet, all walls, inside of glass, plenum below work-tray, and work-tray.
	  B. Prepare Medium 199, supplemented with 10 percent PlasmaPlex, as follows:
	    (1) Attach nonvented spike adaptors to the ends of a Y adaptor. Attach a vented spike adaptor to complete the Y adaptor.
	    (2) In biologic safety cabinet, insert vented spike adaptor into septum cap of PlasmaPlex bottle. Insert a nonvented spike adaptor into spike port of a 1-L pack containing 1 L of Medium 199. Repeat with the second spike and another 1-L pack of Medium 199. Spike into the remaining spike port of each 1-L pack a 2-L transfer pack.

(3) Hang PlasmaPlex bottle from IV pole on SteriCell processor, and hang a 2-L bag on scale hanger. Tare scale.

(4) Open line from the 1-L pack until emptied into the 2-L pack. Open line from the PlasmaPlex bottle until 100 to 120 mL of additional volume is added to bag

(5) Repeat, making up a second pack of medium.

2. STEPS TO PERFORM AFTER SPECIMEN ARRIVAL IN LABORATORY

A. Record time of specimen arrival in laboratory, and general condition of specimen (with respect to clotting/clumping, observable hemolysis, and so on).

B. Hang marrow collection bag in biologic safety cabinet and insert a sampling site adaptor (needle port). Remove, through needle port, samples for colony-forming unit (CFU) assay (3.0 mL), cytospin or smear preparation, WBC/RBC counts and spun hematocrit (Hct) (0.5 mL); and microbiologic assay (7.5 mL).

C. In biologic safety cabinet, connect by spike connection, an empty 2000-mL transfer bag to the marrow collection bag, and clamp the line. Hang the marrow collection bag on the IV pole on the SteriCell processor. Hang empty bag on scale on SteriCell instrument and tare. Open clamp and allow marrow to flow into empty bag. Record weight of marrow (this will approximately equal the volume).

D. Perform WBC count by diluting 20 μL of sample with 180 μL of 3 percent acetic acid solution (1 in 10 dilution). Fill chamber of hemacytometer and count four outer squares.

WBC/mL = Cells in four squares $\times$ 2.5 $\times$ 10^4 $\times$ dilution

Alternatively, Unopette diluters (1:20) for white blood cell counts may be used, and the same formula employed.

E. Stain-cytospin or smear preparations using rapid staining kit (Diff-Quick). Dry slide and perform differential count.

NOTE: *If abnormal cells are present, or if myeloid progenitors are absent, contact attending physician on bone marrow transplant service.*

Compute fraction of mononuclear cells in marrow as:

$$\text{Mononuclear fraction} = \frac{\text{Myeloid precursors} + \text{Erythroid precursors} + \text{Lymphocytes} + \text{Monocytes}}{\text{Total leukocytes counted in smear}}$$

Compute number of mononuclear cells per mL of marrow as:

Mononuclear cells/mL = WBC/mL $\times$ mononuclear fraction

If numbers of mononuclear cells is low and volume of marrow is less than 500 mL, consult with laboratory director about possible switch to Hespan sedimentation protocol.

F. Perform RBC count by diluting 20 μL of sample into 4 mL of physiologic saline (0.9 percent NaCl in water). Fill chamber of hemacytometer and count cells in center square. Note whether cells appear normocytic (approximately 5 RBCs should line up inside smallest squares on Neubauer-type hemacytometer), microcytic, or macrocytic.

$$RBC/mL = \text{Cells in center square} \times 200 \times 10^4$$

Alternately, Unopette diluters (1:200) for erythrocyte counts may be used and the same formula employed.

G. Obtain a spun Hct, and compute the volume of erythrocytes in the marrow as:

$$RBC \text{ volume} = (Hct/100) \times \text{Marrow volume (from step 2C)}$$

Compute the mean corpuscular volume (MCV) of the RBC as:

$$MCV = \frac{(Hct/100)}{RBC/mL}$$

The MCV will be used to compute remaining erythrocyte volumes based on RBC counts, later in the procedure.

3. BUFFY COAT DECISION POINT
   A. *If the red blood cell volume is in excess of 300 mL,* then an initial buffy coat preparation should be performed in the regular gradient bowl set, as described in steps 4A through 5U.
   B. *If the red cell volume is less than 150 mL,* then buffy coat preparation cannot be performed (Bone Marrow Processing Laboratory director should be consulted).
   C. *If the red cell volume is greater than 150 mL but less than 300 mL,* a buffy coat preparation (steps 4A through 5U) should be performed using the Pediatric-Bowl.

4. STERICELL SETUP FOR BUFFY COAT PROCESSING (see Fig. 6–2)
   A. Install a gradient/wash set (or a pediatric gradient/wash set) into the SteriCell processor, as per the operations manual pages 2–4 through 2–9.

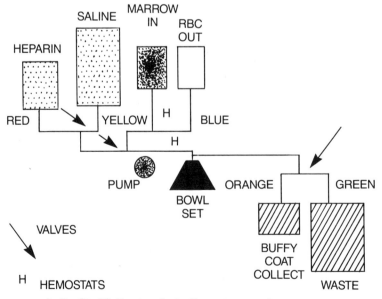

FIGURE 6–2   SteriCell setup for buffy coat processing.

(1) Verify that the chuck O ring is in place and has a light coating of silicone grease. Verify that the chuck screws are loose.

(2) Open SteriCell gradient/wash set (Terumo Cat. No. NCC-902). Holding latham bowl right side up, allow all lines to fall to full extension.

(3) Drape the tubing with bags attached to the right side of the SteriCell processor. Drape the tubing with no bags attached to the left side of the machine.

(4) Tilting the bowl toward the front of the processor, seat the front edge of the bowl into the centrifuge chuck. Then tilt the bowl back, applying even pressure to opposite sides of the shoulder of the bowl to seat it fully in the centrifuge chuck. An audible snap will be heard when the bowl seats fully.

(5) Hold the body of the bowl and tighten the chuck screws in clockwise sequence with the chuck tool. Turn each screw until resistance is felt. Then make a second round, turning each screw until the torque setting on the chuck tool is reached (chuck tool will click).

(6) Turn the bowl 90 degrees so that the GREEN and ORANGE lines (bags attached) are directed away from the control panel, and the BLUE, YELLOW, and RED lines (no bags) are directed *toward* the control panel. Swing the feed tube support arms into place, engage the cam lock, and rotate until it comes to a stop.

(7) Ensure that the bowl can turn freely. If it cannot, remove it and repeat above sequence.

(8) Lead the BLUE inlet tube through the rear slot, then drape to the front of the pump, align in pump using the plastic stops on the tubes, and close the cover of the pump.

(9) Lead the BLUE inlet tube through the blue side of the valve farthest from the control panel. Close the valve by pressing the BLUE button on the control panel, and drape the other inlet tube through the other side of the same valve. Drape the RED inlet tube through the red side of the valve closest to the control panel, then close that valve by pressing either the RED or the YELLOW buttons, and drape the YELLOW inlet tube through the other side of the same valve.

(10) Lead the GREEN outlet line through the green side of the valve on the front of the processor, and hang the attached waste bag to hooks on the side of the machine. Change the position of the front valve by pressing the GREEN or ORANGE buttons on the control panel, and lead the ORANGE outlet tube through the other side of the valve. Hang the collection bag on the scale hanger, and tare.

(11) Close the cover to the centrifuge. Check that all lines not to be used for the next procedure are pinch-clamped, and that all lines which are to be used, are open, and have containers attached to them.

(12) Aliquot aseptically 400 mL Medium 199 into a small SteriCell bag. Add 20 mL preservative-free heparin (1000 U per mL up to a final concentration of 50 U per mL). Attach bag to the RED line on the SteriCell (Fig. 6–1) using the SCD tube welder.

(13) Aseptically spike a bag of normal saline with a SteriCell nonvented spike adaptor. Attach the bag to the YELLOW line using the SCD tube welder (Fig. 6–1).

(14) Aseptically attach a luer-slip transfer adaptor to the needle adaptor on a 600-mL transfer pack. Attach to one of the blue lines using the SCD tube welder, and clamp the line shut with a hemostat (Fig. 6–1).

(15) Attach, using a SCD sterile tube welder, the marrow sample to other of the BLUE lines, and clamp the line shut with a hemostat (Fig. 6–1).

(16) Close the BLUE valve; open the RED valve; and open the GREEN valve.

(17) Set the pump speed to 150 mL per minute and start the pump (press PUMP START/STOP).

(18) Allow heparin solution to fill bowl. When solution enters GREEN line, open the ORANGE valve (which closes the GREEN valve).

(19) Pump additional 50 mL of solution into the ORANGE bag, then stop pump (press PUMP START/STOP), and close ORANGE valve.

(20) Reverse pump by pressing EMPTY button, and start pump.

(21) Pump solution out of bowl until bowl is empty. Record volume of heparin solution in collection bag. Tare scale.

5. BUFFY COAT PROCESSING (Fig. 6–2)

A. *Leave the SteriCell in manual mode.*

B. Open the BLUE valve to the bone marrow and the GREEN valve to the waste bag.

C. Set the centrifuge speed at 4800 rpm and press the CENTRIFUGE START/STOP button.

D. Set the pump to FILL. Set the pump speed to 150 mL per minute. Press the PUMP START/STOP button and allow the centrifuge bowl to fill with bone marrow.

E. After the buffy coat has formed a layer on top of the red cells, and the leading edge of the layer is just below the shoulder of the bowl, reduce the pump speed to 20 mL per minute.

F. When the leading edge of the buffy layer has passed the shoulder of the white inner core (space between inner core and outer wall of bowl is not visible; red light at back of bowl is shining on leading edge of cells), open the ORANGE valve to the product bag (*GREEN valve closes*).

G. Collect cells into the collection (ORANGE line) bag until all of the buffy coat has been collected and red blood cells are starting to enter the bag.

H. Start the timer, and collect cells for 1½ additional minutes (90 seconds) to 2 minutes (120 seconds).

I. Stop the pump (press PUMP START/STOP).

J. Close the ORANGE valve.

K. Clamp the line from the bone marrow bag.

L. Release the clamp on the empty bag line.

M. Close the BLUE valve; open the YELLOW valve; and increase centrifuge speed to 5600 rpm.

N. Reset volume indicator to 0 by pressing EMPTY and then pressing FILL.

O. Set pump speed to 150 mL per minute. Press AGITATE button. Allow red blood cells to wash until 350 mL of saline has been pumped through bowl.

P. Stop washing by pressing AGITATE button again. Stop centrifuge (press CENTRIFUGE START/STOP button).

Q. Open BLUE valve.

R. Reverse the pump direction by pressing EMPTY and make sure that pump speed is set to 150 mL per minute. Push the PUMP START/STOP button to start pump. Run the pump until the bowl is empty, then stop pump.

S. Repeat the procedure starting from step 5B until all of the bone marrow has been processed.

    (1) If the bone marrow runs out before the buffy coat is pushed out of the bowl: Stop the pump by pressing the PUMP START/STOP button; reclamp the branch of the blue line coming from the bone marrow bag; open the line from the red cell collection bag (so that the residual RBC may push the buffy coat out); restart the pump by pressing the PUMP START/STOP button; after the buffy coat is collected *do not change the blue line clamps.*

T. After all of the marrow has been buffy coat processed:

- Open the RED valve, close the BLUE valve.
- Set pump to FILL at 150 mL per minute.
- Pump heparin solution through bowl until it is running into the waste bag.
- Open the ORANGE valve.
- Flush through the collection line with an additional 50 mL of heparinized medium.
- Close the ORANGE valve.
- Set the pump to EMPTY at 150 mL per minute.
- After bowl is completely empty, stop pump (press PUMP START/STOP button).

U. At this point, the buffy coat collection has been completed. Note the volume of the buffy coat (from the scale on the SteriCell instrument and move the buffy coat collection bag into the biologic safety cabinet. Insert a sampling site coupler into the product bag and obtain samples. Perform WBC and RBC counts as described in paragraphs 4A6 and 4A8. Also, make a cytospin or smear preparation and perform a differential analysis.

V. The transfer bag containing the RBC byproduct of the buffy coat is to be labeled and delivered to the blood bank for possible return to the marrow donor.

W. If final product is to be returned directly to the patient, samples should be removed for microbiologic assay and for colony-forming unit–granulocyte-monocyte (CFU-GM) assay. Alternatively, sample processing should continue with gradient separation and wash procedure, or, if indicated, washing should be performed as specified farther on.

6. CELL WASH PROCESS

A. Using SCD sterile tube welder:

- Connect 1 L Medium 199 with PlasmaPlex to RED line.
- Leave remaining saline from preceding parts of procedure on YELLOW line.

- Attach collected Ficoll product cells to BLUE line (it is recommended that the blue line previously used for the RBC byproduct of the Ficoll process be used for these cells).
- Attach empty large SteriCell culture bag to other BLUE line (it is recommended that the blue line previously used for entering buffy coat product or fresh marrow into the gradient separation process be employed for the empty bag). Clamp this line, hang the empty bag on the scale, and tare.

B. Push WASH protocol button *(BLUE valve closes; YELLOW valve opens; and GREEN valve opens)*.

C. Push START/ADVANCE button *(250 mL saline is pumped into bowl; after saline is pumped, BLUE valve opens and cells are pumped into bowl. Display reads: "FIRST CELL LOADING")*.

D. When all the cells have been loaded into the bowl (trailing edge of cells passes Y and entry to pump), press START/ADVANCE *twice* (if display does not read "SECOND CELL LOADING," press START/ADVANCE again until it does). *(Pump stops; centrifuge stops; BLUE valve opens; pump starts; cells in bowl are transferred to bag on BLUE line. BLUE valve closes; RED valve opens; centrifuge starts; 250 mL of Medium 199 is pumped into bowl; BLUE valve opens and cells are pumped into bowl)*.

E. When all the cells are loaded into the bowl a second time, press START/ADVANCE button once *(BLUE valve closes; RED valve opens; centrifuge speed increases to 4900 rpm, Medium 199 is pumped into bowl. Repeated 12 times: Centrifuge increases to 5400 rpm and pauses 2 seconds; centrifuge speed drops to 4900 rpm; wash solution is pumped into bowl(150 mL per minute × 8 seconds); centrifuge speed decreases to 4400 rpm and pauses 8 seconds; pump stops; cycle repeats. After 12 cycles: BLUE valve opens; cells pumped into bag on BLUE line. Repeated 3 times: RED valve opens; BLUE valve closes; 50 mL Medium 199 added to bowl; pump stops, centrifuge stops; BLUE valve opens; 50 mL pumped out of bowl; cycle repeats)*.

F. Cells are ready to be sent to patient, or for distribution into freezing bags. Withdraw samples for final microbiologic analysis (1.5 mL), for CFU assay (1.5 mL) and cytospin or smear preparation (followed by differential analysis), and WBC and RBC counting (0.5 mL) (see steps 4A6 and 4A8).

NOTES

1. SCD sterile tube welder may be used outside of biologic safety cabinet. All connections done with spike fittings must be done inside of cabinet.

2. If desire to perform a gradient (Ficoll) separation after the buffy coat and are using a gradient/wash set (not Pediatric), it may be best to spike the ORANGE line collection bag with two 1-L transfer packs. One pack is for transferring the buffy coat product, and the other is to collect a saline rinse of the original collection bag, thereby leaving it red cell free, for the collection of the subsequent Ficoll separated product.

QUALITY CONTROL

1. Check sterility of operation by setting up aerobic and anaerobic microbiologic culture vials both at the beginning and end of procedure.

2. Check for preservation of hematopoietic cells by CFU assay both at the

beginning and end of procedure. Maintain CFU results on CUMSUM quality control graphical record, and follow up on trends away from mean by verification of proper function of SteriCell on dry run.

3. Perform differential analysis on sample at beginning and end of procedure. Keep a record of percent enrichment and depletion of specific cellular subsets (i.e., granulocytic, monocytic, and so on).

AUTHORS

William E. Janssen, Ph.D.
Bone Marrow Processing and
    Evaluation Laboratory
Bone Marrow Transplant Program
H. Lee Moffitt Cancer Center and
    Research Institute
University of South Florida
12902 Magnolia Dr.
Tampa, FL 33612-9497

Carlos E. Lee, M.T.
Bone Marrow Processing and
    Evaluation Laboratory
Bone Marrow Transplant Program
H. Lee Moffitt Cancer Center and
    Research Institute
University of South Florida
12902 Magnolia Dr.
Tampa, FL 33612-9497

REFERENCES

1. SteriCell Processor: Operating and Maintenance Manual. Terumo Medical Corp., Elkton, MD 21921.
2. Brown, BA: Hematology: Principles and Procedures, ed 4. Lea & Febiger, Philadelphia, 1984, p 33.

Red Blood Cell Sedimentation

HYDROXYETHYL STARCH SEDIMENTATION OF INCOMPATIBLE RED BLOOD CELLS FROM MARROW

DESCRIPTION	Red blood cells are sedimented and removed from bone marrow prior to transplantation. Hydroxyethyl starch (HES) causes the red blood cells to form rouleaux, accelerating the sedimentation. Bone marrow thus processed can be used for transplant of major ABO-incompatible marrow. Other major red cell antigen/antibody incompatibilities between donor and recipient can also be treated in this way.
TIME FOR PROCEDURE	1½ hours per sedimentation
SUMMARY OF PROCEDURE	1. Marrow is delivered to the processing laboratory in one or more transfer packs.
	2. The marrow is pooled and the hematocrit (Hct) adjusted to 25 percent with Hank's balanced salt solution (HBSS).
	3. HES is added to the marrow/HBSS in a 1:7 ratio.
	4. The marrow mix is hung inverted and the red blood cells sedimented.
	5. The red cells are drained into a second transfer pack, leaving leukocytes, platelets, and stem cells suspended in the supernatant plasma/HBSS/HES. Red cell contamination is not more than 1 percent by volume.
	6. The product can be volume reduced by centrifugation or infused.
EQUIPMENT	1. Sterile Connecting Device (SCD) 312 (Haemonetics Corp.)
	2. Heat sealer (Fenwal, Sebra, or other tubing sealer)
	3. Sorval RC3 refrigerated centrifuge
	4. Plasma expressor
	5. Scale
SUPPLIES AND REAGENTS	1. Transfer packs: 2-L, 1-L, 600-mL
	2. HBSS in transfer packs
	3. 500 mL HES
	4. Alcohol preps
	5. Povidone-iodine swabs
	6. Medication injection sites
	7. 5- or 10-mL syringes
	8. 19-gauge needles
	9. Plastic slide clamps
	10. 12 × 75 tubes
	11. Hemostats
	12. Blood culture bottles
	13. Ring stand, IV pole, or other device for inverted suspension of fluids

PROCEDURE

1. Pool marrow into a 2-L transfer pack; heat-seal tubing, leaving 8 to 10 inches of tubing attached to transfer pack.

2. Weigh marrow and record weight.

3. Insert medication injection site into one port of the 2-L pack and clean it with povidone iodine.

4. Label an aerobic and an anaerobic blood culture bottle and clean the tops with alcohol.

5. Mix marrow well and withdraw 5 mL into a 5- or 10-mL syringe.

6. Inject 1 to 2 mL of marrow into each blood culture bottle and put the rest in a labeled 12×75 tube for white cell (WBC) and Hct determination.

7. Obtain WBC count and Hct using the automated cell counter. Record values.

8. Adjust Hct of marrow to 25 percent with HBSS.
   A. Formula:

   $$(1) \quad \frac{\text{Desired Hct (25)}}{\text{Actual Hct}} = \frac{\text{Actual weight}}{\text{Desired final weight (x)}}$$

   (2) Desired final weight $-$ actual weight = Amount of HBSS to add

   B. Using the SCD, attach the tubing of a pack of HBSS to the tubing of a marrow pack.
   C. Place marrow on balance; pinch weld to open flow path and let HBSS flow into marrow pack until desired final weight is reached.
   D. Heat seal tubing.

9. Add one part HES to seven parts marrow/HBSS by volume.
   A. Formula:

   $$\frac{\text{Total weight (vol) of HBSS/marrow}}{7} = \text{Vol of HES to add}$$

   B. Using the SCD, attach the spike of a 1-L transfer pack to the marrow pack. Save the transfer pack.
   C. Spike the HES bag with the marrow bag and pinch weld to open flow path to allow calculated volume of HES to flow into marrow.
   D. After some of the HES has flowed into the marrow, hold the marrow bag upright and squeeze to force air into the HES bag. This will make it possible to determine the HES volume.

10. Heat seal tubing between the two bags.

11. Using the SCD, attach the spikeless 1-L pack to the marrow pack. Mix marrow.

12. Pinch weld to open flow path and allow 1-L pack to fill.

13. Clamp tubing with hemostats.

14. Using the SCD, attach a second 1-L transfer pack to the marrow pack. This will seal off the first 1-L pack.

15. Repeat steps 12 and 13. If marrow remains in original pack, repeat step 14, and then 12 and 13 again.

16. Using the SCD, attach an empty 1-L pack to each 1-L pack containing marrow.

17. *Do not* pinch weld. Hang marrow packs inverted on ring stand.

18. Place plastic slide clamps on tubing between full and empty 1-L packs and pinch the welds to open flow paths.

19. Move the slide clamps so that red blood cells (RBCs) drain slowly into the empty packs.

20. When the red blood cell line is about 1 inch above the outlet ports, clamp tubing with hemostats.

21. Let the red blood cells settle a bit, unclamp and let more red blood cells out. Clamp and unclamp as needed to drain out the most red blood cells, losing the least amount of supernatant, which contains the stem cells.

22. Heat-seal the tubing, leaving no more than 3 inches attached to the supernatant pack.

23. If volume is to be reduced, attach each supernatant pack to a 600-mL transfer pack using the SCD. If not, go to step 27.

24. Transfer the supernatant to the 600-mL packs, leaving the 1-L pack attached. Clamp the tubing with slide clamps.

25. Centrifuge the supernatant at 22°C for 10 minutes at $2419g$ (approximately 3000 rpm in refrigerated centrifuge [RC3]).

26. Express approximately 75 percent of the supernatant into the 1-L packs. Heat seal the tubing and discard the 1-L packs.

27. Connect the bags containing the stem cells, using the SCD.

28. Resuspend cells, pool into a single pack, and weigh. Record weight.

29. Insert medication injection site into pack of stem cells and clean with povidone iodine.

30. Repeat steps 4 through 7 for bacterial culture and WBC count. Hct should be determined using a microhematocrit centrifuge.

31. Calculate the amount of nucleated cells and red blood cells in the original marrow and the stem cell pack. Formulas:

    A. RBC

      (1) $\dfrac{\text{Hct}}{100} \times$ wt of bag contents = Total RBC (g)

      (2) $\dfrac{\text{g RBC}}{1.08}$ = mL RBC

    B. Nucleated cells (use WBC for nucleated cells)

      (1) WBC $\times 10^3 \times$ wt of bag contents $\times 1000$ = Total WBC

      (2) Amount of nucleated cells needed are 2 to 3×10^8 per kg body weight of recipient or wt (kg) $\times 2 \times 10^8$ — weight (kg) $\times 3 \times 10^8$.

32. If more nucleated cells are needed, repeat the procedure: starting with step 8, adjustment of hematocrit to 25 percent using the 2-L RBC bag.

ANTICIPATED RESULTS   Bone marrow for transplant which has red blood cell contamination no higher than 1 percent.

AUTHOR

Sarah F. Donnelly, M.T.(ASCP), S.B.B.
University of Virginia Health
  Sciences Center
Blood Bank and Transfusion
  Services
Charlottesville, VA 22908

REFERENCES

1. Dinsmore, RE, et al: ABH incompatible bone marrow transplantation: Removal of erythrocytes by starch sedimentation. Br J Haematol 54:441, 1983.
2. Warkentin, PI, et al: Transplantation of major ABO-incompatible bone marrow depleted of red cells by hydroxyethyl starch. Vox Sang 48:89, 1985.

MONONUCLEAR CELL PREPARATION

Automated Mononuclear Cell Purification of Marrow with the Fenwal CS3000 and CS3000 Plus

DESCRIPTION	A purified population of mononuclear cells is frequently required for bone marrow manipulation with pharmacologic agents and monoclonal antibodies or cytokines or both. This method isolates mononuclear cells from bone marrow using a Fenwal CS3000 cell separator without the use of density gradient or sedimenting materials. The automated procedure employs a closed, sterile system to recover mononuclear bone marrow cells rapidly in a 200-mL volume with minimal red blood cell and granulocyte contamination. This technique is also useful for preparation of marrow for major ABO-incompatible transplants and for cryopreservation.
TIME FOR PROCEDURE	Approximately 60 minutes to process 1000 mL.

SUMMARY OF PROCEDURE

1. Harvested bone marrow is delivered to the processing laboratory in one or more transfer packs.
2. Anticoagulant citrate dextrose (ACD-A) is added to marrow bag. Final ACD-A concentration is approximately 10 percent.
3. A standard Fenwal apheresis kit is installed on the CS3000 and primed with 1.25 percent human serum albumin in normal saline solution.
4. The instrument is programmed according to the programming chart.
5. The marrow is pumped into the instrument through the inlet line and the plasma/medium automatically removed. The packed red blood cells are diluted with the albumin solution and reprocessed to recover additional mononuclear cells.
6. If desired, the mononuclear fraction can be further purified using the automated density gradient procedure described in this chapter on pp. 158–162.

EQUIPMENT

1. Fenwal CS3000 or CS3000 Plus Blood Cell Separator No. 4R4530 with granulo separation chamber and A-35 collection chamber (Fenwal Laboratories)
2. Electric tube sealer
3. 2 hemostats

SUPPLIES AND REAGENTS

1. Fenwal open apheresis kit No. 4R2210
2. 500-mL bag anticoagulant citrate dextrose formula A (ACD-A)
3. 1000-mL bag 0.9 percent sodium chloride for intravenous (IV) infusion with 50-mL bottle 25 percent human serum albumin added
4. Two 1000-mL transfer packs
5. 1 plasma transfer set with coupler and needle adaptor

6. Two 16-gauge × 1-inch hypodermic needles

7. 2 sampling site couplers

8. Adhesive tape

PROCEDURE   1. INSTALLATION OF APHERESIS KIT (numbers in parentheses refer to Fig. 6–3)

A. Install the kit following the operator's manual and the instruction sheet enclosed with the apheresis kit, with the following modifications:

1. Close the roller clamps on both the inlet (1) and return (2) lines.

2. The ACD line (3) and pump segment are not used. Close the roller clamp on the line and do not connect anything to the line or place the tubing over the roller pump. No adjustment of the ACD delivery wheel is required.

3. Place the SEPARATION container PRBC line into the notch in the GRANULO chamber.

4. Tape the bags into the centrifuge holders to keep them taut.

5. Attach the 1.25 percent albumin/saline solution to the SALINE and VENT lines.

6. Attach a 1000-mL transfer pack to the PLASMA COLLECT line. **NOTE:** *For autologous marrows—A 600-mL transfer pack can be connected to the 1000-mL plasma collection bag to collect albumin/saline for use in preparation of freezing solution.*

7. Do not attach transfer set to the PRBC line (4) until after the completion of the AUTO PRIME.

B. Select procedure 5 with PRIME and RUN switches in AUTO. Set clamp switches to CLOSED and pumps to OFF. (For CS3000 Plus, use special procedure 7.)

C. Press PRIME switch. (For CS3000 Plus, press MODE key, then press START/RESUME key to enter AUTO/PRIME.)

1. At step 2. pause, raise WHOLE BLOOD PUMP (5) handle until inlet light goes out.

2. Close pump handle.

3. Press RESUME and invert AIRTRAP (6) until it is filled with priming solution. Prime using AUTO PRIME according to the operator's manual.

4. This portion of the procedure takes approximately 10 minutes. During this period, reprogram AUTO RUN (section 2) and REINFUSE (section 3).

2. REPROGRAMMING AUTO RUN

NOTE: *If the CS3000 blood cell separator being used has a CPU upgrade or is a CS3000 Plus, follow directions accompanying the instrument to reprogram and store the RUN AND REINFUSE programs. Sections 2, 3, and 4 of this procedure can then be omitted.*

A. Press and hold "hidden C" (the "C" in the name "CS3000" on the front of the instrument) and the RUN switch until the E-2 lamp is illuminated. This enters the RUN reprogramming mode.

B. The two-digit line number (location or L-number) of the computer

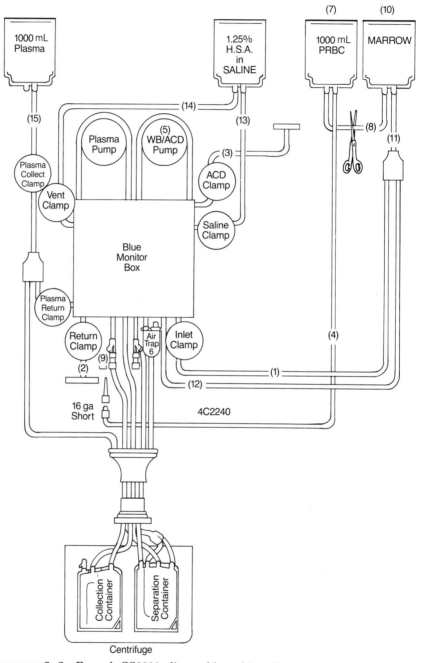

FIGURE 6–3 Fenwal CS3000 disposable tubing kit setup for mononuclear cell concentration.

program is displayed in the STATUS display. This number is increased by pressing E-1 (to increase by 10) or E-2 (to increase by 1). As the line number is increased, the instruction number will be displayed.

C. The four-digit instruction number of a particular line is displayed in the END-POINT display. Instruction numbers can only be changed by simultaneously holding hidden C and pressing the END-POINT key pads.

D. When all instructions have been changed, press RESUME to enter the changed values into the computer memory. It is necessary to enter these numbers before reprogramming REINFUSE.

E. REPROGRAMMING CHART FOR RUN

L#	From	To	L#	From	To
00	0010	0010*	60	0000	0050
01	0220	0140	61	0020	0000
02	0770	0680	62	0000	0010
03	0100	1000	63	0010	0000
04	0500	1000	64	0320	0050
05	0010	0010*	65	0000	0000*
06	0100	0030	66	0000	0000*
07	0000	0000*	67	0000	0000*
08	0640	0000	68	0420	0970
09	0020	0000	69	0000	0800
10	0010	0010*	70	0020	0020*
11	0200	0090	71	0200	1000
12	0770	0680	72	2550	2230
13	0100	1750	73	1020	1020*
14	0500	0000	74	0920	0920*
15	0010	0010*	75	0400	0500
16	0140	0400	76	0610	0810
17	0000	0000*	77	0610	0810
18	0000	0000*	78	0850	0970
19	0000	0000*	79	2050	0680
20	0000	0010	80	2510	2510*
21	0220	0100	81	0030	0030*
22	0770	0680	82	1000	1000*
23	0100	1000			
24	0500	1300			
25	0010	0010*			
26	0050	0120			
27–59	0000	0000*			

*Unchanged.

3. REPROGRAMMING REINFUSE

A. Press and hold "hidden 0" (the last "0" to the right in CS3000 on front of machine) and REINFUSE until the E-2 lamp is illuminated.

B. Reprogram exactly as in sections 2B and 2C. C must be held while reprogramming.

C. When all instructions have been changed, press RESUME to enter the changed values into the computer memory.

D. REPROGRAMMING CHART FOR REINFUSE

L#	From	To	L#	From	To
00	0010	0010*	20	0010	0010*
01	0090	0080	21	0090	0260
02	0260	0640	22	0260	0640
03	0400	0000	23	0500	0000
04	0000	0000*	24	0000	1000
05	1590	2230	25	1590	2230
06	0200	0300	26	0900	0500
07	0000	0000*	27	0000	0000*
08	0000	0000*	28	0000	0320
09	0000	0000*	29	0000	0040
10	0010	0010*	30	0010	0010*
11	0090	0260	31	0080	0260
12	0260	0640	32	0400	0640
13	0400	0000	33	0000	0000*
14	0500	0240	34	0000	1000
15	1590	2230	35	0000	2230
16	0400	0240	36	0450	0150
17	0000	0000*	37 and above unchanged		
			1800000000*		
19	0000	0000*			

*Unchanged.

4. SELECT DRAW RATE
   A. Reset the draw rate to 25 mL per minute by pressing the SET key until illuminated.
   B. Press and hold the END-POINT key pads to set new flow rate at 250 (25 mL per minute).
   C. Press RESUME to enter the new blood flow rate.

5. INSTALL AND PRIME BAG AND TUBING (numbers in parentheses refer to Fig. 6–3)
   A. Label 1 1000-mL transfer bag "PRBC" (7). Enter 1 port of bag with spike of transfer set (4).
   B. Close roller clamp on the transfer set (4).
   C. Place hemostat on PRBC bag tubing between bag and spike (8).
   D. Place a needle on the needle adapter end of the transfer set and aseptically insert the needle into the PRBC line injection site (9) located farthest to the left of the air trap below the blue monitor box. Tape the needle in place.
   E. Open the roller clamp on the transfer set (4) and allow approximately 100 to 200 mL of albumin solution to enter the PRBC bag.
   F. Close roller clamp.
   G. Hang PRBC bag on the second from the right IV hook. Leave this bag hanging so air bubbles do not enter the transfer tubing.

6. CONNECTING MARROW AND FINAL SET UP
   A. Insert sampling site coupler into MARROW bag. If multiple bags are to be processed, connect bags in series.
   B. Spike one port of MARROW bag with coupler from PRBC bag (8), leaving hemostat closed.
   C. Attach 16-gauge × 1-inch needle to apheresis kit inlet line (11).

    D. Open roller clamp on the inlet line (11) and prime completely free of air. Close roller clamp and insert needle into the injection site in the MARROW bag. Tape in place.

    E. If air remains in MARROW bag, while holding bag upright, open hemostat briefly on the tubing between MARROW bag and the PRBC bag (8) and squeeze air into PRBC bag. Replace hemostat.

    F. Place the MARROW bag on the right IV hook and agitate enough to mix the lower portion of the bag without mixing in the fat at the top.

    G. Place a hemostat on the ACD line (12) near the inlet line, as shown in Figure 6–3.

7. AUTOMATIC MARROW PROCESSING

NOTE: *Before beginning automatic processing make sure of the following:*

- *Installation agrees with tubing diagram.*
- *RUN and REINFUSE have been reprogrammed.*
- *Blood flow rate of 25 mL per minute has been selected.*
- *Hemostat is on line between PRBC and MARROW bags (8).*
- *Roller clamp is closed on return (2) and ACD (12) lines.*
- *Roller clamps are open to albumin/saline prime (13) and vent (14) lines and plasma collect (15) line.*

    A. Open roller clamp on inlet (11) line.

    B. Open roller clamp on line to PRBC bag (4).

    C. Press RUN (MODE, then START/RESUME).* Code 84 will appear, and chime will sound.

    D. Press RESUME (START/RESUME).* The centrifuge and pumps will start.

    E. Make sure marrow is entering inlet (1) line from MARROW bag.

    F. Check for fluid entering PLASMA COLLECTION bag (15).

    G. Check with strobe light to see that there are very few bubbles in centrifuge tubing and that they are no longer than 1 inch. Bubbles can be removed by opening door to stop centrifuge and removing air from medical injection sites with a needle and syringe.

    H. Check front panel display to see that inlet flow rate on whole blood pump is about 25 mL per minute.

    I. After plasma appears in the plasma pump lines (approximately 150 to 200 mL processed), reset the optical detector baseline.

For CS3000:

    (1) Press the SET BLOOD FLOW RATE switch until its indicator light illuminates.

    (2) Press the ENTER 2 switch to display the current optical detector voltage in the END POINT display.

    (3) While continuously holding the ENTER 2 switch, press any of the END POINT switches until the RESUME light begins flashing.

    (4) Release the ENTER 2 switch and press the RESUME switch to enter the new optical detector baseline.

For CS3000 Plus:

    (1) Press DISPLAY/EDIT key to display parameters.

    (2) Use up/down arrow keys to display INTERFACE DETECTOR BASELINE in message center.

---

*For CS3000 Plus.

    (3) Press ENTER key to set the values.

    (4) Press DISPLAY/EDIT to exit.

J. No further attention is necessary until the MARROW bag is almost empty. The time for the bag to empty can be calculated as follows:

$$\text{Total volume}/25 \text{ mL/min} = \text{Minutes to load marrow}$$
$$\text{Example: } 1000 \text{ mL}/25 = 40 \text{ min}$$

K. When the MARROW bag is almost empty, begin the second processing of the PRBCs. (Do not allow the fat to enter the tubing.)

    (1) Mix the contents of the PRBC bag, open the hemostat between the PRBC and MARROW bags, and lower empty MARROW bag to permit contents of PRBC to enter.

    (2) Replace hemostat.

    (3) If the MARROW bag is depleted and the centrifuge stops with "STATUS 51 or 70" displayed before step 7K(1) has been performed, transfer packed cells to MARROW bag and press RESUME. For CS3000 Plus, if marrow bag is depleted and centrifuge stops with INLET LINE OCCLUDED alarm, press HALT/IRRIGATE, lower the marrow bag, and permit albumin solution to flush air bubbles back into marrow bag. Transfer PRBCs to the marrow bag and press RESUME.

8. AUTO REINFUSE

A. When the MARROW bag is empty for the second time, press HALT/IRRIGATE, immediately followed by pressing REINFUSE for CS3000 or MODE; START/RESUME for CS3000 Plus..

B. REINFUSE program consists of a 5-minute spin followed by one harvest of the mononuclear cell layer.

C. Processing ends with STATUS 25 displayed.

9. REMOVING MONONUCLEAR CELL PRODUCT

A. Close all roller clamps.

B. The A-35 COLLECTION bag containing the mononuclear cells can be sealed off and removed.

C. If a volume of less than 200 mL is desired:

    (1) Remove plasma collect line (15) from its clamps.

    (2) Lower the PLASMA COLLECTION bag below the centrifuge and place on a scale.

    (3) Open the A-35 bag holder and roller clamp on plasma collect (15) line.

    (4) Approximately 100 mL of supernatant can be removed without loss of cells.

ANTICIPATED RESULTS

The procedure should yield at least 50 percent of the starting mononuclear cells, based on the percentage of mononuclear cells in a slide differential multiplied by the total number of nucleated cells in the product.

NOTES

1. RECOVERY OF MARROW IN AN EMERGENCY: In the event of a power failure or serious instrument malfunction, the bone marrow can be recovered into the PRBC bag in the following manner:

A. Close roller clamps on line to PLASMA COLLECT bag and both roller clamps to PRIME bag.

    B. Lower PRBC and original MARROW bag to bottom of centrifuge and open roller clamp to the plasma transfer set attached to PRBC bag.

    C. Remove the COLLECTION bag from its clamp and hang on the upper hex clamp handle. Permit the contents to siphon through the SEPARATION bag and into the PRBC bag.

    D. The prime solution can be used to flush the lines and bags.

    E. The PRBC bag and the original MARROW bags should be disconnected from the tubing set by removing the needles from the septum at the PRBC injection site and from the septum at the inlet line. The needles should be replaced and left covered.

    F. The MARROW and PRBC bags can then be (1) connected to another CS3000 set for reprocessing or (2) transferred to another bag for storage or additional processing.

2. When reprogramming AUTO RUN, if the RUN light is flashing and RUN is pressed before C, the automatic run procedure will start (or "CODE 84" will appear). If this occurs, press HALT/IRRIGATE to stop the process so that reprogramming can be performed. When RESUME is pressed to complete reprogramming, AUTO RUN will start. Press HALT/IRRIGATE to stop until ready to start the procedure; then press RESUME to begin the automatic run.

3. Do not allow air to enter lines, as this can impede flow into the centrifuge.

4. If flow rate exceeds 25 mL per minute more granulocytes will be collected.

5. This procedure does not remove platelets. Platelets can be removed by (1) centrifuging on the CS3000 at 1000 rpm for 3 to 4 minutes, or (2) centrifuging in a Sorvall RC3 or equivalent at 2000 rpm for 7 minutes.

6. If it is necessary to temporarily interrupt the procedure, the top sliding door can be opened slightly. This will stop the centrifuge and will not affect the yield. To restart the centrifuge, close door and press RESUME.

7. The red blood cell fraction remaining in the PRBC and separation bags can be tranferred to another bag and reinfused to the donor.

8. This procedure can be performed only if the marrow contains at least 150 mL of red blood cells. For smaller marrow collections, irradiated and ABO-incompatible homologous red blood cells may be added.

AUTHORS

Ellen M. Areman, M.L.T., S.B.B.(ASCP)
Bone Marrow Processing Laboratory
Division of Transfusion Medicine
Georgetown University Hospital
Washington, D.C, 20007

Herbert Cullis, B.S.
Fenwal Division
Baxter Healthcare
Deerfield, IL

REFERENCE

1. Areman, E, et al: Automated isclation of mononuclear cells using the Fenwal CS3000 blood cell separator. In Gross, SR and Gee, A (eds): Bone Marrow Purging and Processing. Proceedings of the Second International Symposium on Bone Marrow Purging and Processing. Vol. 33. Progress in Clinical and Biological Research, New York, Alan R Liss, 1990, p 379.

Automated Density Gradient Separation

AUTOMATED FICOLL-HYPAQUE MARROW PROCESSING USING THE COBE 2991

DESCRIPTION	This simplified, automated procedure facilitates processing of marrow for cryopreservation and for ABO-incompatible transplantation. This procedure should be widely applicable (i.e., useful for small as well as large transplant programs) and will produce a product with low numbers of erythrocytes and high numbers of hematopoietic mononuclear leukocytes. This technique uses the density gradient separation properties of Ficoll-Hypaque and the processing capabilities of the COBE 2991 blood cell separator. It uses a simplified, closed sterile system that consistently results in mononuclear leukocyte recoveries of more than 70 percent, with quite low levels of red cell contamination.
TIME FOR PROCEDURE	Approximately 30 minutes to purify up to 400 mL of buffy coat, and an additional 30 minutes to wash the marrow.
SUMMARY OF PROCEDURE	1. The bone marrow buffy coats are pooled into one 600-mL transfer pack.
	2. A processing set is installed in the COBE 2991 blood cell processor.
	3. The machine is set on MANUAL and the pinch valves are bypassed. All lines are clamped by hemostats.
	4. The round processing bag is filled with Ficoll-Hypaque, the centrifuge is turned on, and the bone marrow buffy coat is slowly pumped in.
	5. Mononuclear cells are collected through the RED line into a 600-mL transfer pack.
	6. Granulocytes and red blood cells can be collected into a separate bag if desired.
	7. The mononuclear product is then washed to remove the Ficoll-Hypaque.
EQUIPMENT	1. COBE 2991 blood cell processor
	2. Fenwal hemapheresis pump, Cat. No. 4R4532
SUPPLIES AND REAGENTS	1. 2 COBE 2991 processing sets, Cat. No. 912-647-819
	2. Four 600-mL transfer packs
	3. Plasma exchange set, Fenwal Cat. No. 4C2464
	4. Two 100-mL bottles Ficoll-Hypaque histopaque-1077, Cat. No. H8889, (Sigma Diagnostics)
	5. 1000-mL 0.9 percent sodium chloride for intravenous (IV) injection
	6. 500-mL anticoagulant citrate dextrose solution, formula A (ACD-A) Fenwal Cat. No. 4B7898
	7. 2 plasma transfer sets, Fenwal Cat. No. 4C2243
	8. 8 hemostats
	9. Plasma transfer set with coupler and needle, Fenwal Cat. No. 4C2242
	10. Two 18-gauge $\times$ 1.5 inch needles

PROCEDURE
1. FICOLL-HYPAQUE SEPARATION
   A. Pool buffy coats into a 600-mL transfer pack. Reserve the removed plasma for the wash solution. Transfer 200-mL 0.9 percent normal saline to a 600-mL transfer pack. This saline will be used later to dilute the buffy coat to a desired volume or to rinse the bag, or both. Set aside the remaining 800 mL saline for the wash solution.
   B. Heat seal, near the bag, the attached tubing on the remaining two 600-mL transfer packs. Remove and save the tubing.
   C. Transfer 150-mL Ficoll-Hypaque to one of the transfer packs from step 2 using the plasma transfer set with coupler and needle. Use the 18-gauge needles to vent the bottles.
   D. Install a processing set into the COBE 2991 blood cell processor, according to manufacturer's directions. Set the centrifuge speed at 3000 rpm, superout rate at 100 mL per minute, superout volume at 600 mL. Place the hemapheresis pump on a cart to the operator's right. Thread the plasma exchange tubing through the pump (input at bottom, output at top). The output is connected to the YELLOW line of the COBE 2991 software by inserting the spike on the YELLOW line into one of the female adaptors on the plasma exchange set (outlet line). The second outlet line female adaptor is heat sealed. Bypass all COBE 2991 pinch valves and red cell detector. Set machine for MANUAL operation.
   E. Clamp, with hemostats, all lines including RED, BLUE, PURPLE, GREEN, and YELLOW, and inlet to the processing bag. Hemostat the tubing below both male adaptors on the input plasma exchange set. Attach the pooled buffy coat to one male adaptor and the 200-mL normal saline to the other. Use the coupler from step 2 to spike the saline bag, then insert adaptor. Attach the Ficoll-Hypaque to the BLUE line and the remaining 600-mL transfer pack to the RED line.
   F. Before beginning the Ficoll-Hypaque procedure check all lines to ensure they are properly clamped and make certain the plasma exchange tubing is correctly threaded in the pump.
      (1) RED line: 600-mL transfer pack for collection of final product
      (2) BLUE line: 150-mL Ficoll-Hypaque
      (3) PURPLE line: To be used only to relieve excess pressure
      (4) YELLOW line: Attached to plasma exchange tubing output
      (5) GREEN line: Unattached—used to remove air from system
      (6) Plasma exchange tubing: One of the Y male adaptors attached to buffy coat, the other to 200-mL normal saline
      (7) Hemostats: Attached to RED, BLUE, PURPLE, GREEN, and YELLOW lines, buffy coat, saline, and clear inlet tubing to processing bag
   G. Hang the buffy coat and normal saline on the right-hand metal bar of the COBE 2991. Hang the bags attached to the RED and BLUE lines on the left bar.
   H. Remove hemostats attached to the BLUE line and the inlet tubing to the processing bag to allow the Ficoll-Hypaque to enter. Remove air by pressing START/SPIN then superout. When the Ficoll-Hypaque reaches the multitubing junction simultaneously, clamp the BLUE tubing and press STOP/REST. Clamp tubing to processing bag.
   I. Remove hemostats from the buffy coat bag and the YELLOW and

GREEN lines. To remove the air from the lines, start the pump at 25 mL per minute and remove the GREEN line spike protective cover enough to allow the air to escape. When the buffy coat reaches the multitubing junction, turn the pump off and reclamp the GREEN line. Remove the hemostat from the clear inlet tubing to the processing bag.

J. Press START/SPIN and turn the pump on. Overlay the buffy coat at 25 mL per minute onto the Ficoll-Hypaque. Continue until the buffy coat bag is empty. The bag can be rinsed with saline by removing the hemostat from the saline line and attaching it below the Y. This allows saline to flow into the empty buffy coat bag. Reattach hemostat to saline line after rinsing, then remove hemostat from below the Y. Rinsing can be performed while the pump is either on or off. When the fluid-air interface reaches a point approximately 3 inches above the rotating seal, turn the pump off. Clamp the YELLOW line. Spin an additional 5 to 7 minutes to achieve maximum separation.

NOTE: *The processing set maximum volume is 600 mL. Do not try to pump in more than 450 mL buffy coat/saline rinse.*

K. After the buffy coat has separated, remove the hemostat from the RED line and press SUPEROUT. Collect the plasma and mononuclear layer. Press HOLD and clamp the RED line near the multitubing junction. The granulocytes can be collected into the mononuclear bag or diverted into a separate bag by attaching a transfer pack to the GREEN line and pressing CONTINUE. Continue collecting desired cells; then press HOLD, clamp the GREEN line, and press STOP/RESET. Seal the RED line (and GREEN, if applicable) near the hemostat. Strip the lines and seal.

L. The mononuclear product is now ready for washing.

2. WASHING

A. Transfer 100 mL autologous plasma and 100 mL ACD-A to the 800-mL normal saline bag reserved in step 1 of the Ficoll-Hypaque separation.

B. Install a processing set into the COBE 2991 processor. Load tubing into the red cell detector and pinch valves. Heat seal the BLUE and YELLOW lines. Place a hemostat on the clear tubing just below the red cell detector.

C. Set the machine to MANUAL. Set the centrifuge speed at 3000 rpm, superout rate at 100 mL per minute, and valve selector to V2. The superout volume determines the final product volume. For example, a superout volume setting of 500 mL will leave 100 mL final product in the processing bag. Determine, then set, the superout volume according to desired product volume.

D. Attach the Ficoll-Hypaque product to the RED line and place the bag on the centrifuge. Attach the wash solution to the GREEN line and hang on right-hand metal bar. Press PREDILUTE and allow approximately 200 to 300 mL of wash solution to enter the bag. Press STOP/RESET and hang bag on left-hand side bar.

E. Press BLOOD IN, express any air by pressing AIR OUT, and then press START/SPIN. Spin for 5 minutes.

F. After 5 minutes, press SUPEROUT to allow supernatant to flow into the waste bag. The superout volume should be set at 450 mL for this first wash.

G. After the supernatant stops flowing (approximately 5 minutes) press AGITATE/WASH IN. Continue mixing for 3 minutes; then press START/SPIN. Spin 5 minutes.

   NOTE: *Reset superout volume at this time to desired value.*

H. After 5 minutes press SUPEROUT. Observe when the flow has stopped and press STOP/RESET. Heat seal above and below the rotating seal and remove the processing bag conatining the final product.

ANTICIPATED RESULT	This procedure should yield an average of 69 percent of the starting mononuclear cells (all nucleated white cells except segmented neutrophils), provided no more than 20 percent of the mononuclear cells were lost during the buffy coat preparation.

NOTES

1. The capacity of the COBE 2991 processing set is 600 mL. Never attempt to pump more than this into the set. Do not allow the rotating seal to remain stationary for longer than 3 minutes once fluid has passed through it. If delays occur, clamp all lines, then place the machine in AGITATE WASH IN by pressing in sequence START/SPIN, SUPEROUT, AGITATE WASH IN.

2. The final marrow product can be removed from the processing set through a COBE 2991 Sampling Site and Access Coupler Cat. No. 912-647-903.

AUTHORS

Vicki L. Graves, M.T.(ASCP)
Indiana University Hospital
Indianapolis, IN 46202-5283

Leo J. McCarthy, M.D.
Indiana University Hospital
Indianapolis, IN 46202-5283

Jan Jansen, M.D.
Methodist Hospital
Indianapolis, IN 46204

Denis English, Ph.D.
Bone Marrow Transplant Laboratory
Methodist Hospital of Indiana
1701 N. Senate
MPC, Rm 1417
Indianapolis, IN 46202

BONE MARROW PROCESSING USING THE COBE 2991 CELL PROCESSOR WITH TRIPLE PROCESSING SET

DESCRIPTION	The efficiency of pharmacologic and immunologic marrow purging techniques may be adversely affected by large amounts of red blood cells and polymorphonuclear granulocytes. To reduce these components, a mononuclear cell fraction may be obtained by layering over a density gradient such as Ficoll-Hypaque. This procedure outlines marrow processing done on the COBE 2991 equipped with the triple-processing set.* This set both reduces the processing time and provides a more closed system when compared with the use of multiple single-processing sets.
TIME FOR PROCEDURE	Approximately 2 to 4 hours, for volumes up to 3 L of marrow, to obtain a washed mononuclear cell fraction
SUMMARY OF PROCEDURE	1. The triple processing set is placed on the instrument and prepared for processing.
	2. The marrow is separated into plasma, buffy coat, and red blood cell components. The plasma is collected and removed for use in cryopreservation. Interim buffy coats are collected within the system, as are red cells.
	3. Once all the marrow has been separated, the interim buffy coats are added back to the bowl and spun to yield a final concentrated buffy coat product. This is collected and retained within the system. The packed red cells are removed for immediate autologous reinfusion.
	4. The buffy coat is layered over a Ficoll-diatrizoate density gradient. Granulocytes and remaining red blood cells pass through the Ficoll and the mononuclear cell fraction is collected.
	5. The mononuclear cell fraction is washed with saline in an automated procedure to remove any remaining Ficoll.
EQUIPMENT	1. COBE 2991 cell processor (COBE, Lakewood, CO)
	2. Sebra tube sealer (DuPont, Glenolden, PA)
	3. Timer (Baxter, McGaw Park, IL)
	4. Peristaltic pump (Cole-Parmer, Chicago)
	5. Hemostats (Fisher, Pittsburgh)
SUPPLIES	1. COBE 2991 triple-processing set (COBE, Lakewood, CO)
	2. COBE 2991 double-coupler adaptor (COBE, Lakewood, CO)
	3. Transfer packs, 300 and 600 mL (Baxter-Fenwal, Deerfield, IL)
	4. Transfer sets, double coupler and with needle adaptor (Baxter-Fenwal, Deerfield, IL)
	5. 1000-mL saline bags (hospital pharmacy)
	6. Lymphocyte Separation Media (Organon Teknika, Durham, NC)

---

*Portions of this procedure are copyrighted by COBE Laboratories, Inc., 1990.

7. Sampling site couplers (Baxter-Fenwal, Deerfield, IL)

8. Heparin, 10,000 U per mL (hospital pharmacy)

PROCEDURE   1. BUFFY COAT COLLECTION AND CONCENTRATION

A. Turn on the COBE 2991 and allow to warm up for several minutes. Make initial instrument settings:

- Centrifuge speed (rpm): 3000
- Superout rate (mL/min): 450
- Valve selector: V-2
- Superout volume (mL): 600
- Processing mode switch: MANUAL

B. Install a triple-processing set as in Figure 6–4
  (1) Place the PURPLE and GREEN lines into their respective pinch valves.
  (2) Place the RED and YELLOW lines in the blocks in front of their pinch valves.
  (3) Do *not* put the clear line in the RBC detector.
  (4) Place the other two processing bags on the back of the centrifuge cover.
  (5) Attach a double coupler adaptor to the YELLOW line.
  (6) Close all slide clamps.
  (7) Place hemostats at the locations indicated (Fig. 6–4).
  (8) Press STOP/RESET to close all valves.

C. Under the hood, fill a 300-mL transfer pack with exactly 200 mL of Ficoll-Hypaque.

D. Attach solutions to lines as follows:
  (1) Empty 600-mL transfer pack to one RED line spike; label "Interim B.C."

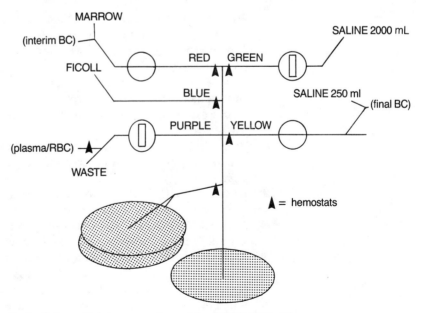

FIGURE 6–4   Setup of triple processing set for COBE 2991 cell processor.

   (2) Ficoll to the BLUE line.

   (3) Empty 300-mL transfer pack to the spike off of the PURPLE waste line; label "Plasma Collection."

   (4) 250-mL saline bag to one YELLOW line spike.

   (5) Empty 300-mL transfer pack to the other YELLOW line spike; label "Final B.C."

   (6) Two 1000-mL saline bags to the GREEN line spikes.

E. When marrow arrives in laboratory, weigh each bag and then attach them together with transfer sets. Remove 1 mL for cell count. Attach to remaining RED line spike.

F. Open up the slide clamp on the RED line leading to the bone marrow bags.

G. Press BLOOD IN. Remove the RED line hemostat and allow the marrow to fill the processing bag.

H. When the flow ceases, press AIR OUT. When all of the air reaches the marrow bag, press BLOOD IN and allow the processing bag to completely fill. Then press STOP/RESET.

I. Reclamp the RED line. Check to make sure the instrument is in MANUAL mode. Press SPIN; set a timer for 5 minutes.

J. When the timer sounds, release the RED line clamp for several seconds to allow the marrow remaining in the tubing to be pushed back up the RED line. Then reclamp the RED line.

K. To collect autologous plasma, perform the following steps:

   (1) Place hemostats on the PURPLE line directly above the waste bag.

   (2) Remove the hemostats on the line leading to the plasma collection bag.

   (3) Press SUPEROUT.

   (4) Collect approximately 300 mL of plasma, then press HOLD.

   (5) Clamp the line to plasma collection bag and unclamp the line to waste bag.

L. Press CONTINUE and express plasma to waste until the buffy coat layer is ½ inch from the inner silver ring. Then press AGITATE-WASH IN.

M. Remove the RED line hemostats and allow the bowl to refill. Then reclamp the RED line.

N. Press SPIN; set a timer for 5 minutes. Remove the plasma collection bag and replace with a 600-mL transfer pack labeled "RBC collection." Place a sampling site coupler in the open port of the plasma collection bag to seal it.

O. When the timer sounds, release the RED line clamp for several seconds to allow the marrow in the tubing to be pushed back up the RED line. Then reclamp the RED line.

P. Press SUPEROUT and express plasma to waste until the buffy coat layer is ½ inch from the inner silver ring.

Q. Press AGITATE-WASH IN. Unclamp the RED line and allow the marrow to refill the bowl, then reclamp the RED line.

R. Press START SPIN; set a timer for 5 minutes.

S. Repeat steps O through R *until the amount of marrow added to the bag in step Q was 200 mL or less. Then proceed directly to step T.*

T. When the timer sounds, perform the following steps:

   (1) Release the RED line hemostats for several seconds, then reclamp.

Press SUPEROUT. When buffy coat is ½ inch from the inner silver ring, press HOLD.

(2) Close the slide clamp on RED line leading to the unprocessed marrow. Then open the slide clamp leading to the "Interim B.C."

(3) Turn the superout rate down to 100 mL per minute.

(4) Place hemostats on the PURPLE line near the main junction.

(5) Remove the hemostats from the RED line.

(6) Press CONTINUE. Collect into the "Interim B.C." bag for 45 to 60 seconds (equal to 75 to 100 mL), then press HOLD.

(7) Reclamp the RED line with hemostats.

(8) Close the slide clamp to the "Interim B.C." bag. Open the slide clamp on the unprocessed marrow line.

(9) Remove the hemostats from the PURPLE line. Replace them on the line immediately above the waste bag. Remove the hemostats on the line leading to the "RBC collection" bag.

(10) Press CONTINUE. Turn the superout rate back up to 450 mL per minute. Collect RBCs until flow stops. Then press AGITATE-WASH IN.

(11) Remove the hemostats from the RED line and allow the bowl to fill with marrow. Then reclamp the RED line.

(12) Place hemostats on the line leading to the "RBC collection" bag. Remove the hemostats leading to the waste bag.

(13) Press START/SPIN; set timer for 5 minutes.

U. Repeat steps O through T until all of the bone marrow has been processed.

V. *On the final bowl fill,* use the interim buffy coat to fill the bowl, as follows:

(1) Allow the unprocessed marrow to drain until the trailing edge reaches the junction with the interim buffy coat bag; then clamp the RED line with hemostats.

(2) Close the slide clamp to the marrow bag, and open the slide clamp to the interim buffy coat bag.

(3) Remove the RED line hemostats and allow the buffy coat to drain into the bowl until the trailing edge reaches the top of the main junction. Then clamp the clear line above the rotating seal with hemostats.

(4) Remove the interim buffy coat bag from the hanger bar and place on the centrifuge lid. Open the slide clamps on the GREEN line saline bags. Press STOP/RESET; then press PREDILUTE. Allow approximately 50 mL of saline into the bag as a rinse; then press STOP/RESET. Rehang the interim buffy coat bag.

(5) Remove the clamp on the clear line. Allow the rinse to drain into the bag until the trailing edge reaches the top of the manifold; then clamp the RED line. Press TUBE LOAD to top off the bowl with saline; then press STOP/RESET.

(6) Press START/SPIN; set timer for *8 minutes.*

W. To collect the final concentrated buffy coat, when the timer sounds, perform the following steps:

(1) Press SUPEROUT and express plasma to waste until the buffy coat is ½ inch from the inner silver ring. Then press HOLD.

(2) Clamp the PURPLE line and unclamp the YELLOW line. Open the slide clamp on the "Final BC" bag.

(3) Press CONTINUE and collect 100 mL by time (60 seconds) or weight.

(4) Press HOLD. Clamp the YELLOW line. Move the clamp on the PURPLE line to directly above the waste bag. Remove the clamp on the line to the "RBC collection" bag.

(5) Turn the superout rate to 100 mL per minute. Press CONTINUE. Collect RBC until the flow ceases, then press STOP/RESET.

(6) Heat seal and remove the used processing bag. Heat seal and remove the RBC collection bag. Apportion the RBCs into units of 300 to 500 mL, label appropriately, and send to blood bank to be irradiated (along with autologous plasma).

2. MONONUCLEAR CELL SEPARATION

A. Load the pump tubing segment on the YELLOW line into the peristaltic pump. After making sure the tubing is occluded in the pump, remove the hemostats from the YELLOW line.

NOTE: *If a buffy coat backup is to be removed, a cell count must be taken at this point and the appropriate volume removed.*

B. Dilute the buffy coat by holding the 250-mL saline bag above the buffy coat bag and then opening the slide clamp. Allow approximately 200 mL of saline into the buffy coat bag; then close the clamp.

C. Make the instrument settings as follows:

• Centrifuge speed (rpm): 2000
• Superout rate (mL/min): 100
• Valve selector: V-2
• Superout volume (mL): 600
• Processing mode switch: MANUAL

D. Load the second processing bag into the centrifuge. *Do not* load the clear line into the RBC cell detector.

E. With hemostats, clamp off the remaining processing bag near the junction.

F. Remove the hemostats from the BLUE line, allowing all the Ficoll-Hypaque to drain into the bowl. Then reclamp the BLUE line.

G. Press START/SPIN. When the bowl is up to speed, press SUPEROUT. Allow the air to be pushed out of the bowl until the Ficoll-Hypaque barely enters the PURPLE line; then press STOP/RESET.

H. Press START/SPIN. When the bowl is up to speed, start the peristaltic pump at a rate of 10 mL per minute. Once the interface is established, the rate may be turned up to 60 mL per minute.

I. Stop the pump when the trailing edge of the fluid reaches the junction with the saline bag. Open the slide clamp and allow the remaining saline to flow into the buffy coat bag. Close slide clamp on saline line.

J. Turn the pump back on and pump the rinse into the bowl until the trailing edge is 2 to 3 inches above the rotating seal.

K. Set a timer for 15 minutes.

L. When the timer sounds, press SUPEROUT. Express the supernatant to the waste bag until the interface is ½ inch from the inner silver ring; then press HOLD.

M. Place hemostats on the clear line just above the junction with the remaining processing bag. Remove the hemostat below the junction.

N. Press CONTINUE and allow the mononuclear cell interface to be collected into the third processing bag. *The volume collected should be determined visually by the operator. Normally 100 to 150 mL is sufficient to ensure complete layer collection.* When the desired volume has been collected, press HOLD.

O. With hemostats, clamp the clear line above the third processing bag. Press STOP/RESET.

3. MONONUCLEAR CELL WASHING

A. Heat seal and remove the processing bag from the bowl. (*Do not* seal off the third processing bag.) Load the third bag (with mononuclear cell fraction) into the bowl. (*Do not* place the clear line in the RBC detector.)

B. Open up the slide clamps leading to the saline bags on the GREEN line.

C. Make instrument settings as follows:

- Centrifuge speed (rpm): 3000
- Superout rate (mL/min): 450
- Minimum agitate time: 70
- Superout volume (mL): 450
- Valve selector: V-2
- Mode selector switch: MANUAL
- Timer 1 (minutes): 2
- Timer 2 (minutes): 3

D. Set the pin board as diagrammed in Figure 6–5:

E. Remove the hemostats from the clear line. Press TUBE LOAD and allow the bowl to fill with saline. When flow ceases, press STOP/RESET.

F. Remove air from the bag by pressing START/SPIN. When the bowl is at speed, press SUPEROUT until fluid almost reaches the PURPLE line; then press STOP/RESET.

G. Press TUBE LOAD, top off the bowl with saline; then press STOP/RESET.

H. Switch the mode selector to AUTO; then press START/SPIN.

I. When the instrument sounds, change the superout volume to 550 mL. Remove the diode pin from the timer 2 column. Press CONTINUE.

J. When the instrument sounds again; press STOP/RESET.

K. Heat seal the processing bag and remove it from the bowl. Under the hood, place a sampling site coupler into the port on the bag and clean

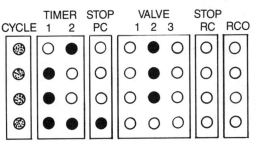

FIGURE 6–5 Pin board settings for bone marrow processing using COBE 2991 and triple processing set.

it with a povidone-iodine swab. Draw the mononuclear cell fraction into a syringe and record the volume.

ANTICIPATED RESULTS	Harvest volumes are calculated on an anticipated minimum return of 10 percent of total nucleated cells. Common values are from 20 to 40 percent. The minimum acceptable number of cells for reinfusion is 0.2×10^8 per kg of patient's weight.

NOTES

1. To collect the final buffy coat in step V, there must be an adequate volume of packed RBCs (200 to 300 mL) in the bowl. If necessary, interim RBCs may be added back to the bowl by spiking onto the RED line.

2. All operators should be thoroughly familiar with the operation of the COBE 2991.

3. For volumes less than 1200 mL it should not be necessary to collect interim buffy coats. The RBCs may be left in the processing bag after final buffy coat collection.

4. Processing should not be started until all of the marrow is in the laboratory. Delays of greater than 3 minutes during the processing may result in rotating seal failure.

5. Care should be taken to ensure an open pathway before pressing SUPER-OUT; failure to do so will result in seal rupture.

6. At no point in the procedure should the clear line be loaded into the RBC detector.

7. After dilution with saline, the final buffy coat volume must not exceed 350 mL.

8. If volume-specific collections are made on a timed basis, the superout rate calibration should be checked beforehand.

9. Care should be taken to ensure the exclusion of air from the rotating seal during centrifugation. The RED line hemostats may be released briefly (1 to 2 seconds) to push such a bubble out of the seal area.

10. All sampling site couplers must be swabbed with povidone-iodine prior to needle entry.

AUTHORS

Charles S. Johnston, M.T.(AMT)
Bone Marrow Transplant Program
University Hospital
Denver, CO 80262

Elizabeth J. Shpall, M.D.
Bone Marrow Transplant Program
University Hospital
Denver, CO 80262

Lisa S. Fox, M.T.(ASCP)
Bone Marrow Transplant Program
University Hospital
Denver, CO 80262

REFERENCES

1. COBE 2991 Model 1 Blood Cell Processor Operations Manual. Cobe Laboratories, 1985.
2. McMannis, J: COBE Guidelines for Bone Marrow Processing at CUHSC Using the COBE 2991 Cell Processor. Personal communication, 1990.
3. Mononuclear cell separation, Cryopreservation Laboratory Procedure Manual, Bone Marrow Transplant Program, Duke University Medical Center, Durham, NC, 1989.

BONE MARROW PROCESSING USING THE HAEMONETICS V-50

DESCRIPTION	Red cell depletion of bone marrow is necessary in both autologous and allogeneic transplants. When preparing cells for cryopreservation for future autologous transplants, the bone marrow volume needs to be reduced and red cells and granulocytes need to be depleted. In allogeneic transplants, in cases of ABO incompatibility, the red cells need to be depleted. We use the Haemonetics V-50 apheresis system to accomplish both tasks. We use two protocols: (1) the bone marrow protocol, which concentrates the bone marrow buffy coat (some granulocytes are lost in the red cell bag); and (2) the Ficoll-Hypaque protocol, which isolates the mononuclear cells. This is accomplished in a sterile, closed cell separation system.
TIME FOR PROCEDURE	60 minutes

SUMMARY OF PROCEDURE

1. Harvested bone marrow is delivered to the laboratory in a bag. Samples are taken for a nucleated cell count, hematocrit (Hct), and other tests and cultures as required.
2. If the packed cell volume (Hct $\times$ total marrow volume) is greater than 300 mL, the bone marrow protocol can be followed. (There needs to be a sufficient red cell volume to displace the buffy cells.) If the packed cell volume is less than 300 mL, the Ficoll-Hypaque protocol is followed. (Ficoll-Hypaque isolates the mononuclear layer.)
3. The 301 kit is loaded into the machine. Saline with 10,000 units of preservative-free heparin per L are added to one of the lines. A 1000-mL and a 600-mL transfer bag are added, as explained in the Haemonetics procedure manual.
4. 6 mL of concentrated sodium citrate per L of marrow are added to the bone marrow. Mix well and attach the bone marrow bag to the 301 kit.
5. The protocol is followed as written in the Haemonetics procedure manual.
6. The product is removed from the apheresis machine and a sample is taken to determine nucleated cell counts, cell recovery, Hct, and so on.

EQUIPMENT

1. Haemonetics V-50 Plus apheresis system
2. Microhematocrit centrifuge

SUPPLIES AND REAGENTS

1. Haemonetics 301 disposable set
2. 1000-mL transfer bag
3. 600-mL transfer bag
4. 500-mL bag of saline (containing 5000 units of preservative-free heparin)
5. 500-mL bottle of Ficoll-Hypaque
6. Sodium citrate concentrate (46.7 percent trisodium citrate)

PROCEDURE

1. Haemonetics
   A. After doing a cell count and measuring Hct on the bone marrow, determine the packed cell volume (Hct $\times$ total marrow volume). If it is

greater than 300 mL, follow the Haemonetics V-50 bone marrow protocol. Add 6 mL of concentrated citrate per L of marrow. Mix well.

(1) Install the 301 kit in the V-50 after inspecting it for kinks or serious imperfections in the plastic.

(2) Secure the bowl in the centrifuge chuck.

(3) Hang the waste bag lower than the outlet tube on the bowl.

(4) Press LOAD to open all of the valves. Place tubing from the waste bag through valve 3. Attach a 600-mL transfer bag on the tubing in valve 2. Clamp off the other extra line in valve 1.

(5) Attach the bone marrow to one spike and a 500-mL bag of saline (with 5000 units of preservative-free heparin) to the other spike of the same Y. Add a 1000-mL transfer bag to the other spike. The spike with the vent on it is extra. Clamp it closed.

(6) Press COMP and the V-50 will display the available component protocols, starting with "PLATELET Y/N." Answer NO until the display reads "LYMPHOCYTE Y/N" and then press YES.

(7) Leave the number of cycles at 08. Press MOD until the display reads "AUTOSURGE—Yes." Press NO. Press MOD again until display reads "RBC VOLUME," then enter 60 (or more if you want to cut more deeply into the red cell layer).

(8) Unclamp the line to the bone marrow and press DRAW. Fill the bowl at a pump speed of 80 mL per minute. When the buffy coat fans over the shoulder of the bowl, the pump speed drops to 20 mL per minute.

(9) Start collecting the cells when the buffy coat fans over the white part of the bowl (before the machine would automatically start collecting). Collect the cells by closing valve 3 and opening valve 2. It will now collect 60 mL into the red cells.

(10) The centrifuge and pumps stop automatically. Close valve 2 (clamping off the bone marrow product bag) and open the line to the 1000-mL transfer bag. In the return mode the machine pumps the processed red cells into this bag. Repeat these steps until all of the marrow has been processed. (On the last pass, if there are not enough red cells to pump out the buffy cells, use the already processed red cells to pump out the bone marrow.)

(11) Remove the bone marrow bag and under the hood take a sample for cell counts and a hematocrit, if necessary. Determine nucleated cell recovery.

B. If the packed cell volume is 240-mL or less, use the Haemonetics V-50 Ficoll-Hypaque protocol.

(1) Install the 301 kit and secure the bowl in the centrifuge as in step A.

(2) Press LOAD to open all valves. Place tubing from the waste bag through valve 3. Attach a 600-mL transfer bag on the tubing in valve 1. Clamp off the extra line in valve 2.

(3) Attach the bone marrow to one spike and a 500-mL bag of saline (and heparin) to the other spike of the same Y. Add the Ficoll-Hypaque to the vented spike and prime the line as far as the pump. Clamp off the Ficoll-Hypaque line. A waste bag can be added to the other spike of the Ficoll-Hypaque Y. Press LOAD to close all valves.

(4) Press COMP and the display reads "PLATELET Y/N." Answer NO until the display reads "MANUAL COMPONENT." Press YES.

(5) Set the RBC volume to 999. Press MOD button and set the centrifuge speed to 3000 rpm.

(6) Open the bone marrow line and press DRAW. Fill the bowl at a rate of 40 mL per minute.

(7) After all of the marrow buffy coat enters the bowl and the marrow bag is washed, add saline to fill the bowl.

(8) Close the wash line, open the Ficoll-Hypaque line and allow the Ficoll-Hypaque to enter at 20 mL per minute. After approximately 50 mL of Ficoll-Hypaque has entered the bowl, stop the pump.

(9) Increase the centrifuge speed to 5600 rpm in 200 rpm increments using the MOD button.

(10) Open the Ficoll-Hypaque line and pump at a speed of 20 mL per minute. When the white cell layer reaches the shoulder of the bowl, open valve 1 and close valve 3. (If the white cells are not easily discernible, start collecting after 200 mL of Ficoll-Hypaque have entered the bowl.)

(11) When the effluent line in valve 1 is clear, close valve 1 and open valve 3. Stop the centrifuge and pumps. The product should be 100 to 150 mL.

(12) The Ficoll-Hypaque can be washed from the marrow using the Haemonetics V-50 wash procedure, or the product bag can be removed from the machine and spun in a regular centrifuge to wash out the Ficoll-Hypaque. Cell counts are done to determine cell recovery.

ANTICIPATED RESULTS

1. The average cell recovery from the bone marrow concentration protocol is 68 percent (± 14 percent).

2. The average cell recovery from the Ficoll-Hypaque protocol is 16.4 percent (± 10.8 percent).

NOTES

1. Concentrated sodium citrate is added to the bone marrow to reduce cell clumping.

2. The air flow detector box on the Haemonetics V-50 must be taped with the bottom of the box down. This allows the pump to go faster.

3. We allow saline to flow into the bowl at the beginning of either procedure to make sure the bowl is properly seated and everything is running smoothly before marrow enters the system.

AUTHORS

Mary Ann Gross, M.T.(ASCP)
Shands Hospital
University of Florida
Gainesville, FL 32610

Charles E. Hutcheson, M.T.(ASCP)
Shands Hospital
University of Florida
Gainesville, FL 32610

REFERENCES

1. Weiner, RS, Richman, CM, and Yankee, RA: Semi-continuous flow centrifugation for the pheresis of immunocompetent cells and stem cells. Blood 49:391, 1977.

2. Johnson, KA, Smith, JW, and Halpern, LN: Automated techniques for mononuclear cell purification using the Haemonetics V-50. European Bone Marrow Transplant Association Meeting, Interlaken, Switzerland. Bone Marrow Transplant 2 (Suppl 1):74, 1987.

3. Haemonetics V-50 Standard Operating Procedure—Bone Marrow Processing. Haemonetics Corp, Braintree, MA.

GRADIENT SEPARATION AND WASHING OF BONE MARROW USING TERUMO STERICELL PROCESSOR

DESCRIPTION	Erythrocytes and granulocytes in the bone marrow are separated according to their density. All separations are performed in a latham bowl, which accentuates normal gravitational forces with centrifugal forces. If the red cell volume of the marrow is large, a buffy coat separation is performed. In buffy coat formation, the nucleated cells in the marrow "float" (by virtue of their lesser density) on top of the red blood cells (RBCs). The nucleated cells are pushed up through and out of the latham bowl by the advancing erythrocyte volume.
	The gradient separation employs a solution of complex sugar (Ficoll) which has a defined density (1.077 g per mL). All of the cells from the buffy coat product, or, if there were insufficient erythrocytes to perform a buffy coat, from the fresh marrow specimen, are loaded into the latham bowl. The density separation solution is then slowly pumped into the bowl. The mononuclear cells in the marrow "float" on the density separation solution, and are lifted up through and out of the bowl, while the erythrocytes and granulocytes, which are of a density greater than 1.077 g per mL, remain in the bottom of the bowl.
	Residual density separation solution (Ficoll-Hypaque) is removed from the mononuclear marrow cells, and they are prepared for infusion (following freezing process when indicated) into the recipient by washing and resuspending in a medium of physiologic salts, vitamins, and amino acids (Medium 199) and human plasma proteins (PlasmaPlex).
TIME FOR PROCEDURE	Approximately 1 to 2 hours from buffy coat decision point (see farther on) to end of wash process.
EQUIPMENT	1. SteriCell processor (Terumo Medical Corp., Elkton, MD)
	2. SteriCell Sterile Connecting Device (SCD) sterile tubing welder
	3. Tube sealer (Sebra)
	4. Hemacytometer (Neubauer ruled)
	5. Timer with sweep second hand
	6. Hemostats (at least 6)
SUPPLIES AND REAGENTS	1. SteriCell gradient/wash set (Terumo Cat. No. NCC-902)
	2. Haemonetics Pedi-Bowl (only required for small RBC volumes)
	3. SteriCell large cell-culture bags (Terumo Cat. No. NCC-910)
	4. Sterile saline, 1-L bag
	5. Ficoll-Hypaque, 1.077 g per mL (Ficoll-Hypaque, Cat. No. 17-0840-03, Pharmacia), 500 mL
	6. Medium 199 with 10 percent PlasmaPlex (PPF), 1 L
	7. 2 SteriCell Y adaptors (Terumo Cat. No. NCC-951)
	8. 2 SteriCell nonvented spike adaptors (Terumo Cat. No. NCC-953)
	9. 2 SteriCell vented spike adaptors (Terumo Cat. No. NCC-954)
	10. 3 percent glacial acetic acid: 97 mL distilled water + 3.0 mL glacial acetic acid or Unopettes for white blood cell (WBC) counting (preferred)
	11. Physiologic saline (0.9 percent) or Unopettes (preferred) for RBC counting

12. Microbiologic assay vials (DuPont Isolators, obtain from central laboratory)

13. Syringes: 3 mL

14. Heparin, sodium, preservative-free, 1000 U/mL and 50 U/mL in Medium 199 (see procedure for making up harvest medium)

PROCEDURE

1. PREPARATIVE STEPS TO PERFORM DAY PRECEDING PROCEDURE
    A. Thoroughly clean biologic safety cabinet with disinfecting agent. Cleaning should include ceiling of cabinet, all walls, inside of glass, plenum below work-tray, and work-tray.
    B. Prepare wash/freeze medium (Medium 199, supplemented with 10 percent PlasmaPlex).

2. INITIAL MEASUREMENTS AND STEPS TO PERFORM AFTER SPECIMEN ARRIVAL IN LABORATORY
    A. Record time of specimen arrival in laboratory, and general condition of specimen (with respect to clotting/clumping, observable hemolysis, and so on).
    B. In biologic safety cabinet, hang marrow collection bag. Insert sampling site coupler into one free spike port, and remove through needle port samples for colony-forming unit (CFU) assay (3.0 mL), cytospin or smear preparation, WBC/RBC counts, and spun hematocrit (Hct) (0.5 mL); and microbiologic assay (7.5 mL distributed as follows: orange top BacTec, 3.0 mL, green top BacTec, 3.0 mL, DuPont Isolator, 1.5 mL).
        (1) Clamp the transfer line on a 2000-mL transfer bag, and spike into the other spike port on the marrow collection bag. Hang marrow collection bag from IV pole on SteriCell instrument. Hang transfer bag on scale on SteriCell, and tare. Open clamp and allow all marrow to flow into transfer bag. Record weight of marrow (this equals approximate volume).
    C. Perform WBC count by diluting 20 μL of sample with 180 μL of 3 percent acetic acid solution (1 in 10 dilution). Fill chamber of hemacytometer and count four outer squares.

    WBC/mL = 1/dilution $\times$ (cells in 4 squares) $\times$ 2.5 $\times$ 10^3

    Alternatively, Unopette diluters (1:20) for WBC counts may be used, and the same formula employed.
    D. Stain cytospin or smear preparations using rapid staining kit (Diff-Quick). Dry slide and perform differential count. *If abnormal cells are present, or if myeloid precursors are absent, contact attending physician on bone marrow transplant service.*
    Compute fraction of mononuclear cells in marrow as:

$$\text{Mononuclear fraction} = \frac{\text{Myeloid precursors} + \text{Erythroid precursors} + \text{Lymphocytes} + \text{Monocytes}}{\text{Total leukocytes counted in smear}}$$

    Compute number of mononuclear cells per mL of marrow as:

    Mononuclear cells/mL = WBC/mL $\times$ Mononuclear fraction

If number of mononuclear cells is low and/or volume of marrow is less than 500 mL, it may be necessary to perform a manual separation procedure.

E. Perform RBC count by adding 20 μL of sample to 3.98 mL of physiologic saline (0.9 percent NaCl in water). Fill chamber of hemacytometer and count cells in five small squares in center square. Note whether cells appear normocytic (approximately 5 RBCs should line up inside smallest squares on Neubauer-type hemacytometer), microcytic, or macrocytic.

$$RBC/mL = \text{Cells in 5 small squares} \times 5 \times 200 \times 10^4$$

Alternatively, Unopette diluters (1:200) for RBC counts may be used, and the same formula should be employed.

F. Obtain a *spun* Hct, and compute the volume of erythrocytes in the marrow as:

$$RBC \text{ volume} = (Hct/100) \times \text{marrow volume (from step 2B1)}$$

Compute the mean corpuscular volume (MCV) of the RBC as:

$$MCV = \frac{Hct/100}{RBC/mL}$$

The MCV will be used to compute remaining RBC volumes based on RBC counts later in the procedure.

3. BUFFY COAT DECISION POINT
   A. *If the red blood cell volume is in excess of 150 mL,* a buffy coat process should be carried out as described in the procedure *Buffy Coat Separation Using Terumo SteriCell Processor.* The resultant buffy coat product can then be separated on the Ficoll-Hypaque gradient.
   B. *If the red cell volume is less than 150 mL,* then buffy coat preparation cannot be performed, and the Ficoll-Hypaque separation procedure should be undertaken directly.

4. STERICELL SETUP FOR FICOLL-HYPAQUE GRADIENT SEPARATION
   A. Install a gradient/wash set into the SteriCell processor, as per the operations manual page 2–4 through 2–9. If a buffy coat preparation has been performed on the marrow using a *large* gradient/wash bowl, then that set may remain in place and be used for the Ficoll-Hypaque separation also. If a buffy coat preparation has not been performed, or if the preparation was performed in a pediatric size bowl, then a new gradient/wash set must be installed as follows:
      (1) Verify that the chuck O ring is in place and has a light coating of silicone grease. Verify that the chuck screws are loose.
      (2) Open SteriCell gradient/wash set (Terumo Cat. No. NCC-902). Holding latham bowl right-side-up, allow all lines to fall to full extension.
      (3) Drape the tubing with bags attached to the right side of the SteriCell processor. Drape the tubing with no bags attached to the left side of the machine.
      (4) While tilting the bowl toward the front of the processor, seat the front edge of the bowl into the centrifuge chuck. Then tilt the

bowl back, applying even pressure to opposite sides of the shoulder of the bowl to seat it fully in the centrifuge chuck. An audible snap with be heard when the bowl seats fully.

(5) Hold the body of the bowl and tighten the chuck screws in clockwise sequence with the chuck tool. Turn each screw until resistance is felt. Then make a second round turning each screw until the torque setting on the chuck tool is reached (chuck tool will click).

(6) Turn the bowl 90 degrees so that the GREEN and ORANGE lines (bags attached) are directed away from the control panel, and the BLUE, YELLOW, and RED lines (no bags) are directed *toward* the control panel. Swing the feed tube support arms into place, engage the cam lock, and rotate until it comes to a stop.

(7) Ensure that the bowl can turn freely. If it cannot, remove it and repeat aforementioned sequence.

(8) Lead the BLUE inlet tube through the rear slot; then drape to the front of the pump, align in pump using the plastic stops on the tubes, and close the cover of the pump.

(9) Lead the BLUE inlet tube through the blue side of the valve farthest from the control panel. Close the valve by pressing the BLUE button on the control panel, and drape the other inlet tube through the other side of the same valve. Drape the RED inlet tube through the red side of the valve closest to the control panel; then close that valve by pressing either the RED or YELLOW buttons, and drape the YELLOW inlet tube through the other side of the same valve.

(10) Lead the GREEN outlet line through the green side of the valve on the front of the processor, and hang the attached waste bag to hooks on the side of the machine. Change the position of the front valve by pressing the GREEN or ORANGE buttons on the control panel, and lead the ORANGE outlet tube through the other side of the valve. Hang the collection bag on the scale hanger and tare.

(11) *Close the cover to the centrifuge. Check that all lines not to be used for the next procedure are pinch-clamped, and that all lines that are to be used are open and have containers attached to them.*

5. BEGIN GRADIENT (FICOLL-HYPAQUE) SEPARATION

A. Using the SCD and appropriate spike connectors, connect the 1-L bag of saline to the YELLOW line, the 500-mL bottle of Ficoll-Hypaque to the RED line, and the buffy coat product (or fresh marrow if no buffy coat performed) bag to one of the BLUE lines. If regular cell collection bag has been removed from the ORANGE line, replace it with a SteriCell small-culture bag.

B. Prime the Ficoll-Hypaque line as follows:

(1) Open the RED valve, close the BLUE valve, and open the GREEN valve.

(2) START the pump and check that the fluid is flowing from the Ficoll-Hypaque bag.

(3) STOP the pump when the fluid gets to the Y at the RED and YELLOW valves.

C. Push the GRADIENT SEPARATION protocol button on the SteriCell control panel. *(YELLOW valve opens; BLUE valve closed; GREEN valve open.)*

D. Push the START/ADVANCE button. *(Pump starts; 250 mL saline is loaded into bowl. After 250 mL of saline is loaded, BLUE line opens and cells are pumped into the bowl.)*

E. When all of the cells have been loaded (trailing edge of cells past the Y at the entry to the pump), press the START/ADVANCE button again. *(RED valve opens; BLUE valve closes; 60 mL of Ficoll-Hypaque is pumped into bowl. Pump stops; centrifuge speed increases from 3000 to 4200 rpm. Pump starts; Ficoll-Hypaque is pumped into bowl; nucleated cell layer begins to be lifted to the top of the bowl.)*

F. When greater than 100 mL of Ficoll has been pumped into the bowl, or a visible cell layer is at the shoulder of the bowl, press START/ADVANCE button again. *(GREEN valve closes; ORANGE valve opens; cells are collected into collection bag.)*

G. When 200 mL of cells (in Ficoll-Hypaque) have been collected or the outlet line leading from the bowl is clear by visual inspection, press the START/ADVANCE button *(pump stops; centrifuge stops; ORANGE valve closes; GREEN valve opens; BLUE valve opens; YELLOW valve opens; waste material is pumped to original bag on BLUE line [should be approximately 270 mL volume]. Bowl Cleaning Step—repeated 3 times: YELLOW valve opens; BLUE valve closes; 50 mL saline is added to bowl. Pump stops; centrifuge stops; BLUE valve opens; YELLOW valve closes, pump starts; 50 mL is pumped out of bowl; cycle repeats).*

H. At this point the gradient separation procedure is finished. The SteriCell will indicate on its control panel that it is back in manual mode. Inspect the bowl to ensure that it is empty of all fluid. If it is not, set pump to EMPTY, check that BLUE valve is open, GREEN valve is open, and start pump. Run pump until bowl is empty; then press STOP.

I. Determine volume of Ficoll-Hypaque separated product from SteriCell instrument scale and add 2 mL heparin (1000 U/mL) through the needle port. This will inhibit clot formation owing to residual clotting factors.

J. Collect samples from the product bag and perform WBC counts as described in step C. Prepare cytospin or smear slides for differential analysis.

6. CELL WASH PROCESS
   A. Using SCD sterile tube welder:
      (1) Connect 1-L Medium 199 with PlasmaPlex to RED line.
      (2) Leave remaining saline from preceding parts of procedure on YELLOW line.
      (3) Attach collected Ficoll-Hypaque separated product cells to BLUE line (it is recommended that the BLUE line previously used for the RBC byproduct of the Ficoll process be used for these cells).
      (4) Attach empty large SteriCell culture bag to other BLUE line (it is recommended that the BLUE line previously used for entering buffy coat product or fresh marrow into the gradient separation process be employed for the empty bag). Clamp this line, hang the empty bag on the scale, and tare.

B. Push WASH protocol button *(BLUE valve closes; YELLOW valve opens; GREEN valve opens)*.

C. Push START/ADVANCE button *(250 mL saline is pumped into bowl; after saline is pumped, BLUE valve opens and cells are pumped into bowl; Display reads: "FIRST CELL LOADING")*.

D. When all the cells have been loaded into the bowl (trailing edge of cells passes Y and entry to pump), press START/ADVANCE *twice* **(if the display does not read "SECOND CELL LOADING," press START/ADVANCE again until it does).** *(Pump stops; centrifuge stops; BLUE valve opens; pump starts; cells in bowl are transferred to bag on BLUE line. BLUE valve closes; RED valve opens; centrifuge starts; 250 mL of Medium 199 is pumped into bowl; BLUE valve opens and cells are pumped into bowl.)*

E. When all the cells are loaded into the bowl a second time, press START/ADVANCE button once *(BLUE valve closes; RED valve opens; centrifuge speed increases to 4900 rpm, Medium 199 is pumped into bowl. Repeated 12 times: centrifuge increases to 5400 rpm and pauses 2 seconds; centrifuge speed drops to 4900 rpm; wash solution is pumped into bowl (150 mL per minute $\times$ 8 seconds); centrifuge speed decreases to 4400 rpm and pauses 8 seconds; pump stops; cycle repeats. After 12 cycles: Product collection step—BLUE valve opens; cells pumped into bag on BLUE line. Repeated 3 times: RED valve opens; BLUE valve closes; 50 mL Medium 199 added to bowl; pump stops, centrifuge stops; BLUE valve opens; 50 mL pumped out of bowl; cycle repeats)*.

F. Cells are ready to be sent to patient or for distribution into freezing bags (adjust volume to approximately 247 mL). Withdraw samples for:
   (1) Final microbiologic analysis (1.5 mL)
   (2) CFU assay (1.5 mL)
   (3) Cytospin or smear preparation (followed by differential analysis) and WBC and RBC counting (0.5 mL)
   (4) Liquid nitrogen storage for future testing needs (two vials at 1.5 mL each)
   See paragraphs C and E.

NOTE   SCD sterile tube welder may be used outside of biologic safety cabinet. All connections done with spike fittings must be done inside of cabinet.

AUTHORS

William E. Janssen, Ph.D.
Bone Marrow Processing and
   Evaluation Laboratory
Bone Marrow Transplant Program
H. Lee Moffitt Cancer Center and
   Research Institute
University of South Florida
12902 Magnolia Dr.
Tampa, FL 33612-9497

Carlos E. Lee, M.T.
Bone Marrow Processing and
   Evaluation Laboratory
Bone Marrow Transplant Program
H. Lee Moffitt Cancer Center and
   Research Institute
University of South Florida
12902 Magnolia Dr.
Tampa, FL 33612-9497

REFERENCES   1. Terumo Medical Corp.: SteriCell Processor, Operating and Maintenance Manual, August 1990, Elkton, MD.
2. Brown, BA: Hematology: Principles and Procedures, ed 4. Lea & Febiger, Philadelphia, 1984, p 33.

AUTOMATED BONE MARROW PROCESSING AND DENSITY GRADIENT SEPARATION USING THE FENWAL CS3000

DESCRIPTION	This procedure describes a method for purifying bone marrow mononuclear cells in an automated fashion. Although originally developed for processing of autologous bone marrow prior to cryopreservation, it may also be used for processing of major ABO-incompatible bone marrow or any bone marrow requiring elimination of most of the red blood cells (RBCs).
	After the marrow suspension has been concentrated in the Fenwal CS3000, density gradient separation is performed based on a method developed by Dr. Abe Lin and colleagues. This method involves underlaying the mononuclear cell concentrate in the A35 collection chamber with Ficoll-Hypaque medium during centrifugation in order to further reduce red cell and granulocyte contamination in the bone marrow mononuclear cell suspension.
	Although designed as a two-part method, the mononuclear cell concentration can be done as a separate procedure if a larger degree of red cell and granulocyte contamination in the end product can be tolerated. The packed RBC volume is 2 to 3 mL after the density gradient separation.
TIME FOR PROCEDURE	Approximately 100 minutes.
SUMMARY OF PROCEDURE	1. Mononuclear cell concentration: See "Automated Mononuclear Cell Purification of Marrow with the Fenwal CS3000 and CS3000 Plus" earlier in this chapter. The bone marrow suspension is loaded into the granulo separation chamber, with removal of most of the red blood cells and many of the granulocytes into a packed RBC fraction, while the mononuclear cells are pumped from the granulo separation chamber into the A35 collection chamber. A second pass is carried out by loading the packed RBC fraction back into the granulo separation chamber.
	2. Automated density gradient separation: The A35 collection chamber is isolated by clamping off the input and output of the granulo separation chamber. With the centrifuge operating, Ficoll-Hypaque density gradient medium is pumped into the A35 collection chamber to underlay the mononuclear cell concentrate. Mononuclear cells are flushed from the A35 collection chamber into a transfer pack, leaving most of the red blood cells and granulocytes packed in the chamber.
	3. Wash: After flushing the red cells and granulocytes from the plastic pack in the A35 chamber into a waste bag, the marrow mononuclear cells are loaded into the A35 chamber and washed with a large volume of Hank's balanced salt solution (HBSS), and resuspended in an appropriate medium for infusion, further processing, or cryopreservation.
EQUIPMENT	1. Fenwal CS3000 cell separator with granulo separation chamber and A35 collection chamber (Fenwal Division, Baxter Healthcare)
	2. Scale and balance bags
	3. Heat sealer
	4. Sterile connection device (SCD) (Terumo/Haemonetics)

SUPPLIES AND REAGENTS

1. Fenwal open system apheresis kit for CS3000 (Fenwal Cat. No. 4R2210)
2. Three-lead blood recipient sets (Fenwal Cat. No. 4C2210), with roller clamps closed before using
3. Blood component recipient set (Fenwal Cat. No. 4C2100)
4. Y connector (Cutter 812-70)
5. 2 to 4 600-mL transfer packs (Fenwal Cat. No. 4R2024)
6. Three 2000-mL transfer packs (Fenwal Cat. No. 4R2041)
7. Two 1000-mL bags normal saline (Kendall-McGaw Y94-001-769)
8. 19-gauge sterile needles (Monoject)
9. 300 mL sterile Ficoll-Hypaque (Whittaker Bioproducts, Walkersville, MD) in a 300-mL PL732 transfer pack (Fenwal Cat. No. 4R2111)
10. 1000-mL PL732 transfer pack (Fenwal Cat. No. 4R2110) containing 1000 mL sterile tissue culture medium or HBSS without calcium, magnesium, or phenol red (Whittaker Bioproducts), supplemented as desired (this will be the wash and the final resuspension fluid)
11. Plastic tape
12. Hemostats

PROCEDURE

1. SETUP OF APHERESIS KIT: When planning to perform this procedure after "Automated Mononuclear Cell Purification of Marrow with the Fenwal CS3000 and CS3000 Plus," the following change is necessary in the setup of the apheresis kit:
   A. Attach the straight portion of a Y connector to the plasma return line.
   B. Attach two 600-mL transfer packs to the arms of the Y connector (Fig. 6-6).

2. COMPLETION OF MONONUCLEAR CELL PURIFICATION
   A. Immediately after the centrifuge slows to a halt, change the RUN toggle switch to MANUAL and press the RUN button to restart the device in manual control. If "CODE 25" has appeared in the status display before this step is accomplished, a power-down procedure will have to be performed in order to restart in manual control.

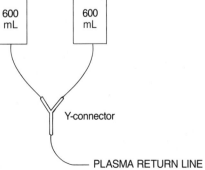

FIGURE **6-6** Modification of CS3000 tubing kit setup for density gradient separation.

Power-Down Procedure

1. Turn the power off and switch the PRIME and RUN toggle switches to MANUAL. Set all the toggle switches for clamps to the close position. Turn the manual pump controls to the stop position and turn the flow rate controls fully counterclockwise.
2. Turn the power back on and press the PRIME button.
3. Press RESUME to clear the five or six codes that will appear.
4. When the RUN button begins to flash, start the manual procedure by pressing RUN and then RESUME.

B. The marrow concentrate is now ready for density gradient separation.

3. AUTOMATED DENSITY GRADIENT SEPARATION PROCEDURE

A. Set procedure switch to 5. Press RESUME.
B. Open VENT and RETURN to clear the vent bubble trap of red cells.
C. Close VENT and RETURN.
D. Fill the Ficoll-Hypaque bubble trap. Prime the Ficoll-Hypaque line into a waste receptacle. Aseptically attach the Ficoll-Hypaque set to the component-rich plasma (CRP) injection port.
E. Lower the marrow bag to the floor. Open PLASMA COLLECT. Excess saline and plasma will now siphon out of the chamber and into the original marrow bag.
F. Close PLASMA COLLECT when approximately 40 to 80 mL of effluent have been collected or when cellular components appear in the collection chamber line.
G. Place a hemostat on the packed red blood cell (PRBC) line below the box. Open the centrifuge door and resuspend the cells.
H. Place a hemostat on the CRP line below the injection port.
I. Open the Ficoll-Hypaque roller clamp.
J. Press RESUME. Turn the plasma pump to 0 (fully counterclockwise). Open PLASMA RETURN. Put plasma pump forward to 10 mL per minute. Cells are now being underlayed with Ficoll.
K. Continue to underlay with Ficoll-Hypaque until "CODE 52" is displayed. Stop plasma pump. Close PLASMA RETURN.
L. Press RESUME. Remove hemostat from PRBC line. Open VENT.
M. Start centrifuge. Open the plasma pump platen to allow Ficoll-Hypaque to fill A35 chamber as it expands; then close. Open PLASMA COLLECT.
N. Put plasma pump forward to 4 mL per minute. (A faster rate may lead to RBC contamination.)
O. After 20 mL of Ficoll-Hypaque has entered the chamber, switch the hemostat from the 600-mL collection bag to the waste bag. Ficoll-Hypaque and mononuclear cells will now begin collecting in the collection bag.
P. Place a hemostat directly below the Y on the plasma return line leading to the blue monitor box to prevent any sedimentation of cellular precipitates in this line.
Q. Continue the collection process until a distinct clear layer appears below the cellular layer in the collection bag.
R. Stop the plasma pump. Close VENT and PLASMA COLLECT. Heat seal the collection bag containing the cells, placing the seal close to the bag. Stop the centrifuge.

S. Heat-seal the Ficoll-Hypaque set, leaving about 6 inches of line above the injection port. The Ficoll-Hypaque bag may now be disposed.

T. To one of the leads of the three-lead set attach the 1000-mL bag of wash solution (HBSS), and to another lead attach a 1000-mL bag of normal saline. Prime the three-lead set with the normal saline, and then connect the main line of the set, using the SCD, to the 6 inches of tubing left above the CRP injection port. Have all clamps closed at this point.

U. Before proceeding to the wash, the A35 chamber must be rinsed free of red cells. To do this:

    (1) Lower the waste bags to the floor. Open PLASMA COLLECT. Open the centrifuge door. Remove the plastic pack from the A35 chamber and squeeze the contents of the bag out.

    (2) Close PLASMA COLLECT. Open the three-lead main line and saline line. Put plasma pump forward to 88 mL per minute. Allow 30 to 60 mL of saline to enter the bag. Then stop the plasma pump.

    (3) Open PLASMA COLLECT. Squeeze the contents out of the bag. Close PLASMA COLLECT.

    (4) Repeat steps U1 through U3 three to five times or until all of the red cells have been removed from the bag. Then replace the bag into the chamber.

V. Fill the rinsed bag with saline as follows: Place a hemostat on the PRBC line just below the box. Open PLASMA RETURN. Put plasma pump forward to 88 mL per minute until "CODE 52" appears. Stop plasma pump and close PLASMA RETURN. Remove the hemostat from the PRBC line. Press RESUME and open VENT.

W. Attach the cell bag to the three-lead set. Dilute with 300 to 400 mL of saline.

X. Establish an open line to the saline. Start the centrifuge. Open the pump platen. After the chamber has expanded (wait several seconds), close the pump platen.

Y. Put plasma pump forward and reduce flow rate to 60 mL per minute.

Z. Simultaneously open the cell line and close the saline line.

AA. After the bag containing cells empties, rinse with saline. (Open roller clamp to saline and hold cell bag below saline bag.)

BB. Finish by washing with 1 L of media (HBSS with 1 mL DNAse), by closing roller clamp on normal saline line and opening clamp on HBSS line.

CC. Stop the plasma pump. Close all clamps. Stop the centrifuge.

DD. Remove the marrow cell bag from the A35 chamber by heat sealing, leaving a 4- to 6-inch tail. Discard all disposables. Place the procedure switch on 1. Change the prime and run switches to the AUTO position.

EE. The marrow cells, in a volume of about 200 mL, are now ready for further processing (purging) or for cryopreservation.

ANTICIPATED RESULTS

In 40 autologous bone marrows and six allogeneic marrows processed by this method, the mononuclear cell yield was 70 to 95 percent after the mononuclear cell concentration. After density gradient separation, the mean mononuclear cell yield was 56 percent, with a range of 30 to 70 percent. The red cell volume is 15 to 40 mL after the mononuclear cell concentration, but only 2 to 4 mL after both procedures. The marrow concentrate is in a final volume of 200 mL after completion of the density gradient separation.

AUTHORS

Charles S. Carter, B.S.
Special Services Laboratory
Department of Transfusion
   Medicine
National Institutes of Health
Bethesda, MD 20892

Holly Goetzman, M.T.(ASCP)
Special Services Laboratory
Department of Transfusion
   Medicine
National Institutes of Health
Bethesda, MD 20892

Elizabeth J. Read, M.D.
Department of Pathology
University of Utah Medical Center
Salt Lake City, UT 84132

REFERENCES

1. Carter, CS, et al: Use of a continuous-flow cell separator in density gradient isolation of lymphocytes. Transfusion 27:362, 1987.
2. Muul, LM, et al: Development of an automated closed system for generation of human lymphokine activated killer (LAK) cells for use in adoptive immunotherapy. J Immunol Methods 101:171, 1987.
3. Carter, CS, et al: Semi-automated processing of autologous bone marrow for transplantation (abstr). Transfusion 29:6S, 1989.
4. Fenwal CS3000 Mononuclear Cell Processing System: Protocols for investigation. Fenwal Division, Baxter Healthcare Corp., Deerfield, IL, 1991.

T-CELL DEPLETION TO PREVENT GRAFT-VERSUS-HOST DISEASE FOLLOWING ALLOGENEIC BONE MARROW TRANSPLANTATION

7

Commentary by RICHARD CHAMPLIN and KYOUNG LEE

NONIMMUNOLOGIC
T-Cell Depletion of Bone Marrow by
    Treatment with Soybean Agglutinin and
    Sheep Red Blood Cell Rosetting
Counterflow Centrifugation
   Lymphocyte Depletion of Bone Marrow
      Grafts Using Elutriation
   Centrifugal Elutriation for Lymphocyte
      Removal
Methylprednisolone and Vincristine

Treatment of Bone Marrow in HLA-
    Mismatched Bone Marrow Transplants
T-Cell Depletion of SBA— Cells by
    Adherence on the AIS-Cellector–T Cell
IMMUNOLOGIC
Bone Marrow Purging of T Lymphocytes
    with $T_{10}B_9$ Monoclonal Antibodies and
    Complement
Ex Vivo Immunotoxin-Mediated T-Cell
    Depletion

Graft-versus-host (GVH) disease is a major complication of allogeneic bone marrow transplantation.[1-5] Two forms of GVH have been recognized—acute and chronic. Acute GVH disease typically occurs within 3 months of transplantation and results from immunocompetent donor cells present in the donor bone marrow reacting against recipient (host) tissues.[2] Chronic GVH disease generally has an indolent presentation developing 3 months to 1 year following transplant with protean clinical features resembling scleroderma and abnormal regulation of immunity.[6]

Several approaches have been evaluated to prevent GVH disease. Most patients have received immunosuppressive drugs for several months following transplantation using methotrexate, cyclosporine, cyclophosphamide, corticosteroids, antithymocyte globulin, or combinations of these drugs.[7-12] Despite these treatments, acute GVH disease develops in 20 to 60 percent of recipients receiving transplants from HLA-identical donors and is fatal in a proportion of affected patients.[13] From 25 to 60 percent of patients surviving for more than 6 months develop chronic GVH disease.[6] The risk of acute GVH disease is substantially higher following transplantation of HLA-nonidentical bone marrow[14] or bone marrow from phenotypically identical unrelated donors.[15]

Although numbers of cell populations are present in the lesions of acute and chronic GVH disease, the process is dependent on the presence of T lymphocytes. Depletion of these putative effector cells from the donor bone marrow prior to transplantation is an effective means of reducing the incidence and

163

severity of both acute and chronic GVH disease across both major and minor histocompatibility differences.[16-18]

Several techniques have been proposed for ex vivo depletion of T lymphocytes from human bone marrow prior to transplantation, including soybean lectin agglutination,[19] E-rosette formation,[20] centrifugal elutriation,[21] treatment with cytotoxic drugs or corticosteroids,[22,23] or separation using anti–T-cell antisera or monoclonal antibodies. Anti–T-cell antibodies have been used alone,[24-26] with complement,[27-32] conjugated to toxins such as ricin (immunotoxins),[33] or bound to magnetic beads with depletion in a magnetic field.[34]

Ex vivo treatment of donor bone marrow with single or multiple anti–T-cell lymphocyte antibodies alone has been ineffective to reduce substantially the incidence of GVH disease indicating that opsonization of T cells, at least with these antibodies, is insufficient to prevent GVH disease.[24-26] Techniques that lyse or physically eliminate T lymphocytes from the donor bone marrow before transplantation have been more effective. Most studies have used murine or rat monoclonal anti–T-cell antibodies and complement. A variety of antibodies have been used, either alone or in combination. Combinations of multiple antibodies have generally produced a greater elimination of T lymphocytes than treatment with a single antibody. In addition, repeating several antibody-complement treatments may further improve the efficacy of depletion.[35] Optimal techniques are capable of a three- to four-log reduction (99.90 to 99.99 percent) of T lymphocytes. Unfortunately, each cycle of in vitro treatment results in some loss of hematopoietic stem cells and it is uncertain whether multiple treatments lead to superior clinical results.

Monoclonal antibodies directed to one or more T-cell antigens have been used, including the E-rosette receptor (CD2), as well as CD3, CD5, CD6, and CD8. These antibodies are nonreactive with hematopoietic progenitors such as colony-forming unit—granulocyte, macrophage (CFU-GM); burst-forming unit—erythroid (BFU-E); and colony-forming unit—granulocyte, erythroid, macrophage, megakaryocyte (CFU-GEMM); and the antibody-complement-treated marrow can restore hematopoiesis following transplantation. Techniques that effectively deplete T lymphocytes have uniformly reduced the incidence and severity of GVH disease in recipients of HLA-identical transplants.[36] Zero to fifteen percent of patients develop greater than grade 2 acute GVH disease after T-cell–depleted transplants; if GVH disease occurs it is usually mild in severity. This is a notable advance, as no other form of treatment has substantially affected the development of GVH disease.

However, depletion of T lymphocytes has also been associated with adverse clinical effects. The risk of graft failure is approximately 2 percent in recipients receiving transplants for leukemia, using unmodified bone marrow from an HLA-identical sibling donor. In contrast, 10 to 20 percent of patients receiving T-lymphocyte–depleted bone marrow transplants have had graft failure.[27,31,37] Graft failure has occurred in two clinical patterns; some patients fail to have any evidence of initial engraftment, whereas others have initial hematologic recovery only to experience late graft failure leading to marrow aplasia.

Most cases of graft failure following T-cell–depleted transplants are due to immunologic rejection.[38] In some well-studied cases, host T lymphocytes that react against donor major or minor histocompatibility antigens have been described.[38-40] Less commonly, natural killer (NK) cells have been implicated.[41,42] T cells from the donor marrow may be necessary in some patients to eradicate residual recipient immunocompetent cells that survive the pre-transplant chemotherapy-irradiation preparative regimen by a limited GVH response. Alternatively, growth factors or other products produced by T cells may facilitate engraftment. It is unlikely that injury to hematopoietic stem cells by the T-cell–depletion procedure is responsible because transplantation of autologous T-cell–depleted bone marrow is uncommonly associated with graft failure.

Recent clinical and experimental data indicate that an important immune-mediated graft-versus-leukemia (GVL) effect may occur following allogeneic bone marrow transplantation.[43–46] The mechanisms of the GVL effect and the cell populations mediating this process are incompletely understood. T-cell clones reactive with human leukemia cells have been described,[47] and lymphokine-activated killer (LAK) and NK cells may also contribute.[48,49]

Clinical data indicate a critical role for the GVL effect to prevent recurrence of leukemia following allogeneic bone marrow transplantation. Rarely, patients with leukemia have been reported who achieve remission after development of acute GVH disease[50] or after infusion of donor lymphocytes.[51] Recipients who develop GVH disease have a lower incidence of leukemia relapse than patients without GVH disease.[43–46] This antileukemic effect correlates best with the presence of chronic GVH disease. The impact of acute GVH disease is less striking, but the lowest rate of relapse occurs in patients with both acute and chronic GVH disease. Patients with acute or chronic myelogenous leukemia (AML or CML) receiving transplants from identical twin donors have a significantly higher risk of relapse than those receiving allogeneic bone marrow transplants.[45,46] Conversely, patients receiving transplants from unrelated donors who have a significantly higher rate of GVH disease have been reported to have a lower risk of leukemia relapse than those receiving transplants from HLA-identical siblings.[15]

T-cell depletion is associated with a substantial increase in the risk of leukemia relapse, presumably owing to loss of the GVL effect[27,31,52]; as a net result, the benefit of reducing GVH disease is largely offset by graft failure and leukemia relapse so that disease-free survival is not improved. The increased risk of leukemia relapse is most striking for patients with CML. Approximately 12 percent of patients with CML in chronic phase receiving unmodified HLA-identical bone marrow transplants relapse, compared with a relapse rate of more than 50 percent with T-cell–depleted transplants.[53] This marked probability rate of relapse is present even if compared with unmodified allograft recipients without signs of GVH disease, which suggests an effect of T cells independent of GVH disease. Unlike patients with acute leukemia in remission, those in chronic phase receive transplants when the leukemic clone is fully expanded and hematopoiesis is almost exclusively leukemic in origin. Relapse of chronic phase CML may be due to competitive repopulation of host-derived hematopoiesis, and T cells may be critical to prevent this process. This high relapse rate with T-cell–depleted transplants indicates that viable leukemia cells survive the preparative regimen and are capable of reestablishing the disease. Growth of these leukemic cells is presumably suppressed by the GVL effect, which is at least partially mediated by T lymphocytes. It is uncertain whether the GVL effect can be distinguished from GVH disease in humans. It is also unknown whether the same or different cell populations mediate each process.

As indicated, the risk of acute GVH disease is highest in patients receiving HLA-nonidentical or unrelated donor transplants. In this setting, T-cell depletion is an effective means to reduce the incidence and severity of GVH disease.[19,54,55] Graft failure has been a greater problem in these cases, occurring in 20 to 50 percent of cases. There continues to be a risk of severe GVH disease, particularly if detectable T cells are present following treatment of the donor bone marrow. It is notable, however, that some successful transplants have been performed from haploidentical donors, a setting in which transplantation of unmodified marrow is rarely successful. The best results are reported for children with severe combined immunodeficiency disease who have received successful transplants using T-cell–depleted bone marrow from an HLA-haploidentical parental donor.[56] Results have been less encouraging for patients with leukemia—particularly adults.

A number of approaches have been considered to improve clinical results of T-cell–depleted transplants for leukemia. As indicated, the major problems are graft failure and recurrent leukemia. One approach is to employ an intensified pretransplant preparative regimen in the hope of overcoming resistance to engraftment and providing greater antileukemic activity. Although preliminary data suggest that administration of a higher dose of total body irradiation (13.5 to 15.75 Gy) may be associated with a lower risk of graft failure, toxicity is also increased.[37,55] It is possible that a less effective depletion technique that spares a small number of T lymphocytes may allow engraftment and still reduce GVH disease. There is considerable interest in the use of monoclonal antibody-toxin immunoconjugates (immunotoxins)[57] to target therapy specifically to lymphoid or leukemic cells or use of bone-seeking radionuclides[58] or antibody-radionuclide immunoconjugates[59] to localize delivery of radiation to the bone marrow or lymphoid tissue without adding further systemic toxicity. Controlled studies are necessary to determine if T-cell depletion will improve disease-free survival in HLA-nonidentical or unrelated donor transplants.

Graft failure has been a problem with all methods of T-cell depletion including antibody-complement treatment, immunotoxins, and lectin agglutination. Preliminary data in a small series of patients suggest that antibodies of more limited specificity (which do not encompass all T cells) may posssibly be associated with a higher rate of engraftment, and that more complete T-cell depletion increases the risk of graft failure.[32] Encouraging results have recently been reported using subtotal T-cell depletion (approximately 1.5 logs) in combination with post-transplant systemic treatment with cyclosporine or anti-CD5 ricin immunotoxin for HLA-mismatched and unrelated donor transplants.[54]

It is uncertain whether distinct cell populations can be identified that mediate the GVL effect and GVH disease. T-cell clones or LAK and NK cell populations capable of mediating an antileukemic effect raise the possibility of infusing allogeneic effector cells after transplant to enhance immune antileukemia activity.[60,61] Similarly, the use of hematopoietic growth factors may facilitate engraftment or monocyte-macrophage antileukemic mechanisms.[62–64] Controlled trials are necessary to evaluate whether these agents will improve transplant outcome.

It is conceivable that different cellular subsets are responsbile for GVH disease and GVL effect. CD4-positive T cells recognize antigens presented with class II MHC antigens.[65] CD8-positive lymphocytes recognize antigens present in the context of class I loci. In murine models, CD4-positive cells primarily mediate acute GVH disease in MHC class II disparate recipients, whereas CD8-positive cells are responsible for GVH disease in class I disparate transplant mice.[3,66] Depletion of the CD8-positive cytotoxic-suppressor subset of T lymphocytes is sufficient to reduce or prevent GVH disease in most donor-recipient murine strain combinations that are MHC compatible but mismatched for minor histocompatibility loci. Selective depletion of CD8-positive cells in combination with post-transplant cyclosporine has recently been evaluated in humans; this approach resulted in a reduced rate of acute GVH disease in HLA-matched sibling grafts without an increase in leukemia relapse in preliminary studies.[67] For patients with CML, the actuarial incidence of equal to or greater than grade 2 acute GVH disease was 22 percent in the CD8-depleted group compared with 5 percent in historic control subjects receiving pan T-cell depletion and 58 percent with unmodified marrow transplants. The actuarial rate of leukemia relapse was 65 percent following pan T-cell depletion but none of the patients transplanted using CD8-depleted bone marrow or unmodified marrow have relapsed.[68] These data need confirmation in larger studies with more extended follow-up, but this suggests that GVH disease and the GVL effect may possibly be separated. Improved methods to selectively induce or enhance the GVL effect following T-cell– or T-subset–depleted transplants may be possible.

In conclusion, the use of T-lymphocyte–depleted bone marrow transplants has reduced the risk of GVH disease, a major complication of bone marrow transplantation but is associated with other problems. A number of techniques appear to have similar efficacy, and it is not possible to determine an optimal depletion method from the data avilable. It may be advisable to retain a small number of T cells in the graft to facilitate engraftment and maintain the GVL effect. At least in the setting of HLA-identical transplants, an incomplete reduction of T lymphocytes may still be effective in reducing GVH disease. HLA-mismatched transplants have posed a much greater problem; despite T-cell depletion of the donor bone marrow, moderate to severe GVH disease may occur and graft failure is still more frequent. More effective treatment regimens both before and after transplant must still be developed, to ensure engraftment and prevent leukemia relapse.

REFERENCES

1. Thomas, ED, et al: Bone marrow transplantation. N Engl J Med 192:832, 1975.
2. Glucksberg, H, et al: Clinical manifestation of graft-versus-host disease in human recipients of marrow from HLA matched sibling donors. Transplantation 18:295, 1974.
3. Korngold, R and Sprent, J: T-cell subsets and graft-versus-host disease. Transplantation 44:335, 1987.
4. Ferrara, J and Burakoff, SJ: The pathophysiology of acute graft-vs-host disease in a murine bone marrow transplant model. Marcel Dekker, New York, 1990, p 9.
5. Grebe, SC and Streilein, JW: Graft-versus-host reactions: A review. Adv Immunol 22:119, 1976.
6. Sullivan, KM, et al: Late complications after bone marrow transplantation. Semin Hematol 21:53, 1984.
7. Gale, RP, et al: Risk factors for acute graft-versus-host disease. Br J Hematol 67:397, 1987.
8. Ramsay, NKC, et al: A randomized study of the prevention of acute graft-versus-host disease. N Engl J Med 306:392, 1982.

9. Deeg, HJ, Storb, R, and Thomas, ED: Cyclosporine as prophylaxis for graft-versus-host disease: A randomized study in patients undergoing marrow transplantation for acute nonlymphoblastic leukemia. Blood 65:1325, 1985.

10. Doney, KD, et al: Failure of early administration of antithymocyte globulin to lessen graft-versus-host disease in human allogeneic marrow transplant recipients. Transplantation 31:141, 1981.

11. Forman, SJ, et al: A prospective randomized study of acute graft-versus-host disease in 107 patients with leukemia: methotrexate/prednisone versus cyclosporine/prednisone. Transplant Proc 21:2605, 1987.

12. Storb, R, et al: Methotrexate and cyclosporine compared with cyclosporine alone for prophylaxis of acute graft-versus-host disease after marrow transplantation for leukemia. N Engl J Med 12:729, 1986.

13. Martin, PJ, et al: A retrospective analysis of therapy for acute graft-versus-host disease: Initial treatment. Blood 76:1464, 1990.

14. Beatty, PG, et al: Marrow transplantation from related donors other than HLA-identical siblings. N Engl J Med 313:765, 1985.

15. Gajewski, JL, et al: Bone marrow transplantation using unrelated donors for patients with advanced leukemia or bone marrow failure. Transplantation 50:244, 1990.

16. Okunewick, JP: Review of the effects of anti-T-cell monoclonal antibodies on major and minor GvHR in the mouse. In Baum, S (ed). Experimental Hematology Today. Springer-Verlag, New York, 1985.

17. Vallera, DA, et al: Bone marrow transplantation across major histocompatibility barriers in mice: Effect of elimination of T cells from donor grafts by treatment with monoclonal Thy-1.2 plus complement or antibody alone. Transplantation 31:218, 1981.

18. Ferrara, J and Burakoff, SJ: The pathophysiology of acute graft-vs-host disease in a murine bone marrow transplant model. Marcel Dekker, New York, 1990, p 9.

19. Reisner, Y, et al: Transplantation for acute leukemia with HLA-A and B nonidentical parental marrow cells fractionated with soybean agglutinin and sheep red blood cells. Lancet 2:327, 1981.

20. Dicke, KA, Van Hofft, JIM, and Van Bekkum, DW: The selective elimination of immunologically competent cells from bone marrow and lymphatic cell mixtures. Transplantation 6:562, 1968.

21. de Witte, T, et al: Depletion of donor lymphocytes by counterflow centrifugation successfully prevents acute graft-versus-host disease in matched allogeneic marrow transplantation. Blood 67:1302, 1986.

22. Prentice, HG, et al: Remission induction with adenosine-deaminase inhibitor 2'-deoxycoformycin in thy-lymphoblastic leukemia. Lancet 1:170, 1980.

23. Korbling, M, et al: 4-hydroperoxycyclophosphamide: A model for eliminating residual human tumor cells and T-lymphocytes from the bone marrow graft. Br J Haematol 52:89, 1982.

24. Prentice, HG, et al: Use of anti-T cell monoclonal antibody OKT-3 to prevent graft-versus-host disease in allogeneic bone marrow transplantation for actue leukemia. Lancet 1:700, 1982.

25. Filipovich, AH, et al: Pretreatment of donor bone marrow with monoclonal antibody OKT-3 for prevention of acute graft-versus-host disease in allogeneic histocompatible bone marrow transplantation. Lancet 1:1266, 1982.

26. Martin, JP, Hansen, JA, and Thomas, ED: Preincubation of donor bone marrow cells with a combination of murine monoclonal anti T-cell antibodies without complement does not prevent graft-versus-host disease after allogeneic marrow transplantation. J Clin Immunol 4:18, 1984.

27. Mitsuyasu, R, et al: Depletion of T-lymphocytes for prevention of graft-versus-host disease: A prospective randomized trial. Ann Intern Med 105:20, 1986.

28. Prentice, HG, et al: Depletion of T-lymphocytes in donor marrow prevents significant graft-versus-host disease in matched allogeneic leukemia marrow transplant recipients. Lancet 1:472, 1984.

29. Slavin, S, et al: Elimination of graft-versus-host disease in matched allogeneic leukemic transplant recipient using CAMPATH-1. Adv Exp Med Biol 186:813, 1985.

30. Trigg, ME, et al: Depletion of T cells from human bone marrow with monoclonal antibody CT-2 and complement. J Biol Respir Mod 3:406, 1984.

31. Maraninchi, D, et al: Impact of T-cell depletion on outcome of allogeneic bone marrow transplantation for standard-risk leukemias. Lancet 2:175, 1987.

32. Soiffer, RJ, et al: Reconstitution of T-cell function after CD6-depleted allogeneic bone marrow transplantation. Blood 75:2076, 1990.

33. Filipovich, AH, et al: *Ex vivo* treatment of donor bone marrow with anti-T cell immunotoxins for prevention of graft-versus-host disease. Lancet 1:469, 1984.

34. Frame, JN, et al: T cell depletion of human bone marrow. Comparison of Campath-1 plus complement, anti-T cell ricin A chain immunotoxin, and soybean agglutinin alone or in combination with sheep erythrocytes or immunomagnetic beads. Transplantation 47:984, 1989.

35. Bast, RC, et al: Elimination of leukemic cells from human bone marrow using monoclonal antibody and complement. Cancer Res 43:1389, 1983.

36. Champlin, R: T-cell depletion to prevent graft-versus-host disease after bone marrow transplantation. Hematol Oncol Clin North Am 4:687, 1990.

37. Martin, PJ, et al: Effects of *in vitro* depletion of T cells in HLA-identical allogeneic marrow grafts. Blood 66:664, 1985.

38. Martin, PJ: The role of donor lymphoid cells in allogeneic marrow engraftment. Bone Marrow Transplant 6:283, 1990.

39. Kernan, NA, et al: Graft failure after T-cell-depleted human leukocyte antigen identical marrow transplants for leukemia: I. Analysis of risk factors and results of secondary transplants. Blood 74:2227, 1989.

40. Voogt, PJ, et al: Rejection of bone marrow graft by recipient-derived cytotoxic T-lymphocyte against minor histocompatibility antigens. Lancet 335:131, 1990.

41. Nakamura, H and Gress, RE: Graft rejection by cytolytic T-cells: Specificity of the effector mechanism in the rejection of allogeneic marrow. Transplantation 49:453, 1990.

42. Murphy, WJ, et al: An absence of T-cells in murine bone marrow allografts leads to an increased susceptibility to rejection by natural killer cells and T-cells. J Immunol 144:3305, 1990.

43. Weiden, PL, et al: Antileukemic effect of chronic graft-versus-host disease: Contribution to improved survival after allogeneic marrow transplantation. N Engl J Med 304:1529, 1981.

44. Sullivan, KM, et al: Graft-versus-host disease as adoptive immunotherapy in patients with advanced hematologic neoplasms. N Engl J Med 320:828, 1989.

45. Gale, RP and Champlin, RE: How does bone marrow transplantation cure leukemia? Lancet 2:28, 1984.

46. Horowitz, MM, et al: Graft-versus-leukemia reactions after bone marrow transplantation. Blood 75:555, 1990.

47. Sosman, JA, et al: Specific recognition of human leukemic cells by allogeneic T cells: II. Evidence for HLA-D restricted determinants on leukemic cells that are crossreactive with determinants present on unrelated nonleukemic cells. Blood 75:2005, 1990.

48. Delmon, L, et al: Characterization of antileukemia cells' cytotoxic effector function. Implications for monitoring natural killer responses following allogeneic bone marrow transplantation. Transplantation 42:252, 1986.

49. Hauch, M, et al: Anti-leukemia potential of interleukin-2 activated natural killer cells after bone marrow transplantation for chronic myelogenous leukemia. Blood 75:2250, 1990.

50. Higano, CS, et al: Durable complete remission of acute nonlymphocytic leukemia associated with discontinuation of immunosuppression following relapse after allogeneic bone marrow transplantation: A case report of a probable graft-versus-host leukemia effect. Transplantation 50:175, 1990.

51. Kolb, HJ, et al: Donor leukocyte transfusions for treatment of recurrent chronic myelogenous leukemia in marrow transplant patients. Blood 76:2462, 1990.

52. Marmont, A, et al: International Bone Marrow Transplant Registry (in press).

53. Goldman, JM, et al: Bone marrow transplantation for chronic myelogenous leukemia in chronic phase: Increased risk of relapse associated wtih T-cell depletion. Ann Intern Med 108:806, 1988.

54. Ash, RC, et al: Successful allogeneic transplantation of T-cell-depleted bone marrow from closely HLA-matched unrelated donors. N Engl J Med 332:485, 1990.

55. Bozdech, M, et al: Transplantation of HLA-haploidentical T-cell depleted marrow for leukemia: Addition of cytosine arabinoside to the transplant conditioning prevents rejection. Exp Hematol 13:1201, 1985.

56. Reisner, Y, et al: Transplantation for severe combined immunodeficiency with HLA-A, B, D, Dr incompatible parental marrow cells fractionated by soybean agglutinin and sheep red blood cells. Blood 61:341, 1983.

57. Vallera, DA, et al: Monoclonal antibody toxin conjugates for experimental graft-versus-host disease prophylaxis. Transplantation 36:73, 1983.

58. Appelbaum, FR, et al: Antibody-radionuclide conjugates as part of a myeloblative preparative regimen for marrow transplantation. Blood 73:2202, 1989.

59. Appelbaum, FR, et al: Myelosuppression and mechanism of recovery following administration of Samarium-EDTMP. Antibody Immunoconjugates and Radiopharmaceuticals 1:263, 1988.
60. Slavin, S, et al: The graft-versus-leukemia (GVL) phenomenon: Is GVL separable from GVHD. Bone Marrow Transplant 6:155, 1990.
61. Hauch, M, et al: Anti-leukemia potential of interleukin-2 activated natural killer cells after bone marrow transplantation for chronic myelongenous leukemia. Blood 75:2250, 1990.
62. Munn, DH, Garnick, MB, and Cheung, N-KV: Effects of parenteral recombinant human macrophage colony-stimulating factor on monocyte number, phenotype, and antitumor cytotoxicity in nonhuman primates. Blood 75:2042, 1990.
63. Blazar, BR, et al: Enhanced survival but reduced engraftment in murine recipients of recombinant granulocyte/macrophage colony-stimulating factor following transplantation of T-cell-depleted histoincompatible bone marrow. Blood 72:1148, 1988.
64. Blazar, BR, et al: Improved survival and leukocyte reconstitution without detrimental effects on engraftment in murine recipients of human recombinant granulocyte colony-stimulating factor after transplantation of T-cell-depleted histoincompatible bone marrow. Blood 74:2264, 1989.
65. Sprent, J, et al: Functions of purified L3T4+ and Lyt-2+ cells in vitro and in vivo. Immunol Rev 91:195, 1986.
66. Korngold, R and Sprent, J: Variable capacity of L3 T4+ T cells to cause lethal graft versus host disease across minor histocompatibility barriers in mice. J Exp Med 165:52, 1987.
67. Champlin, R, et al: Selective depletion of CD8+ T-lymphocytes for prevention of graft-versus-host disease after allogeneic bone marrow transplantation. Blood 76:418, 1990.
68. Champlin, RE, et al: Retention of graft-versus-leukemia using selective depletion of CD8-positive T-lymphocytes for prevention of graft-versus-host disease following bone marrow transplantation for chronic myelogenous leukemia. Transplant Proc 23:1695, 1991.

NONIMMUNOLOGIC

T-Cell Depletion of Bone Marrow by Treatment with Soybean Agglutinin and Sheep Red Blood Cell Rosetting

DESCRIPTION	T cells may be depleted from bone marrow using a sequential treatment of agglutination with soybean agglutinin followed by removal of residual T cells by rosetting with treated sheep erythrocytes. Hematopoietic precursors are concentrated by this procedure in approximately 6 percent of the original cell number, accompanied by a loss of the majority of mature blood elements, including granulocytes, natural killer (NK) cells, B cells, and T cells, with a 2- to 3-$\log_{10}$ depletion of T cells. Graft-versus-host (GVH) disease is significantly reduced in allogeneic HLA-matched and mismatched bone marrow transplantation using this procedure.
TIME FOR PROCEDURE	7 to 10 hours
SUMMARY OF PROCEDURE	1. Erythrocytes are removed from the harvested bone marrow by unit gravity sedimentation with 3 percent gelatin in normal saline. Red blood cell (RBC)–depleted bone marrow (unseparated population) is washed on a COBE 2991 cell washer with phosphate-buffered saline (PBS) plus 1 percent human serum albumin (HSA), and concentrated to 1.5 to 4.0 $\times$ 10^8/mL in PBS.
	2. The unseparated population is agglutinated with an equal volume of soybean agglutinin (SBA) at 2 mg/mL. The nonagglutinated (SBA$-$) cells, which contain the hematopoietic precursors, are separated from the agglutinated (SBA$+$) cells on 5 percent bovine serum albumin (BSA) gradients at unit gravity. To remove the SBA the cells are washed with the competitive sugar galactose on a COBE 2991 cell washer and resuspended in M-199 tissue culture medium. The SBA$+$ cells are washed sequentially with 0.2 M galactose and M-199, then subjected to 3000-rad irradiation with a cesium source and maintained on ice until final washing with lactated Ringer's solution with 1 percent HSA.
	3. The SBA$-$ cells are rosetted with a 2 percent solution of 2-aminoethylisothiouronium bromide hydrobromide (AET)–treated sheep erythrocytes (E-AET). The residual sheep erythrocyte receptor–bearing T cells are separated on Ficoll-Hypaque gradients, yielding an SBA-E$-$ population at the interface. The SBA-E$-$ cells are washed with lactated Ringer's solution on a COBE 2991 cell washer.
	4. Samples are taken of the unseparated SBA$-$ and SBA-E$-$ for analysis of cell number, rosette-positive cells, clonable T cells, hematopoietic precursors, and sterility.
EQUIPMENT	1. COBE Blood Cell Processor, No. 2991, COBE Laboratories
	2. Fenwal Plasma Extractor, No. 4R4414, Fenwal Division, Baxter Healthcare
	3. Coulter Counter ZM No. 901, Coulter Electronics or other cell counter

4. Sorvall T6000 Table Top Centrifuge, Rotor No. H 1000B, Sorvall Division, DuPont

5. Ficoll rack (see Notes)

SUPPLIES AND REAGENTS

1. 2000-mL transfer pack with coupler (Fenwal 4R2041)
2. Six 1000-mL transfer packs with couplers (Fenwal 4R2032)
3. 6 plasma transfer sets with two couplers (Fenwal 4C2243)
4. 3 COBE 2991 blood cell processor processing sets
5. 4 blood bag injection sites
6. Forty 50-mL conical centrifuge tubes, clear polystyrene, Corning No. 25339
7. Fifty 50-mL conical centrifuge tubes, opaque polypropylene, Falcon No. 2070
8. Twelve 30-mL, disposable, sterile syringes
9. Seventeen 60-mL, disposable, sterile syringes
10. Five 60-mL catheter-tip, disposable syringes
11. 10-mL, disposable, sterile syringe
12. Twenty-four 18-gauge 1½-inch sterile needles
13. Three 15-gauge 1½-inch sterile needles
14. Two 19-gauge 3½-inch sterile, disposable, spinal needles, quincke type point
15. Two 490-cm^2 disposable sterile roller bottles, Corning No. 25130
16. Lectin soybean agglutinin, No. L1010, Vector Laboratories
17. Gelatin powder, No. 2124-01, J. T. Baker Company
18. Lymphoprep, Nyegaard Company, Oslo, Norway, distributed by Accurate Chemical
19. Sheep red blood cells in Alsever's solution, No. CS-113U, Colorado Serum Company (sheep cells are tested for sterility and shipped fresh weekly)
20. 2-Aminoethylisothiouronium bromide hydrobromide (AET), No. A5879, Sigma Chemical Company
21. Heparin sodium injection, USP, 1000 units/mL, preservative-free, Squibb-Marsam, Inc.
22. Penicillin-streptomycin solution (100 ×), No. 600-5140 AG, Gibco
23. Human serum albumin, 25 percent (New York Blood Center)

MEDIA

1. 1000-mL bag PBS without calcium and magnesium with 10 mL penicillin-streptomycin (P/S)
2. 1000-mL bag PBS without calcium and magnesium with 10 mL (P/S) and 50 mL 25 percent HSA added
3. 1000-mL bag PBS with 0.2 M D-galactose to which has been added 10 mL (P/S) and 50 mL 25 percent HSA
4. 1000-mL bag medium-199 (M-199) with 10 mL (P/S) and 50 mL 25 percent HSA added
5. 1000-mL bag lactated Ringer's solution, injection grade, USP, with 10 mL (P/S) and 50 mL 25 percent HSA added

6. 1000-mL bag lactated Ringer's solution, injection grade, USP, with 50 mL 25 percent HSA added

7. 500-mL bag lactated Ringer's solution, injection grade, USP, with 25 mL 25 percent HSA added

8. 500-mL bottle PBS with 5 mL (P/S) added

9. 500-mL bottle PBS with 0.2 M D-galactose, with 5 mL (P/S) added

10. Two 500-mL bottles PBS with 5 percent bovine serum albumin (BSA), with 5 mL (P/S) added to each bottle

11. Four 500-mL bags physiologic saline for injection, USP

PROCEDURE

1. RBC SEDIMENTATION: Optimal agglutination with SBA requires that the nucleated bone marrow cells first be separated from the majority of the RBCs. The procedure that follows is a 1g sedimention with 3 percent gelatin in transfusion grade normal saline (see Notes for other RBC-depletion methods).

A. Harvest bone marrow, mix with saline and preservative-free heparin at a final concentration of 5 to 7 units per mL, and filter sequentially through 300- and 200-mesh stainless steel filters. It is delivered to the processing laboratory in a single 2000-mL transfer pack.

B. Insert a sterile injection site into the transfer pack and inject an additional 5 mL of isotonic preservative-free heparin per 500 mL of marrow. Withdraw a small aliquot of marrow for cell count and sterility assays.

C. Drain bone marrow into previously prepared 1000-mL transfer packs containing 500 mL of 3 percent gelatin in normal saline. Divide equally 1 L of marrow by draining simultaneously into two 1000-mL gelatin transfer packs via a side port. Connect the central port of each 1000-mL bag to a single empty 2000-mL transfer pack, and clamp the lines. The contents of the 1000-mL bags are mixed thoroughly and the bags are hung with ports upright in a Fenwal plasma extractor in a laminar flow hood (Fig. 7–1).

D. Allow the mixture to settle, usually for 20 minutes or until the RBC portion occupies approximately 20 percent of the total volume in the bag and there is a definite interface between the white blood cell (WBC)–rich plasma and the sedimented RBCs. Express the RBC-depleted portion into the attached 2000-mL blood bag via the transfer sets. Stop collecting this leukocyte-rich plasma just before the RBC layer enters the tubing. Pinch the tubing shut with a hemostat and clamp. The majority of nucleated cells (usually more than 60 percent) in the marrow are recovered from a single sedimentation. Negligible numbers of hematopoietic precursors are lost in the sedimented RBCs, which are highly depleted of low-density cells. When the patient weighs more than 40 kg, a second sedimentation is required to increase the cell yield. The second sedimentation is done by adding both RBC sediments to a single bag of 500-mL gelatin and repeating the sedimentation as described previously.

E. Install a sterile, disposable processing set in the COBE 2991. Attach the washing reagents (numbers 1 and 2 in Media), previously prepared in sterile 1-L transfer bags, by the spike adapters. Load the unseparated

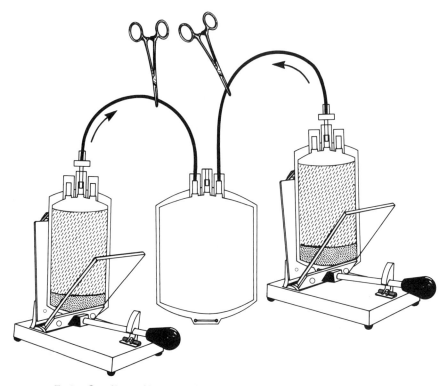

FIGURE 7–1 One liter of harvested marrow is mixed in two 500-mL aliquots with 500 mL of 3 percent gelatin in saline, and each sedimentation bag is connected to a 2-L supernatant bag as illustrated. Sedimentation is allowed to proceed in two Fenwal plasma extractors for 20 minutes until there is a definite line between the sedimented RBCs and the leukocyte-rich plasma. Then the hemostats are released on the tubing to the supernatant bag, and the leukocyte-rich plasma containing the unseparated cell population is extruded into the supernatant bag. The sedimentation bags are clamped and the RBC sediment from the two bags pooled into another 1-L bag containing 500 mL of gelatin. After a second sedimentation, which is usually shorter than 20 minutes, the second leukocyte-rich plasma is pooled with the first, and the cells washed on a COBE 2991 cell washer, as described in the text.

cells into the 2991 through the pink line into the 600-mL donut-shaped bag in the centrifuge bowl of the machine. Remove the air from the system and clear the tube lines by running washing reagent into the bag. Centrifuge the marrow at 2000 rpm for 3 minutes. Super-out the supernatant into the waste bag at 300 mL per minute for 1 minute, 45 seconds. Load the remaining cell mixture into the donut, centrifuge, and remove the supernatant. When all of the cell mixture has been run into the donut and spun down, wash the cell pellet once with PBS+P/S, spinning at 2000 rpm for 3 minutes. Follow by two washes with PBS+P/S containing 1 percent normal HSA.

F. After the final wash and removal of supernatant, clamp the donut off and cut away from the rest of the processing set. Transfer the bag to the biohazard hood and attach a sterile injection site to the donut. Remove the cell suspension with a syringe and place in 50 mL conical tubes. Rinse the bag with 100 mL PBS+P/S. Centrifuge the cells at 1800 rpm for 8 minutes. After this centrifugation, combine the pellets into one tube and resuspend to a total volume of 50 mL with PBS+P/S. Note that the cells are resuspended in PBS+P/S without HSA.

G. Determine the total number of nucleated cells recovered and the percent recovery from the harvested bone marrow. RBC:WBC ratio is established by counting an unlysed sample and subtracting the number of nucleated cells per milliliter from the total number of cells per milliliter, then dividing by the number of nucleated cells per milliliter. Ratios of 6:1 to 2:1 are usually seen. Higher RBC:WBC ratios sometimes result in larger agglutinins for which additional dilution of the cell mixture is indicated (see farther on). The cell mixture is adjusted to 150 to 400×10^6 per mL nucleated cells with PBS+P/S. A sample (15×10^6) is withdrawn for quality control assays.

2. AGGLUTINATION WITH SBA: Soybean agglutinin binds to N-acetylgalactosamine residues which are expressed on RBCs, monocytes, granulocytes, B cells, and T cells.[1] Agglutination with SBA reduces total T-cell numbers by 1 $\log_{10}$, taking primarily CD4-positive T cells. Too rapid or too large agglutination can result in trapping of the nonagglutinated (SBA−) cells, resulting in loss of hematopoietic precursors. Agglutination that is slow and fine can result in excessive numbers of small agglutinins remaining in the 5 percent BSA gradients. Accordingly, a test agglutination is done.

A. Set out sixteen 40-mL aliquots of 5 percent BSA in PBS+P/S in 50-mL polystyrene (clear) conical tubes, prepared earlier. Remove with suction any air bubbles at the surface.

B. Do a test agglutination in a 10-mL round-bottom disposable tube. Add 1 mL of cell suspension to 1 mL of soybean agglutinin (2 mg per mL in PBS). Gently agitate, observing the progress of the agglutination. After 1 to 3 minutes of incubation and gentle shaking, layer the contents on the 5 percent BSA gradient, placing the tip of the pipette right at the interface and layering very slowly. If the agglutination is too rapid and the agglutinins too large, decrease the cell concentration by adding PBS+P/S to the suspension. If the agglutination is too slow and fine, the cell concentration may be increased. In practice, it is difficult to increase the cell concentration at this point without extensive cell loss due to clumping. Therefore, the lectin:cell ratio is increased by using 1.5 to 2.0 mL SBA to each milliliter of cell suspension.

C. To agglutinate the remaining cells in bulk, add 6 mL of lectin and 6 mL of the cell suspension to a sterile T75 tissue culture flask (Fig. 7–2). Tilt the flask to spread the mixture on the surface of the flask and agitate gently along a horizontal plane. After the incubation, layer the mixture (total volume of 12 mL) alternately onto two 5 percent BSA gradients.

Allow the agglutinated mixture to settle on the BSA gradients for 5 to 10 minutes. The large agglutinins will fall rapidly to the bottom of the tube, while the small agglutinins will settle more slowly. After an extended period, the SBA− cells will begin to fall as well. Therefore, the SBA− cells must be harvested from the gradient after the small agglutinins have settled but before the unagglutinated cells begin to settle out. Remove the top layer of the gradient with a 25-mL pipette, taking the SBA− cells and harvesting to the 10-mL mark the gradient on the tube. Take care to avoid any clumps. Pool the SBA− cells into a sterile, disposable tissue culture roller bottle (Corning, 490

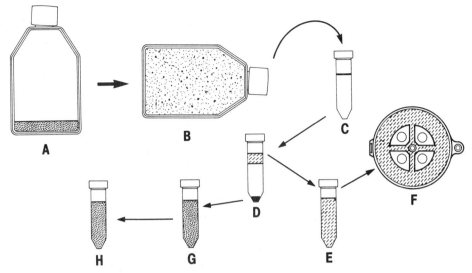

FIGURE 7–2 Bulk SBA agglutination is performed in T75 tissue culture flasks by combining 6 mL of unseparated marrow with 6 mL of SBA at 2 mg per mL (A). The agglutination is carried out for 3 to 5 minutes with constant agitation (B). The agglutinins are layered onto 5 percent BSA gradients (C), where the agglutinated SBA+ cells fall to the bottom and the nonagglutinated SBA− cells float on the top (D). The SBA− cells are pooled, allowing large agglutinins to settle to the bottom (E) and washed with 0.2 M galactose on the COBE 2991 cell washer, as described (F). The SBA+ cells are pooled (G) and washed with 0.2 M galactose and irradiated with 3000 rad (H).

cm^2). Take care not to disturb the bottle, so that any agglutinins collected with the SBA− cells can settle out to the bottom.

Collect the SBA+ cells from the bottom of the BSA gradients. Combine these into three or four 50-mL centrifuge tubes containing 25 mL of 0.2 M galactose in PBS+P/S. Spin at 1800 rpm for 8 minutes. Wash once again with 0.2 M galactose in PBS+P/S. Wash once with M-199+P/S. Resuspend the SBA+ cells in a total of 50 mL of M-199+P/S. Irradiate with 3000 rad and place on ice.

D. Collect the SBA− cells from the tissue culture flask, avoiding the clumps which settle to the bottom. Connect a 1000-mL transfer pack via its endogenous coupler to the barrel of a 60-mL catheter-tip syringe. Using a 25-mL pipette, transfer the cell suspension to the syringe from the collection flask, taking care not to stir up the agglutinins that have settled to the bottom. Spin the last 10 mL left in the flask 30 seconds to pellet the agglutinins and add the supernatant to the bag. Rinse the syringe with galactose.

E. Load the cells into a new sterile processing set in the COBE 2991 as described previously. After spinning down to a pellet, wash the SBA− cells twice with 0.2 M galactose in PBS+1 percent HSA+P/S and then once with M-199+1 percent HSA+P/S. All spins are at 2000 rpm for 3 minutes.

F. After the final wash and removal of the supernatant, clamp the donut off and cut away from the rest of the processing set. Connect a sterile injection site adapter to the donut. Remove the cell suspension with a syringe and place in 50 mL polypropylene conical tubes. Rinse the bag with 100 mL of M-199+P/S. Do a cell count and determine the total number of cells recovered, the percent recovery from the previous step and from the starting count. Remove a small (15×10^6) sample for assays.

3. ROSETTING SBA− CELLS: The nonagglutinated SBA− are depleted of 90 percent of the original number of CD2-positive (sheep RBC-receptor) cells, and greatly enriched for hematopoietic precursors. Additional T-cell depletion techniques can be applied to remove the residual CD2-positive cells. We have shown that a single round of rosetting with AET-treated sheep RBCs[2] is equivalent to the previously reported two-cycle rosetting method[3] and that the number of remaining clonable T cells correlates with the occurrence of grade 1 and 2 GVH disease in HLA-matched recipients.[4] We describe here the procedure for a single round of rosetting.

   A. Adjust SBA− cells in M-199 to 2.5×10^6 per mL with 2 percent AET-treated sheep RBCs and 10 percent absorbed fetal calf serum (FCS). The rosette mix is aliquoted into 50-mL polypropylene tubes and centrifuged at 1000 rpm for 10 minutes. The rosetting tubes are incubated on ice for 1 hour.

   B. After incubation, draw off the supernatant to the 25-mL mark with suction. Resuspend the pellets slowly and carefully by gently inverting the tubes until the pellet is resuspended. Take a 25-μL sterile sample of the cell suspension from at least two tubes to determine the percent of rosettes in the mixture. Layer the cell suspension onto 20 mL of Ficoll-Hypaque aliquoted into 50-mL clear polystyrene tubes using a plexiglass Ficoll rack (Fig. 7–3). Spin at $400g$ for 25 minutes.

   C. After centrifuging the Ficoll gradients, collect the interfaces, trying not to take up any red cells. Collect the SBA-E− cells into a 1000-mL blood bag for washing on the COBE 2991 blood cell processor. Wash the cells with 1 L of lactated Ringer's solution containing 1.0 percent normal HSA+P/S. Finally, wash the cells once with lactated Ringer's solution containing 1.0 percent normal HSA without P/S. All centrifugations are at 2000 rpm for 3 minutes. Adding more spins or increasing the centrifuge speed at this point results in clumping of the cells in the donut.

   D. Remove the cells from the donut as above into 50-mL polypropylene tubes, rinsing the bag with 100 mL of lactated Ringer's solution containing 1.0 percent normal HSA without P/S. Spin the cells at 1500 rpm for 8 minutes. Combine the pellets in lactated Ringer's solution containing 1.0 percent normal HSA without P/S. Do a cell count and remove 15×10^6 cells for assays.

   E. Wash the SBA+ cells separately while the SBA-E− cells are being washed. Remove any large clumps that may have formed in the SBA+ fraction. Wash the SBA+ cells four times with lactated Ringer's solution containing 1.0 percent normal HSA without P/S. Centrifuge at 1500 rpm for 6 minutes. Resuspend in lactated Ringer's solution containing 1.0 percent normal HSA without P/S.

   F. Load the SBA-E− cells and the SBA+ cells each into 60-mL syringes using a 19-gauge spinal needle to remove the cells from the centrifuge tubes. The volume for resuspension is dependent on the weight of the recipient, ranging from 25 mL for infants to 50 mL for adults. Label

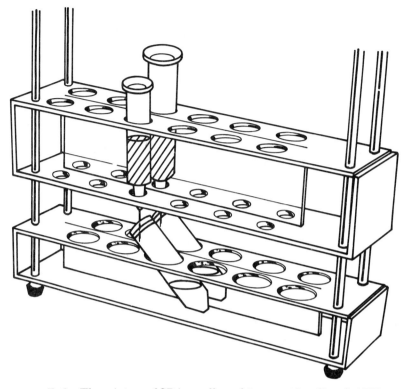

FIGURE 7–3 The mixture of SBA− cells and 2 percent irradiated, AET-treated sheep RBCs with 10 percent absorbed FCS is distributed into 50-mL centrifuge tubes, centrifuged at $400 \times g$ for 10 minutes, and incubated on ice for 1 hour. These multiple rosetting tubes may be layered onto polystyrene centrifuge tubes containing 15 mL of Ficoll-Hypaque by use of the illustrated rack. Twelve sterile syringes fitted with 18-gauge needles are loaded into the rack (six 60-mL syringes in the back row and six 30-mL syringes in the front row). After the hour incubation, one half of the supernatant is removed from each tube and the pellets are then gently resuspended. The mixture is poured into the syringes, which then drip onto the Ficoll-Hypaque gradients, preserving a good interface.

syringes with the cell fraction and cell dose. Attach irradiation stickers to the SBA+ cell fraction. The SBA-E− graft is administered to the patient following infusion of the irradiated SBA+ cells.

4. ASSAYS FOR GRAFT QUALITY
   A. Count cells on a Coulter ZM, adjusted for standard nucleated cells counts. At each successive purification, calculate the percentage recovery and projected recovery for the next step (see table under Anticipated Results).
   B. Evaluate hematopoietic precursors in the unseparated and SBA-E− populations by a modification of the 7-day agar assay[4] and/or the 14-day methylcellulose assay. Figure the total number of clonogenic units at each step in the separation, and calculate percentage recovery.
   C. Set analytic rosettes on the unseparated and SBA-E− cell fractions by mixing one to two 5×10^6 cells with rosetting mixture, centrifuging at 1000 rpm for 5 minutes, and incubating overnight at 7°C. Rosettes

are calculated after microscopic examination of at least 200 cells. Rosettes in SBA− cells are calculated from 25-μL samples taken from at least two tubes of resuspended SBA-E− cells.

ANTICIPATED RESULTS

The following are results of 87 T-cell depletions done over a 5-year period, in which data exist for hematopoietic precursor recovery and/or T-cell frequency by limiting dilution assays for each cell population.

	Unseparated*	SBA−	SBA-E−
Percent recovery cell number from prior step	66.3 ± 17.6	22.0 ± 10.0	47.6 ± 14.8
Percent rosettes	15.9 ± 7.0	6.0 ± 3.5	0.0 ± 0.1
Percent recovery from unseparated			
CFU-GM	100.0	83.0 ± 55.1	60.8 ± 32.8
7-day agarose assay			
CFU-GM	100.0	58.7 ± 25.2	46.2 ± 22.4
14-day methylcellulose assay			
BFU-E	100.0	205.8 ± 248.1	154.8 ± 237.7

*Mean ± standard deviation.

NOTES

1. RBC depletion of harvested bone marrow was originally done with sedimentation with hetastarch, a standard technique used to deplete RBCs prior to administering ABO-incompatible grafts. However, the variability in sedimentation time from donor to donor (0.5 to 2.0 hours) prompted us to use the gelatin method. Ficoll-Hypaque density gradient separation is used as an initial step in some centers prior to agglutination. This greatly reduces the number of agglutination tubes needed, and results in smaller, more finely dispersed agglutinins that settle more slowly through the BSA (Friedrich, personal communication). For this reason, we continue to use gelatin RBC depletion.

2. Reisner and associates[5] have reported a faster E-rosetting method which eliminates the hour incubation on ice. Additionally, the SBA− cells are suspended with the E at 15×10^6 per mL, resulting in a reduction in the number of rosetting tubes.

AUTHORS

Nancy H. Collins, Ph.D.
Memorial Sloan-Kettering Cancer
  Center
1275 York Avenue
New York, NY 10021

Sharon A. Bleau, M.S.
Memorial Sloan-Kettering Cancer
  Center
1275 York Avenue
New York, NY 10021

Nancy A. Kernan, M.D.
Memorial Sloan-Kettering Cancer
  Center
1275 York Avenue
New York, NY 10021

Richard J. O'Reilly, M.D.
Memorial Sloan-Kettering Cancer
  Center
1275 York Avenue
New York, NY 10021

REFERENCES

1. Reisner, Y, et al: Enrichment for CFU-C from murine and human bone marrow using soybean agglutinin. Blood 69:360, 1982.
2. Pellegrino, MA, et al: Enhancement of sheep red blood cell human lymphocytes rosette forma-

tion by sulfhydryl compound 2-amino ethylisothiouronium bromide. Clin Immunol Immuno-pathol 3:324, 1975.

3. Kernan, NA, et al: Quantitation of T lymphocytes in human bone marrow by a limiting dilution assay. Transplantation 40:317, 1985.

4. Kernan, NA, et al: Prevention of GVHD in HLA-identical marrow grafts by removal of T cells with soybean agglutinin and SRBCs. Bone Marrow Transplant 2:13, 1987.

5. Reisner, Y, Friedrich, W, and Fabian, IA: A shorter procedure of preparation of E-rosette bone marrow for transplantation. Transplantation 42:312, 1986.

Counterflow Centrifugation

LYMPHOCYTE DEPLETION OF BONE MARROW GRAFTS USING ELUTRIATION

DESCRIPTION	Acute graft-versus-host (GVH) disease remains a prominent cause of morbidity and mortality after allogeneic bone marrow transplantation. Depletion of T lymphocytes from bone marrow allografts results in a significant decrease in the incidence and severity of acute GVH disease. Counterflow centrifugation elutriation (CCE) provides a rapid and reproducible separation of large numbers of cells without impairing cell function or yield. The separation is based on the differences in the size and density of the cells. Before the elutriation is performed, a buffy coat concentrate must be prepared to reduce the volume and number of red cells present in the harvested marrow. This buffy coat concentrate is then processed using either the Beckman JE-10X or J5.0 elutriation rotor. Cell fractions are collected based on the medium flow rates (LOAD [70 mL per minute], 110 mL per minute, 140 mL per minute, and ROTOR OFF [R/O]). The R/O fraction is collected by stopping the rotor while maintaining medium flow. This fraction is progenitor cell enriched, lymphocyte depleted, as well as containing the largest cells loaded into the chamber. Since elutriation medium is infusion compatible, the R/O fraction can be transfused immediately. Automated cell counts and leukocyte differentials are then performed on all fractions. A second product is prepared so that the patient receives a predetermined total lymphocyte dose. Calculations take into account the residual lymphocytes already infused in the R/O fraction and determine the volume of the 140 mL per minute fraction necessary to obtain the correct lymphocyte dose (e.g., 5.0×10^5 lymphocytes/kg [ideal body weight]). In cases when the entire 140 mL per minute fraction is not sufficient, the 110 mL per minute fraction supplies the additional lymphocytes.
TIME FOR PROCEDURE	The actual elutriation procedure takes 40 minutes. However, time is required for the preparation of the buffy coat concentrate, instrument setup, and cell differentials.
SUMMARY OF PROCEDURE	1. Buffy coat concentrate is prepared. 2. Cells are filtered (170 μm) into the sample bag attached to the pump. 3. Total red cells and volume are standardized. 4. Calibration of the balance is checked. 5. Cells are loaded into the chamber. 6. Medium flow rate is increased as per procedure and fractions collected. 7. Fractions are sampled and cell counts performed. 8. R/O fraction is infused. 9. Cell differentials are performed. 10. The appropriate amount of the remaining fraction(s) are prepared for infusion (based on lymphocyte dose).
EQUIPMENT	1. Beckman centrifuge (Beckman J-6M) 2. Rotor and associated hardware (Beckman JE-10X or J5.0)

3. Chambers (Beckman 354649 [JE-10X] or 356940 [J5.0])

4. Sample reservoir (70-mL) (Beckman 335197)

5. Sample reservoir (30-mL) (Beckman 335213)

6. Pressure gauge (Beckman 340148)

7. Pumps (Masterflex 900-197)

8. Quick load pump heads (Masterflex 7021-24)

9. Balance (Mettler PM 4600)

10. Ultrasonic cleaner (Bransonic B3200-R2)

11. 3 burette clamps and stand

12. Torque screwdriver

13. Cell counter

14. Microscope

15. Laminar flow hood

16. Heat sealer

17. IV pole

18. Test tube rack

19. Clamps

20. Computer (used to calibrate flow rates)*

SUPPLIES AND REAGENTS

1. Elutriation medium† (Whittaker 04-440L)

2. Blood spike adaptor (for medium) (Whittaker 01886)

3. Masterflex silicone tubing (Cole-Parmer 6411-14)

4. Masterflex silicone tubing (Cole-Parmer 6411-16)

5. Blood filter (Abbott 9143)

6. 2000-mL transfer pack (Fenwal 4R2041)

7. 1000-mL transfer pack (Fenwal 4R2031)

8. 600-mL transfer pack (Fenwal 4R2023)

9. Y blood component recipient set (Fenwal 4C2196)

10. Plasma transfer set (Fenwal 4C2240)

11. Sampling site coupler (Fenwal 4C2405)

---

*Flow rates are calculated by the change in the weight of the transfer pack as a function of time. A density correction factor of 1.004 g per mL is used to correct mass to volume. The pumps are calibrated before each clinical procedure. A program was written in Microsoft BASIC to run on an IBM PC compatible computer (IBM Corporation, Boca Raton, FL). Contact authors for information concerning the computer program. The computer must be interfaced to a Mettler PM4600 Delta Range Balance (Mettler Instruments, Greifensee, Switzerland). The interface cable is available from Mettler as an option.

†Elutriation medium is not designed for long-term cell storage. However, it will maintain short-term viability and cell size differences, prevent clumping, and reduce the sheer forces encountered during CCE. Elutriation medium consists of physiologic saline (0.9 percent), D-glucose (1 mg per mL) and disodium ethylenediaminetetraacetic acid (EDTA, 0.3 mM or 100 mg per L). The final pH is set at 7.2 to prevent platelet clumping while the osmolality of the final product is adjusted to 290 ± 10 mOsm. Albumin is added immediately before use (20 mL of albumin per L of medium [0.5 g per percent final concentration]). The anticoagulant EDTA was chosen because it chelates all remaining divalent cations present from albumin or damaged cells or both.

12. Female adaptor (extension tube) (Baxter K50)

13. Calcium chloride (10 percent)

14. Human albumin (25 percent)

PROCEDURE

The data accrued during elutriation are entered onto a Lotus 1-2-3 spreadsheet to facilitate graft calculations and future analyses. Cell counts and recovery data for the buffy coat concentrate and the various CCE fractions as well as leukocyte differentials are entered. The amount of red cells and plasma needed to standardize the buffy coat product (refer to Separation Procedure for details) can be calculated along with the amount of the 140 mL per minute and if necessary 110 mL per minute fractions needed to compose a graft containing 5×10^5 lymphocytes per kg (ideal body weight).

- Create a worksheet for the patient using the Lotus spreadsheet. Type in the patient and donor information. Print the worksheet in order to record all information when the computer is moved to the basic program to calibrate and monitor the balance.
- From the harvested marrow, obtain a gross weight and set aside a 3-mL sample. Mix the bag well before sampling. Place 1 mL of the sample in an aerobic blood culture bottle and 0.2 mL in a tube for red and white cell counts and differentials. Follow the count procedure described in Appendix 1 on page 194 to obtain appropriate dilutions for red and white cell counting.
- Prepare a buffy coat concentrate using the Haemonetics Model 30 or comparable procedure (refer to Chapter 6 on buffy coat concentration).
- The temperature of the elutriation medium does have a significant effect on the elutriation profile. Remove elutriation medium from the refrigerator the evening before the procedure. If this was not done, place the medium in a 37°C incubator. Add 20 mL of 25 percent human albumin per L of medium, and check the pH before use.
- Clean and sterilize the equipment that is used for the procedure before the day of the elutriation procedure. The equipment has been divided into five working units. The sterilization procedure is described next.

1. PRE-ELUTRIATION STERILIZATION PROCEDURE
    A. Unit 1: Media Line
        (1) Attach 20 inches of Silastic tubing (No. 16) to the right side of the pressure gauge by pushing the plastic hex connector over the tubing. Insert the plastic tubing adapter and loosely screw the hex connector onto the pressure gauge.
        (2) Attach 6 inches of tubing (No. 16) to the left side of the pressure gauge, as previously described.
        (3) Screw the cap of the large 70-mL reservoir over the stopper (stopper should have long and short needles with luer-lock adapters through it). Attach the other end of the 6-in tubing to the luer-lock adapter on the long needle.
        (4) Attach 3 inches tubing (No. 16) to the luer-lock adapter on the short needle. Insert the stopper loosely into the medium reservoir.
        (5) Use 4- × 4-inch nonsterile gauze to wrap exposed tubing ends. Secure the gauze with ethylene oxide indicator tape (½ inch for gas sterilization). Wrap in disposable drape (17 × 19 inches), and tape. Place in pouch (12 × 15 inches).
        (6) Label with sticker "Unit 1 Bone Marrow Elutriation."

B. Unit 2: Sample Line
   (1) Screw the cap of the small 30-mL sample reservoir over the stopper (stopper should have long and short needles with luer-lock adapters through it).
   (2) Attach 30 inches of tubing (No. 14) to the short needle of the small 30-mL sample reservoir. To the other end of the 30 inches of tubing attach a female adapter (remove the female adapter from the end of an extension tube).
   (3) Attach 3 inches of tubing (No. 16) to the long needle. To the other end of the 3 inches of tubing attach the short arm of a Y fitting.
   (4) Attach 40 inches of tubing (No. 16) to the long arm of the Y fitting. Attach an inlet connector with an O-ring to the other end of the 40 inches of tubing.
   (5) Wrap the exposed adapters on the tubing ends and the exposed arm of the Y fitting with 4- × 4-inch nonsterile gauze. Secure the gauze with ethylene oxide indicator tape (½ inch for gas sterilization). Wrap in disposable drape (17 × 19 inches), and tape. Place in pouch.
   (6) Label with sticker "Unit 2 Bone Marrow Elutriation."
C. Unit 3: Chamber
   (1) Place the gasket between the chamber parts in proper position (make sure all holes line up). Insert wooden applicator sticks into the chamber screw holes to keep the chamber lined up.
   (2) Loosely screw the inlet tubing (long piece) into the outer hole of the chamber. The outlet tubing (short piece) should be loosely screwed into the center hole.
   (3) Wrap the chamber with elastic bandage or gauze and secure with tape (make sure inlet and outlet tubings are not bent).
   (4) Wrap the tubing ends with 4- × 4-inch nonsterile gauze and secure with autoclave indicator tape. Wrap in disposable drape (17 × 19 inches).
   (5) Wrap the four screws with washers in separate gauze and secure with indicator tape. Place the chamber and screws into a pouch.
   (6) Label with sticker "Unit 3 Bone Marrow Elutriation."
D. Unit 4: Rotor
   (1) Inspect the black seal and lap it, if necessary, to remove scratches or imperfections in contact surface (see manual). Position the black seal on top of the spring in the center of the rotor.
   (2) Partially screw down the seal housing onto the bearing assembly. Set the bearing assembly on the rotor shaft and tighten while pushing down on entire assembly.
   (3) Loosely attach bypass tubing to both connections.
   (4) Cap the scavenger line with gauze and secure with autoclave indicator tape. Cover the entire bearing assembly with two pieces of 4- × 4-inch gauze, and secure with indicator tape.
   (5) Label a piece of indicator tape on the outer edge of the rotor with "Unit 4 Bone Marrow Elutriation."
   (6) Place the plastic cap in a separate bag. Label with indicator tape and "Cap."
E. Unit 5: Collection Tubing
   (1) Attach the inlet connector with an O-ring into the end of a piece

of 35 inches of tubing (No. 16). To the other end attach the long end of a Y fitting.

(2) Add 3-inch pieces of tubing to the Y fitting. Add another Y fitting to the end of one of the pieces of tubing. Repeat this until four Y fittings are in sequence. Add a 6-inch piece of tubing to the last Y fitting. Add 3-inch pieces of tubing to all remaining arms of the Y fittings.

(3) Wrap all exposed tubing ends with gauze and secure with autoclave indicator tape. Wrap in disposable drape (17 × 19 inches) and tape. Place in pouch.

(4) Label with sticker "Unit 5 Bone Marrow Elutriation."

Sterilization: Units 1 through 5 are delivered to the sterile processing facility. Units 1 and 2 are sterilized by ethylene oxide and aerated (gas sterilization). Units 3, 4, and 5 are sterilized by autoclaving (steam sterilization).

2. ASSEMBLY (JE-10X) (Fig. 7–4)

A. Work in a sterile hood and wear gloves when assembling the system. Unwrap the outside drape of unit 4 (rotor). Use this wrap to prepare a sterile field for subunit assembly.

B. Open the wrap of unit 3 and place the chamber next to the rotor.

C. Unwrap the screws and sparingly lubricate the threads of screws with Spinkote (supplied with rotor) lubricant.

D. Remove the wooden applicator sticks from the holes in the chamber. Place the four screws (with washers in place) into these holes.

E. Tighten the screws in a clockwise direction using a torque screwdriver set to 8 inch-lb or with a hex wrench (supplied with rotor). Once resistance is felt, turn opposing screws one-quarter turn until torque screwdriver clicks and all screws are tight.

F. Tighten the inlet and outlet tubing by hand. Then tighten an additional one-quarter turn with a $\frac{5}{16}$-inch wrench.

G. Remove the inner second wrap from the rotor. Attach the outlet tubing (from center hole of chamber) to the lower rotor hole. Attach the inlet tubing similarly (the two pieces of tubing should cross). Tighten all tubing connections (including the bypass tubing) by one-quarter turn with a $\frac{5}{16}$-inch wrench.

H. Place the chamber in the rotor chamber bucket. Insert the buckets and counter balances into the rotor. Check that the reflector tape that triggers the strobe unit is in position on the bottom of the rotor.

I. Check that the sensor, strobe, and window are in the correct position (see instruction manual). Place the rotor in the centrifuge, making sure that the height of the chamber equals the height of the strobe wire shield.

J. Unwrap unit 1 and place the stopper in the reservoir tube and screw on the black cap (check for proper needle placement and that there are no cracks in the polycarbonate tube).

K. Tighten the hexagonal tubing connector to the pressure gauge. Place the reservoir and pressure gauge into the burette clamps. The reservoir should be placed in the clamp with the black cap down.

L. Unwrap unit 2 and place the stopper in the reservoir and screw on the black cap (check for proper needle placement). Place the reservoir in

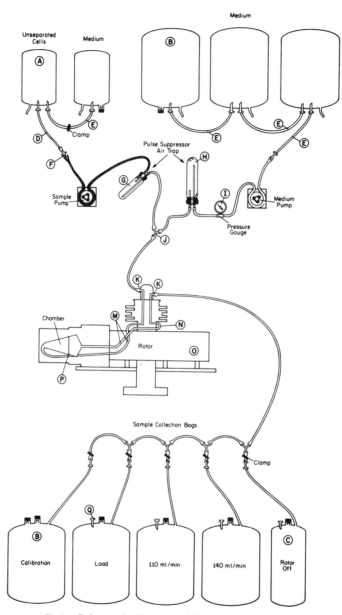

FIGURE 7–4   Schematic diagram of the clinical elutriation system used for lymphocyte depletion. The system uses either the Beckman JE-10X rotor depicted here or the newer J5.0. Letter codes: 600-mL sample bag (A), 2000-mL container of medium or cells (B), 1000-mL transfer bag for Rotor Off fraction (C), sample (D) and medium (E) transfer sets, female (F) adaptor, 30-mL (G) and 70-mL (H) air traps, pressure gauge (I), Y fitting (J), inlet/outlet connector with O-ring (K), inlet-outlet (M) and bypass (N) tubing assembly, JE-10X elutriation rotor (O) and standard chamber (P), sampling site couplers (Q). (Adapted from the Beckman JE-10X instruction manual with the permission of Beckman Instruments, Inc., Spinco Division, Palo Alto, CA.)

the proper clamp. The reservoir should be placed in the clamp with the black cap up at a 45-degree angle.

M. Feed the small tubing into the lower pump (to conserve space the pumps can be positioned on top of each other) and the large tubing (from unit 1) into the upper pump. The Quick-load pump heads can be used for either size tubing. Check for proper orientation of the tubing in the pump heads.

N. Remove the wrap from the arm of the Y fitting and attach it to the short tube leading from the large reservoir. Insert the inlet tubing through the stopper and bracket hole at the rear of the centrifuge.

O. Unwrap unit 5 and thread the short tubings through the test tube rack. The outlet tubing should be inserted through the stopper and bracket hole toward the front of the centrifuge.

P. Insert sampling site couplers into three 2-L transfer packs and label them "load," "110," and "140." Add 0.8 mL $CaCl_2$ per L to the bags (0.8 mL into "load" and "140"; 1.6 mL into "110"). This restores calcium chelated by EDTA in elutriation medium and extends viability through further sample manipulation. Since the R/O fraction is infused immediately, the addition of calcium is not necessary. Insert a sampling site coupler into a 1-L transfer pack and label "R/O." Label a 2-L transfer pack "calibration" and weigh each bag (denote weight on bag). Insert the couplers from the transfer packs into the tubing of unit 5 in the order "calibration," "load," "110," "140," and "R/O" (left to right with "calibration" bag closest to the centrifuge). Label all of the bags with the donor's name.

Q. Clamp all tubings (except "calibration") with hemostat clamps.

R. Remove the cover from the seal housing of rotor. Place the black cap over the seal housing. Insert the metal tubing connectors for inlet tubing (upper hole) and outlet tubing (lower hole) into the seal housing (connectors click into place). Turn the black cap into place. Using the "T" wrench (supplied), loosen the housing. Push down on housing and retighten.

S. Remove the gauze from the scavenger line and attach to a low suction line. Pull the tubing leading out from the centrifuge tight (no slack should be in the lines).

3. PRIME

A. Connect two 600-mL transfer bags. Add a roller clamp to close the line. Seal off the extra tubing. Place a sampling site coupler and the spike end of a needle adaptor transfer set into one of the bags. Attach the needle adaptor at the other end of the transfer set into the coupler on the spike of the medium container. Allow approximately 250 mL of medium to enter the 600-mL transfer pack, making sure the roller clamp between bags is closed. Once the bag is filled, attach the bags to the sample line using the needle adaptor end of the plasma transfer set.

B. Connect the two 4-L carboys of medium to each other using a Y blood component recipient set. Hang both containers on IV poles and connect them to the medium line.

C. Open the roller clamps on the medium line and turn the medium pump on low (check that the medium is flowing in the proper direction). Clamp the outlet line on the small reservoir and fill two thirds of the large reservoir. In order to fill this reservoir, it must be temporarily inverted.

    D. Remove the clamp from the tubing near the small reservoir. Turn on the sample pump and fill one third of the small reservoir. Turn off the pump and reclamp the line.

4. AIR PURGE

    A. Turn on the medium pump and purge all inlet lines of air bubbles by tapping the tubing (air under pressure in the spinning rotor will add back pressure and can interfere with separation).

    B. Turn the rotor by hand and allow air to exit the rotor. Remove the chamber from the bucket and tilt it up to allow air to exit (tap slightly to dislodge air from the sides of the chamber).

    C. Use fingers to clamp the outlet tubing and spin the rotor until the pressure rises to 5 psi. Release the tubing and allow air to exit. Repeat the procedure as needed.

    D. Turn on the centrifuge and enter the settings: Rotor: 3.2, Speed: 150 rpm, Time: 5.000 hours, Temp: 20°C.

    E. Start the centrifuge and repeat the finger-clamp purge. When the finger clamp is released, pressure should return to baseline.

    F. Increase the speed to 2040 rpm and repeat the finger-clamp purge. Check for any tubing or connection leaks.

    G. Let the centrifuge stop and check for leaks in the chamber and rotor tubings.

5. CALIBRATION

    A. Allow the centrifuge to reach the targeted speed before beginning the calibration procedure. If it fails to reach the speed of 2040, then turn the centrifuge off and try to bring it up again. Look through the strobe hole for liquid formation, which may indicate system leaks. If medium is seen, determine where the leak is and tighten the appropriate connection.

    B. Locate BASIC program in computer. Key in the appropriate command to locate the flow program. A welcome should appear on the screen, followed promptly by "PRESS SPACE TO START." After pressing the space bar, flow data should appear on the screen. If the message "PLEASE TURN BALANCE ON" remains in the upper left hand corner of the screen, either the balance has not been turned on or it has not been interfaced correctly. Check the cable. The flow rate should appear on the screen. (This procedure may change if different BASIC language versions are used to run the program.)

    C. Key in C for calibration mode. This measures the flow rate at a number of different pump settings and performs a linear regression analysis of flow rate versus pump setting. Enter the maximum pump setting and the number of points to be monitored. Follow the prompts on the screen ("SET PUMP TO _____") to calibrate the flow rate for the medium pump. Once the medium pump is calibrated, the desired flow rates (50, 110, 140) can be typed in and the appropriate settings will appear. The medium pump should deliver 50 mL per minute for the load fraction, followed by 110 mL per minute and 140 mL per minute.

    D. Set the medium pump to deliver 50 mL per minute. Remove the clamp on the sample line and turn on the sample pump. Follow the calibration procedure to calibrate the sample pump. The sample pump should deliver 20 mL per minute while the medium pump delivers 50 mL per minute (a total of 70 mL per minute for the LOAD fraction). Turn the sample pump off and place a clamp back on the outlet line from the small reservoir. Run any excess medium (used for sample pump calibration) from the transfer bag back into the attached 600-mL bag and close the roller clamp near the sample bag. Close the roller clamp between the sample bag and the pump.

E. After the calibration is complete, the centrifuge can be left at 2040 rpm until the marrow is ready to be loaded. If there will be a long delay, the centrifuge and medium pump can be turned off and the pumps will remain calibrated.

6. SEPARATION PROCEDURE

A. Obtain a tare weight on the empty 600-mL sample bag. Transfer the buffy coat cells into this transfer bag using a blood filter. Obtain the gross weight and then remove 0.7 mL for cell counts, sterility, differentials, and cell culture. Use the Lotus worksheet to determine how much plasma and residual (red blood cell concentrate obtained from the buffy coat procedure) to add. The loaded product should contain 175 mL (total) and 1.6×10^{11} total red blood cells. The total leukocyte count will vary.

B. Turn the medium pump on (if needed) and set it to deliver 50 mL per minute. Turn the centrifuge on (if needed) and set the speed to 2040 rpm. Open the roller clamp between the sample bag and the pump. Set the sample pump at the 20 mL per minute position. Remove the clamp on the outlet line of the small reservoir and turn on the sample pump. Move the clamp from the LOAD line to the CALIBRATION line. Marrow will enter the system. When 10 mL of marrow remains in the sample bag, open the line from the 600-mL medium bag to rinse the bag and flush the remaining marrow from the bag. Set a timer for 3 minutes.

C. At the end of the 3 minutes, turn the sample pump off and clamp the outlet tubing from the small reservoir. Remove the clamp from the 110 line and clamp the LOAD line. Start the timer (set at 18.06 minutes) and increase the flow to the 110 setting (increase one increment on the pump speed control every second).

D. Place the 110 bag on the balance. Check the flow rate.

E. At the end of the 18.06 minutes, remove the clamp from the 140 line and clamp the 110 line. Start the timer (set at 7.12 minutes) and increase the flow to the 140 setting.

F. Place the 140 bag on the balance. Check the flow rate.

G. At the end of the 7.12 minutes, remove the clamp from the R/O line and clamp the 140 line. Turn the centrifuge off and start the timer (set at 2.36 minutes).

H. At the end of the 2.36 minutes, turn the medium pump off and clamp the R/O line.

I. Obtain gross weights on all of the bags. Heat seal each bag and withdraw the appropriate volumes for counts and testing. Samples can be pulled from the bags (after the individual fraction is collected and weighed) while the procedure is in progress.

J. Label the R/O fraction and issue to the physician for infusion.

K. Perform cell counts on all of the fractions. One milliliter of the 140 fraction should be added to an aerobic blood culture bottle. Cell counts should be entered in the computer. The spreadsheet should contain a section that lists the amount of cells and medium (90 percent TC-199 and 10 percent autologous plasma) needed for cytospins. Cytospins (5×10^5 cells) should be prepared at 600 rpm for 6 minutes. The slides can be stained using an automated hematology stainer. Differentials (500 cell) are performed on the R/O, and 140 fractions. Lymphocytes and others (other myeloid cells plus plasma cells) are counted. This is followed by myeloid cells:erythroid cells (M:E) ratio. The differential results should be entered into the worksheet. The amount of additional marrow (140 fraction) to be infused is calculated. It may be necessary to add some of the 110 fraction to the graft, and then a 110 differential should be preformed.

L. If the volume of the second half of the graft is greater than 300 mL, transfer the appropriate volume to a 600-mL bag and centrifuge in a Sorvall RC-3B at 1400 rpm (500 $\times$ g) for 10 minutes at 20°C. After centrifugation, the marrow should be placed in a plasma expressor and medium removed to yield a final volume of approximately 200 mL. Weigh the final product and record the volume. Label the marrow and issue it to a physician for infusion.

MODIFIED INSTRUCTIONS FOR USE OF THE J5.0 ROTOR (Fig. 7–5)

7. PRE-ELUTRIATION STERILIZATION PROCEDURE
   A. Unit 1: Media line: Follow steps 1 through 6 for the JE-10X rotor.
   B. Unit 2: Sample line: Follow steps 1 through 6 for the JE-10X rotor except that there is *no* inlet connector required.
   C. Unit 3: Chamber
      (1) Place the gasket on the upper chamber half and insert all nipples completely into the alignment holes. Position the lower half of the chamber such that the single dots (etched into right side of chamber sections) are together. Insert wooden applicator sticks into the chamber screw holes to keep the chamber parts together.
      (2) Turn the chamber over and place two hexagonal nuts into the holes in the upper half of the chamber and secure with tape.
      (3) Cut a short piece of gauze to place over the transfer tube holes in top of the chamber and affix with tape.
      (4) Wrap the chamber completely with elastic bandage or gauze and secure with indicator tape.
      (5) Wrap the chamber screws in separate gauze and secure with indicator tape.
      (6) Place the chamber and screws in pouch.
      (7) Label with sticker "Unit 3 Bone Marrow Elutriation."
   D. Unit 4: Seal Assembly
      (1) Inspect the black seal and lap if necessary (see JE-10X rotor). Place the seal (flat side down) into the recessed area of the lower plate. Insert the spring into the seal guide and seat on the black seal.
      (2) Examine the bearing assembly O-rings and ensure that the retaining clip is securely seated in its groove.

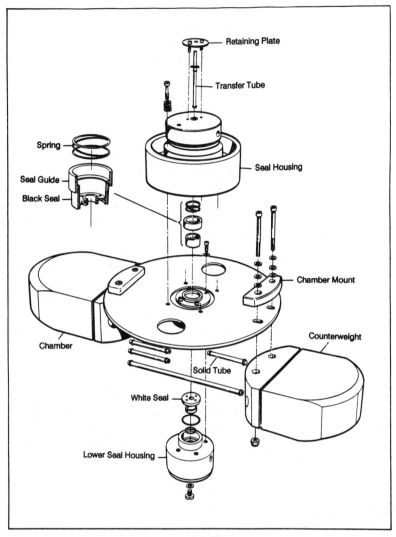

FIGURE 7–5 The Beckman J5.0 elutriator chamber and housing assembly. An accurate schematic of the totally autoclavable chamber assembly, which slips into the J5.0 rotor body via bayonet fittings (see text for a detailed description of rotor setup). (Adapted from the Beckman J5.0 instruction manual with the permission of Beckman Instruments, Inc., Spinco Division, Palo Alto, CA.) Please note that only the single-chamber configuration is shown. For use of two chambers in series (not described in text), please refer to the explicit instructions in the J5.0 manual.

(3) Carefully lower the bearing assembly onto the lower plate. Push down gently and tighten the screws. Loosen all screws one turn.

(4) Invert the assembly and insert both short hollow transfer tubes into the pair of holes in the transfer hub. Insert the short solid transfer tube into the single hole in the opposite side of the hub.

(5) Cover the transfer tubes and hub with gauze and secure with tape.

(6) Invert the assembly and cover both the inlet (side) and outlet (top) tubes with gauze. Secure with indicator tape. Wrap the

        entire bearing assembly and secure with indicator tape and label with sticker "Unit 4 Bone Marrow Elutriation."

E. Unit 5: Collection Tubing: Follow steps 1 through 4 for the JE-10X rotor, except that there is *no* outlet connector required.

        Sterilization: Units 1 through 5 are handled the same as the JE-10X rotor.

8. ASSEMBLY (J5.0)

A. Work in a sterile hood and wear gloves when assembling the system. Unwrap unit 4 and tighten the screws on the bearing assembly.

B. Unwrap unit 3 and place the chamber next to the bearing assembly.

C. Unwrap the screws and lubricate the threads of the screws with Spin-kote. Remove the applicator sticks from the chamber.

D. Place the two chamber screws into the appropriate holes in the chamber. Tighten the screws in a clockwise direction until finger tight.

E. Invert the bearing assembly and remove the gauze covering the transfer tubes. Orient the chamber such that the side with the tape is facing up. Remove the gauze from the chamber head and carefully slide the transfer tubes into the chamber head.

F. Insert the long transfer tube into the second hole from the top of the chamber. Carefully slide the transfer tubes into the head of the counterweight.

G. Invert the assembly.

H. Align the chamber mount over the holes above the counterweight. Insert the two short screws and tighten.

I. Align the second mount over the chamber. Carefully insert the two long screws and tighten. Remove the tape from the bottom of the chamber.

J. Loosen all four chamber mount screws one-half turn.

K. Place the rotor over the spindle in the centrifuge and tighten the center screw.

L. Lower the chamber assembly into the rotor. Retaining cones (bayonet fitting) will snap into place securing the assembly to the rotor. (To remove the assembly, press the cones toward the center of the rotor.)

M. Attach the retaining cable to the bearing assembly.

N. Check that the sensor, strobe, and window are in the correct position.

O. Unwrap unit 1 and place the stopper in the reservoir tube and screw on the black cap (check for proper needle placement and that there are no cracks in the polycarbonate tube).

P. Tighten the hexagonal tubing connector to the pressure gauge. Place the reservoir and pressure gauge in the burette clamps. The reservoir should be placed in the clamp with the black cap down.

Q. Unwrap unit 2 and place the stopper in the reservoir and screw on the black cap (check for proper needle placement). Place the reservoir in the proper burette clamp. The reservoir should be placed in the clamp with the black cap up at a 45-degree angle.

R. Feed the small tubing into the lower pump (to conserve space the pumps can be positioned on top of each other) and the large tubing (from unit 1) into the upper pump. The Quick-load pump heads can be used for either size tubing. Check for proper orientation of the tubing in the pump heads.

S. Remove the wrap from the arm of the Y fitting and attach it to the short tube leading from the large reservoir. Insert the inlet tubing through the stopper and bracket hole at the rear of the centrifuge.

T. Unwrap unit 5 and thread the short tubings through the test tube rack. The outlet tubing should be inserted through the stopper and bracket hole toward the front of the centrifuge.

U. Insert sampling site couplers into three 2-L transfer packs and label them "load," "110," and "140." Add 0.8 mL $CaCl_2$ per L to the bags (0.8 mL into "load" and "140"; 1.6 mL into "110"). This restores calcium chelated by EDTA in elutriation medium and extends viability through further sample manipulation. Because the R/O fraction is infused immediately, recalcification is not necessary. Insert a sampling site coupler into a 1-L transfer pack and label "R/O." Label a 2-L transfer pack "calibration" and weigh each bag (denote weight on bag). Insert the couplers from the transfer packs into the tubing of unit 5 in the order "calibration," "load," "110," "140," and "R/O" (left to right with "calibration" bag closest to the centrifuge). Label all bags with the donor's name.

V. Place clamps on all of the tubings except "calibration."

W. Remove the gauze from the inlet port on the rotor assembly and connect the input line. Repeat for the outlet tubing.

X. Pull the tubing lines leading out from the centrifuge tight (no slack should be in the lines).

9. PRIME: Follow steps 1 through 4 for the JE-10X rotor.

10. AIR PURGE
A. Turn the medium pump on and purge all of the air bubbles from the inlet lines by tapping the tubing.
B. Turn the rotor by hand and allow air to exit the rotor.
C. Use your fingers to clamp the outlet tubing and spin the rotor until the pressure rises to 5 psi. Then release the tubing and allow air to exit. Repeat the procedure as needed.
D. Turn on the centrifuge and enter the following settings: Rotor: 5.2; Speed: 150 rpm; Time: 5.000 hours; Temp: 20°C.
E. Start the centrifuge and repeat the finger-clamp purge. When the finger clamp is released, pressure should return to baseline.
F. Increase the speed to 3000 rpm and repeat the finger-clamp purge. Check for any tubing or connection leaks.
G. Let the centrifuge stop and check for leaks in the chamber and rotor tubing.

11. CALIBRATION
A. The centrifuge should be spinning at 3000 rpm before beginning the calibration procedure. Look through the strobe window for liquid formation, which may indicate system leaks. If medium is seen, determine where the leak is and tighten the appropriate connection.
B. Follow steps 2 through 5 for the JE-10X rotor.

12. SEPARATION PROCEDURE: Follow steps 1 through 12 for the JE-10X rotor, except that run speed is 3000 rpm.

APPENDIX 1: SUGGESTED DILUTIONS FOR CELL COUNTS

  A. HARVEST SPECIMEN

    (1) Add 20 μL of the specimen to 10 mL of Isoton (Coulter Diagnostics, Hialeah, FL).

    (2) Remove 100 μL from container 1 and add this to 9.90 mL of Isoton. Obtain cell count without Zap-oglobin II (Coulter).

    (3) Add Zap-oglobin to container 1, and count.

  B. BUFFY COAT SPECIMEN

    (1) Add 20 μL of the specimen to 10 mL of Isoton.

    (2) Remove 100 μL from container 1 and add this to 9.90 mL of Isoton. Obtain cell count without Zap-oglobin.

  C. RESIDUAL SPECIMEN

    (1) Add 20 μL of the specimen to 10 mL of Isoton.

    (2) Remove 100 μL from container 1 and add this to 9.90 mL of Isoton. Obtain cell count without Zap-oglobin.

    (3) Add Zap-oglobin to container 1, and count.

  D. LOAD SPECIMEN

    (1) Add 20 μL of the specimen to 10 mL of Isoton.

    (2) Remove 1 mL of container 1 and add this to 9.00 mL of Isoton. Obtain count without Zap-oglobin.

    (3) Add Zap-oglobin to container 1, and count.

  E. FRACTION 110 SPECIMEN

    (1) Add 20 μL of the specimen to 10 mL of Isoton. Obtain count without Zap-oglobin.

    (2) Add 200 μL of the specimen to 10 mL of Isoton. Obtain count with Zap-oglobin.

  F. FRACTION 140 SPECIMEN: (1) Add 200 μL of the specimen to 10 mL of Isoton. Obtain a count without Zap-oglobin. (2) Add Zap-oglobin and obtain another count.

  G. R/O SPECIMEN: (1) Add 20 μL of the specimen to 10 mL of Isoton. Obtain a count without Zap-oglobin. (2) Add Zap-oglobin and obtain another count.

ANTICIPATED RESULTS Results involving the first 40 patients who received CCE lymphocyte-depleted bone marrow are shown.

Fraction	TOTAL CELLS		DIFFERENTIAL			CFU-GM ($\times 10^6$)
	Nucleated ($\times 10^9$)	RBC ($\times 10^{10}$)	Lymph	Blast	Other	
Harvest	32.0 ($\pm$1.1)	391.2 ($\pm$20.1)	16.2 ($\pm$1.8)	2.0 ($\pm$0.3)	76.1 ($\pm$2.7)	Not done
Buffy coat	14.2 ($\pm$0.6)	14.5 ($\pm$0.7)	20.3 ($\pm$1.5)	3.4 ($\pm$0.6)	68.7 ($\pm$2.9)	20.9 ($\pm$9.0)
70 mL/min	5.0 ($\pm$0.3)	11.7 ($\pm$0.7)	89.0 ($\pm$1.8)	1.0 ($\pm$0.3)	6.6 ($\pm$1.4)	3.6 ($\pm$3.6)
110 mL/min	1.6 ($\pm$0.1)	2.8 ($\pm$0.1)	50.9 ($\pm$3.9)	1.7 ($\pm$0.3)	25.4 ($\pm$2.9)	2.2 ($\pm$1.2)
140 mL/min	0.9 ($\pm$0.1)	0.5 ($\pm$0.1)	49.5 ($\pm$5.6)	3.2 ($\pm$0.6)	33.5 ($\pm$7.7)	0.9 ($\pm$1.0)
Rotor Off	6.7 ($\pm$0.3)	0.0 ($\pm$0.0)	0.3 ($\pm$0.1)	5.2 ($\pm$1.1)	88.8 ($\pm$1.8)	13.0 ($\pm$8.2)

AUTHORS

Janice M. Davis, M.T. (ASCP),
  S.B.B.
Cell Processing Laboratory
The Johns Hopkins Oncology Center
Baltimore, MD 21205

Stephen J. Noga, M.D., Ph.D.
The Johns Hopkins Oncology Center
Baltimore, MD 21205

Christopher J. Thoburn
The Johns Hopkins Oncology Center
Baltimore, MD 21205

Albert D. Donnenberg, Ph.D.
The Johns Hopkins Oncology Center
Baltimore, MD 21205

Scott D. Rowley, M.D. (FACP)
The Fred Hutchinson Cancer
  Research Center
Seattle, WA 98104

REFERENCES

1. Gao, IK, et al: Implementation of a semiclosed large scale counterflow centrifugal elutriation system. J Clin Apheresis 3:154, 1987.
2. Noga, SJ: Elutriation: New technology for separation of blood and bone marrow. Lab Med 19(4):234, 1988.
3. Noga, SJ, Donnenberg, AD, and Santos, GW: The use of elutriation to purge lymphocytes from human bone marrow. Bone Marrow Transplant 2(Suppl 2):18, 1987.
4. Noga, SJ, et al: Using elutriation to engineer bone marrow allografts. Prog Clin Biol Res 333:345, 1990.
5. Wagner, JE, et al: Bone marrow graft engineering by counter-flow centrifugal elutriation. Results of a phase I-II clinical trial. Blood 75(6):1370, 1990.
6. Noga, SJ, et al: Lymphocyte dose modification of the bone marrow allograft using elutriation. In Gee, A (ed): Bone Marrow Processing and Purging—a Practical Guide. CRC Press, New York, p 175, 1991.

CENTRIFUGAL ELUTRIATION FOR LYMPHOCYTE REMOVAL

DESCRIPTION	One of the consequences of allografting bone marrow is graft-versus-host (GVH) disease. The cells responsible for GVH disease include natural killer (NK) cells and T lymphocytes. To lessen the severity of GVH disease, bone marrow can be manipulated to remove lymphocytes prior to transplantation.
	Using a sterile closed system, the bone marrow is subjected to opposing forces in an elutriation chamber that allows large numbers of cells to be sorted according to size. Rotating the chamber at high speed creates one force (centrifugal); this forces the cells to the outside of the spinning chamber. Pumping media through the chamber creates the counterflow force on the cells. The counterflow force pushes the cells toward the inside of the chamber. By overcoming the centrifugal force (centrifuge rpms), which is constant, with increasing counterflow force (media flow rates), on the cells, the desired cell fractions can be purified and forced from the chamber to be collected as an isolated population.
TIME FOR PROCEDURE	60 minutes
SUMMARY OF PROCEDURE	1. Harvested bone marrow is delivered to the processing laboratory in a 2000-mL blood bag.
	2. Using the Haemonetics V-50 and 301 cell wash and separation kits, the mononuclear cells are harvested, according to the Haemonetics bone marrow concentration protocol. Then, using a new 301 kit, neutrophils and red blood cells (RBCs) are removed according to the Haemonetics Ficoll-Hypaque protocol. Other methods of mononuclear cell purification may also be used.
	3. The mononuclear product is then washed to remove the leftover Ficoll-Hypaque. Then the mononuclear cells are resuspended in the elutriation media.
	4. The cells distribute according to size in the rotating chamber, and are pushed out of the chamber in order of their size (smaller to larger), by changing the flow rate of the media through the elutriation chamber.
	5. As the cells are forced out of the chamber by the flowing media, separation of the fractions is accomplished by manually opening or closing three-way stopcocks to collect the desired fractions into 600-mL transfer bags.
EQUIPMENT	1. Beckman model J-6B centrifuge with a JE5.0 rotor system
	2. Masterflex peristaltic pump model 900-197 fitted with 7021-20 Quick-release pump head
	3. Elzone model 280 PC by Particle Data interfaced with a personal computer
	4. Haemonetics V-50 outfitted with a 301 cell separation kit (or comparable cell separator)
SUPPLIES AND REAGENTS	1. 2 Fenwal plasma transfer sets 4C2240
	2. Masterflex silicone tubing 6411-16
	3. 2 Pharmaseal three-way stopcocks with extension tube K52L

4. 4 Mallinckrodt three-way stopcock with male luer-lock adapter 91037

5. 4 Fenwal 600-mL transfer pack container with needle adapter

6. Fenwal 2000-mL transfer pack with coupler

7. 20 to 30 tuberculin syringes with 20-gauge needles

8. 20 to 30 blood cell counting vials

9. Isotonic blood cell counting fluid

10. Ethylenediaminetetraacetic acid (EDTA) (tetra sodium salt)

11. Hank's balanced salt solution (HBSS) without calcium or magnesium

12. Human serum albumin

13. Sodium bicarbonate

PROCEDURE

1. Steam sterilize the entire elutriation assembly, including the tubing harness, prior to use. After sterilization, the three-way stopcocks, media bag, and transfer bags are sterilely attached to the tubing harness.

2. Calibrate the media pump for the elutriation before use by utilizing the calibration line (Fig. 7–6) on the tubing harness to deliver the pumped media to a graduated cylinder. The pump speed adjustment knob is used to determine what settings will result in a media delivery rate of 70, 110, and 140 mL per minute, respectively.

3. Calibrate the Elzone particle analyzer using latex calibration beads and the particle data calibration protocol.

4. Using the Haemonetics V-50 outfitted with a 301 kit and the Haemonetics bone marrow concentration protocol, concentrate the marrow buffy cells.

5. Further purify the concentrated marrow following the Haemonetics Ficoll-

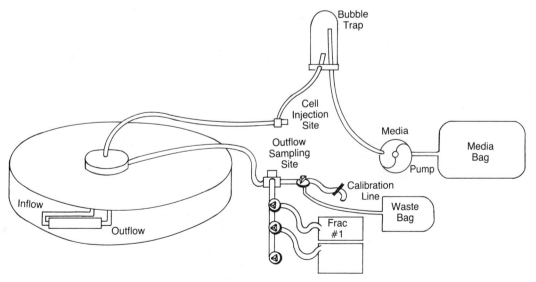

FIGURE 7–6 Beckman JE5.0 rotor system and attachments for bone marrow elutriation.

Hypaque protocol. The bone marrow is processed for Ficoll-Hypaque separation of mononuclear cells on the Haemonetics V-50.

6. Wash the Ficoll-Hypaque product to remove Ficoll-Hypaque from the cells and to deplete the product of platelets. Washing is performed by placing the product into 250-mL conical centrifuge tubes and diluting with a $1\times$ HBSS containing 1 percent human serum albumin, then centrifuging at 180g for 10 minutes. The supernatant is aspirated and the cell pellets are resuspended and combined into one of the conical tubes. The cells are diluted once again with HBSS with 1 percent human serum albumin and centrifuged at 120g.

7. Aspirate the supernate to leave a volume of cells and media that will be 30 to 40 mL in volume. The cell suspension is then aspirated into a syringe.

8. Use a small sample of these purified cells to generate a cell-sized histogram on the Elzone particle analyzer. This histogram is the reference against which to compare cells being sized as they come off the elutriator.

9. With the rotor on, at 2040 rpm, and media flowing through the entire system at a flow rate of 70 mL per minute, cells are ready to be injected. Turn the three-way stopcocks so as to collect the flowing media into fraction 1 (lymphocyte) bag. The rubber puncture pad is sterilized with Betadine prior to cell injection. The syringe containing the cells is fitted with a 20-gauge needle, which is inserted into the rubber puncture pad, and the cells are injected slowly into the rotor inlet tubing.

10. When all the cells are introduced into the chamber, take a sample from the outflow side rubber puncture pad by first wiping with Betadine, then inserting a tuberculin syringe fitted with a 20-gauge needle and aspirating a few drops of the outflow media. This sample is then analyzed on the Elzone particle analyzer. The size of the particles being carried out of the chamber can thus be quantitated. The smallest particles are removed first. These are any platelets, RBCs, and cell fragments.

11. To begin eluting the larger cell populations, gradually increase the media pump speed over 20 to 30 minutes up to 140 mL per minute, frequently removing a sample of the outflowing media and analyzing the sample for cell size. When the cell-sized histogram indicates that the very first monocytes are being eluted (Fig. 7–7), adjust the three-way stopcock assembly so as to collect the outflowing media into fraction 2 (monocytes/stem cells) bag. The elutriation rotor is now turned off, allowing the media flow to flush the chamber of any remaining cells.

12. Spin each fraction in a 250-mL flask. The cell pellets are then resuspended in physiologic saline.

13. Count and analyze a sample from each bag with monoclonal antibodies including T3, T11, M3, Leu12.

14. Quantitate the number of T3-positive cells in fractions 1 and 2. Lymphocytes from fraction 1 are added to fraction 2 to achieve a T3-positive cell dose of 1.5×10^6 per kg body weight.

15. Put the final marrow transplant into a 60-mL syringe or a 600-mL transfer bag (depending on volume).

16. Perform colony-forming assays on fractions 1 and 2.

17. Perform aerobic and anaerobic bacterial cultures on both fractions.

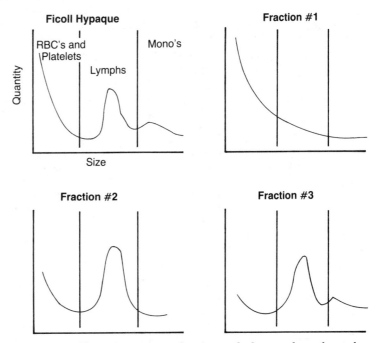

FIGURE 7–7 Representative Elzone histograms showing peak changes throughout elutriation of bone marrow.

ANTICIPATED RESULTS	The post–Ficoll-Hypaque cell population numbers should be roughly equally distributed between lymphocytes and monocytes. The variances among patients are so great that any hard and fast guidelines about cell recovery, purity, and so on, are impossible to make; however, this table contains a compilation of averages from our T-lymphocyte depletions:

AVERAGES FROM CELLS PLACED ON ELUTRIATOR

		MARKER POSITIVE FOR		
		T3	B1	M3
Cell recovery	85.8 ± 16			
Lymphocyte fraction	45.9 ± 21	53 ± 10	14 ± 7	4.5 ± 4
Stem cell fraction	49.5 ± 14	4.5 ± 4.8	6 ± 8	18 ± 8
GFU-GM in stem cell peak	83% ± 23			

NOTES	The elutriation chamber and tubing harness have many junctions and fittings that tend to collect air bubbles. The introduction of air into the rotor during the elutriation procedure can cause major problems with the ability of the system to conduct fluids. Take the precaution to pinch and then release the flexible tubing to free any air bubbles from the system before you inject the cells.

AUTHORS

Mary Ann Gross, M.T. (ASCP)
Shands Hospital
University of Florida
Gainesville, Florida 32610

Charles E. Hutcheson, M.T. (ASCP)
Shands Hospital
University of Florida
Gainesville, Florida 32610

REFERENCES

1. Weiner, RS and Shah, VO: Purification of human monocytes: Isolation and collection of large numbers of peripheral blood monocytes. J Immunol Methods 36:89, 1980.
2. Mason, RR and Weiner, RS: Application of the Beckman JE-6B Elutriator system (R) in the isolation of human monocyte subpopulations. Scand J Hematol 34:5, 1984.
3. Zucali, JR, et al: Two stage separation of immature and mature T lymphocytes from myeloerythroid clonogenic bone marrow cells by elutriation centrifugation. Transfusion 27:148, 1987.
4. Noga, SJ, et al: Rapid separation of whole human bone marrow aspirates by counterflow centrifugation elutriation. Transplantation 43:438, 1986.
5. Noga, SJ: Elutriation: New technology for separation of blood and bone marrow. Lab Med 19:234, 1988.

Methylprednisolone and Vincristine Treatment of Bone Marrow in HLA-Mismatched Bone Marrow Transplants

DESCRIPTION	Histocompatible related or unrelated donors are available for fewer than 50 percent of all patients with lethal immunohematologic disorders who might be effectively treated with bone marrow transplants. For those patients who lack histocompatible donors, bone marrow transplant has been undertaken following depletion of alloreactive T cells by various methods to prevent lethal graft-versus-host (GVH) disease. However, delayed immunologic reconstitution, graft failure, and, in some cases, GVH disease continue to be the problems with such procedures. The ideal procedure would be to eliminate or modulate alloreactive T cells while preserving those cells that facilitate the engraftment process by producing hematopoietic growth factors (cytokines) and those cells that reconstitute the immune system without increasing the risk of GVH disease. We have used methylprednisolone and vincristine to treat bone marrow in vitro to modify its T-cell responses. In vitro treatment of bone marrow with methylprednisolone (MP) and vincristine (VCR) depletes or modulates T cells as observed by T-cell immunophenotype, in vitro proliferative responses, and cytokine (interleukin-2) production. This procedure has a greater effect on CD4-positive cells than on CD8-positive cells; and further, the in vitro alloreactive responses are affected more than other lymphoproliferative responses.

TIME FOR PROCEDURE	Approximately 1.5 hours, including incubation time and washes, but excluding Ficoll-Hypaque and media preparation time.

SUMMARY OF PROCEDURE	1. Ficolled, washed bone marrow mononuclear cells are suspended at 60×10^6 per mL in RPMI 1640 with 10 percent fetal calf serum.
	2. MP and VCR are prepared.
	3. A 30-minute incubation in a 37°C waterbath; a 10-minute incubation on ice; and two washes at 4°C are performed.
	4. Cells are resuspended in TC-199 medium with 5 percent human serum albumin.

EQUIPMENT	This procedure requires no special equipment.

SUPPLIES AND REAGENTS	1. 50-mL polystyrene centrifuge tubes, sterile
	2. 15-mL polystyrene snap cap tubes, sterile
	3. Sterile transfer pipettes
	4. 1-mL sterile pipettes
	5. 5-mL sterile pipettes
	6. 10-mL sterile pipettes
	7. Container for liquid waste

8. 3-mL syringes

9. Green (21-gauge) needles

10. 1-mL syringe with needle

11. 250-mL plastic beaker with ice

12. Timers

13. 500-mL RPMI 1640 with 25 mM Hepes buffer with L-glutamine (Whittaker Bioproducts, Inc., 8830 Biggs Ford Rd., Walkersville, MD 21793-0127)

14. 1 X Alpha Medium (Gibco Laboratories, Life Technologies, Inc., Grand Island, NY 14072)

15. TC-199 Medium (Gibco Laboratories, Life Technologies, Inc., Grand Island, NY 14072)

16. Penicillin/streptomycin (P/S) (Gibco Laboratories, Life Technologies, Inc., Grand Island, NY 14072)

17. Glutamine (GLN) (Gibco Laboratories, Life Technologies, Inc., Grand Island, NY 14072)

18. Fetal calf serum (FCS) (Cell Culture Laboratories, Cleveland, OH 44128)

19. 40-mg vial, MP (Hem 19 Methypred Sodium Succinate Vial 40-mg) (The Upjohn Company, Kalamazoo, MI 49001)

20. 1-mg per mL vial, VCR (Quad Pharmaceuticals, Inc., Indianapolis, IN 46268); store at 4°C

PREPARATION

1. Cells obtained from Ficoll-Hypaque centrifugation are washed and suspended in RPMI 1640 with P/S, GLN, and 10 percent FCS.

2. Suspend cells at 50 to 60×10^6 per mL (60×10^6 optimal)

3. MP, 40 mg per mL, a lyophilized powder in a two-tier vial, with powder at bottom and diluent containing benzyl alcohol on top
   A. Prepare MP: Use a 3-mL syringe with a green (21-gauge) needle. Remove as much factory diluent as possible. Be careful not to push separation plug into powder. Volume is 1 mL.
   B. Replace diluent with 1 mL 1 X Alpha medium. Push vial cap to allow 1 X Alpha medium to mix with MP powder. Dissolve powder completely. It is necessary to shake vial several times to thoroughly dissolve powder. Remove MP from vial. Put in a 3-mL snap cap tube. This is a 40 mg per mL solution.

4. VCR, 1 mg per mL, liquid
   A. Prepare VCR: VCR is a 1 mg per mL solution. Using a 1-mL syringe, remove VCR and add to 9 mL of 1 X Alpha medium. This makes a 1:10 working solution.

5. RPMI 1640, culture medium
   A. 10 percent FCS, 100 U per mL penicillin, 100 μg per mL streptomycin, 0.29 mg per mL GLN.

PROCEDURE

1. Following Ficoll-Hypaque centrifugation, suspend bone marrow mononuclear cells in RPMI-1640 at a concentration of 60×10^6 cells per mL. Place 5 mL of this cell suspension in 50-mL polystyrene tube (higher cell number is avoided to prevent cell compaction during incubation and to effectively

Cells at 60 $\times 10^6$ mL	Remove RPMI Supernatant	Add MP (40 mg/mL)	Add VCR (1:10 working solution)
1 mL	85 μL	75 μL	10 μL
2 mL	170 μL	150 μL	20 μL
5 mL	425 μL	375 μL	50 μL

wash MP and VCR at the completion of incubation). Spin the cell suspension at 1200 to 1500 rpm for 10 minutes. Remove an amount of supernatant equal to the volume of MP and VCR to be added.

2. After removing RPMI, resuspend cells in remaining RPMI, add appropriate volumes of MP and VCR. Mix thoroughly. For example,

3. At final solution there are 60×10^6 cells, 3 mg MP, and 1 μg VCR in each mL.

4. MP-VCR INCUBATION
   A. 30 minutes in 37°C waterbath, agitate tubes every 5 minutes.
   B. After incubation place tube in ice for 10 minutes.
   C. Wash twice at 4°C with RPMI.
   D. Suspend cells in a known volume, make cell count and viability with trypan blue.
   E. Reserve cells for CFU-GM and CFU-GEMM assays, mixed lymphocyte culture (MLC), and mitogen response.
   F. Resuspend in TC-199 medium with 5 percent human serum albumin at a 40×10^6 nucleated cells per mL for reinfusion to patient.

ANTICIPATED RESULTS

Mean cell recovery following incubation with MP and VCR and washes should be greater than 75 percent. Viability should be greater than 95 percent. Cytofluorometric analysis for identification of the number of T cells and T-cell subsets will reveal no difference before and after MP and VCR except for a decrease in the intensity of fluorescence of CD4-positive cells. Following MP and VCR treatment, there will be a decrease in proliferative responses to 30 to 50 percent of control values when the bone marrow is stimulated with mitogens. There will also be a reduction in response to 4 to 20 percent of untreated cells when treated cells are exposed to a pool of allogeneic cells. Interleukin-2 production by the treated cells can be expected to drop to less than 5 percent of the control value after treatment with MP and VCR.

AUTHORS

Neena Kapoor, M.D.
Ohio State University
Pediatric Bone Marrow
  Transplantation Program
Columbus OH 43210

Eric X. Beck
Ohio State University
Pediatric Bone Marrow
  Transplantation Program
Columbus OH 43210

Arnalda Lanfranchi, Ph.D.
Ohio State University
Pediatric Bone Marrow
  Transplantation Program
Columbus OH 43210

REFERENCES

1. Kapoor, N, et al: Effect of ex vivo treatment with methylprednisolone and vincristine on bone marrow lymphohematopoietic cells. Proceedings of the Third International Symposium of Bone Marrow Purging and Processing, San Diego, 1991 (abstr).

2. Kapoor, N, et al: Effect of ex vivo treatment with methylprednisolone and vincristine on bone marrow lymphohematopoietic cells. Exp Hematol 19:567, 1991.

3. Lanfranchi, A, et al: T cell depletion from histocompatible bone marrow graft for congenital lethal disorders (in preparation).

4. Kapoor, N, Tutschka, PJ, and Copelan, EA: Bone marrow purging with glucocorticoids. In Gross, S, Gee, A, and Worthington-White, DA (eds): Bone marrow purging and processing. Progr Clin Biol Res 333:39, 1990.

IMMUNOLOGIC

T-CELL DEPLETION OF SBA— CELLS BY ADHERENCE ON THE AIS CELLECTOR–T CELL

DESCRIPTION	Residual T cells may be removed from SBA— cells by adherence on a polystyrene device to which monoclonal antibodies to the T-cell antigens CD5 and CD8 have been covalently bound. Treatment by this panning method results in specific loss of T cells without loss of high-density cells and additional nonspecific cell loss. The number of cells recovered after adherence is significantly greater than with rosetting, with similar T-cell frequencies to the rosetted marrow. Total $\log_{10}$ T-cell depletion is less than SBA-E— because of the higher cell dose; however, the incidence of graft-versus-host (GVH) disease has not been significantly increased in patients receiving SBA-CD5— and SBA-CD8— grafts. This method has proven to have significant advantages in ease of operation, use of closed systems, and standardization.

TIME FOR PROCEDURE	3 hours

SUMMARY OF PROCEDURE	1. SBA— cells are suspended in 0.5 percent Gamimune in phosphate-buffered saline (PBS) without calcium and magnesium and incubated at room temperature for 15 minutes.
	2. SBA— cells are added to previously washed CELLector-T cell devices at 5×10^6 per mL in PBS without calcium and magnesium with 1 mM ethylenediaminetetraacetic acid (EDTA) and incubated at room temperature according to manufacturer's directions (60 minutes for T-624, 30 minutes per side for T-3000).
	3. Nonadherent cells are removed and washed with lactated Ringer's solution for administration to patient.
	4. Samples are removed for analysis of sterility, cell number, 2-aminoethylisothiouronium bromide, hydrobromide–treated sheep erythrocytes (E-AET) clonable T cells, and hematopoietic precursors.

EQUIPMENT	1. AIS CELLector–T cell T-624 or T-3000, with tubing sets and connectors as supplied by manufacturer, Applied Immune Sciences, Inc., Menlo Park, CA.
	2. COBE 2991 cell washer (Cobe, Lakewood, CO)

SUPPLIES AND REAGENTS	1. Sterile PBS, without calcium and magnesium with 1 mM EDTA
	2. Sterile heat-inactivated 0.5 percent Gamimune in PBS
	3. 1000-mL and 600-mL transfer packs (Fenwal)
	4. Plasma transfer sets, coupler-needle adaptor

5. Lactated Ringer's solution (Abbott Laboratories)
6. COBE 2991 cell washing kit

PROCEDURE

1. PRIMING CELLectors
    A. Remove the CELLectors from plastic bags, noting that the sterility indicator is red-orange.
    B. Rinse the CELLectors three to five times with saline, according to manufacturer's instructions, using vacuum via the attached drain set. Make sure that the device remains level and the active surface does not dry out.
    C. Store the activated device with saline (100 mL for the T-624, 265 mL for the T-3000) on a level nonvibrating surface while cells are being prepared.

2. ADHERENCE OF SBA− CELLS
    A. After washing on the COBE 2991 cell washer, SBA− cells are suspended into 50 mL of 0.5 percent Gamimune in PBS for a 15-minute incubation.
    B. SBA− cells are counted and the number of devices to be used for adherence calculated. T-624 containers have a maximum cell load of 5×10^8 cells and the T-3000 a maximum cell load of 2×10^9 cells.
    C. SBA− cells are loaded into devices through one port of the three-way stopcock either by syringe or from a transfer pack containing the SBA− cells adjusted to 5×10^6 per mL in PBS without calcium (Ca^{2+}) and magnesium (Mg^{2+}), and with 1 mM EDTA. Additional PBS without $Ca^{2+}Mg^{2+}$ is added to make up to volume (100 mL for T-624 and 265 mL for T-3000).
    D. Devices are incubated on a level, nonvibrating surface at room temperature. The T-624 is incubated for 60 minutes, with gentle resuspension of cells after 30 minutes. The T-3000 device is incubated for 30 minutes on the first side and 30 minutes on the second side. If double passage is required, the cells are transferred via tubing to the second device by gravity flow, followed by a second room temperature incubation.
    E. The nonadherent cells are collected from the devices after gentle resuspension by gravity flow into a transfer pack. T-624 devices are rinsed twice with 20 mL each of PBS without Ca^{2+} and Mg^{2+}. The resultant SBA-CD5− and SBA-CD8− cells are washed twice with lactated Ringer's solution supplemented with penicillin and streptomycin, and once with antibiotic-free Ringer's on the 2991 cell washer.
    F. The SBA-CD5− and SBA-CD8− cells are collected into 50 mL of antibiotic-free lactated Ringer's solution and counted. Samples are removed for quality control assays: sterility, hematopoietic precursor recovery, limiting dilution assays for T cells, and rosetting. The SBA-CD5− and SBA-CD8− graft is administered to the patient following infusion of the irradiated SBA+ cells.

ANTICIPATED RESULTS

The following are the mean ± standard deviation of nine consecutive depletions of T cells from SBA− cell population by adherence on the CD5/CD8 CELLector–T cell.

	SBA−(CD5/CD8)
Number cells recovered $\times 10^9$	1.92 ± 0.84
Percent from SBA−	81.16 ± 8.11
Percent from harvested marrow	7.73 ± 2.97
Percent E$^+$	0.97 ± 0.93
T-cell frequency by LDA*	$1/816.79 \pm 1/703.01$
Log$_{10}$ T-cell depletion from unseparated	2.37 ± 0.33
CFU-GM recovery as percent of unseparated	62.9 ± 45.0
BFU-E recovery as percent of unseparated	68.55 ± 67.37

*Limiting dilution assay.

NOTES

1. T-cell depletion by this method is specific for cells bearing the CD5 and/or CD8 antigens. Thus, the number of residual CD4 cells is higher in these grafts than in SBA-E− grafts. Additionally, residual rosette-positive cells detected in the nonadherent are CD56-bearing NK cells.

2. Serial transfer of cells from one T-624 to a second T-624 can be complicated by the appearance of air locks in the tubing during the two 20-mL wash steps, which stop the flow of cells into the second device. Air locks can be avoided by closing the stopcock before the tubing fills with air. If air locks are introduced, tubing strippers can be used to reestablish flow.

AUTHORS

Nancy H. Collins, Ph.D.
Memorial Sloan-Kettering Cancer
  Center
New York, NY 10021

Richard J. O'Reilly, M.D.
Memorial Sloan-Kettering Cancer
  Center
New York, NY 10021

Jane Lebkowski, Ph.D.
Applied Immune Sciences, Inc.
Menlo Park, CA 94025-1109

Thomas Okarma, Ph.D., M.D.
Applied Immune Sciences, Inc.
Menlo Park, CA 94025-1109

REFERENCES

1. Collins, NH, et al: Depletion of T lymphocytes from soybean lectin agglutinin treated bone marrow with the AIS T-Cellector. J Cell Biochem S14A:292, 1990.
2. Collins, NH, et al: T cell depletion of allogeneic bone marrow grafts by soybean lectin agglutination and adherence on CD5/CD8 AIS Cellector-T cell. Laboratory evaluation, accepted, American Society of Hematology, 32nd Annual Meeting, Boston, December, 1990.

BONE MARROW PURGING OF T LYMPHOCYTES WITH $T_{10}B_9$ MONOCLONAL ANTIBODIES AND COMPLEMENT

DESCRIPTION	Prevention of severe graft-versus-host (GVH) disease in patients undergoing bone marrow transplantation from HLA-nonidentical or unrelated donors is not easily achieved without high risk of graft failure. In these patients larger doses of donor T cells are not tolerated despite rigorous postgrafting GVH disease prophylaxis, whereas infusion of marrow extensively depleted of T lymphocytes precludes stable engraftment. Incomplete purging of T cells from donor bone marrow with anti–T-cell monoclonal antibody $T_{10}B_9$ and complement minimizes the risk of graft rejection offering a partial protection against acute severe GVH disease. This procedure has been effectively used in bone marrow transplantation across the histocompatibility barrier.
TIME FOR PROCEDURE	Time necessary for purging a mononuclear bone marrow cell fraction is approximately 4 hours.

SUMMARY OF PROCEDURE

1. Mononuclear cells (MNCs) separated from harvested bone marrow are suspended in RPMI and incubated with anti-CD3 monoclonal antibody $T_{10}B_9$.

2. The incubation is followed by two 45-minute cycles of cell exposure to rabbit serum complement.

3. Residual bone marrow cells are washed and resuspended in HBSS mixed with human serum albumin for infusion into the patient.

EQUIPMENT

1. One or two centrifuges accommodating 50-mL conical tubes and 250-mL centrifuge bottles, programmed to spin the tubes at 400g, 20°C, and the bottles at a minimum of 8000g (preferably 12,000 to 15,000g), 4°C

2. Tube rotator or rocker platform capable of accommodating at least 20 conical 50-mL centrifuge tubes

3. Laminar flow hood

SUPPLIES AND REAGENTS

1. 50-mL conical disposable centrifuge tubes, polypropylene (Falcon 2098)

2. 250-mL autoclavable centrifuge bottles, polycarbonate (Nalgene 3122-0250)

3. 1000-mL Erlenmeyer flask, polypropylene (Nalgene 4102-1000)

4. 30-mL and 60-mL plastic syringes and 18-gauge hypodermic needles

5. 0.22-μm syringe filter (Millipore SLGV 025LS) used to sterilize nuclease solution

6. Two to four 500-mL serum filters, 0.22 μm pore size (Nalgene 162-0020) used to sterilize complement

7. Three-way disposable syringe stopcock with male luer-lock adapter (Pharmaseal)

8. Sterile plastic pipettes: 1-, 2-, 25-, and 50-mL sizes

9. RPMI 1640 supplemented with 10 percent fetal bovine serum, 2 mM glutamine, 100 U penicillin per mL, and 100 μg streptomycin per mL (RPMI)

10. Hank's balanced salt solution (HBSS) without calcium and magnesium

11. Human serum albumin

12. Nuclease, micrococcal (Sigma N 3755): A stock solution is made by dissolving 500 units nuclease in 25 mL of RPMI and sterilizing it by filtration; sterilized nuclease can be stored at $-30°C$

13. Rabbit serum complement (Pelfreeze) pretested for lack of toxicity against peripheral blood cells and hematopoietic progenitors as well as for ability to lyse T cells in conjunction with $T_{10}B_9$. Complement is stored at $-70°C$. It should be thawed immediately before purging procedure. Do not reuse unspent portion of thawed complement as its activity may be significantly reduced.

14. $T_{10}B_9$ in ascites form (the ascites contains on the average 1.5 mg per mL of IgM protein). This anti-CD3 murine monoclonal antibody of IgM class reacts selectively with normal peripheral blood T cells and mature medullary thymocytes and activates rabbit complement but is not mitogenic. The target antigen is an 80- to 90-kd protein located at the T-cell receptor site. The antibody was originally developed in the laboratory of John S. Thompson.

PROCEDURE

The procedure is carried out under a laminer flow hood.

1. PREPARATION OF COMPLEMENT
   A. Thaw an adequate portion of complement under cold running water. This takes 20 to 30 minutes.
   B. Centrifuge thawed complement in 250-mL bottles for 20 minutes at $8000g$ (or more), 4°C. Remove the top film of lipid by suction with a plastic pipette.
   C. Sterilize complement by filtration under vacuum using 500-mL serum filters, and store on ice.

2. T-CELL DEPLETION
   A. In 1000-mL plastic Erlenmeyer flask suspend bone marrow MNCs in RPMI at a concentration of 3×10^7 cells per mL. After reserving 2 mL of the suspension for quality control add to the flask 2 percent (v/v) of $T_{10}B_9$ in ascites form. Incubate the flask on ice for 30 minutes.
   B. Add to the flask an equal volume of complement supplemented with 0.4 U per mL of nuclease, and distribute 35-mL portions of the mixture among 50-mL plastic tubes. Rotate the tubes for 45 minutes at room temperature.
   C. Sediment cells by centrifugation at $400g$ for 10 minutes; discard the supernatant.
   D. Resuspend cells in each tube in 35 mL of RPMI mixed with an equal volume of complement and supplemented with 0.2 U per mL of nuclease. Repeat the 45-minute incubation cycle with rotation at room temperature.
   E. Sediment cells by centrifugation at $400g$ for 10 minutes.
   F. Pool all cells into two 50-mL centrifuge tubes. Wash them three times using 45 mL per tube of HBSS containing 2 percent human serum albumin.
   G. Pool all cells into one 50-mL tube, wash them once in 45 mL of HBSS plus 5 percent human albumin, and, after sedimentation, resuspend in the same medium to a volume of 25.5 mL. Reserve 0.5-mL sample for quality control.
   H. Transfer the remaining suspension with a pipette into a 60-mL syringe

with plunger removed, connected via the stopcock with a second 60-mL syringe. Aspirate the contents of the first syringe into the second syringe. Rinse carefully the centrifuge tube and the first syringe with additional 25 mL of HBSS plus 5 percent albumin and aspirate into the second syringe. Disconnect the syringe from the stopcock, secure with a covered needle and deliver for transfusion into the patient.

ANTICIPATED RESULTS

The procedure should remove 98 to 99.7 percent (1.7 to 2.5 logs) of T cells from the MNC fraction of harvested bone marrow as defined functionally by limiting dilution analysis. More than 80 percent of other viable cells present in the original MNC fraction are usually recovered. Hematopoietic progenitors remain unaffected by the procedure.

NOTE

To obtain quality control for the efficiency of T-cell depletion immediately after purging, phenotypic T-cell analysis is used. There should be less than 1 percent of CD3-positive cells within the depleted bone marrow fraction; $T_{10}B_9$ does not block binding of OKT3 or Leu-4 to cell membrane.

AUTHORS

Ewa Marciniak, M.D.
Dept. of Medicine
University of Kentucky Medical Center
Lexington, KY 40536

P. Jean Henslee-Downey, M.D.
Dept. of Medicine
University of Kentucky Medical Center
Lexington, KY 40536

Kelvin Bailey, B.S.
Dept. of Medicine
University of Kentucky Medical Center
Lexington, KY 40536

John S. Thompson, M.D.
Dept. of Medicine
University of Kentucky Medical Center
Lexington, KY 40536

REFERENCES

1. Marciniak, E, et al: Laboratory control in predicting clinical efficacy of T cell-depletion procedures used for prevention of graft-versus-host disease: Importance of limiting dilution analysis. Bone Marrow Transplant 3:589, 1988.
2. Thompson, JS, et al: Antigens common to monocytes and endothelial cells. In McCullough, J and Sandler, GS (eds): Advances in Immunology: Blood Cell Antigens and Bone Marrow Transplantation. Allan R. Liss, New York, 1984, p 169.

EX VIVO IMMUNOTOXIN-MEDIATED T-CELL DEPLETION

DESCRIPTION

A variety of immunologic and pharmacologic procedures have been evaluated for the specific lysis of human T lymphocytes from bone marrow inocula. In this procedure, we describe the purging of T cells from bone marrow using a ricin A chain conjugated to an F(ab')$_2$ fragment of a murine anti-CD5 monoclonal antibody (MAb), ST1 (Sanofi Reserche, Montpellier, France). Intact ricin consists of two disulfide-linked 30-kd subunits.[1] The ricin A chain appears to bind to and inactivate eukaryotic ribosomes, inhibiting protein synthesis and resulting in cell death. The ricin B chain binds to galactosyl residues which are ubiquitously expressed on the cell surface and allows transport of the ricin A chain into the cell. ST1-IT has been constructed by coupling the F(ab')$_2$ fragment of anti-CD5 MAb to ricin A chain alone, thus eliminating the need to block galactosyl residues to achieve specificity of binding.

CD5 is a 67-kd molecule expressed on the surface of the majority of mature CD3-positive T cells, but not on natural killer cells, a small proportion of CD3- and CD8-positive T cells, or a proportion of those T cells that express the $\gamma\delta$ T-cell receptor.[2] Anti-CD5 MAb induces CD5 capping and internalization into the cell, and thus immunotoxin (IT) coupled to the anti-CD5 MAb is endocytosed and delivered into the cytoplasm of the cell. The anti-CD5 MAb fragment confers specificity to the ricin A chain toxin. The relative efficacy of Fab, F(ab')$_2$, and whole Ig preparations of MAb coupled to immunotoxin depends in part on the target antigen and thus cytotoxicity and binding should be determined for each potential antigen and each immunotoxin. This comparison for CD5 has been studied in detail by Derocq and Chiron and their colleagues.[3-5]

Immunotoxin depletion of T cells from the bone marrow inocula offers several advantages over MAb plus complement protocols. Immunotoxin purging is, in general, more rapid and less labor intensive. It involves less manipulation of the bone marrow, and thus less opportunity for contamination. Furthermore, IT preparations can be standardized, unlike baby rabbit complement which must be individually tested for nonspecific cytotoxicity.

TIME FOR PROCEDURE

Approximately 3 hours are required to prepare bone marrow mononuclear cells by density gradient separation, described subsequently. If bone marrow is processed on the Fenwal CS3000 this step can be eliminated (see Chapter 6). Approximately 30 to 45 minutes are required both for counting and for resuspending the bone marrow mononuclear cells and for calculating, preparing, and adding the reagents for incubation. The incubation with ST1-IT is 2 hours, after which samples are removed for evaluation of efficacy of T-cell depletion.

SUMMARY OF PROCEDURE

1. Bone marrow is harvested from the donor and processed either automatically using a Fenwal CS3000 cell separator (see Chapter 6) or manually by density gradient separation (see farther on).

2. The mononuclear cells or buffy coat are counted and appropriately resuspended.

3. The reagents for incubation are calculated, prepared, and added to the bone marrow inocula. The incubation must be carried out at a basic pH, buffered against the acidity of the IT preparation.

4. The marrow is incubated with ST1-IT (or other appropriately tested MAb-IT preparation) for 2 hours at 37°C on a rocker platform. Aliquots of marrow are removed before and after incubation for evaluation of efficacy of T-cell depletion (see Chapter 11).

EQUIPMENT	1.	Centrifuge
	2.	Rocker platform (Bellco Biotechnology, Vineland, NJ, or equivalent)
	3.	37°C warm room

SUPPLIES AND REAGENTS

1. 500 mL Hank's balanced salt solution (HBSS) $1\times$ with phenol red (Whittaker Bioproducts, Inc., Walkersville, MD)

2. 2 bottles human serum albumin (HSA) 25 percent, 50 mL (Armour Pharmaceutical Co., Kankakee, IL, or equivalent)

3. 100-mL bottles lymphocyte separating medium (LSM) (Organon Teknika, Durham, NC) (specific gravity 1.077 to 1.080), 100-mL bottle containing 9.4 g sodium diatrizoate and 6.2 g Ficoll-Hypaque, sterile filtered, or equivalent. For non-nucleated cell removal, 12 mL is needed for each 35 mL marrow.

4. 20 mL ammonium chloride (5 mEq per mL) Injection, USP (Abbott Laboratories, N. Chicago, IL)

5. RPMI-1640 with L-glutamine and without sodium bicarbonate (Gibco Laboratories, Grand Island, NY)

6. 500 mL THAM Solution (Tromethamine) Injection (each 100 mL contains tromethamine 3.6 g or 30 mEq, approximately) (Abbott Laboratories, N. Chicago, IL)

7. ST1-Ricin (Sanofi Reserche) reconstituted in 5 mL 25 percent HSA; 10^{-6} M ricin A chain initial concentration, 10^{-8} M ricin A chain final concentration

8. Transfer pack unit with coupler (Fenwal Laboratories, Deerfield, IL) (600-mL bag [code 4R2033] for small volumes or pediatric patients; 1000-mL bag [code 4R2032] for larger volumes or adult patients)

9. Plasma transfer sets (Code 4C2240) (Fenwal Laboratories, Deerfield, IL)

10. Sampling site couplers (Code 4C2405) (Fenwal Laboratories, Deerfield, IL)

11. 1000-mL sterile water for irrigation, USP (Abbott Laboratories, N. Chicago, IL) (*use bottle,* discard sterile H_2O)

12. 38-mm screw cap adapter (Abbott Laboratories, N. Chicago, IL)

13. Hand sealer (Code 4R4417) (Fenwal Laboratories, Deerfield, IL)

14. Hand sealer clips (Code 4R4418) (Fenwal Laboratories, Deerfield, IL)

15. Hemacytometer (Reichert-Jung, Cambridge Instruments Inc., Buffalo, NY, or equivalent)

16. Trypan blue stain 0.4 percent (Gibco Laboratories, Grand Island, NY), diluted 1:10 for use

17. 4 percent acetic acid

18. Needles, plasticware

PROCEDURE

1. BONE MARROW HARVEST: Bone marrow is harvested into either (a) D_5^- lactated Ringer's solution or (b) RPMI-1640 medium without sodium bicarbonate (Gibco, Grand Island, NY) to which 100 U per mL preservative-free heparin (Abbott Laboratories, Organon Laboratories, or other supplier) has been added. For each kilogram recipient body weight, approximately 15 mL bone marrow is harvested from the donor by multiple aspirations from the anterior and/or posterior iliac crests. Bone marrow is filtered (Fenwal) or, alternatively, passed through a course wire mesh and subsequently transferred to either 600- or 1000-mL transfer pack units (Fenwal).

2. CELL CONCENTRATION: If the total volume of bone marrow exceeds 300 mL (for all patients except pediatric patients weighing less than 20 kg), it must be concentrated prior to treatment. Bone marrow is transported to the blood bank at room temperature. It is concentrated on an IBM 2991 blood cell processor (see Chapter 6), to a total volume of 50 to 200 mL.

3. INITIAL BONE MARROW DILUTION: Pour off 50 mL HBSS into one sterile 50-mL conical tube. Pour concentrated bone marrow into 50-mL conical tubes. Then distribute 60 to 75 mL concentrated bone marrow into each 500-mL bottle of HBSS, approximately 1:6 or 1:10 dilution, usually requiring two to three bottles. Rinse conical tubes by pouring 25 mL reserved sterile HBSS into tubes, then add back to bottle.

4. PRE–FICOLL-HYPAQUE CELL COUNT: Although it is not crucial to know the starting concentration, cells must be reserved for cell count. (We count these cells later, during first wash after Ficoll-Hypaque.)
   A. Shake HBSS bottles for even cellular distribution.
   B. Using a 1-mL sterile pipette, take off 100-μL aliquot from each bottle and place in small plastic tube.
   C. Cell count dilution: 100 μL cells
                            100 μL media
                            100 μL trypan blue
                            100 μL 4 percent acetic acid
   D. Using hemacytometer, count cells. Derive average number of cells per mL; multiply by volume in each bottle.

5. FICOLL-HYPAQUE BONE MARROW
   A. Distribute 35 mL diluted bone marrow in HBSS into 50-mL conical tubes. Underlayer each 35 mL marrow with 12 mL LSM.
   B. Centrifuge at 1500 rpm ($400g$) for 20 minutes. During this centrifugation, distribute and underlayer with LSM the second bottle of diluted bone marrow, if there is one.
   C. Remove interface.
      (1) Aspirate media to 20-mL mark, leaving approximately 10 mL serum above the interface, using a sterile 5-mL plastic pipette connected to a 2-L Erlenmeyer vacuum flask.
      (2) Remove interface using sterile 10-mL plastic pipette so that there is little red color remaining. White buffy coat (interface) should now be removed.

(3) Transfer interface to 50-mL conical tubes. When all buffy coats have been removed, equalize volumes in 50-mL conical tubes.

(4) Centrifuge at 1200 rpm for 8 minutes.

D. Wash and combine pellets.

(1) Prepare HBSS with 0.5 percent HSA or 500 mL HBSS plus 10 mL HSA (25 percent). This will be known as "wash media."

(2) From conical tubes containing spun buffy coats, aspirate media leaving 5 mL residual media containing cell pellet.

(3) Combine cell pellets from two conical tubes to one by resuspending first pellet using a sterile plastic 10-mL pipette and transferring to second tube already containing pellet in 5 mL; resuspend second pellet using same pipette. (Same pipette should be used sequentially to combine all cell pellets from a single centrifuge spin. This minimizes cell loss by adherence to plastic.)

(4) Rinse first tube with 10 mL of wash media; combine with second tube.

(5) Fill second tube to 50 mL with wash media.

(6) Centrifuge at 1200 rpm for 10 minutes.

(7) Over three washes, transfer and combine cell pellets from approximately 10 tubes to 1 final tube by repeating previous steps 2 through 6.

(8) With final single pellet, aspirate and discard as much media as possible without removing any cells. In the end, this should be done using a sterile plastic pipette, not the vacuum flask.

6. RESUSPENSION OF FINAL PELLET

A. Fill a sterile 50-mL conical tube with 50 mL RPMI-1640 with L-glutamine and without sodium bicarbonate.

B. With a 10-mL sterile plastic pipette, add 30 mL RPMI-1640 media to the 50-mL conical tube with pellet. Cap tube and tilt tube up and down. When cell pellet appears to be resuspended, uncap tube and add remaining 20 mL media. Again, cap tube and mix well by inversion.

7. POST–FICOLL-HYPAQUE COUNT

A. Volume is 50 mL.

B. To count: Dilute 100 μL of cells into 400 μL media (1:5 dilution). From this dilution take 100 μL of cells. Add to this cell suspension 100 μL media, 100 μL trypan blue, and 100 μL 4 percent acetic acid, and count as done earlier. (Remember to multiply calculated cell concentration by factor of 5 to compensate for initial 1:5 dilution.)

C. Calculate cell recovery: Post–Ficoll-Hypaque count divided by pre-Ficoll-Hypaque count, multiplied by 100. Average recovery is 20 to 50 percent.

D. Calculate cell dose: Post–Ficoll-Hypaque cell count divided by recipient's weight in kilograms. (Average cell dose is approximately 1 $\times$ 10^8 cells per kg; cell dose is usually higher for children.)

8. CALCULATION OF REAGENTS FOR TREATMENT

A. Treatment concentration: 2 $\times$ 10^7 cells per mL. Therefore, total post–Ficoll-Hypaque cell count divided by 2 $\times$ 10^7 cells per mL equals total treatment volume in mL.

B. *For example, for 100-mL treatment volume:*

HSA 5% (from a vial of 25% HSA)*	20 mL
NH$_4$Cl (1:250)	0.4 mL
THAM (start at 5%)	5 mL
ST1-Ricin (1%)	1 mL
	26.4 mL reagents
	+ 50.0 mL marrow (present volume)
	76.4 mL

100.0 mL − 76.4 mL = 23.6 mL media (RPMI-1640)

*The HSA stock is 25%; so, to calculate the necessary volume, take 5% of the treatment volume × 4 (or simply 20% of the treatment volume).

9. ADDING REAGENTS AND TAKING SAMPLES
   A. Remove sterile H$_2$O from Sterile Water for Irrigation container (container itself is large and sterile).
   B. Add volume of RPMI-1640 media to sterile container to reach treatment volume (in previous example, 23.6 mL).
   C. Add cells in 50 mL volume with RPMI-1640 without sodium bicarbonate; rinse tube.
   D. Add HSA, NH$_4$Cl, then THAM (THAM must be last).
   E. Remove 700 μL to measure pH. Optimize pH, approximately 7.5 to 8.0. (Make it a little basic because immunotoxin will cause slight decrease in pH.) For example, 7.84 final pH with 5 percent THAM.
   F. Remove "pre" sample for later evaluation of efficacy of T-cell depletion (see Chapter 11) by removing 1.5 to 2 mL to small sterile plastic tube (labeled "pre"); this sample will be rocked alongsíde the main volume.
   G. Add immunotoxin:
      (1) Use one vial for every 5 mL of immunotoxin to be added.
      (2) Add 5 mL HSA (25 percent) to reconstitute immunotoxin vial to 10^{-6} M ricin A chain.
      (3) Add immunotoxin to cells to reach a final concentration of 10^{-8} M ricin A chain (1 percent of treatment volume).
   H. Remove 700 μL for pH determination; record.
   I. Remove "post" sample by removing 1.5 to 2 mL to small sterile plastic tube, appropriately labeled; incubate along with main volume.

10. TRANSFER OF CELLS FROM STERILE CONTAINER TO TRANSFER PACK
   A. Label transfer pack with name of patient, date, and other required information.
   B. Attach screw cap adapter to treatment container.
   C. Attach transfer pack to adapter.
   D. Pour cell solution to transfer pack. Transfer pack must be dependent.
   E. Tie knot in tubing and/or crimp tube with crimper (hand sealer clips and hand sealer).

11. INCUBATION
   A. Incubate 2 hours at 37°C on rocker platform (gentle motion).
   B. Take sample at end of incubation for final pH determination. This must be done by going into the bag with a 1-mL syringe through one port, being very careful not to puncture the wall of the bag.

12. PREPARE CELLS FOR FUNCTIONAL ASSAYS
    A. Centrifuge "pre" and "post" laboratory samples (at 1200 rpm for 4 to 5 minutes). Freeze supernatant from "post" sample in labeled freezing vial (label "rescue sample," date, patient name). Freeze at −70°C for long-term storage. Remove supernatant from "pre" sample and discard supernatant. Resuspend "pre" and "post" cell pellets in RPMI-1640/20 percent FCS.
    B. Rescue sample can be used later to see if ST1-IT was active; that is, if it is able to kill CD5-positive tissue culture cells (e.g., Jurkat cells). This would be necessary if it was determined that efficacy of T-cell depletion was poor. If it is late, may transfer cells to T flask and incubate in 10 mL RPMI-1640 plus 20 percent FCS overnight. Set up functional assays next day. If time permits, functional assays can be set up that evening.

13. INFUSION OF TREATED MARROW INTO THE PATIENT
    A. Patient may be premedicated with acetaminophen and diphenhydramine hydrochloride 30 to 60 minutes before infusion.
    B. Within 1 hour following the end of incubation, treated marrow is infused into the patient intravenously through a needle of minimum bore 18 gauge over 30 minutes. No filter should be used.

ANTICIPATED RESULTS

Cell recovery after density gradient separation is typically 25 to 40 percent, although there is no change in the number of CFU-E or CFU-GM bone marrow progenitors observed. We achieve approximately 95 percent depletion of T cells by FACS analysis, by PHA-induced proliferation, and by limiting dilution analysis of proliferating T cells. For evaluation of efficacy of T-cell depletion, see Chapter 11.

NOTES

1. All procedures should be carried out in a laminar air flow hood or in a closed system (i.e., Fenwal transfer pack).
2. TO ENSURE MAXIMUM EFFICACY OF ST1-IT TREATMENT:
    A. Maintain pH greater than 7.6 at beginning of incubation. If pH is greater than 8.2, bone marrow progenitors may be damaged. Do not add excess THAM.
    B. Maintain hematocrit (Hct) at less than or equal to 3 percent. If Hct exceeds 3 percent, dilute bone marrow with appropriate volume of medium (RPMI-1640 plus 5 percent HSA) prior to addition of reagents for incubation. Calculate reagents based on final volume.
    C. Maintain cell concentration at 2×10^7 cells per mL. If cell concentration exceeds this limit, dilute bone marrow with medium as previously described.
    D. Maintain NH_4Cl concentration at 20 mM. Higher concentrations may be toxic.
    E. Shake well on rocker platform during incubation to ensure even distribution of the immunotoxin.
3. If the volume of bone marrow is too great for reinfusion into the patient, centrifuge at the end of the 2-hour incubation and remove appropriate volume. This is particularly critical for pediatric patients.
4. Late reinfusion of the bone marrow (owing to prolonged incubation in NH_4Cl) may be toxic to bone marrow progenitors.

AUTHOR

Barbara E. Bierer, M.D.
Hematology-Oncology Division
Brigham and Women's Hospital
Div. of Pediatric Oncology
Dana-Farber Cancer Institute
Room 1610B
44 Binney St.
Boston, MA 02115

REFERENCES

1. Olsnes, S and Pihl, A: Different biological properties of the two constituent peptide chains of ricin, a toxic protein inhibiting protein synthesis. Biochemistry 12:3121, 1973.
2. Bierer, BE, et al: Phenotypic and functional characterization of human cytolytic cells lacking expression of CD5. J Clin Invest 81:1390, 1988.
3. Derocq, J-M, et al: Comparison of the cytotoxic potency of T101 Fab, F(ab')$_2$ and whole IgG immunotoxins. J Immunol 141:2837, 1988.
4. Derocq, J-M, et al: Rationale for the selection of ricin A-chain anti-T immunotoxins for mature T cell depletion. Transplantation 44:763, 1987.
5. Chiron, M, et al: Sensitivity of fresh leukemic cells to T101 ricin A-chain immunotoxin: A comparative study between Fab fragment and whole Ig conjugates. Leuk Res 13:491, 1989.

8 | PURGING TECHNIQUES IN AUTOLOGOUS TRANSPLANTATION

Commentary by SCOTT D. ROWLEY and
JANICE M. DAVIS

The necessity for and efficacy of in vitro purging is controversial in autologous bone marrow transplantation. Purging of autologous bone marrow grafts refers to the removal of tumor cells contaminating the harvested bone marrow product. In theory, small quantities of viable tumor cells in the graft (minimal-residual disease), protected from the intensive marrow-lethal induction regimen administered to the patient, are capable of causing disease relapse, thereby negating the potential benefit of dose-intensive therapy.[1] However, there is little evidence that purging is necessary for successful autologous transplantation, and numerous autologous transplant trials involving purging have been based on theoretical considerations. For example, the fact that patients with acute leukemia in second or subsequent remission rarely are cured with standard induction regimens suggests that bone marrow grafts harvested from these patients almost certainly will contain leukemic cells. An

218

extension of this argument is that for patients with acute leukemia in remission (less than 5 percent blasts on microscopic examination of a marrow aspirate), a graft consisting of 1 to 2×10^{10} cells could contain up to 1×10^8 tumor cells. Yet, similar numerical arguments against the need for purging have also been proposed.[2] Moreover, others have argued that the number of patients required to prove the efficacy (and, therefore, necessity) of purging in rigorous, randomized trials may exceed the available resources, and that the utility of purging may therefore never be proven to any reasonable degree of certainty.[3] All of these arguments are based on assumptions of questionable validity about the probability of residual disease, relapse, and purging efficacy. In actuality, the question regarding the need for purging is more complex than the preceding numerical arguments portray. Evidence for the effectiveness and necessity of in vitro purging in some patient groups is accumulating, as will be discussed. This evidence, however, also illustrates the difficulty in generalizing the advantage of purging for large diagnostic groups (e.g., patients with acute leukemia in remission), because the risk for marrow contamination can vary greatly for patients with similar diagnoses. Rather, selection of appropriate therapy for well-defined groups of patients based on the probability of residual disease is becoming the primary issue. Factors such as diagnosis, previous therapy, and timing of harvesting and transplantation all influence the likelihood of residual disease, and must be accounted for in clinical trials of purging. Obviously, purging efficacy can never be proved in studies of patients with little risk of residual bone marrow disease.

Regardless, many diseases that show steep dose-response curves, and therefore are amenable to dose-escalation therapies such as autologous transplantation, are diseases of the marrow or diseases that frequently involve the marrow at some stage in their natural history (Table 8–1). For these diseases, purging may be important. Conversely, for diseases that rarely involve the marrow, purging would be of no value, especially if the toxicity incurred as a result

Table 8–1 CLASSIFICATION OF DISEASES ACCORDING TO BONE MARROW INVOLVEMENT

Diseases of the Bone Marrow
(Purging Probably Important for Control of Residual Disease)
Acute leukemia
Chronic leukemia*
Multiple myeloma

Diseases Frequently Metastatic to Bone Marrow
(Purging Possibly Important in Defined Circumstances)
Non-Hodgkin's lymphoma
Hodgkin's disease
Breast cancer
Melanoma
Neuroblastoma

Diseases Rarely Metastatic to Bone Marrow
(Purging Probably Contributes Little to Transplant Results)
Ovarian cancer
Testicular cancer
Glioblastoma

*Uncertain for chronic *myeloid* leukemia.

of the in vitro manipulation (e.g., a higher graft failure rate or increased mortality from prolonged aplasia) exceeded the maximal possible benefit achieved by a lower probability of disease relapse. Purging, regardless of technique, is not without toxicity. It is in those diseases in which the theoretical benefit of purging is marginal that its use can most easily be challenged. At this time, no one should justify purging for any disease with the simple argument that purging is harmless and adds no risk to the patient's treatment.

A number of approaches for in vitro marrow purging have been studied in preclinical models of disease.[4] The in vitro treatment of the marrow graft allows the use of agents or doses that could cause unacceptable, nonhematopoietic (extramedullary) toxicity in the host. For example, escalation of cyclophosphamide doses will rapidly increase the probability of hemorrhagic myocarditis, without causing irreversible marrow failure.[5] Yet bone marrow incubation in vitro with 4-hydroperoxycyclophosphamide (4-HC) can result in aplasia durations measured in months.[6-10] Likewise, the dose of methylprednisolone sodium succinate (10 mM) used in a recent phase I trial is 10,000-fold greater than the plasma level achievable by intravenous administration to patients.[11] Two major purging techniques—immunologic and pharmacologic—have been developed in preclinical and clinical research. [Physical techniques, such as separation by density or by differences in cryopreservation survival,[12,13] do not appear adequate to achieve the 8 logs (10^8 cells) of tumor depletion theoretically necessary.] Immunologic techniques take advantage of tumor-specific or normal differentiation antigens not found on hematopoietic stem cells. The malignant cells can then be removed or destroyed (or, with "positive selection" using stem cell antigens, the hematopoietic stem cells concentrated[14,15]) by magnetic separation or the addition of complement or toxins. Judicious selection of antibodies and other reagents should avoid normal hematopoietic progenitor cell toxicity. Pharmacologic purging relies on a differential sensitivity between the malignant and normal cells. The greater the difference between the normal and malignant cell dose-response curves, the more likely that a given agent or combination of agents will achieve adequate tumor cell kill without undue normal cell cytotoxicity.

Timing of harvesting and transplantation may affect the patient's tumor burden and, therefore, the need for in vitro purging (Table 8–2). Intensive treatment of the patients either before or after transplantation (i.e., in vivo purge[16])

Table 8–2 STRATEGIES TO ELIMINATE MINIMAL-RESIDUAL DISEASE

Before Bone Marrow Harvesting
In vivo purge
  Intensive induction-consolidation regimens

At Harvesting
Peripheral blood hematopoietic progenitor cells
In vitro purging

After Bone Marrow Transplantation
In vivo purge
  Immune modulation
  Sequential autologous marrow tranplantation

may eliminate or reduce minimal residual disease to curative levels while avoiding the need for in vitro purging. Purging is required only if the graft contains sufficient quantities of tumor cells to cause relapse after transplantation. In the treatment of acute myelogenous leukemia (AML), for example, several groups have reported durable post-transplant remissions without purging of the grafts.[17-20] Generally, however, these patients received transplants after several cycles of intensive consolidation. The transplant may have served as an additional, intensive consolidation cycle. Intensive consolidation has been shown to improve the disease-free survival of patients with AML entering first remission.[21-23] Also, the administration of several consolidation cycles in the treatment of AML requires several months. Therefore, those patients who relapse early during therapy are excluded from transplant trials, leaving a group of patients with potentially less aggressive disease. (Comparison of results between phase II trials obviously requires that patient selection also be rigorously compared.) Gorin and colleagues,[24] for example, reported a multi-institutional trial of AML for the European Bone Marrow Transplant Group that purging may provide a survival advantage for patients transplanted in first remission. The advantage of purging, however, a 41 percent decrease in probability of relapse, was only found in those patients receiving transplants within 6 months of achieving remission. Purging, therefore, may be most important for patients at high-risk of relapse.* At present, there are no generally accepted, clinically relevant predictive tests to determine if minimal-residual disease remains in the harvested graft and should be purged before transplantation, although this is an obvious area of interest.

Minimal-residual disease may also be treatable after transplantation. Such an approach would treat disease that escaped the in vitro purge and was reinfused, as well as residual disease in the host surviving the preparative regimen. Evidence supporting this approach includes the different probabilities of relapse for patients classified by the presence or absence of graft-versus-host (GVH) disease after allogeneic transplantation. The lower relapse rate for patients experiencing GVH disease has led to the concept of a graft-versus-leukemia (GVL) effect.[25-30] Some groups are experimentally inducing GVH disease in their autologous recipients in an attempt to achieve a similar immunologic effect.[31,32] Considering that patients undergoing autologous transplantation probably cannot achieve relapse-free survivals greater than that of recipients of syngeneic transplants (without tumor contamination of the graft, but also without GVH disease, leading to about a 50 percent relapse rate in acute leukemia), post-transplant therapy could have a profound effect on the relapse rate after autologous transplantation. This approach may be even more important for patients treated for lymphoma or solid tumors. Post-transplant relapses in these patients usually occur at previous sites of disease,[33-37] suggesting that the tumor survived the preparative regimen and was not reintroduced with the graft. Therefore, postgrafting immunotherapy (such as with

*An alternate explanation is that patients receiving transplants after longer intervals may have had higher levels of residual disease, and the purging technique used may not have been adequate to kill the contaminating tumor cells. Therefore, no difference in probability of relapse would be found between recipients of purged or unpurged grafts. The heterogeneity of the patient population would have also prevented the authors from discerning any possible delay in relapse as a result of the partial purging.

induced GVH disease,[31,32] lymphokine-activated killer (LAK) cells,[38,39] interferon treatment,[40] or antibody infusion[41]) may supplement the preparative regimens, which are generally already at the limits of tolerable drug dosages.*

The evidence supporting the efficacy of purging is indirect. First, it is possible to clone in vitro tumor cells from samples of bone marrow harvested for autologous transplantation.[44–47] Second, investigators have reported miliary osseous metastases in several patients after transplantation with unpurged bone marrow for the treatment of non-Hodgkin's lymphoma and breast cancer.[48,49] At Johns Hopkins, one patient given a transplant with a 4-HC–purged graft for non-Hodgkin's lymphoma developed miliary pulmonary metastases 3 months after transplantation; a second patient, similarly treated for breast cancer, developed miliary osseous metastases 4 months after transplantation (also suggesting that purging may not be 100 percent effective). Third, we demonstrated a dose response for our patients with AML, using CFU-GM survival after purging as a measure of cytotoxicity.[43] The more cytotoxic the 4-HC effect, the higher the probability of relapse-free and overall disease-free survival. Fourth, we have also demonstrated that the sensitivity to 4-HC of leukemic cells cloned in vitro (colony-forming unit—leukemic, or CFU-L) predicted the disease-free survival of patients transplanted for acute leukemia.[45] Finally, as discussed earlier, Gorin and associates[24] reported an improved probability of disease-free survival for recipients of purged grafts if the marrow was harvested within 6 months of achieving a remission. The arguments against this evidence are that tumor cells clonable in vitro may not represent tumor stem cells capable of causing relapse; reports of widespread metastases shortly after autografting are anecdotal (and widespread metatases could conceivably result from immune dysfunction from the transplant procedure); there is no correlation between CFU-L and CFU-GM sensitivity to 4-HC; the in vitro CFU-L sensitivity to 4-HC could actually be reflecting the sensitivity to cyclophosphamide (used in our preparative regimens) of the residual disease in the host; and finally the European trial was not randomized, and therefore subject to selection bias.

In the absence of properly designed, controlled trials to determine the efficacy of purging in any defined population, the decision to purge must therefore balance the theoretical benefits against the morbidity resulting from delayed or partial hematologic or immunologic engraftment. We believe the evidence in support of purging for acute leukemia is most compelling and, for our patients, justifies the prolonged aplasia resulting from the intensive 4-HC purging of those grafts. Although the evidence to support purging for our patients with non-Hodgkin's lymphoma is less compelling, this group, in balance, also has less toxicity (less prolonged aplasia) from the in vitro purge (Figs. 8–1 and 8–2).[50]

---

*The importance of timing, especially for acute leukemia, raises the question of whether some patients should have marrow stored for later use in the event of disease relapse. We have not advocated this approach at Johns Hopkins primarily because of the rapidly changing (and, it is hoped, improving) purging techniques. Unless purging techniques are developed that can be applied to marrow after thawing, the patient may receive a graft treated with outdated methods. Second, we have not yet found a significant difference in outcome (in either probability of relapse or engraftment kinetics) for patients with acute leukemia transplanted in first compared with second remission,[42,43] suggesting that there is no advantage to using marrow harvested in first remission.

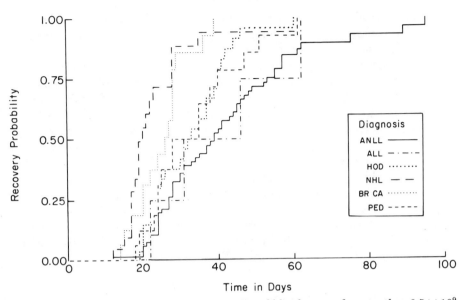

FIGURE 8–1   Probability of achieving a peripheral blood count of greater than 0.5×10^9 granulocytes per L after marrow reinfusion for patients classified by diagnosis. (From Rowley, SD, et al.,[50] with permission.)

It must be understood that purging is only one aspect of the in vitro processing involved in autologous bone marrow transplantation. Initial concentration steps to collect buffy coat and light-density cells and subsequent cryopreservation techniqes may profoundly affect the efficacy of the purge or the kinetics of engraftment. Our previously described 4-HC dose-response in dis-

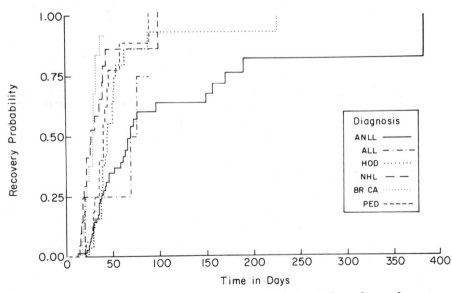

FIGURE 8–2   Probability of achieving platelet transfusion independence after marrow reinfusion for patients classified by diagnosis. (From Rowley, SD, et al.,[50] with permission.)

ease-free survival resulted from varying erythrocyte contamination of the buffy coat, with, consequently, varying inactivation of the drug.[10,43] Treatment of density gradient separated cells has decreased the variance in CFU-GM survival, although at the expense of an additional step in the marrow processing.[51] Poor cryopreservation technique may also limit the extent to which the marrow can be purged. Gorin suggested that freeze-thaw survival of CFU-GM less than 50 percent of fresh could result in engraftment failure.[52] We also found that poor freeze-survival of CFU-GM from 4-HC–treated grafts predicted a delay in engraftment.[53] Surprisingly, despite the widespread use of dimethyl sulfoxide (DMSO) for bone marrow cryopreservation, the cost in terms of hematopoietic progenitor cell loss and delayed engraftment from cryopreservation of autologous marrow grafts has not been well defined.[54] Alternate cryoprotectants may improve the freeze-survival of hematopoietic progenitors.[55] If the cryopreservation technique itself causes severe progenitor cell loss, this limits the rigor of the in vitro purge, unless the purging technique itself has absolutely no toxicity to the hematopoietic progenitor cells in the graft.

CURRENT APPROACHES

Pharmacologic Techniques

Antineoplastic drugs administered to humans produce greater tumor cell than normal cell kill, thereby achieving a therapeutic ratio in their effect. The more sensitive the tumor, or the more selective the agent, the greater is the therapeutic ratio. In vitro purging with pharmacologics similarly depends on a therapeutic ratio between the intended tumor cell target and the normal hematopoietic progenitor and accessory cells necessary for lymphohematopoietic engraftment of the patient (Table 8–3). In vitro purging with pharmacologics has an advantage over direct administration to patients: extramedullary (nonhematopoietic) toxicities are not of concern in in vitro purging, assuming that the agent used can be removed or decreased to acceptable, nontoxic levels before reinfusion. Therefore, the time-dose exposure during purging can be much greater than that achieved by direct patient administration, even accounting for the generally short incubation times used with in vitro purging. Just as dose intensity is the justification for using marrow-lethal preparative regimens with autologous bone marrow transplantation for dose-sensitive tumors,[56] dose intensity is also important for in vitro purging. Effective purging

Table 8–3 CRITERIA FOR AN EFFECTIVE PURGING AGENT

Little, or nonlimiting, hematopoietic cell toxicity
In vitro dose-concentration severalfold higher than achievable in vivo
Differential cytotoxicity between normal and malignant cells
Tumor cytotoxicity not cell-cycle–dependent
Ability to remove or inactivate agent before marrow reinfusion
Short incubation duration

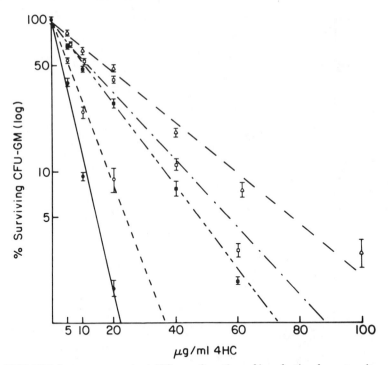

FIGURE 8–3   CFU-GM dose response to 4-HC as a function of incubation hematocrit: ● _____ ●, 0 percent; ○ . . . ○, 1 percent; ■ __ __ __ ■, 5 percent; □ __ __ __ □, 10 percent △ ____ ____ △, 20 percent. The respective regression equations are y = 1.98–0.091 × (n = 46, r = −0.98); y = 1.99–0.057 × (n = 36, r = −0.95); y = 1.98–0.027 × (n = 52, r = −0.98); y = 1.94–0.022 × (n = 69, r = −0.94); y = 1.98–0.017 × (n = 62, r = −0.97). All correlation coefficients are significant at p < 10⁻⁶. (From Jones, RJ, et al.,[10] with permission.)

requires that the drug concentration(s) used be severalfold higher than those attained by direct patient administration, which limits purging to agents with acceptable hematopoietic toxicity profiles.

The most widely used drugs are activated oxazaphosphorines such as 4-HC and mafosfamide. These drugs are derivatives of cyclophosphamide not requiring hepatic metabolism for activity.[57] 4-HC spontaneously decomposes in water to 4-hydroxycyclophosphamide, releasing hydrogen peroxide; mafosfamide similarly decomposes. 4-Hydroxycyclophosphamide is the common intermediate for 4-HC, mafosfamide, and cyclophosphamide. No differences in metabolism of these drugs exist after the formation of this intermediate. The major pathway of drug inactivation, differential sensitivity of normal versus malignant cells, and possibly drug-resistance, is via the formation of carboxyphosphamide, catalyzed by cellular aldehyde dehydrogenase. This enzyme is present in varying amounts in mature and immature blood and bone marrow cells.[56–58] Thus, variation in the erythrocyte and nucleated cell concentrations during the in vitro purge will result in variation in drug effect (Figs. 8–3 and 8–4; again, emphasizing the importance of cell isolation techniques preceding the actual purge procedures).[10,43,50]

Activated cyclophosphamides are toxic to normal myeloid progenitor cells, although a range in sensitivity exists with the more primitive progenitors being

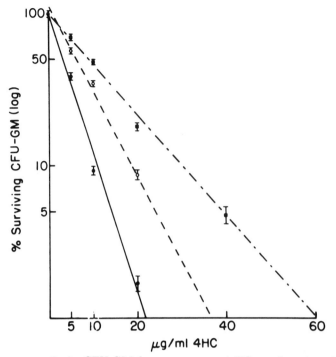

FIGURE 8–4 CFU-GM dose response to 4-HC as a function of the incubation concentration of mononuclear bone marrow cells; ● ————— ●, 5 × 10⁶ cells per mL; ○ — — — ○, 10 × 10⁶ cells per mL; ■ _ _ _ ■, 20 × 10⁶ cells per mL. The respective regression equations are y = 1.98–0.91 × (n = 46, r = −0.98); y = 2.04–0.057 × (n = 40, r = 0.99); y = 2.0–0.034 × (n = 39, 4 = −0.98). All correlation coefficients are significant at < 10⁻⁶. (From Jones, RJ, et al.,[10] with permission.)

less sensitive.[59,60] Autologous transplantation with 4-HC- or mafosfamide-purged grafts results in prolonged aplasia. Patients receiving transplants for AML at Johns Hopkins currently experience median times to granulocyte and platelet recoveries of about 45 and 86 days, respectively.[51] The survival of CFU-GM through the purge averages less than 1 percent,[51] with about a 10-day prolongation in aplasia for each 10-fold (1 log) decrease in CFU-GM quantity.[9] The cytotoxicity to normal myeloid cells may be exacerbated by previous chemotherapy, as the kinetics of engraftment are shorter for patients with other diagnoses (see Figs. 8–1 and 8–2). Patients with non-Hodgkin's lymphoma, for example, have about 4 percent CFU-GM survival, experience median granulocyte and platelet aplasias of 23 and 29 days, respectively,[51] and require about one-half the blood product support of AML patients,[61] despite receiving grafts purged with identical doses of 4-HC.

For patients with AML, there is little leeway for additional toxicity. With the already prolonged aplasia duration associated with this disease, further escalation of 4-HC cytotoxicity would dramatically increase the probability of engraftment failure. (Of further interest, patients with prolonged aplasia after 4-HC–purged autografting frequently fail to respond to recombinant human GM-CSF[62] possibly because the more mature myeloid progenitors have been depleted by the in vitro purge, and therefore cannot be rescued by the use of this cytokine.) This degree of toxicity requires that purge technique (including cell isolation and cryopreservation steps) be meticulous, to avoid additional progenitor cell loss from the already damaged graft. Again, attention must be given to the other aspects of graft processing and cryopreservation, to ensure uniformity of techniques and to minimize any additional unwanted toxicity. With activated cyclophosphamide purging, simple tests of graft viability such as dye exclusion or cell quantification cannot be used because the cytotoxicity is not immediately expressed. Only progenitor cell (CFU-GM) cultures have been shown to predict engraftment kinetics and therefore serve as a clinically meaningful, quality control measure in the laboratory.[9]

Other drugs have been studied in preclinical models of purging or clinical transplant trials. Etoposide (VP-16), vincristine, methylprednisolone, daunomycin, cisplatin, and others have all been shown in preclinical models to achieve greater tumor than normal cell cytotoxicity,[63-65] but when compared none have been as effective in these preclinical models as 4-HC.[66,67] Comparative clinical trials have not been reported. Recently, several transplant programs have pursued clinical purging with combinations of drugs[12,68] or combinations of drugs and immunologic purging techniques.[69] In some preclinical models, the addition of other drugs to 4-HC may decrease the normal cell toxicity (antagonism to 4-HC effect), while enhancing tumor cell kill (synergism), thereby dramatically increasing the therapeutic ratio.[46,70,71]

In general, preclinical evaluations of pharmacologic purging agents compared the cytotoxicity to tumor-derived cell lines with the cytotoxicity to human bone marrow cell cultured in vitro. However, the therapeutic ratio directly defined by these experiments does not validate clinical trials because there is no correlation of cell line kill with purging efficacy. Also, the degree of kill achieved varies with the model chosen, with several "logs" difference between cell lines in the number of cells killed. The real value in cell line experiments is the development of purging technique, defining approximate drug concentrations, duration of incubation, and effects of other incubation parameters such as contaminating cell populations (e.g., erythrocytes for 4-HC), or timing and sequence of cotreatment with other agents.

Immunologic Techniques

In theory, immunologic purging using monoclonal antibodies should avoid all hematopoietic cell toxicity, thereby achieving an effective purge with little risk of engraftment delay or failure. Monoclonal antibodies can be targeted against tumor-specific antigens or cell-differentiation antigens not shared by the more primitive cells responsible for lymphohematopoietic engraftment. Thus a differential between malignant and normal cells is established by the presence or absence of cell surface antigens. This approach has been most attractive for the treatment of nonmyeloid leukemias and nonhematopoietic malignancies such as breast cancer and neuroblastoma. Immunologic purging has also been used successfully for T-cell depletion of allogeneic grafts, to decrease the risk of GVH disease.

A variety of clinical protocols have been reported for both allogeneic and autologous bone marrow transplantation.[72-74] Antibodies used depend on the cell target but include antibodies to B-cell, T-cell, myeloid, and neuroblastoma determinants. However, the major conceptual differences between immuno-purging protocols are the techniques used to remove or kill the tumor cells. Several techniques have been developed. Incubation with complement is most effective if the antibody is of IgM isotype or if the expected antigen density on the target cell is high enough to achieve adequate activation of complement. Rabbit complement is frequently used because many of the antibodies bind human complement poorly. Alternatively, the antibody can be fixed to magnetic beads (or similar solid phase material) for physical separation. A third technique used is the conjugation of a toxic molecule such as the A chain of ricin to the antibody. Antibody bound to the cell surface is endocytosed, with concomitant ingestion of the toxin and cell death. The development of antibodies to antigens specific for early myeloid progenitors allows the "positive selection" of hematopoietic stem cells from the marrow.[14,15] These techniques are all designed to handle large volumes of cells, facilitating the clinical use of immunologic purging techniques.

The major difficulty with immunologic purging is the heterogeneity of antigen expression on malignant cells.[75] Cells expressing low levels of antigens are not likely to be killed by this approach, even with several cycles of purging. To overcome this, many centers purge with multiple antibodies, each targeted to a different antigen, not just different epitopes of the same antigen.[76] Additional cycles of purging may increase the efficiency of complement-mediated purging;[76] use of automated cell-processing devices with the continuous addition of fresh complement and removal of spent reagents may similarly enhance the efficacy of the purge.[74] Another problem may be that the antigenic profile of the malignant stem cell may differ from that of the majority of malignant cells present in the harvested marrow. Thus, purging may be aimed at inconsequential targets. Finally, blocking cell populations, complement-mediated hematopoietic cell toxicity, and variability in complement potency are all problems that must be resolved before actual patient accrual on a particular clinical trial. For the processing laboratory, immunopurging requires quality control of a number of reagents not used in pharmacologic purging.

More so than with pharmacologic purging, there is no evidence that immunologic purging in autologous bone marrow transplantation is effective. This is not to suggest that immunologic purging is necessarily inadequate. It has been suggested by one transplant group that the relatively unsatisfactory results after autologous transplantation with immunopurged grafts for acute lymphoblastic leukemia (ALL) are difficult to interpret because of possibly inadequate preparative regimens used in those trials.[69] Immunologic purging for T-cell depletion of allogeneic grafts removes only about 95 to 99.9 percent of T cells.[77,78] Theoretically, this "2–3 logs" depletion may not be adequate for optimal autografting, if "8 logs" of clonogenic tumor are present (although in actual use, single drug purges are also unlikely to achieve "8 logs" of kill,[11,46] further suggesting that this degree of purging is not necessary for optimal transplantation). Although comparable disease-free survivals to pharmacologic purging have been reported for immunologic purging in the treatment of AML,[74] the possibility of selection biases between these phase II trials, of course, cannot be discounted. In preclinical models, the combined immunopharmacologic purging approaches appear to achieve much greater levels of tumor kill than immunologic (or single-drug pharmacologic) techniques alone.

SPECIFIC PROTOCOLS

Pharmacologic Purging

Several different drugs—4-HC, mafosfamide, etoposide, and combinations of 4-HC or etoposide with other drugs—are specified in the pharmacologic purging protocols included in this chapter. Otherwise, the protocols are remarkably similar. These protocols treat either bone marrow buffy coat or density gradient–separated cells with fresh drug for a specified period, followed by removal of the drug with the supernatant or by more rigorous washing. Experience in clinical trials with these protocols varies. The 4-HC protocols (or similar protocols) have been used in phase I and II trials,[6,7,79,80] and is currently being used in a phase III intergroup cooperative trial comparing intensive consolidation therapy with autologous transplantation in the treatment of patients with AML in first complete remission. Likewise, mafosfamide in fixed or adjusted doses has been used in phase II trials.[8,24,81] 4-HC has recently been approved by the Food and Drug Administration (FDA) for use in purging autologous marrow from patients with AML. Phase I or II clinical experience with etoposide as a single agent has not yet been published. We recently completed a phase I trial of the 4-HC, vincristine, methylprednisolone combination,[11] providing some baseline data.

The major difference in these protocols, then, involves the concentration of the purging agent. The protocol of Rizzoli and colleagues advocates adjusted-dose purging, with the adjustment based on ex vivo cultures of hematopoietic progenitors. The protocols of Yao and Chao suggest treating buffy coat cells with 60 μg per mL of 4-HC, whereas those of Davis and Rowley suggest a 4-HC dose of 100 μg per mL for buffy coat cells and 60 μg per mL for density gradient–separated cells. The rationale for adjustment of drug doses when using alkylating agents is to achieve maximal tumor cell cytotoxicity while minimizing normal cell damage. Diagnosis is a major predictor of aplasia duration (see Figs. 8-1 and 8-2) after 4-HC purging, possibly because of the differing chemotherapeutic induction regimens previously administered.[50] In general, treatment of buffy coat cells with 100 μg per mL is probably at the limits of tolerance for patients with AML (median time to achieve 0.5×10^9 granulocytes per L, 39 days) while patients with non-Hodgkin's lymphoma (NHL) (median time to achieve 0.5×10^9 granulocytes per L, 19 days) could receive grafts treated with much higher concentrations of drugs.[9] (Effective 4-HC and mafosfamide concentrations can also be affected by the red blood cell content of the incubation mixture,[59] hence the focus on this parameter in these protocols.)

The clinical experience with 4-HC and mafosfamide is extensive, and phase I and II trials have been published. Experience with other drugs listed in these protocols is much more limited. Detailed phase I data have not been published for any of these other protocols. Therefore, doses listed should be viewed as suggestions only, and investigators adopting these protocols should discuss available clinical experience with the protocol authors.

The combination drug purge by Oldenburg and Stiff and the etoposide-purging protocol by Ciobanu and associates call for cryopreservation using a cryoprotectant solution of DMSO, hydroxyethyl starch (HES), dextrose, and human serum albumin.[58] Addition of HES probably allows for a decrease in

DMSO concentration, which should correspondingly decrease direct DMSO-induced progenitor cell toxicity, as well as infusion-related toxicities to the patient.[82] This technique has not been compared in clinical trials with cryopreservation with 10 percent DMSO. Cryopreservation survival affects the engraftment kinetics of 4-HC–purged grafts, so changes in any aspect of these protocols, including the cryopreservation technique specified, should be considered with caution.

Immunologic Purging

The techniques listed in this section involve different antibodies for different diseases. Again, the major conceptual differences between these protocols involve the techniques used for the separation of the target cells from the remainder of the marrow.

The protocols by Yao and Negrin and by Schwarz and colleagues use baby rabbit complement to lyse target cells. The latter developed the continuous flow of fresh complement into the incubation mixture (and removal of spent reagents from the mixture) by performing the immunopurge in an apheresis device. Thus, they appear to have achieved maximal target cell lysis without requiring several cycles of antibody-complement treatment. The other immunopurging protocols all depend on the physical separation of target cells. Magnetic beads coated with antibodies reactive to the monoclonal antibodies used in the purge are added to the cells after the cells have been treated with the monoclonal antibodies and excess antibody washed from the mixture. The mixture is then passed through a strong magnetic field and the target cells depleted from the graft. Again, these protocols call for only one pass to deplete the tumor cells, as opposed to the multiple passes usually employed in complement-mediated purging. The advantage of physical separation is that this avoids the use of a biologic agent (complement), thus somewhat simplifying the purge procedure (and possibly achieving greater uniformity). Also, the target cells are not destroyed but can be removed from the beads if desired. To account for variable expression of antigens on the target cells, these protocols use multiple antibodies directed against different antigens. All protocols involve treatment of density gradient–separated grafts.

Both Shimazaki and Shpall and their associates combine the immunopurge with 4-HC treatment of the marrow. The quantity of 4-HC used by Shimazaki and colleagues is low compared with the pharmacologic purges discussed earlier, but they add sedimenting agents to the buffy coat collection step to enhance erythrocyte depletion and extend the incubation time to 60 minutes. The cytotoxicity resulting from the pharmacologic purge can be assayed by progenitor cell culture separate from any cytotoxicity from the immunomagnetic purge and should be part of the laboratory quality control steps. The order of incubation appears important in these two protocols. Shimazaki demonstrated that 4-HC did not alter the antigen expression of the cells in their preclinical model; this is obviously an aspect that must be verified before any modification of the technique is attempted. Shpall found less CFU-GM toxicity but equal tumor cytotoxicity when the 4-HC preceded the immunopurge.[83]

OTHER CONSIDERATIONS

All these protocols are lacking quality control sections. The adjusted-dose mafosfamide protocol relies on in vitro "blast" colony formation, but correlation of this assay with engraftment kinetics has not been documented.[84] Likewise, enumeration of committed progenitor cells after 4-HC purging may not correlate with engraftment and therefore may serve as quality control if optimal culture techniques are not used.[9] At a minimum, any laboratory involved in in vitro pharmacologic purging should have quality control measures for postpurge engraftment potential and for sterility. All calculations should be independently checked before drug addition. Worksheets should be designed so that review of calculations is simplified. Cell quantities, treated and frozen, should be recorded. Cell viability (e.g., by trypan blue dye exclusion) has little value, as pharmacologic agents do not immediately kill. Any of these quality control measures is virtually worthless, however, if the processing laboratory members do not monitor patient engraftment kinetics and survival after transplantation and correlate this information with the laboratory results of the in vitro purge.

The issues of quality control are much more complex for the immunologic purging protocols. Potency, safety (lack of hematopoietic stem cell toxicity), pyrogenicity, and sterility of antibodies, complement, and other reagents are the responsibility of the processing laboratory. Extensive preclinical testing of reagents and practice are important before actual use of any technique.

The protocol by Yao and Nelson raises the issue of microbiologic contamination of the graft. Their protocol calls for the addition of antibiotics at the start of processing, presumably because of the open collection of light-density cells. Although low levels of contamination may be common as a result of the open, percutaneous harvesting technique used,[85] life-threatening infections have been reported in conjunction with open processing.[86] All marrows should be cultured after processing. Contaminated marrows should be discarded, however, only after serious consideration of the ramifications to the patient, especially considering that patients appear to tolerate low levels of bacterial contamination. Contamination may also occur during the processing; hence the addition of povodone-iodine to the laboratory waterbaths suggested by Shpall. At the least, bone marrow microbiologic studies are required to monitor laboratory practices. These studies may also assist in the care of the autograft recipient, if clinical infection occurs.

No standards currently exist for bone marrow processing facilities. This does not condone deviation from good laboratory practices, however. Open processing techniques should be discouraged, for example, if alternatives are available. In this regard, some aspects of these protocols can be adapted to replace similar techniques in other protocols. Separation of buffy coat cells in transfer packs or using automated devices can probably replace the use of open centrifuge tubes. Automated devices are also probably the most effective technique for washing grafts, and avoid the risk of centrifuging transfer packs containing spikes from sampling site couplers. Our laboratory purchases tissue culture media packaged in containers that can be directly attached to our cell washers, avoiding the need for first transferring media to blood transfer packs. We can also directly spike our media bottles after replacing the original cap with a commercially available septum. Personnel involved in processing bone marrow must be familiar with blood bank practices. A familiarity with pharmacy techniques is also valuable when manufacturing the reagents listed in these protocols.

REFERENCES

1. Santos, GW, Yeager, AM, and Jones, RJ: Autologous bone marrow transplantation. Annu Rev Med 40:99, 1989.
2. Schultz, FW, Martens, ACM, and Hagenbeek, A: The contribution of residual leukemic cells in the graft to leukemia relapse after autologous bone marrow transplantation: Mathematical considerations. Leukemia 3:530, 1989.
3. Appelbaum, FR and Buckner, CD: Overview of the clinical relevance of autologous bone marrow transplantation. In Goldstone, AH (ed): Clinical Haematology. WB Saunders, London, 1986, p 1.
4. Gross, S, Gee, AP, and Worthington-White, DA (eds): Bone Marrow Purging and Processing. Wiley-Liss, New York, 1989.
5. Friedman, OM, Myles, A, and Colvin, M: Cyclophosphamide and related phosphoramide mustards. Advances in Cancer Chemotherapy 1:143, 1979.
6. Kaizer, H, et al: Autologous bone marrow transplantation in acute leukemia: A phase I study of in vitro treatment of marrow with 4-hydroperoxycyclophosphamide to purge tumor cells. Blood 65:1504, 1985.
7. Yeager, AM, et al: Autologous bone marrow transplantation in patients with acute nonlymphocytic leukemia, using ex vivo marrow treatment with 4-hydroperoxycyclophosphamide. N Engl J Med 315:141, 1986.
8. Gorin, NC, et al: Autologous bone marrow transplantation using marrow incubated with Asta Z 7557 in adult acute leukemia. Blood 67:1367, 1986.
9. Rowley, SD, et al: CFU-GM content of bone marrow graft correlates with time to hematologic reconstitution following autologous bone marrow transplantation with 4-hydroperoxycyclophosphamide purged bone marrow. Blood 70:271, 1987.
10. Jones, RJ, et al: Variability in 4-hydroperoxycyclophosphamide activity during clinical purging for autologous bone marrow transplantation. Blood 70:1490, 1987.
11. Rowley, SD, et al: Phase I study of combination drug purging for autologous bone marrow transplantation. J Clin Oncol, 1991 (in press).
12. Dicke, KA, et al: Autologous bone-marrow transplantation in relapsed adult acute leukaemia. Lancet 1:514, 1979.
13. Hagenbeek, A and Martens, ACM: Cryopreservation of autologous marrow grafts in acute leukemia: survival of in vitro clonogenic leukemic cells and normal hemopoietic stem cells. Leukemia 3:535, 1989.
14. Berenson, RJ, et al: Antigen CD34+ marrow cells engraft lethally irradiated baboons. J Clin Invest 81:951, 1988.
15. Berenson, RJ, et al: Stem cell selection—clinical experience. In Gross, S, Gee, AP, and Worthington-White, DA (eds): Bone Marrow Purging and Processing. Wiley-Liss, New York, 1989, p 403.
16. Spinolo, JA, et al: Strategies for the clinical application of autologous bone marrow transplantation in acute leukemia. In Gale, RP and Champlin, RE (eds): Bone Marrow Transplantation: Current Controversies. Alan R. Liss, New York, 1989, p 149.
17. Burnett, AK, et al: Transplantation of unpurged autologous bone marrow in acute myeloid leukemia in first remission. Lancet 2:1068, 1984.
18. Lowenberg, B, et al: Transplantation of non-purified autologous bone marrow in patients with AML in first remission. Cancer 12:2840, 1984.
19. McMillan, AK, et al: High-dose chemotherapy and autologous bone marrow transplantation in acute myeloid leukemia. Blood 76:480, 1990.
20. Löwenberg, B, et al: Autologous bone marrow transplantation in acute myeloid leukemia in first remission: results of a Dutch prospective study. J Clin Oncol 8:287, 1990.
21. Vaughn, WP, Karp, JE, and Burke, PJ: Two-cycle timed-sequential chemotherapy for adult acute nonlymphocytic leukemia. Blood 64:975, 1984.
22. Wolff, SN, et al: High-dose cytosine arabinoside and daunorubicin as consolidation therapy for acute nonlymphocytic leukemia in first remission: A pilot study. Blood 65:1407, 1985.

23. Wolff, SN, et al: High-dose cytarabine and daunorubicin as consolidation therapy for acute myeloid leukemia in first remission: Long-term follow-up and results. J Clin Oncol 7:1260, 1989.

24. Gorin, NC, et al: Autologous bone marrow transplantation for acute myelocytic leukemia in first remission: A European survey of the role of marrow purging. Blood 75:1606, 1990.

25. Weiden, PL, et al: Anti-leukemia effect of chronic graft-versus-host disease. Contribution to improved survival after allogeneic marrow transplantation. N Engl J Med 304:1529, 1981.

26. Weiden, PL, et al: Antileukemic effect of graft-versus-host disease in human recipients of allogeneic marrow grafts. N Engl J Med 300:1068, 1979.

27. Weisdorf, DJ, et al: Allogeneic bone marrow transplantation for acute lymphoblastic leukemia in remission: Prolonged survival associated with acute graft-versus-host disease. J Clin Oncol 5:1348, 1987.

28. Butturini, A, Bortin, MM, and Gale, RP: Graft-versus-leukemia following bone marrow transplantation. Bone Marrow Transplant 2:233, 1987.

29. Kersey, JH, et al: Comparison of autologous and allogeneic bone marrow transplantation for treatment of high-risk refractory acute lymphoblastic leukemia. N Engl J Med 317:416, 1987.

30. Sullivan, KM, et al: Graft-versus-host disease as adoptive immunotherapy in patients with advanced hematologic neoplasms. N Engl J Med 320:828, 1989.

31. Jones, RJ, et al: Induction of graft-versus-host disease following autologous bone marrow transplantation. Lancet 2:754, 1989.

32. Talbot, DC, et al: Cyclosporine-induced graft-versus-host disease following autologous bone marrow transplantation in acute myeloid leukaemia. Bone Marrow Transplant 6:17, 1990.

33. Phillips, GL, et al: Treatment of resistant malignant lymphoma with cyclophosphamide, total body irradiation, and transplantation of cryopreserved autologous marrow. N Engl J Med 310:1557, 1984.

34. Jones, RJ, et al: High dose cytotoxic therapy and bone marrow transplantation for relapsed Hodgkin's disease. J Clin Oncol 8:527, 1990.

35. Freedman, AS, et al: Autologous bone marrow transplantation in B-cell non-Hodgkin's lymphoma: Very low treatment-related mortality in 100 patients in sensitive relapse. J Clin Oncol 8:784, 1990.

36. Gulati, SC, et al: Autologous bone marrow transplantation for patients with poor-prognosis lymphoma. J Clin Oncol 6:1303, 1988.

37. Williams, SF, et al: High-dose consolidation therapy with autologous stem cell rescue in stage IV breast cancer. J Clin Oncol 7:1824, 1989.

38. van den Brink, MRM, et al: Lymphokine-activated killer cells selectively kill tumor cells in bone marrow without compromising bone marrow stem cell function in vitro. Blood 74:354, 1989.

39. Long, GS, et al: Lymphokine-activated killer (LAK) cell purging of leukemic bone marrow: Range of activity against different hematopoetic neoplasms. Bone Marrow Transplant 6:169, 1990.

40. Meyers, JD, et al: Prophylactic use of human leukocyte interferon after allogeneic marrow transplantation. Ann Intern Med 107:809, 1987.

41. Wagner, JE, et al: Systemic monoclonal antibody therapy for eliminating minimal residual leukemia in a rat bone marrow transplant model. Blood 73:614, 1989.

42. Yeager, AM, et al: Autologous bone marrow transplantation in acute nonlymphocytic leukemia: studies of ex vivo chemopurging with 4-hydroperoxycyclophosphamide. In Gale, RP and Champlin, RE (eds): Bone Marrow Transplantation: Current Controversies. Alan R. Liss, New York, 1988, p 157.

43. Rowley, SD, et al: Efficacy of ex vivo purging for autologous bone marrow transplantation in the treatment of acute nonlymphoblastic leukemia. Blood 74:501, 1989.

44. Uckun, FM, et al: Use of a novel colony assay to evaluate the cytotoxicity of an immunotoxin containing pokeweed antiviral protein against blast progenitor cells freshly obtained from patients with common B-lineage acute lymphoblastic leukemia. J Exp Med 163:347, 1986.

45. Miller, CB: Correlation of occult leukemia drug sensitivity with relapse after autologous bone marrow transplantation. Blood 78:1125, 1991.

46. Jones, RJ, et al: In vitro evaluation of combination drug purging for autologous bone marrow transplantation. Bone Marrow Transplant 5:301, 1990.

47. Estrov, Z, et al: Detection of residual acute lymphoblastic leukemia cells in cultures of bone marrow obtained during remission. N Engl J Med 315:538, 1986.

48. Vaughan, WP, et al: Early leukemia recurrence of non-Hodgkin lymphoma after high-dose anti-neoplastic therapy with autologous marrow rescue. Bone Marrow Transplant 1:373, 1987.

49. Peters, WP, et al: High-dose combination cyclophosphamide (CPA), cisplatin (cDDP) and carmustine (BCNU) with bone marrow support as initial treatment for metastatic breast cancer: Three–six year follow-up. Proc Am Soc Clin Oncol 9:31, 1990.

50. Rowley, SD, et al: Analysis of factors predicting speed of hematologic recovery after transplantation with 4-hydroperoxycylophosphamide-purged autologous bone marrow grafts. Bone Marrow Transplant 7:183, 1991.

51. Rowley, SD, et al: Density-gradient separation of autologous bone marrow grafts before *ex vivo* purging with 4-hydroperoxycyclophosphamide. Bone Marrow Transplant 6:321, 1990.

52. Gorin, NC: Collection, manipulation and freezing of haemopoietic stem cells. In Gladstone, AH (ed): Clinics in Haematology. WB Saunders, London, 1986, p 19.

53. Rowley, SD, Piantadosi, S, and Santos, GW: Correlation of hematologic recovery with CFU-GM content of autologous bone marrow grafts treated with 4-hydroperoxycyclophosphamide. Culture after cryopreservation. Bone Marrow Transplant 4:553, 1989.

54. Fahy, GM: The relevance of cryoprotectant "toxicity" to cryobiology. Cryobiology 23:1, 1988.

55. Stiff, PJ, et al: Autologous bone marrow transplantation using unfractionated cells cryopreserved in dimethylsulfoxide and hydroxyethyl starch without controlled-rate freezing. Blood 70:974, 1987.

56. Frei, III P and Canellos, GP: Dose: A critical factor in cancer chemotherapy. Am J Med 88:585, 1980.

57. Sladek, NE: Metabolism of oxazaphosphorines. Pharmacology and Therapeutics 37:301, 1988.

58. Helander, A and Tottmar, O: Cellular distribution and properties of human blood aldehyde dehydrogenase. Alcoholism: Clinical and Experimental Research 10:71, 1986.

59. Sahovic, EA, et al: Role for aldehyde dehydrogenase in survival of progenitors for murine blast cell colonies after treatment with 4-hydroperoxycyclophosphamide *in vitro*. Cancer Res 48:1223, 1988.

60. Gordon, MY, Goldman, JM, and Gordon-Smith, EC: 4-Hydroperoxycyclophosphamide inhibits proliferation by human granulocyte-macrophage colony-forming cells (GM-CFC) but spares more primitive progenitor cells. Leuk Res 9:1017, 1985.

61. Davis, J, et al: Blood component use in autologous bone marrow transplantation (ABMT) (abstr). Transfusion 29:60S, 1989.

62. Neumanaitis, J, et al: Use of recombinant human granulocyte-macrophage colony-stimulating factor in graft failure after bone marrow transplantation. Blood 76:245, 1990.

63. Peters, RH, et al: In vitro synergism of 4-hydroperoxycyclophosphamide and cisplatin: Relevance for bone marrow purging. Cancer Chemother Pharmacol 23:129, 1989.

64. Chang, T-T, et al: Comparative cytotoxicity of various drug combinations for human leukemic cells and normal hematopoietic precursors. Cancer Res 47:119, 1987.

65. Gulati, SC, et al: Comparative regimens for the *ex vivo* chemopurification of B cell lymphoma-contaminated marrow. Acta Haematol 80:65, 1988.

66. Blaauw, A, et al: Potential drugs for elimination of acute lymphatic leukemia cells from autologous bone marrow. Exp Hematol 14:683, 1986.

67. Auber, ML, et al: Evaluation of drugs for elimination of leukemic cells from the bone marrow of patients with acute leukemia. Blood 71:166, 1988.

68. Gulati, SC, et al: Autologous bone marrow transplant using 4-HC, VP-16 purged bone marrow for acute nonlymphoblastic leukemia. Bone Marrow Transplant 4:116, 1989.

69. Uckun, FM, et al: Autologous bone marrow transplantation in high-risk remission T-lineage acute lymphoblastic leukemia using immunotoxins plus 4-hydroperoxycyclophosphamide for marrow purging. Blood 76:1723, 1990.

70. De Fabritiis, P, et al: Efficacy of a combined treatment with ASTA-Z 7654 and VP16-213 *in vitro* in eradicating clonogenic tumor cells from human bone marrow. Bone Marrow Transplant 2:287, 1987.

71. Chang, TT, et al: Synergistic effect of 4-hydroperoxycyclophosphamide and etoposide on a human promyelocytic leukemia cell line (HL-60) demonstrated by computer analysis. Cancer Res 45:2434, 1985.

72. Ramsay, N, et al: Autologous bone marrow transplantation for patients with acute lymphoblastic leukemia in second or subsequent remission: Results of bone marrow treated with monoclonal antibodies BA-1, BA-2, BA-3 plus complement. Blood 66:508, 1985.

73. Ritz, J, et al: Autologous bone marrow transplantation in CALLA-positive acute lymphoblastic leukemia after *in vitro* treatment with J5 monoclonal antibody and complement. Lancet 2:60, 1982.

74. Ball, ED, et al: Autologous bone marrow transplantation for acute myeloid leukemia using monoclonal antibody-purged bone marrow. Blood 75:1199, 1990.

75. Gee, AP, et al: Selective loss of expression of a tumor-associated antigen on a human leukemia cell line induced by treatment with monoclonal antibody and complement. J Natl Cancer Inst 78:29, 1987.

76. LeBien, TW, et al: Utilization of a colony assay to assess the variables influencing elimination of leukemic cells from human bone marrow with monoclonal antibodies and complement. Blood 65:945, 1985.

77. Prentice, HG, et al: Use of anti-T cell monoclonal antibody OKT3 to prevent acute graft-versus-host disease in allogeneic bone-marrow transplantation for acute leukaemia. Lancet 1:700, 1982.

78. Filipovich, AH, et al: Pretreatment of donor bone marrow with monoclonal antibody OKT3 for prevention of acute graft-versus-host disease in allogeneic histocompatible bone-marrow transplantation. Lancet 1:1266, 1982.

79. Rosenfeld, C, et al: Autologous bone marrow transplantation with 4-hydroperoxycyclophosphamide purged marrows for acute nonlymphocytic leukemia in late remission or early relapse. Blood 74:1159, 1989.

80. Lenarsky, C, et al: Autologous bone marrow transplantation with 4-hydroperoxycyclophosphamide purged marrows for children with acute non-lymphoblastic leukemia in second remission. Bone Marrow Transplant 6:425, 1990.

81. Körbling, M, et al: Disease-free survival after autologous bone marrow transplantation in patients with acute myelogenous leukemia. Blood 74:1898, 1989.

82. Davis, J, et al: Toxicity of bone marrow graft infusions. Transfusion 12:551, 1987.

83. Anderson, IC, et al: Elimination of malignant clonogenic breast cancer cells from human bone marrow. Cancer Res 49:4659, 1989.

84. Gordon, MY, et al: Colony formation by primitive haemopoietic progenitors in cocultures of bone marrow cells and stromal cells. Br J Haematol 60:129, 1985.

85. Rowley, SD, et al: Bacterial contamination of bone marrow grafts intended for autologous and allogeneic bone marrow transplantation: Incidence and clinical significance. Transfusion 28:109, 1988.

86. Henslee, J, et al: Prevention of early gram positive (gm+) septicemia in autologous bone marrow transplant (ABMT) patients (PTS) (abstr). Proc Am Soc Clin Oncol 3:100, 1984.

NONIMMUNOLOGIC

TREATMENT OF BUFFY COAT CELLS WITH 4-HYDROPEROXYCYCLOPHOSPHAMIDE

DESCRIPTION	Successful autologous marrow transplantation is limited by the possible presence of residual marrow tumor cells even when a clinical complete remission is achieved. Physical, pharmacologic, and immunologic techniques have been used to try to separate these tumor cells from the marrow hematopoietic stem cells. The procedure uses a cyclophosphamide derivative, 4-hydroperoxycyclophosphamide (4-HC), at 100 μg per mL to purge tumor cells from the marrow. The purged marrow is then frozen (see appropriate procedure) and the patient is treated with marrow-lethal chemotherapy with or without total body irradiation. The purged marrow is thawed and infused to rescue the patient from the chemotherapy.
TIME FOR PROCEDURE	Approximately 1 hour for the drug incubation and wash after buffy coat cells are collected
SUMMARY OF PROCEDURE	1. Bone marrow is harvested. 2. Buffy coat cells are collected. 3. Backup cells are removed. 4. Red blood cell concentration is adjusted when necessary. 5. Cells are incubated with 4-HC, centrifuged, and frozen.
EQUIPMENT	1. 37°C waterbath 2. Laminar flow hood 3. Cell counter 4. Balance 5. Heat sealer
SUPPLIES AND REAGENTS	1. 2000-mL transfer pack (Fenwal 4R2041) 2. 1000-mL transfer pack (Fenwal 4R2031) 3. 600-mL transfer pack (Fenwal 4R2023) 4. 300-mL transfer pack (Fenwal 4R2014) 5. Lifecell septum and cap (Fenwal 4C2471) 6. Sampling site couplers (Fenwal 4C2405) 7. 4-HC (Nova Pharmaceutical Co.) 8. Administration set (Cutter 20-5614) 9. TC-199 (Gibco 320-1151) 10. 0.22-μm Millipore filter (Millipore SLGS02505) 11. 16-gauge needles 12. 60-mL luer-lock syringes 13. Alcohol wipes

PROCEDURE

1. Prepare a buffy coat concentrate from the harvested marrow. Obtain a specimen for the following:
   A. Nucleated cell count
   B. Hematocrit (Hct)
   C. Progenitor cell assays
   D. Sterility

2. Determine the number of nucleated cells per kg patient weight present in the buffy coat concentrate. The following guidelines should be used to determine how to separate the marrow into primary and secondary (backup) fractions.
   A. The buffy coat is split: two thirds of the marrow is treated at 100 μg per mL and one third is untreated.
   B. The recommended number of cells for primary treatment should be 3.0×10^8 per kg with backup of at least 0.7×10^8 per kg.
   C. If the two thirds–one third division causes the primary to be less than 3×10^8 per kg, then the primary will be adjusted if possible to 3.0×10^8 per kg. Some patients may not have enough cells to allow for an untreated backup graft. The final decision is made by the medical director.

3. Determine the total number and volume of cells to be treated as the primary and backup. Transfer the appropriate volume (volume = cells per kg $\times$ patient weight $\div$ buffy coat cells per mL) of backup cells into properly labeled freeze bags and place them in the refrigerator. The cells that are to be treated should be placed in a 200-mL transfer pack.

   NOTE: *All bags must be labeled with the patient's name, hospital number, and the type of treatment.*

4. Determine the total volume of the incubation mixture.

   Total volume = Total number of cells/fraction $\div$ 2.0×10^7 cells/mL

5. Determine the incubation Hct.

   Buffy coat Hct $\times$ primary cell volume $\div$ total incubation volume

   The incubation Hct should be between 5 and 10 percent. Red cells obtained during the buffy coat procedure should be added to the product to increase the Hct when necessary.

   To determine how much RBC concentrate to add perform the following calculation:

   mL RBC to be added = (desired Hct $\times$ total incubation volume)
   $-$ (primary cell volume $\times$ buffy coat Hct)

   After the addition of red cells, obtain a sample for a repeat cell count and Hct. The count and volume obtained after the red cell addition should be used to determine the volume of reagents for the actual incubation, as shown here.

   Total volume = Total number of cells/fraction $\div$ 2.0×10^7 cells/mL
   mL plasma = Total volume $\times$ 0.2
   mg 4-HC = Total volume $\times$ 100 μg/mL $\div$ 1000 μg/mg

$$\text{mL 4-HC} = \text{mg 4-HC} \div 10 \text{ mg/mL (4-HC stock concentration)}$$
$$\text{mL media} = \text{Total volume} - \text{plasma volume} - \text{cell volume} - \text{4-HC volume}$$

6. Add the correct volume of autologous plasma to the incubation bag.

7. The appropriate number of media bottles (TC-199) are stoppered using the Lifecell septums and caps.

8. Using an administration set and by weighing the bag on the balance, add the correct amount of TC-199 media. This may be syringed into the bag if the volume is small.

9. Place the bag in the 37°C waterbath and allow the cells to remain for 10 minutes before the addition of the 4-HC.

10. The 4-HC (200-mg vial) should be reconstituted in 20 mL of room temperature TC-199 media. This results in a solution containing 10 mg 4-HC per mL. Refer to package insert for details.

11. The appropriate amount of dissolved 4-HC is added to the incubation bag through a 0.22-μm filter attached to a syringe.

12. Mix the incubation bag, obtain a sample to determine the actual incubation Hct and cell count, and set a timer for 30 minutes. The ports of the bag should not be immersed in the water; they should be taped to the side of the waterbath. Mix the bag every 5 minutes.

13. After the 30-minute incubation, the cells should be transferred to 600-mL bags. If the incubation volume is greater than 600 mL, enter the incubation bag with a 300-mL bag, then enter this 300-mL bag with two other 600-mL bags. Allow the cells to fill the final 600-mL bags (this ensures that when the bags are centrifuged there are no spikes in them).

14. Centrifuge the 600-mL bags at 4°C for 10 minutes at 2900 rpm ($2170g$) in the centrifuge. After centrifugation, place the bags in the plasma expressor. Connect a 600-mL transfer bag to the port and remove as much media as possible without losing cells.

15. Combine the cells into one bag. Record the final volume.

16. Mix the final product and obtain samples for:

   A. Cell count
   B. Progenitor cell assays
   C. Differentials
   D. Sterility

17. Freeze the graft according to standard procedure.

ANTICIPATED RESULTS

This procedure should result in the recovery of more than 80 percent of the cells that were treated. The recovery of colony-forming units–granulocyte, macrophage (CFU-GMs) should be approximately 1 percent and will vary according to patient diagnosis and Hct of the incubation mixture.

Janice M. Davis, M.T.(ASCP),
Cell Processing Laboratory
The Johns Hopkins Oncology Center

Scott D. Rowley, M.D., FACP
The Fred Hutchinson Cancer

REFERENCES

1. Yeager, AM, et al: Autologous bone marrow transplantation in patients with acute nonlympho-cytic leukemia, using ex vivo marrow treatment with 4-hydroperoxycyclophosphamide. N Engl J Med 315:141, 1986.
2. Jones, RJ, et al: Variability in 4-hydroperoxycyclophosphamide activity during clinical purging for autologous bone marrow transplantation. Blood 70:1490, 1987.
3. Rowley, SD, et al: Efficacy of ex vivo purging for autologous bone marrow transplantation in the treatment of acute nonlymphoblastic leukemia. Blood 74:501, 1989.

TREATMENT OF DENSITY GRADIENT–SEPARATED CELLS WITH 4-HYDROPEROXYCYCLOPHOSPHAMIDE

DESCRIPTION	Successful autologous marrow transplantation is limited by the possible presence of residual marrow tumor cells even when a clinical complete remission is achieved. Physical, pharmacologic, and immunologic techniques have been used in an attempt to separate these tumor cells from the marrow hematopoietic stem cells. This procedure uses a cyclophosphamide derivative, 4-hydroperoxycyclophosphamide (4-HC), at 60 μg per mL to "purge" tumor cells from the marrow. Additionally, red blood cells are removed from the cell mixture to reduce the variability of colony-forming unit—granulocyte, macrophage (CFU-GM) survival. The purged marrow is then frozen (see appropriate procedure) and the patient is treated with marrow-lethal chemotherapy with or without total body irradiation. The purged marrow is thawed and infused to rescue the patient from the chemotherapy.
TIME FOR PROCEDURE	Approximately 1 hour for the drug incubation and wash. This time does not include the time required to collect the buffy coat cells and perform the density gradient separation.
SUMMARY OF PROCEDURE	1. Bone marrow is harvested. 2. Buffy coat cells are collected. 3. Backup cells are removed. 4. Cells are further separated using a density gradient. 5. Cells are incubated with 4-HC, washed with cold medium, and frozen.
EQUIPMENT	1. 37°C waterbath 2. Laminar flow hood 3. Heat sealer 4. COBE 2991 or other cell washer 5. Cell counter
SUPPLIES AND REAGENTS	1. 2000-mL transfer pack (Fenwal 4R2041) 2. 1000-mL transfer pack (Fenwal 4R2031) 3. 600-mL transfer pack (Fenwal 4R2023) 4. 300-mL transfer pack (Fenwal 4R2014) 5. Sampling site couplers (Fenwal 4C2405) 6. Lifecell septum and cap (Fenwal 4C2471) 7. 4-HC (Nova Pharmaceutical Co.) 8. Administration set (Cutter 20-5614) 9. TC-199 (Gibco 320-1151) 10. RPMI-1640 (4-L container) (Whittaker 12-167L) 11. 0.22-μm Millipore filter (Millipore SLGS02505) 12. 16-gauge needles 13. 60-mL luer-lock syringes

14. Alcohol wipes

15. Software for washing device

PROCEDURE

1. Prepare a buffy coat concentrate from the harvested marrow. Obtain a specimen for the following:
   A. Nucleated cell count
   B. Hematocrit (Hct)
   C. Progenitor cell assays
   D. Sterility

2. Determine the number of nucleated cells per kg patient weight present in the buffy coat concentrate. The primary fraction will be red cell depleted by density gradient separation and treated with 4-HC. The secondary (backup) fraction will be untreated.
   A. The recommended number of cells for the backup fraction is at least 0.7×10^8 per kg.
   B. The remainder of the buffy coat cells (preferably more than 1.5×10^8 cells per kg) should be processed using a density gradient–separation technique. Some patients may not have enough cells to allow for an untreated backup graft. The final decision is made by the medical director.

3. Determine the total number and volume of cells present in the primary and backup. Transfer the appropriate volume (volume = cells per kg × patient weight ÷ buffy coat cells per mL) of backup cells into properly labeled freeze bags and place them in the refrigerator. The cells that are to be further processed should be transferred to a 600-mL transfer pack.

   NOTE: *All bags must be labeled with patient's name, hospital number, and the type of treatment.*

4. After the light-density cells are collected, they are washed with RPMI media and resuspended in a final volume of approximately 50 mL. Cell counts are performed to determine the number of cells to be treated. Cell culture specimens should be obtained. Determine the volume of reagents using the following calculations:

$$\text{Total volume} = \text{Total number of cells/fraction} \div 2.0 \times 10^7 \text{ cells/mL}$$
$$\text{mL plasma} = \text{Total volume} \times 0.2$$
$$\text{mg 4-HC} = \text{Total volume} \times 60 \ \mu g/mL \div 1000 \ \mu g/mg$$
$$\text{mL 4-HC} = \text{mg 4-HC} \div \text{4-HC stock concentration (mg/mL)}$$
$$\text{mL media} = \text{Total volume} - \text{plasma volume} - \text{cell volume} - \text{4-HC volume}$$

5. Add the correct volume of autologous plasma to the incubation bag.

6. The appropriate number of TC-199 media bottles are stoppered using the Lifecell septums and caps.

7. Using an administration set and by weighing the bag on the balance, add the correct amount of TC-199 media. This may be syringed into the bag if the volume is small.

8. Place the bag in the 37°C waterbath and allow the cells to remain for 10 minutes before the addition of the 4-HC.

9. The 4-HC (20-mg vial if available) should be reconstituted in 20-mL of room temperature TC-199 media. Refer to the package insert for details.

10. The dissolved 4-HC is added to the cells using a 0.22-μm filter attached to a syringe (to deliver small volumes of drug: filter the drug into a sterile tube, remove the appropriate amount using 1-mL syringes and add the drug to the cells).

11. After the 4-HC is added, mix the incubation bag and obtain a sample to determine the actual incubation cell count. Set a timer for 30 minutes. The ports of the bag should not be immersed in the water. They may be taped to the side of the waterbath. Mix the bag every 5 minutes.

12. After the 30-minute incubation, the cells should be washed on the COBE 2991 (or an equivalent device) with 1.5 L of *cold* RPMI media containing 2 percent autologous *irradiated* (greater than 1500 rad) plasma.

13. The COBE wash procedure is as follows:
    A. Attach the cells to the RED line and fill the bowl. The RPMI media should be attached to the GREEN line and the remainder of the bowl should be filled with media before beginning the program. The operator control panel should be set as follows:

Centrifuge Speed	Super-Out Rate	Agitate Time	Super-Out Volume	Valve Selector
3000	450	80	450*	N/A

*At the start of the last cycle, change the super-out volume (SOV) to 600.

- Spin Time 1: 2 minutes
- Spin Time 2: N/A
- Auto/Manual: Auto

    B. The board should be set as follows:

Timer*	PC	Valve	SOV
X O	O	O X O	450
X O	O	O X O	450
X O	X	O O O	600

*X = a peg in the slot; O = no peg in the slot.

14. After the cells are washed, resuspend the product and obtain the final specimens as follows:
    A. Cell count
    B. Progenitor cell assays
    C. Differentials
    D. Sterility

15. Freeze the graft according to standard procedure.

ANTICIPATED RESULTS	This procedure should result in the recovery of more than 80 percent of the cells that were treated. The recovery of colony-forming units—granulocyte, macrophage (CFU-GMs) should be approximately 1 percent and will vary according to patient diagnosis.

AUTHORS

Janice M. Davis, M.T.(ASCP), S.B.B.
Cell Processing Laboratory
The Johns Hopkins Oncology Center
Baltimore, MD 21205

Scott D. Rowley, M.D., FACP
The Fred Hutchinson Cancer Research Center
Seattle, WA 98104

REFERENCES

1. Rowley, SD, et al: Density-gradient separation for 4-hydroperoxycyclophosphamide purging of autologous bone marrow grafts. In Gross, SR and Gee, A (eds): Bone Marrow Purging and Processing. Proceedings of the Second International Symposium on Bone Marrow Purging and Processing, vol 333. Progress in Clinical and Biological Research. Alan R. Liss, New York, 1990, p 369.
2. Jones, RJ, et al: Variability in 4-hydroperoxycyclophosphamide activity during clinical purging for autologous bone marrow transplantation. Blood 70:1490, 1987.
3. Rowley, SD, et al: Efficacy of ex vivo purging for autologous bone marrow transplantation in the treatment of acute nonlymphoblastic leukemia. Blood 74:501, 1989.

MARROW PURGING WITH MAFOSFAMIDE AT INDIVIDUALLY ADJUSTED DOSE

DESCRIPTION

Autologous bone marrow transplantation (ABMT) after high-dose cytotoxic therapy has been widely used as a treatment for acute leukemias, lymphomas, and solid tumors.[1-3] Because of the possibility that the reinfused marrow may be contaminated with residual malignant cells responsible for leukemic relapse after ABMT,[4] in vitro marrow purging with pharmacologic agents has been proposed to achieve elimination of residual neoplastic cells from the graft.[5,6] The most widely used agents for chemical purging are active metabolites of cyclophosphamide such as 4-hydroperoxycyclophosphamide (4-HC) and the more stable compound mafosfamide (Asta-Z 7557). Although the efficacy of marrow purging is still controversial, recently reported data demonstrate an improved clinical outcome in leukemic patients receiving purged autografts as compared with those transplanted with unpurged marrow.[7,8] The rationale for in vitro marrow purging is based not only on a supposed difference in sensitivity between leukemic and normal progenitor cells to active metabolites of cyclophosphamide but also on the activation of immunologic mechanisms with potential antileukemic effects.[9]

By means of clonogenic assays, it has been demonstrated that, similar to the other metabolites of cyclophosphamide, mafosfamide inhibits the in vitro growth of pluripotent (colony-forming unit—granulocyte, erythrocyte, macrophage, megakarocyte [CFU-GEMM]) and lineage-restricted progenitor cells (burst-forming unit—erythroid [BFU-E] and colony-forming unit—granulocyte, macrophage [CFU-GM]), as well as leukemic clonogenic cells (acute myelogenous leukemia colony-forming unit [AML-CFU]).[10-12] However, no selectivity could be demonstrated by assaying the toxicity of mafosfamide toward primary cultures of normal and leukemic cells,[12] even using as a target the pluripotent progenitor CFU-GEMM. In contrast to pluripotent and committed progenitors, the early progenitor cells such as the stroma-adherent blast colony-forming cells (blast-CFC) are spared by mafosfamide at concentrations known to be completely inhibitory to the growth of normal, as well as leukemic progenitor cells, and can be considered the least sensitive progenitors to mafosfamide.[13]

Hematopoietic and immunologic reconstitution following ABMT occurs even when the CFU-GM and the more primitive CFU-GEMM are no longer detectable in the grafted marrow.[14] This evidence implies that the conventional in vitro clonogenic assays do not allow the growth of the cell type responsible for marrow repopulation after ABMT. Several alternatives to these conventional assays such as the stroma-adherent blast-CFC assay have now been proposed to detect early hematopoietic progenitors that closely predict (or are responsible for) marrow repopulation after transplantation.[15]

The availability of a reliable in vitro assay for a class of early progenitors such as blast-CFC, which (a) is spared by mafosfamide—that is, shows a difference in sensitivity to mafosfamide as compared with normal and leukemic progenitors and (b) closely predicts the marrow repopulating ability of the graft, prompted us to establish a two-step procedure for marrow purging based on the evaluation of mafosfamide effect at an early level of hematopoietic ontogeny. The first step consists of an in vitro test evaluating in each patient the cytotoxic effect of the drug at the level of blast-CFC. Using this test the dose of mafosfamide that spares 50 percent of blast-CFC may be calculated. For the second step marrow is harvested and purged ex vivo with the dose of mafosfamide extrapolated from the in vitro test.

This procedure implies at least two theoretical advantages. First, the possibility of an individual adjustment of the dose, related not only to physiologic differences within progenitor cell compartments of different patients but also to chemotherapy-induced damages. Second, the possibility of using a dose of mafosfamide able to induce the maximal antileukemic effect combined with the necessity to spare—at least in part—an early class of progenitors reflecting marrow repopulating ability.

TIME FOR PROCEDURE	1. Step 1: Approximately 7 hours to perform the in vitro test aimed at evaluating individual sensitivity to mafosfamide
	2. Step 2: Approximately 60 minutes to purge marrow harvest

SUMMARY OF PROCEDURE

1. Ten to 14 days before marrow harvest, a sample of bone marrow is collected and the sensitivity of blast-CFC[13] to increasing concentrations of mafosfamide evaluated in each patient by means of an in vitro clonogenic assay for the stroma-adherent blast-CFC.

2. Harvested marrow is delivered to the processing laboratory in 250-mL centrifuge bottles.

3. Buffy coat is obtained and the cell concentrations adjusted at 20×10^6 per mL. If the hematocrit (Hct) value is 1 to 2 percent, step 4 is performed; otherwise, buffy coat is again centrifuged until Hct is reduced to less than 5 percent.

4. Marrow is purged with mafosfamide at the concentration extrapolated by the preharvest in vitro test.

5. Marrow cells are cryopreserved.

EQUIPMENT

No specific equipment is required.

SUPPLIES AND REAGENTS

1. 250-mL centrifuge bottles (Nalgene, Rochester, NY)
2. 50-mL centrifuge tubes
3. Medium 199
4. Mafosfamide (Asta Pharma AG, Bielefeld, Germany)
5. Laminar air flow
6. Waterbath

PROCEDURE

1. INDIVIDUAL EVALUATION OF SENSITIVITY TO MAFOSFAMIDE
   A. Preparation of stromal layer for blast-CFC growth
      (1) Obtain normal bone marrow from consenting donors by aspiration from the posterior iliac crest.
      (2) Isolate light-density mononuclear cells (MNCs) by centrifugation (30 minutes, $400g$, 4°C) on a Ficoll-Hypaque density gradient (d = 1.077 g per mL).
      (3) Wash and resuspend MNCs (5×10^5 per mL) in alpha-medium supplemented with 15 percent fetal bovine serum and 2×10^{-6} M methylprednisolone.

      (4)   Plate 1-mL aliquots in 35-mm petri dishes and incubate at 37°C in a humidified atmosphere supplemented with 5 percent CO_2.

      (5)   Feed the cultures weekly by complete replacement of medium and serum until confluent. Usually, confluence is reached after 3 to 4 weeks, and the stromal layers can be used to support blast-CFC growth for 3 to 4 weeks.

  B.   In vitro cell treatment

      (1)   Obtain from consenting patients bone marrow cells to be evaluated for their sensitivity to mafosfamide, by aspiration from the posterior iliac crest.

      (2)   Separate buffy coat cells by centrifugation at $1300g$ for 10 minutes.

      (3)   Count the cells and adjust their concentration at 2×10^7 per mL with a Hct level under 5 percent.

      (4)   Divide buffy coat cells into five aliquots and incubate with concentrations of mafosfamide ranging from 30 to 150 μg per mL, in steps of 30 μg.

      (5)   Incubate each sample for 30 minutes in the 37°C waterbath with frequent agitation.

      (6)   Incubate the cells for 5 minutes in ice-cold water to stop the reaction, and wash twice.

      (7)   Separate MNCs by centrifugation on a Ficoll-Hypaque gradient (density 1.077 g per mL) at $400g$ for 30 minutes at 4°C.

      (8)   Obtain nonadherent MNCs by incubation (37°C, 5 percent CO_2) of marrow cells (5×10^6 per mL), suspended in RPMI-1640 medium with 10 percent FBS for 120 minutes in 25-cm² plastic tissue culture flasks.

      (9)   Carefully harvest nonadherent MNCs, wash, and resuspend (5×10^5 per mL) in alpha-medium supplemented with 15 percent FBS and 2×10^{-6} M methylprednisolone.

  C.   Blast-CFC assay

      (1)   Add untreated and mafosfamide-treated nonadherent MNCs (5×10^5 per mL) to confluent stromal layers and incubate for 2 hours to allow attachment of cells giving rise to blast-CFC.

      (2)   Wash the stromal layer and overlay with 1 mL 0.3 percent agar in alpha-medium supplemented with 15 percent FBS and 2×10^{-6} M methylprednisolone.

      (3)   Incubate cultures for 5 days in a humidified 5 percent CO_2 atmosphere at 37°C.

      (4)   Aggregates of at least 20 blast cells are scored as blast-CFC.

      (5)   Four plates per experiment are scored for each data point, and the results are expressed as the mean $\pm$ 1 SEM.

      (6)   Mafosfamide concentrations resulting in 50 percent inhibition of colony formation (ID_{50}) are calculated for each experiment by extrapolating from a least-square linear regression line relating the mafosfamide concentration to the percentage of blast-CFC inhibition.

2.   MARROW HARVEST: Harvested marrow—usually 4.0×10^8 cells per kg patient weight—is delivered to the processing laboratory in 250-mL centrifuge bottles.

3. MANUAL PREPARATION OF THE BUFFY COAT
    A. Centrifuge harvested marrow (1300g, 15 minutes, 4°C) and remove autologous plasma.
    B. Transfer pelleted marrow resuspended by manual agitation, into 50-mL Falcon tubes. Wash each 250-mL bottle once to completely recover nucleated cells.
    C. Centrifuge marrow (1300g, 15 minutes, 4°C), aspirate the nucleated cells, and transfer them in 50-mL Falcon tubes.
    D. Repeat step C two or three times.
    E. Following the last centrifugation, pool all the buffy coat cells and adjust the volume of the cell suspension at 100 mL with autologous plasma.
    F. After carefully mixing the cells, obtain samples for cell count, cell culture, differentials, Hct.

4. MARROW PURGING WITH MAFOSFAMIDE
    A. Determine the number of nucleated cells per kg patient weight present in the buffy coat.
    B. Split the buffy coat: treat two thirds of the marrow with mafosfamide at individual adjusted-dose and leave one third untreated.
    C. The recommended number of cells for purging is 3.0×10^8 per kg with a backup of at least 0.7×10^8 kg. Some patients may not have enough cells to allow for an untreated backup graft.
    D. Transfer the appropriate volume of backup cells (volume = cells per kg $\times$ patient weight $\div$ buffy coat cells per mL) into a labeled tissue culture flask and place in the refrigerator. Place the cells that are to be treated with mafosfamide in a roller bottle.
    E. Determine the volume of reagents using the following calculations:

Total volume	= Total number of cells to be purged $\div 2 \times 10^7$ per mL
Total amount of mafosfamide (mg)	= Total volume $\times$ mafosfamide (μg/mL) concentration inducing 50 percent inhibition of blast-CFC growth $\div 1000$ μg/mL
Total volume of mafosfamide (ml)	= mg of mafosfamide $\div$ 10 mg per mL
Medium 199 (mL)	= Total volume $-$ cell volume $-$ mafosfamide volume

    F. Determine the incubation Hct as follows:

    Buffy coat Hct $\times$ cell volume $\div$ total incubation volume

    The incubation Hct should be between 1 and 2 percent, otherwise the purging procedure should be stopped and the buffy coat again centrifuged to reduce Hct to the desired values.
    G. Add the correct volume of medium to the roller bottle.
    H. Place the cell suspension in the 37°C waterbath for 10 minutes before adding mafosfamide.
    I. Reconstitute the mafosfamide (50 mg per vial) with 5 mL of tissue cul-

ture medium, resulting in a solution containing 10 mg mafosfamide per mL.

J. Add the dissolved mafosfamide to the cell suspension through a 0.22-μm filter attached to a syringe.

K. Carefully mix the roller bottle and aspirate a sample to determine the actual Hct and cell count.

L. Incubate the roller bottle for 30 minutes at 37°C in a waterbath with agitation every 5 minutes.

M. After 30 minutes place the roller bottle in ice-cold water for 5 minutes to stop the reaction.

N. Transfer the cell suspension in 50-mL Falcon tubes and centrifuge (1300g, 10 minutes, 4°C).

O. Aspirate as much of the medium as possible without losing cells. Then, resuspend the cells in autologous plasma, and pool.

P. Carefully mix the cell suspension and obtain samples for:
   (1) Cell count
   (2) Cell culture
   (3) Differentials
   (4) Hct
   (5) Sterility

5. CRYOPRESERVATION: After resuspending (4×10^7 per mL) in autologous irradiated plasma (55 percent), medium-199 (35 percent), and dimethyl sulfoxide (10 percent), freeze marrow cells according to the standard procedure.

ANTICIPATED RESULTS	The in vitro test performed before harvesting marrow for ABMT should provide the concentration of mafosfamide inducing 50 percent of blast-CFC formation. By harvesting 4.0×10^8 cells per kg patient weight, the manual preparation of buffy coat should yield 3.0×10^8 cells per kg for purging and a backup of 0.7×10^8 cells per kg. The procedure for marrow purging—including incubation with mafosfamide and the subsequent centrifugation—results in a cell loss of 1 to 1.5×10^9 nucleated cells. Therefore, the anticipated number of cells (3×10^8 per kg body weight) should be increased by 1 to 1.5×10^9 before purging to compensate for cell loss.
NOTES	Carefully control cell concentration (2×10^7 per mL), Hct value (less than 5 percent), and waterbath temperature (37°C) before purging marrow. A Hct value ranging from 1 to 2 percent is recommended.

AUTHORS

Lina Mangoni
Dept. of Hematology
Bone Marrow Transplantation Unit
University of Parma
Parma, Italy

Carmelo Carlo-Stella
Dept. of Hematology
Bone Marrow Transplantation Unit
University of Parma
Parma, Italy

Vittorio Rizzoli, M.D.*
Dept. of Hematology
Bone Marrow Transplantation Unit
University of Parma
Parma, Italy

---

*To whom correspondence concerning this manuscript should be addressed.

REFERENCES

1. Yeager, AM, et al: Autologous bone marrow transplantation in patients with acute non-lymphocytic leukemia, using ex vivo marrow treatment with 4-hydroperoxycyclophosphamide. N Engl J Med 315:141, 1986.

2. Armitage, JO: Bone marrow transplantation in the treatment of patients with lymphoma. Blood 73:1749, 1989.

3. Spitzer, G, et al: High-dose combination chemotherapy with autologous bone marrow transplantation in adult solid tumors. Cancer 45:3075, 1980.

4. Schultz, FW, Martens, ACM, and Hagenbeek, A: The contribution of residual leukemic cells in the graft to leukemia relapse after autologous bone marrow transplantation: Mathematical considerations. Leukemia 3:530, 1989.

5. Sharkis, SJ, Santos, GW, and Colvin, OM: Elimination of acute myelogenous leukemic cells from marrow and tumor suspension in the rat with 4-hydroperoxycyclophosphamide. Blood 55:521, 1980.

6. Rizzoli, V, et al: Autologous bone marrow transplantation for acute leukemia: optimal timing and mafosfamide treatment. In Dicke, KA, et al (eds): Autologous bone marrow transplantation. Proceedings of the fourth international symposium. Houston, University of Texas M.D. Anderson Cancer Center, 1989, p 13.

7. Rizzoli, V and Mangoni, L: Pharmacological-mediated purging with mafosfamide in acute and chronic myeloid leukemias. In Gross, SR, Gee, AP, and Worthington-White, DA (eds): Bone Marrow Purging and Processing. Alan R. Liss, New York, 1990, p 21.

8. Gorin, NC, et al: Autologous bone marrow transplantation for acute myelocytic leukemia in first remission: A European survey of the role of marrow purging. Blood 75:1606, 1990.

9. Skorski, T, et al: The kinetic of immunologic and hematologic recovery in mice after lethal total body irradiation and reconstitution with syngeneic bone marrow cells treated or untreated with mafosfamide (Asta Z 7654). Bone Marrow Transplant 3:543, 1988.

10. Rowley, SD, Colvin, M, and Stuart, RK: Human multilineage progenitor cell sensitivity to 4-hydroperoxycyclophosphamide. Exp Hematol 13:295, 1985.

11. Herve, P, Tamayo, E, and Peters, A: Autologous stem cell grafting in acute myeloid leukemia: technical approach of marrow incubation in vitro with pharmacological agents (prerequisite for clinical applications). Br J Haematol 53:683, 1983.

12. Kluin-Nelemans, HC, et al: No preferential sensitivity of clonogenic AML cells to Asta-Z-7557. Leuk Res 8:723, 1984.

13. Gordon, MY, et al: Colony formation by primitive haemopoietic progenitors in cocultures of bone marrow cells and stromal cells. Br J Haematol 60:129, 1985.

14. Kaizer, H, et al: Autologous bone marrow transplantation in acute leukemia: A phase I study of in vitro treatment of marrow with 4-HC to purge marrow cells. Blood 65:1504, 1985.

15. Gordon, MY, et al: Haemopoietic stem cell subpopulations in mouse and man: Discrimination by differential adherence and marrow repopulating ability. Bone Marrow Transplantation 5(Suppl 1):6, 1990.

ETOPOSIDE PURGING OF MARROW HARVESTED FROM PATIENTS WITH ACUTE LEUKEMIAS, LYMPHOMAS, OR SOLID TUMORS

DESCRIPTION	In vitro treatment of remission bone marrow has been shown to be highly effective in eliminating acute nonlymphocytic leukemia cells without prohibitive destruction of normal hematopoietic stem cells. This method describes the treatment of marrow harvest buffy coat with etoposide at a concentration of 50 μM, for 1 hour at 37°C and a nucleated cell concentration of 2×10^7 per mL.
TIME FOR PROCEDURE	Approximately 90 minutes
SUMMARY OF PROCEDURE	1. Harvested bone marrow is delivered to the processing laboratory in one or more transfer packs.
	2. Marrow buffy coat is obtained using either manual or machine (COBE 2991) blood cell processing.
	3. Three fourths of the buffy coat cell content, or a minimum of 2×10^8 nucleated cells per kg, are set aside for ex vivo etoposide treatment. The untreated marrow will be frozen without further processing.
	4. Marrow to be purged is diluted to a cell concentration of 2×10^7 nucleated cells per mL (final concentration) in 20 percent autologous plasma (irradiated to 30 Gy or 3000 Gy). Hematocrit (Hct) in this admixture must be adjusted to be in the 5 to 10 percent range.
	5. Etoposide (molecular weight 588) is added to achieve a final concentration of 50 μM (29.4 μg per mL).
	6. Treated marrow bag is incubated at 37°C for 1 hour in a waterbath.
	7. Following immediate cooling to 4°C, the purged marrow is washed twice with normal saline containing 2 percent autologous irradiated plasma.
	8. Treated marrow is frozen at a final concentration of 40 to 80 $\times 10^6$ nucleated cells per mL in 10 percent dimethyl sulfoxide (DMSO) and 20 percent autologous irradiated plasma.
EQUIPMENT	1. 37°C waterbath
	2. Laminar flow hood
	3. Sebra heat sealer
	4. Mettler balance
SUPPLIES AND REAGENTS	1. 2000-mL transfer packs (Fenwal 4R2041)
	2. Two 600-mL transfer packs (Fenwal 4R2023)
	3. Sampling site couplers (Fenwal (4C2405)
	4. Administration set (Cutter 20-5614)
	5. Etoposide 20 mg per mL stock solution (Bristol Laboratories)
	6. DMSO multidose containers (Cryoserv)
	7. One 500-mL tissue culture media (RPMI-1640)
	8. Two 1-L bags normal saline
	9. 15-gauge needles

10. 60-mL luer-lock syringes

11. Alcohol wipes

12. 3-mL syringe

13. Freeze bags (250-mL capacity) (Fenwal Cryocyte PL269)

14. Sorvall RC-3B centrifuge (or equivalent refrigerated centrifuge)

PROCEDURE   1. INCUBATION WITH ETOPOSIDE

A. Based on counts obtained from the buffy coat, determine the number of nucleated cells per kilogram. Use the following guidelines to determine how to treat the marrow. The final decision is made by the medical director.

   (1) The recommended total number of cells is at least 2.5×10^8 per kg.

   (2) The division should be three-fourths treated at 50 μM etoposide and one-fourth untreated.

   (3) The minimum number of cells acceptable for primary etoposide treatment is 2.0×10^8 per kg.

   (4) If a three-fourths/one-fourth division causes the primary to be less than 2.0×10^8 per kg, then the primary will be adjusted to be 2.0×10^8 per kg. The backup marrow should be at least 5.0×10^7 per kg.

B. Determine the total number and volume of cells to be treated as the primary and to be frozen untreated as backup. Transfer the appropriate volume of backup cells into a properly labeled freeze bag. Place the freeze bag in the refrigerator at 4°C. The cells that are to be treated as the primary should be placed in a 2000-mL transfer pack if they are not in one already.

NOTE: *All bags should be labeled with patient's name, hospital number, and the type of incubation—that is, "primary" or "backup."*

C. Determine the volume of reagents using the following calculations:

$$\text{Total volume} = \text{Total number of cells per fraction} \div 2.0 \times 10^7 \text{ cells per mL}$$
$$\text{mL plasma} = \text{Total volume} \times 0.2$$
$$\text{mL media} = \text{Total volume} - \text{mL plasma} - \text{mL cells}$$
$$\text{mg etoposide} = \text{Total volume} \times \mu\text{g/mL etoposide} \div 1000 \ \mu\text{g per mg}$$

NOTE: *After dilution of the buffy coat with autologous plasma and RPMI medium, the final red cell hematocrit (Hct) must be between 5 and 10 percent. If the Hct is less than 5 percent, additional autologous red blood cells must be added to achieve that Hct level.*

D. Call the pharmacy and request the amount of etoposide needed.

E. Add the correct volume of autologous plasma to the incubation bag.

F. Using an administration set and weighing the bag on the Mettler balance, add the correct amount of media. Specific gravity of the media is considered to be 1.000.

G. Add the etoposide using a 3-mL syringe.

H. Mix the incubation bag and place in a 37°C waterbath for 60 minutes. The port of the bag should not be immersed in the water. The bag may be taped to the side of the waterbath. Mix the bag every 5 minutes.

2. WASH CELLS AFTER INCUBATION BY MANUAL OR AUTO-MATED TECHNIQUE

A. Manual washing

(1) Transfer the incubated cells into 600-mL transfer bags. If the incubation volume is greater than 600 mL, enter the incubation bag with a 600-mL bag, then enter this 600-mL bag with two other 600-mL bags. Allow the cells to fill the final two 600-mL bags. (When the bags are centrifuged the first time there should not be a spike in them.)

(2) Centrifuge the 600-mL bags at 4°C for 10 minutes at 3000 rpm (2230g) in the RC-3B Sorvall centrifuge.

(3) After centrifugation, place the bags in the plasma expressor. Connect a 600-mL transfer bag to the port and remove as much of the media as possible without losing cells.

(4) Fill each 600-mL bag containing purged marrow with normal saline to submaximal capacity (550 mL).

(5) Repeat steps 12 and 13 for a total of two washings.

(6) Combine the cells from similar incubation treatments into one freeze bag. Record the final volume.

(7) Mix the freeze bag well and obtain 1.2 mL for the following:
  (a) Sterility
  (b) Cell count and Hct
  (c) Cytospin or differential

(8) Freeze both purged and backup bone marrow at a final concentration of 40 to 80 $\times$ 10^6 nucleated cells per mL, in 10 percent DMSO and 20 percent irradiated (30 Gy) autologous plasma.

(9) Place purged and backup marrow in freezing frames in a horizontal position in a −80°C freezer.

(10) Move after 24 hours the frozen frames to a −135°C electrical freezer or a liquid nitrogen freezer.

B. Automatic washing

(1) Use the COBE 2991 Processing Set II (No. 912647-910), make the fluid connections as follows:
  (a) RED line: Diluted purged bone marrow
  (b) GREEN line: 1 L normal saline
  (c) PURPLE line: Waste products
  (d) BLUE and YELLOW lines: To be clamped

(2) Centrifuge marrow for 5 minutes using the following parameters of the manual settings:
  (a) Centrifuge speed (rpm): 3000
  (b) Super-out rate (mL/min): 450
  (c) Minimum agitate time: Not applicable (N/A)
  (d) Super-out volume (mL): 650
  (e) Spin timer 1 and 2: N/A
  (f) Auto/Manual: Manual
  (g) Red cell over-ride: N/A

(3) Wash marrow twice with normal saline, each time allowing 2 minutes minimum agitate time.

(4) After collection of washed purged marrow proceed as in steps 16 through 19.

ANTICIPATED RESULTS	The technique will result in 10 to 15 percent loss of nucleated cells from the purged material.

AUTHOR:

Niculae Ciobanu, M.D.
Montefiore Medical Center
Bronx, NY 10467

REFERENCES

1. Ciobanu, N, et al: Etoposide as an in vitro purging agent for the treatment of acute leukemias and lymphomas in conjunction with autologous bone marrow transplantation. Exp Hematol 14:626, 1986.
2. Lazarus, H, et al: High dose polychemotherapy (BCNU, Cisplatin, VP-16) with or without involved field radiotherapy (IFRT) and autologous bone marrow transplant (ABMT) for relapsed or refractory lymphoma. Blood 74(Suppl 1):617A, 1989.

PURGING OF LEUKEMIC CELLS FROM AUTOLOGOUS BONE MARROW WITH CYTOSINE ARABINOSIDE AND ETOPOSIDE

DESCRIPTION	Although a marrow may look normal histologically, a typical patient in first remission still has a leukemic body burden of 10^8 to 10^9 leukemic cells. As bone marrow collection removes 1 percent of the total marrow, an autologous transplant could involve the reinfusion of 10^6 to 10^7 leukemic cells, potentially enough to cause a relapse. Using a combination of cytosine arabinoside (ara-C) and etoposide (VP-16), the leukemic cells can be purged from the marrow ex vivo. The treated marrow is then reinfused after lethal chemoradiotherapy, leading to normal hematopoietic recovery.
TIME FOR PROCEDURE	Approximately 6 hours
SUMMARY OF PROCEDURE	1. Bottles for washes and dilutions are prepared. 2. Buffy coat with bottle A is initially diluted. 3. Reserve supply of marrow is removed and cryopreserved. 4. Remaining cells are diluted to 550 mL with bottle B. 5. Drugs are prepared and added. 6. Marrow is transferred into 37°C shaking waterbath for 1 hour. 7. Drugs are eliminated. 8. Cells are washed twice. 9. Final dilution takes place. 10. Cryopreservation is performed.
EQUIPMENT	1. COBE 2991 cell separator 2. Heat sealer 3. 37°C shaker waterbath 4. −80°C freezer 5. Plasma extractor 6. Centrifuge with large-volume buckets
SUPPLIES AND REAGENTS	1. Three 500-mL bottles RPMI-1640 (Whittaker, Inc.) 2. Five 250-mL evacuated bottles (Abbott Laboratories) 3. 19-g × ⅝-inch butterfly infusion set (Abbott Laboratories) 4. Four 60-mL disposable syringes 5. 1 Unit AB-negative (or autologous) plasma 6. Twenty 16-g hypodermic needles 7. 5 sampling site couplers (Fenwal) 8. 5-mL vial of preservative-free, sodium injection, USP heparin (1000 U per mL) (Squibb-Marsam, Inc.) 9. Five 10-mL disposable syringes 10. 5 venting needles

11. 6 plasma transfer sets (Fenwal)
12. Two 600-mL plasma transfer packs with coupler (Fenwal)
13. Ten 600-mL plasma transfer packs with needle adaptor (Fenwal)
14. CharterMed 4403-2 freezing bag triplicate set (Charter Med, Inc.)
15. 5-mL vial VP-16, 20 mg per mL (Bristol Myers)
16. Three 2-g vials Ara-C (Upjohn)
17. 30-mL preservative-free sterile water (Whittaker, Inc)
18. 4- × 4-inch gauze sponges (Johnson and Johnson)

PROCEDURE

1. PREPARATION OF BOTTLES FOR WASHES/DILUTIONS
   A. Transfer of RPMI-1640 into five 250-mL evacuated bottles
      (1) Attach a 19-g × ⅞-inch butterfly infusion set to a 60-mL disposable syringe.
      (2) Remove the plunger from the syringe and discard.
      (3) Pour sterile RPMI-1640 directly into the open syringe. When the syringe is full, plunge the butterfly needle into a 250-mL evacuated bottle.
      (4) The bottle will begin to fill. As it does, replenish the supply of RPMI-1640 in the 60-mL syringe. Continue to add RPMI to the syringe until the volume in the bottle is approximately 250 mL.
      (5) Repeat this process until each of the five bottles is filled with approximately 250 mL RPMI.
   B. Addition of fresh frozen plasma
      (1) Obtain 1 U AB-negative fresh frozen plasma.
      (2) Using a 60-mL syringe, add 50 mL of plasma to four of the prepared bottles of RPMI, leaving one bottle without plasma. In lieu of the AB-negative plasma, autologous plasma can be used.
   C. Addition of heparin
      (1) Using a 10-mL syringe, add 1 mL of sodium injection, USP, preservative-free heparin (1000 U per mL) to each of the five bottles.
   D. The contents of the five prepared bottles should now be as follows:

   Bottle A: 250 mL RPMI + 50 mL plasma
                                  + 1 mL heparin → Initial dilution
   Bottle B: 250 mL RPMI + 50 mL plasma
                                  + 1 mL heparin → Initial dilution
   Bottle C: 250 mL RPMI + 50 mL plasma
                                  + 1 mL heparin → First wash
   Bottle D: 250 mL RPMI + 50 mL plasma
                                  + 1 mL heparin → Second wash
   Bottle E: 250 mL RPMI + 1 mL heparin → Final dilution

   E. Vent each bottle with a venting needle.
   F. Insert the spiked end of a Fenwal plasma transfer set into each bottle.
   G. Attach a 16-g needle to each needle adaptor of the plasma transfer sets.
   H. Keep the bottles on ice until ready for use.

2. INITIAL DILUTION OF THE BUFFY COAT
   A. Collect the buffy coat from the cell separator (volume approximately 150 mL) into a 600-mL plasma transfer bag. Once collected, seal the bag and insert a Fenwal sampling site coupler.

B. Insert the needle from bottle A into the sampling site coupler. Allow the RPMI/plasma to flow into the bag and dilute the collected buffy coat cells. Empty the entire bottle into the bag.

C. At this point, the volume in the buffy coat bag should be approximately 450 mL. Perform a cell count and remove one third of the total cells for cryopreservation *without treatment* using our DMSO/hydroxy-ethyl starch (HES) cryoprotectant, as described in Chapter 9. These cells will act as a reserve supply of marrow for the unusual possibility that the treated marrow fails to engraft.

D. Further dilute the remaining two thirds to a final volume of 550 mL (determined by weight) with bottle B.

3. PREPARATION OF DRUGS

A. Use a combination of two commercially available drugs (Ara-C and VP-16) for the bone marrow purging. The drugs should be reconstituted and diluted immediately before use.

(1) *VP-16:* Etoposide (Veepesid; Bristol Myers) is diluted to a total volume of 20 mL in RPMI-1640 at room temperature. Our current dose is 30 μg per mL or 0.9 mL of drug (20 mg per mL) in the 600-mL final volume.

(2) *Ara-C:* Cytosine arabinose (2-g vials; Upjohn) is diluted with pre-servative-free sterile water to give a final volume of 20 mL (10 mL each vial). If necessary, warm the vials to 37°C for 10 minutes to completely dissolve the drug.

B. Draw the drugs into syringes and inject into the plasma transfer bag containing the bone marrow. The volume in the bag should now be 600 mL.

C. Mix thoroughly.

4. TRANSFER INTO 37°C WATERBATH

A. Once the drugs have been added, split the marrow into two new 600-mL plasma transfer bags (300 mL each).

(1) The marrow can be drained through the sampling site coupler via a 600-mL transfer bag with needle adaptor. It can also be drained through the available port via a 600-mL transfer bag with spike coupler.

B. Seal off both bags and insert sampling site coupler into each. Place them into a shaking 37°C waterbath, and allow the cells and drugs to incubate for 1 hour. Mix thoroughly by hand at 15-minute intervals.

5. POST-TREATMENT WASHING

A. After 1 hour remove the bags from the shaking 37°C waterbath.

B. Firmly pack the bags (ports up) into large volume centrifuge buckets using 4- × 4-inch gauze pads as packing material.

C. Balance the buckets and centrifuge for 15 minutes at 2300 rpm (1035g) at 4°C with the *brake off*.

D. After centrifugation, carefully remove one bag without tipping and place it into a plasma extractor.

E. Slowly extract the plasma through the sampling site coupler via a 600-mL transfer pack with 16-gauge needle attached. Continue extracting until the cell layer is within 3 inches from the top of the bag. Remove the transfer line and discard plasma.

F. Remove the second bag from the centrifuge bucket and likewise extract the supernatant.

6. FIRST WASH
   A. One of the cell-containing transfer packs and bottle C are now added to the second cell-containing transfer pack as follows:
      (1) Empty bottle C into one of the bags containing cells via its sampling site coupler.
      (2) Mix this bag thoroughly and, in turn, empty it into the second cell-containing bag via a plasma transfer set with 16-gauge needle attached.
      (3) At this point, all the cells should be in a single plasma transfer pack suspended in bottle C media.
   B. Firmly pack the bag into a centrifuge bucket using 4- × 4-inch gauze pads. Counter balance with 600-mL plasma transfer packs filled with water and pack in a similar manner.
   C. Centrifuge for 15 minutes; 2300 rpm at 4°C; *brake off.*
   D. After centrifugation, carefully remove the bag and place it into a plasma extractor. Slowly remove plasma, as previously done in step 5E (via a 600-mL plasma transfer pack with 16-gauge needle attached).

7. SECOND WASH
   A. Empty bottle D into the cell-containing transfer pack via its sampling site coupler.
   B. Mix thoroughly.
   C. Firmly pack the bag into a centrifuge bucket and counter balance as in step 6B.
   D. Centrifuge for 15 minutes; 2300 rpm at 4°C; *brake off.*
   E. Carefully remove bag and extract plasma as in step 5E (via 600-mL transfer pack with 60-gauge needle attached).

8. FINAL DILUTION
   A. Dilute the treated cells to a final volume of 300 mL (determined by weight) with bottle E.
   B. The cells are now ready for cryopreservation using our DMSO-HES cyroprotectant as described in Chapter 9.

ANTICIPATED RESULTS	1. Overall cell yields after processing are in range of 80 to 85 percent.
	2. Colony-forming unit—granulocyte, macrophage (CFU-GM) and burst-forming unit—erythroid (BFU-E) assays are done before- and after-purge and for our current VP-16 and Ara-C doses (30 μg per mL and 10 mg per mL) total loss of CFU-GM/BFU-E is about 95 percent.
	3. Engraftment is delayed by about 7 days compared with unpurged transplants.
NOTES	1. A total dose of 4 to 6 × 10^8 cells per kg must be collected from the patient in the operating room, such that enough is available for cryopreservation of an untreated reserve supply.
	2. If another cryopreservation method is used, it would have to be evaluated in vitro before clinical use.

AUTHORS

David H. Oldenburg
Section of Hematology/Oncology
Loyola University Medical Center
Maywood, IL 60153

Patrick J. Stiff, M.D.
Section of Hematology/Oncology
Loyola University Medical Center
Maywood, IL 60153

REFERENCES

1. Stiff, PJ and Koester, AR: *In vitro* chemoseparation of leukemic cells from murine bone marrow using VP16-213: Importance of stem cell assays. Exp Hematol 15:263, 1987.
2. Stiff, PJ, Marks, L, and Dvorak, K: *Ex vivo* chemopurification of bone marrow using VP16 and cytosine arabinoside. Blood 70 (Suppl 1):324, 1987.

IMMUNOLOGIC

Monoclonal Antibodies with Complement

MANUAL AUTOLOGOUS BONE MARROW PURGING USING MONOCLONAL ANTIBODIES AND COMPLEMENT

DESCRIPTION	In autologous bone marrow transplantation, there is a possibility that clonogenic tumor cells could be present in the marrow graft. Upon reinfusion of this marrow into the patient, these cells could contribute to a relapse of the underlying malignancy. In an attempt to remove these cells, the marrow will be treated with a panel of monoclonal antibodies (MAb) and newborn rabbit complement prior to cryopreservation.
TIME FOR PROCEDURE	Approximately 4 hours from receiving buffy coat to freezing.
SUMMARY OF PROCEDURE	1. Mature granulocytes and red cells are removed first by Ficoll-Hypaque (Lymphoprep) procedure.
	2. Mononuclear cells (MNCs), adjusted to 2×10^7 per mL, are incubated with MAb(s) on ice for 30 minutes.
	3. DNAse and newborn rabbit complement are added and incubated at 37°C for 60 minutes.
	4. Cells are pelleted by centrifugation and incubation is repeated with MAb(s) and then complement.
	5. Cell pellet is resuspended in autologous plasma and frozen as usual.
EQUIPMENT	1. Ice bucket
	2. Centrifuge
	3. Waterbath
SUPPLIES AND REAGENTS	1. Mouse ascites (sources of monoclonal antibodies); purified and titered
	2. Newborn (3 to 4 weeks old) rabbit complement, sterile pooled
	3. DNAse I (add saline to resuspend to 5×10^4 U per mL)
	4. Lymphoprep, Ficoll-Sodium metrizoate, endotoxin-free, density 1.077
	5. 600-mL transfer packs
	6. 250-mL sterile centrifugation tubes
	7. Saline media:

- 1 mL penicillin, final 100 U per mL: 10^6 U per bottle, reconstituted with 10 mL saline, frozen in 1-mL aliquots, 10^5 units each
- 1 mL streptomycin sulfate, final 100 μg per mL: 1.0-g bottle reconstituted with 10 mL saline and frozen in 1-mL aliquots
- 1.5 mL sodium bicarbonate: 8.4 percent (1.0 mEq per mL) sodium bicarbonate aliquoted and frozen; final 1.5 mEq per L
- 4 mL human serum albumin (25 percent HSA): final 1 percent HSA

PROCEDURE

1. Check whether the patient is allergic to penicillin. Calculate the minimum number of nucleated cells required to be purged for this patient: 2×10^8 per kg.

2. Bone marrow buffy coat cells are adjusted to 400 mL with autologous plasma. Save 1 mL for polymerase chain reaction (PCR) or other appropriate assays and test as prepurge specimen.

3. Save autologous plasma for freezing: High-speed spin, then store clear plasma at 4°C.

4. Label 16 50-mL tubes. Dispense 25 mL of Lymphoprep into each tube.

5. Gently overlay marrow onto Lymphoprep at 45-degree angle.

6. Centrifuge at 17°C, 1300 rpm, for 30 minutes. No brake is used.

7. Suction off the supernatant slowly until approximately 10 mL supernatant is above the interface. Collect the interface with a 10-mL pipette into two 250-mL tubes for the first wash, each containing 100 mL saline media. Leave the pipette in a 15-mL tube. The drippings in the tube can be used for prepurge tissue culture.

8. Use a 60-mL syringe and 14-gauge cannula to resuspend cell pellets. Wash one more time in a 250-mL tube.

9. Resuspend cells to 100 mL and do a cell count. Calculate the total MNCs.

10. Calculate the incubation volume (V):

$$V = \frac{\text{Total MNCs}}{2 \times 10^7}$$

11. Adjust volume to (V − V/8) by adding (V − 100 − 2V/100 − V/8) mL saline media. Mark the tube at this level for the next cycle of incubation.

12. Check with the physician which MAbs are to be used according to patient's diagnosis. Add MAb(s) at proper dilution(s), incubate on ice for 30 minutes with occasional mixing.

13. Start thawing complement, bury in ice immediately after only a small icicle is left in the bottle. Prepare DNAse by adding saline to the vial.

14. At the end of 30 minutes, add DNAse and (V/8) mL complement. Incubate the tube at 37°C waterbath for 60 minutes with occasional mixing.

15. Pellet cells and save 2 mL supernatant to check MAb saturation.

16. Resuspend cells to the marked level (V − V/8) mL, and repeat MAb and complement incubations.

17. Resuspend cells in clear autologous plasma. Save 1 mL for cell count, differential, tissue culture, PCR, and sterility test.

18. Freeze as usual in two bags.

ANTICIPATED RESULTS

1. The recovery of MNCs should be at least 70 percent from the buffy coat at freezing stage.

2. The supernatant should demonstrate positive indirect immunofluorescence test results, indicating a saturation of MAb.

3. The tumor signal(s) should be absent in the postpurge PCR specimens.

4. The tissue culture (CFU-GM) results of prepurge and postpurge specimens are equivalent.

NOTE	The incubation (250-mL) tube is sealed with parafilm strip when put on ice or in the waterbath.

AUTHORS	Jean T. Yao, M.S., S.B.B.(ASCP) Blood Bank Methodist Medical Center 221 N.E. Glen Oak Ave. Peoria, IL 61636	Robert Negrin, M.D. Hematology Dept. Stanford University Hospital 300 Pasteur Dr. Stanford, CA 94035

AUTOMATED PURGING OF BONE MARROW USING MONOCLONAL ANTIBODIES AND COMPLEMENT

DESCRIPTION	Prior to transplantation of autologous bone marrow collected from patients with acute myelogenous leukemia (AML) it may be important to purge the marrow of residual leukemic cells. This method uses monoclonal antibodies and complement to purge the marrow before freezing. The automated procedure uses the Haemonetics V-50 cell processor and employs a closed system to ensure end-product sterility. The final end product is also free of granulocytic contamination.
TIME FOR PROCEDURE	Approximately 2 to 3 hours for each treatment done, depending on the starting cell number available
SUMMARY OF PROCEDURE	1. Mononuclear cells purified by Haemonetics V-50 cell processor are washed and counted.
	2. Cell mixture is transferred to 600-mL transfer pack. Monoclonal antibodies (at predetermined amounts) are added and incubated for 15 minutes at room temperature with continuous mixing.
	3. The cell wash and separation set is loaded into the Haemonetic V-50, and the necessary software modifications are made.
	4. The machine is programmed, and the cell-antibody mixture is added to the centrifuge bowl.
	5. The complement (C′) solutions are added to the cell mixture over 60 minutes.
	6. The treated mononuclear cells are transferred to a transfer pack. This final product is washed and cryopreserved.
EQUIPMENT	1. Haemonetics V-50 Cell Processor, Haemonetics Corporation
	2. Sterile Connecting Device, Haemonetics Corporation
	3. Hematron Dielectric Sealer, Fenwal (4R4330)
	4. Gambro WD2 Welding Device, Scientific, Inc.
	5. Rate Control Freezer, Kryo 10 Series (Planer Biomed)
SUPPLIES AND REAGENTS	1. Haemonetics cell wash and separation set (List 301)
	2. 300-mL transfer pack
	3. Two 600-mL transfer packs
	4. Two 150-mL transfer packs
	5. Custom pack obtained from Haemonetics (sterile anticoagulant line from Haemonetics apheresis set, List 603)
	6. Large apheresis bowl (List 5811)
	7. Cell harvest bowls
	8. Sampling site couplers
	9. Gambro haemofreeze bags (Gambro DF200-2)
	10. 250-mL conical tubes (Corning 25350)
	11. Rabbit complement (Pel-Freeze)

12. Dimethyl sulfoxide (DMSO), Cryoserv

13. Deoxyribonuclease I (DNAse), Sigma D4513

14. Human serum albumin (5 percent), Baxter

15. Monoclonal antibodies: PM-81 (CD15) and AML-2-23 (CD14), Medarex

PROCEDURE

1. INSTALLATION OF APHERESIS SET
   A. Using aseptic technique, attach either a cell harvest bowl, or a large apheresis bowl to the cell wash and separation set (List 301). The size of the bowl used is determined by the number of cells being treated.
   B. Over-ride the donor safety features of the V-50 by placing a water-filled drip chamber in the air detector and by taping down the monitor box.
   C. If the cell harvest bowl is being used, the V-50 must be modified so that the pediatric adapter (containing the bowl) can be placed in the centrifuge well.
   D. Using the sterile connecting device, remove the drip chamber from the custom pack line. Also, use the sterile connecting device to attach a 300-mL transfer pack to the line at valve 2 and a 600-mL transfer pack to the reinfusion line (see Fig. 8–5 for the proper attachment of these transfer bags). Place a clamp on the line leading to the 600-mL transfer pack.
   E. Load the modified software into the V-50, using standard procedures.
   F. Using the sterile connecting device, attach the cells to be treated to the apheresis set, as shown in Figure 8–5. Clamp the line until ready for use.

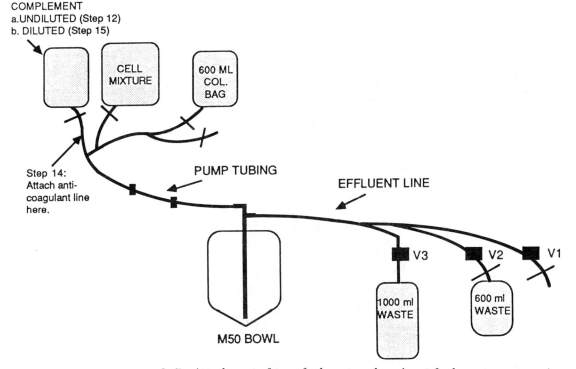

FIGURE 8–5 Attachment of transfer bags to apheresis set for bone marrow purging using the Haemonetics V-50. (From Dartmouth Hitchcock Medical Center.)

G. Using the sterile connecting device, attach the modified custom pack (anticoagulant) line to the apheresis set, as shown in Figure 8–5; clamp until ready for use.

2. PROGRAMMING
   A. The display now reads "SELECT PROTOCOL." Press COMP to select a component collection.
   B. Press NO at the "PLATELETS? Y/N" prompt.
   C. Press NO at the "PLTS/PLASMA? Y/N" prompt.
   D. Press NO at the "PLTS/GRAN? Y/N" prompt.
   E. Press NO at the "GRANULOCY? Y/N" prompt.
   F. Press NO at the "LYMPHOCY? Y/N" prompt.
   G. Press ENTER at the "MANUAL COMPONENT" prompt.
   H. At the "SET RBC VOLUME" prompt, press 999, then ENTER.
   I. At the "NO. OF CYCLES" prompt, press 99, then ENTER.
   J. The V-50 now displays "READY MANUAL 999 M."

3. PURGING
   A. Mononuclear cell fraction: Mononuclear cells are isolated by Ficoll-Hypaque density gradient centrifugation from a buffy coat fraction on the Haemonetics V-50. During the processing autologous plasma is isolated, which is then irradiated and added to the freezing medium just before cryopreservation.
      (1) Wash cells in RPMI-1640 containing 10 U per mL heparin (preservative-free) and centrifuge at 1500 rpm at room temperature.
      (2) Count cells and transfer to 600-mL transfer pack containing 0.5 percent human serum albumin and 10 U per mL DNAse.
   B. Monoclonal antibody treatment: The maximum number of cells to be treated in a small or large bowl is 2.5×10^9 and 3.75×10^9, respectively. Depending on the cell number, either one or more treatments are performed. For example, if 5×10^9 cells are to be treated then the cell mixture is divided and two treatments (2.5×10^9 cells each) are performed consecutively using the same small bowl. If two machines are available then the treatments could be run simultaneously.
      (1) Add monoclonal antibodies at 10 U per 10^6 cells (based on quality control results).
      (2) Incubate the suspension at room temperature for 15 minutes with continuous gentle mixing on a mechanical platform.
      (3) Load cells into the Haemonetics V-50 centrifuge bowl at a rate of 40 mL per minute.
   C. Complement treatment
      (1) When the cells have been completely added to the bowl, use the sterile connecting device to attach the bag of undiluted complement to the line where the cells were attached.
      (2) Add the undiluted complement (42 mL for a small bowl and 60 mL for a large one to achieve a 1:6 dilution based on quality control results) to the bowl at a rate of 40 mL per minute.

         NOTE: *Once fluid is seen in the effluent line, open valve 2 and close valve 3. This diverts the spent complement from the air-plasma bag (where it would be mixed with the treated cells when the bowl is emptied) to the waste collection bag.*

(3) Once all the complement has entered the bowl, press STOP and set two timers, one for 10 minutes and one for 60 minutes.

(4) Using the sterile connecting device attach the bag of diluted complement (17 mL C′ in 83 mL RPMI-1640) to the anticoagulant (custom pack) line; place the line in the pump tubing. Keep the bag of complement, and as much tubing as possible, on ice during the remaining 50 minutes of complement infusion.

(5) When the 10-minute timer rings, start the centrifuge and allow it to run for approximately 2 to 3 minutes to separate the cells from the liquid portion of the mixture.

(6) Add the complement to the bowl at 40 mL per minute; when the complement begins to enter the bowl, decrease the pump speed to 20 mL per minute. This corresponds to a flow rate of approximately 2 mL per minute.

(7) Continue adding the complement until the second timer rings, at which time all the complement should have been added to the bowl. Check the volume of complement remaining when there are 15 minutes left on the treatment; if necessary the pump speed can be increased to allow all the complement to be added to the bowl before the 50 minutes are up. If all the complement is in prior to the completion of the treatment, keep the bowl spinning until 50 minutes have elapsed.

(8) At the end of the treatment press RETURN and collect the treated cells in the 600-mL collection bag.

(9) Remove the bag from the apheresis set, determine the total volume and remove a sample for white count and differential.

D. Marrow freeze down

(1) Wash cells in cold RPMI-1640 after complement treatment.

(2) Apply a sampling site coupler to the port near the top of the freezing bag.

(3) Add 30-mL or less to each bag at a concentration of 30 to 60 × 10^6 cells per mL.

(4) Cool down the mixture to 0 to 4°C and add an equal volume of freezing medium (20 percent DMSO plus 40 percent autologous plasma in RPMI). Do not allow marrow cells to be exposed to DMSO at temperatures greater than the freezing point any longer than absolutely necessary.

(5) Remove large air bubbles from the bag by aspirating with a 16-gauge needle attached to a 60-mL syringe.

(6) Place the bags in freezing envelopes to flatten the cell suspension to a thin layer.

(7) Place bags in a precooled (4°C) controlled-rate freezer. The temperature is dropped at a rate of 2°C per minute until −60°C.

(8) Remove freezing envelopes, transfer bags to holding racks and place in liquid nitrogen.

ANTICIPATED RESULTS

1. All of the cells after treatment should be mononuclear cells.

2. The expected percent recovery after purging ranges from 50 to 80 percent of the number of cells treated.

NOTES	1. If a large bowl is used it is necessary to add 30 mL of packed irradiated red blood cells to the cell-antibody mixture prior to adding to the bowl. If this is not done the mononuclear cells will be trapped in the groove at the bottom of the bowl.
	2. If more than one treatment is being done (because of large cell number) the same setup can be used for each one, but a new collection bag for the treated cells must be added each time. If multiple treatments are being done using a large bowl, the additional cells need to be added only to the first treatment.
	3. Only the anticoagulant pump is used.
	4. Ensure that the proper clamps are open or closed prior to the start of each phase.

AUTHORS

Lamia M. Schwarz, B.S.
Dartmouth-Hitchcock Medical
  Center
Hanover, NH 03756

Miriam F. Leach, M.T.(ASCP),
  S.B.B.
Dartmouth-Hitchcock Medical
  Center
Hanover, NH 03756

Alix L. Howell, Ph.D.
Dartmouth-Hitchcock Medical
  Center
Hanover, NH 03756

Edward D. Ball, M.D.
University of Pittsburgh
Pittsburgh Cancer Institute
Pittsburgh, PA 15213

REFERENCES

1. Ball, ED, et al: Autologous bone marrow transplantation for acute myeloid leukemia using monoclonal antibody-purged bone marrow. Blood 75:1199, 1990.
2. Howell, AL, et al: Continuous infusion of complement by an automated cell processor enhances cytotoxicity of monoclonal antibody sensitized leukemia cells. Bone Marrow Transplant 4:317, 1989.

Immunomagnetic Purging of Neuroblastoma Cells from Autologous Bone Marrow

DESCRIPTION	The propensity of neuroblastoma to metastasize to the marrow, combined with the limited ability to detect marrow infiltration, has resulted in the development of a variety of methods for purging in this disease. The most widely used approach has been that of immunomagnetic cell removal, in which the target neuroblasts are identified using a panel of tumor-directed mouse-derived monoclonal antibodies and then are mixed with antimouse immunoglobulin (IgG)–coated paramagnetic microspheres, which will selectively bind to the neuroblasts. The bead-coated tumor cells, together with any unbound microspheres, can then be separated by passage of the marrow through a magnetic field. This technique was originally described by Treleaven and associates.[1] The following modification has been used at the University of Florida to purge more than 100 marrows.

TIME FOR PROCEDURE	Approximately 3 to 4 hours from receipt of nucleated cell population to initiation of cryopreservation

SUMMARY OF PROCEDURE	1. Harvested bone marrow is received in the laboratory, and a nucleated cell population is prepared by (a) erythrocyte sedimentation, (b) Ficoll-Hypaque density cushion centrifugation, or (c) buffy coat isolation. All methods have been used successfully; however, (a) is used routinely.
	2. The nucleated cells are incubated at 4°C with a panel of five monoclonal antineuroblastoma antibodies and washed extensively to remove unbound antibody.
	3. Paramagnetic microspheres coated with sheep antimouse IgG are incubated with the marrow at 4°C with gentle mixing.
	4. The mixture of beads and marrow is passed through a sterile chamber placed in a magnetic field generated by an array of permanent magnets.
	5. The treated marrow is cryopreserved for subsequent transplantation.

EQUIPMENT	1. Erytrenn plasma separator (used for nucleated cell enrichment) (Biotest)
	2. Refrigerated (4°C) centrifuge (Sorval RT6000 or equivalent)
	3. Magnetic separation chamber, including peristaltic pump and permanent magnet array
	4. Magnetic separator for bead washing (MPC-1, Dynal, Inc)
	5. End-over-end rotator, variable speed (Rototorque, Cole Parmer Instrument)
	6. Plasma extractor (Fenwal 4R4414, Baxter Healthcare)

SUPPLIES AND REAGENTS	1. Medium-199 (special order) with Earle's salts and L-glutamine, without phenol red (Gibco BRL Life Technologies)
	2. Hespan, 6 percent Hetastarch in 0.9 percent sodium chloride injection (du Pont Pharmaceuticals)
	3. 0.9 percent sodium chloride, injection USP (Baxter 2B1323, Baxter Healthcare)

4. Plasma protein fraction, 5 percent solution, heat treated (NDC 0053 775301, Armour Pharmaceutical)

5. Dynabeads M450 coated with sheep antimouse IgG (Dynal)

6. Antineuroblastoma antibodies (Provided courtesy of Dr. John Kemshead, Paediatric and NeuroOncology Laboratory, Imperial Cancer Research Fund, Frenchay, Bristol, England. A panel of five reagents is used: 5.1.H11, UJ127.11, Thy-1, M340, and UJ13A)

7. Sterile syringes: 60-mL (10 to 20); 10-mL (1); and 5-mL (3 to 4)

8. Sterile hypodermic needles: 16-gauge × 1 inch

9. Sterile serologic pipettes: 25-mL (20 to 25); 10-mL (10)

10. 2 portable Pipet-Aid pipette pumps with tissue culture nosepiece (Drummond Scientific)

11. Sterile polypropylene centrifuge tubes, conical bottom: 50-mL (2 to 7) No. 62-547-004; 15-mL (2 to 4) No. 62-554-002 (Sarstedt)

12. Transfer packs: 600-mL (3 to 8) No. 4R2023; 300-mL (10 to 20) No. 4R-2014; Plasma transfer sets: 6 to 10 No. 4C2240; 2 No. 4C2243; and 2 No. 4C2244 (Fenwal Division, Baxter Healthcare)

13. Sampling Site Couplers: 10 to 15 No. 4C2405 (Fenwal Division, Baxter Healthcare)

14. Sterile filter, 0.2-μm pore size Acrodisc (No. 4191, Gelman Industries)

15. Sterile Pasteur pipettes

16. Line stripper/sealer (No. H5508; clips, No. H5C119; Medicore)

17. Alcohol swabs

18. Ice baths

PROCEDURE

The following procedure was developed for the treatment of pediatric volumes of bone marrow (200 to 750 mL). The nucleated cell separation procedure that is described was therefore performed manually. For larger volumes, automated separation methods can be used, as described in Chapter 6.

1. DAY PRIOR TO PURGE
   A. Assemble two purging chambers in separate trays, and autoclave.
   B. Aseptically transfer 180 mL medium-199 into two 300-mL transfer packs and refrigerate.
   C. Label the following with the patient's name and hospital number:
      (1) Three 600-mL transfer packs with the lines sealed off with clips
      NOTE: *This is to be used for the nucleated cell separation.*
      (2) 600-mL transfer pack with lines *not* sealed off
      NOTE: *This is to be used as reservoir for marrow cells and beads.*
      (3) 4 300-mL transfer packs with lines sealed off with clips
      NOTE: *This is to be used for collection of nucleated cells after erythrocyte sedimentation.*
      (4) 4 freezing packs (e.g., Cryocyte containers [Baxter])
      (5) 8 marrow sampling tubes for colony-forming units, and other tests, as required (e.g., Sarstedt 2-mL cryopreservation tubes)
      (6) 2 sets blood culture tubes (for sterility testing)
   D. Clean and disinfect laminar flow hoods and centrifuges.

2. DAY OF PURGE PROCEDURE—BEFORE ARRIVAL OF MARROW: *All procedures are performed using aseptic technique in a laminar flow safety cabinet.*
    A. Place the following in the laminar flow hood:
        (1) 500-mL bag sterile saline
        (2) 500-mL pack of Hespan
        (3) Aliquots of medium-199 previously prepared
        (4) 250-mL bottle plasma protein fraction (PPF)
        (5) Two 500-mL bottles of medium-199
        (6) 70-mL bottle dimethyl sulfoxide (DMSO) (Cryoserve)
        (7) Syringes: twenty 60-mL and one 10-mL
        (8) 16-gauge needles
        (9) Tube sealer
    B. Prepare four 50-mL syringes of Hespan; label and set aside.
    C. Supplement each 500-mL bottle of medium-199 with 55 mL plasma protein fraction, mix, and aliquot 200 mL into each of five sterile containers (e.g., tissue culture flasks) for cell washing. Label "medium-199/PPF" and refrigerate.
    D. To one 180-mL bag of medium-199 (prepared previously), add 20 mL plasma protein fraction. Label and set aside.

        NOTE: *This will be used to prime the magnetic separation chamber.*

    E. Using a sampling site coupler and syringe, to one 180-mL pack of medium-199 add 50 mL DMSO slowly with mixing. Allow the mixture to cool and add 50 mL plasma protein fraction while mixing. Remove 30 mL in a syringe for the "dummy" freezing bag. Aliquot the remainder as follows:
        (1) 30 mL into four 60-mL syringes
        (2) 10 mL into a 10-mL syringe
        (3) 5 mL into a 5-mL syringe
        (4) 1 mL into a 3-mL syringe

        NOTE: *These can be used to provide an exact volume of freezing medium equivalent to the processed marrow volume.*

    F. Prepare the dummy freezing bag for the programmable freezer. Add 30 mL of the freezing medium prepared in step E to 30 mL of the medium-199/PPF prepared in step D. Label and refrigerate.

3. DAY OF PURGE PROCEDURE—UPON ARRIVAL OF MARROW
    A. Check label on marrow pack for patient's name, birth date, hospital number, date, and time of collection, as well as any other appropriate information. Gently mix marrow by inversion. If the marrow contains a large amount of fat, an inverted spin may be required prior to further manipulation (see Chapter 6).
    B. Determine marrow volume by weight, and divide marrow equally in 100- to 250-mL aliquots into 600-mL transfer packs. Attach a presealed 300-mL transfer pack to the center port of the 600-mL pack (used to harvest the nucleated cells) and a sampling site coupler to the outer port (used to add the Hespan).

        Transfer of the marrow can be achieved most easily by connecting the marrow pack to the empty 600-mL transfer pack via a three-way stopcock with attached 60-mL syringe. *Retain a 6-mL sample for sterility testing, as in step E.*

C. Multiply the volume of marrow in milliliters in the aliquot by 0.2 to obtain the volume of Hespan in milliliters that should be added to the pack. Add the appropriate volume of Hespan from the previously prepared syringes, using a sampling site coupler. Mix gently, and hang the pack, sampling ports downward, in the Erytrenn apparatus. Additional packs can be hung temporarily in the Fenwal plasma extractor.

D. Incubate the packs for 30 minutes at ambient temperature.

E. Aliquot the 6-mL marrow sample for prepurge testing as follows:
   (1) 1 mL for sterility testing (twice)
   (2) 2.5 mL for immunofluorescent detection of tumor cells
   (3) 1 mL for colony forming assays
   (4) 0.25 mL for total nucleated cell counts

F. Remove antineuroblastoma antibodies from $-70°C$ freezer and thaw.

G. Collect supernatant cell fraction from marrow using the Erytrenn device. The bag should be clamped off approximately 1 cm below the red blood cell/supernatant interface, rotated, and the supernatant collected into the attached 300-mL transfer pack after removal of the sealing clip. The line should be stripped and resealed. Refrigerate the harvested cells until all the packs have been harvested.

   In the case of marrows with a low nucleated cell count but a high hematocrit, it may be advisable to repeat the Hespan sedimentation step to increase the cell yield. This is accomplished by replacing the volume of supernatant removed from the sedimented red cells, with an equal volume of sterile saline, and readding Hespan to the mixture.

H. Centrifuge the nucleated cell packs at $600g$ for 10 minutes at 4°C. Hang the packs in the Fenwal plasma extractor and attach a plasma transfer set to the center port (roller clamp closed), and a 300-mL transfer pack to the side port. Use the extractor to express the supernatant medium from the cell pack into the attached 300-mL bag.

   Once the supernatant is removed, collect the cells, using the center line, into 50-mL centrifuge tubes. Residual cells can be flushed from the bag using 10 to 20 mL of the supernatant medium that was collected into the attached 300-mL pack. Each pack should be flushed twice.

I. Fill each centrifuge tube to the 45 or 50-mL mark with medium-199/PPF and centrifuge at $600g$ for 10 minutes at 4°C. Aspirate and discard the supernatants, and pool the cells to a single tube. Bring the volume to 45 to 50 mL with medium-199/PPF and repeat the centrifugation.

J. The final packed cell volume should be 10 to 25 mL. If less than 10 mL the volume can be increased by the addition of *washed* red cells remaining from the Hespan sedimentation step.

K. The antineuroblastoma monoclonal antibodies are mixed and filtered through a 0.2-μm pore sterilizing filter. For purging of an average volume (200 to 750 mL) pediatric marrow, Dr. Kemshead has recommended the following amounts of each antibody:
   (1) 0.5 mg each of UJ13A and 5.1.H11
   (2) 1.0 mg each of Thy-1, UJ127.11, and M340
   These concentrations are in excess of those required to sensitize all neuroblastoma cells in an overtly infiltrated pediatric marrow, while allowing a comfortable safety margin. It is recommended that marrows

that are contaminated with more than about 2 percent neuroblasts should not be purged without substantial changes to the procedure.

L. Add the sterile antibody mixture in a volume not to exceed the packed cell volume. Mix the cells by gentle swirling, and incubate on ice for 30 minutes, mixing every 5 minutes.

M. The number of beads that should be added to the marrow should be in the range of 40 to 75 beads per *tumor* cell. Assuming that marrows are harvested in remission, and that a 2 percent infiltration of neuroblasts can be readily detected, sufficient beads should be added to achieve the desired bead to neuroblastoma cell ratio, based on an assumed 2 percent infiltration. The following formula can be used:

Required number of beads = Total number nucleated cells
$\times$ 0.02 $\times$ required bead-to-neuroblastoma cell ratio

The beads are supplied at a concentration of approximately 4×10^8 per mL; this should be checked for each bottle by counting a well-mixed aliquot withdrawn aseptically.

Because the beads are supplied in buffer containing a preservative, they must be washed before use. The required volume should be withdrawn aseptically into a 50- or 15-mL centrifuge tube, and the beads collected by exposure to the MPC-1 magnetic separator for at least 3 minutes. The supernatant is aspirated and discarded and the pellet resuspended in 10 mL medium-199/PPF.

The collection and washing procedures are repeated until the beads have been washed with at least 4×10 mL medium-199/PPF. The final bead pellet should be resuspended in 5 mL of that buffer, and kept on ice until required.

N. Following incubation of the marrow and antibodies, bring the volume in each tube to 45 to 50 mL with medium-199/PPF and pellet the cells by centrifugation at 600g for 10 minutes at 4°C (for optimal washing it is preferable to split the marrow at this stage into two aliquots in 50-mL tubes). This procedure is repeated until the cells have been washed with at least 4×40 mL buffer. The final volume in each tube is adjusted to 40 mL.

O. Divide the bead suspension between the two tubes containing the marrow cells. The tubes are capped tightly and the tops secured with Parafilm. To minimize ingestion of beads by phagocytic cells, the marrow is chilled by placing the tubes in a plastic pouch containing crushed ice. This pouch is placed on the end-over-end rotator and gently mixed (2 to 4 rpm) for at least 30 minutes at 4°C.

P. During the incubation procedure the marrow separation chamber is assembled and primed. The second chamber is retained as a backup.

NOTE: *The magnetic separation apparatus is produced at the University of Florida, and investigators who wish to use the system are required to be trained. Detailed instructions on assembly have not therefore been provided, as they would be confusing in the absence of the apparatus. The design of the system has been described previously in detail, and is shown diagrammatically in Figure 8–6. Other magnetic separation systems have been commercially produced by Baxter Healthcare Corporation and Dynal, Inc., for in vitro research applica-*

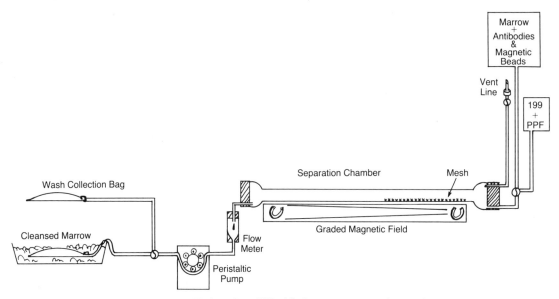

FIGURE 8–6   University of Florida immunomagnetic purging system.

tions. Briefly, the Florida system consists of a low-ceilinged Lexan chamber of rectangular cross-section that is placed in contact with a series of samarium-cobalt permanent magnets. Upstream from the chamber are three lines, one of which is an air vent (to permit easy draining of the system); the second of which is connected to a transfer pack containing medium-199/PPF, for priming the system; and the third of which is connected to the transfer pack containing the bone marrow and beads.

Downstream there is a small in-line flow meter, a peristaltic pump to draw the marrow through the system, and a transfer pack on ice for collection of the purged sample. Prior to connection of the marrow pack, the entire system is primed with medium-199/PPF, taking care to remove any air bubbles.

Q. Following incubation, remove the marrow from the ice pouch and dry the tubes thoroughly. The cells are then transferred to a 600-mL transfer pack. Care must be taken at this stage not to disrupt bead/tumor cell complexes. For this reason, transfer is achieved by pouring the marrow from the tubes into the barrel of a 60-mL syringe that is connected, via a female luer connector, to the transfer pack (i.e., without the use of a hypodermic needle). The tubes are each rinsed with 5 mL medium-199/PPF, the washings pooled to the transfer pack, and the line stripped and sealed.

R. Place the transfer pack containing the marrow in an insulated box containing cold packs; this helps to maintain a stable temperature during processing. The pack is then connected to the separation chamber, and the peristaltic pump started. A flow rate of 1.5 mL per minute is routinely used.

In the case of large volumes of marrow (i.e., more than 750 mL at harvest) when more than 200 mg beads are used, it may be necessary to debulk the marrow of some of the beads before running it through the chamber. This avoids any possible blocking of the main separation chamber and can be achieved by placing the marrow pack in contact with a sheet magnet before turning on the pump. In either case, the bulk of the separation in the main chamber occurs as the marrow passes over the first three magnets. Cells and beads will be seen accumulating in this area.

S. Once the marrow has been processed through the chamber, stop the pump, and strip and seal the line to the collection pack. Although the chamber could be drained of marrow by using the vent line to admit air, it is preferable to flush the cells from the chamber by running fluid from the priming pack (connected at the input) through the system. This prevents the formation of an air-fluid interface at the magnet surface, which could shear beads from the magnets. This step increases the volume of the marrow, but the volume can be reduced, if required, by centrifugation prior to freezing.

The processed marrow is aliquoted, via a sampling site coupler and syringes, into 30- to 40-mL aliquots in prelabeled freezing bags. *A 4- to 6-mL sample is also taken for postpurge testing, as described previously.*

Add an equal volume of freezing medium (prepared previously) to the bags with mixing, and freeze the marrow according to the protocol in use at the institution.

ANTICIPATED RESULTS	1. Immunomagnetic purging for neuroblastoma routinely gives a 50 to 70 percent recovery of the original nucleated cell count, with excellent retention of colony-forming unit–granulocyte, macrophage (CFU-GM). Cell viabilities, by dye exclusion, are 95 to 100 percent. The treated marrow is capable of producing full hematopoietic reconstitution with a mean engraftment time of approximately 40 days.
	2. Although it is difficult to quantitate purging efficiency in the clinical situation, this method has been shown to be capable of depleting 3 to 5 logs of neuroblastoma cells in model experiments. Routine examination of postpurge marrow using indirect immunofluorescence has demonstrated effective removal of up to an 11 percent infiltration to the limits of detection of the assay.
NOTES	1. Although immunomagnetic purging is now a widely used technique, it requires careful optimization of treatment conditions. These depend on the antibodies selected, cell numbers and concentrations, flow rates, and so on. For this reason, the method described earlier should be regarded as an outline only, and not a standard operating procedure.
	2. Any center contemplating using this approach is strongly cautioned to determine optimal conditions in its own laboratory. All clinical procedures are required to have been preapproved by the United States Food and Drug Administration.

AUTHORS

Adrian P. Gee, Ph.D.
Adjunct Associate Professor
Dept. of Pediatrics
University of Florida
Gainesville, FL 32610

and
Senior Scientist
Baxter Healthcare Corp.
3015 S. Daimler
Santa Ana, CA 92705

Samuel Gross, M.D.
Professor and Chief
Pediatric Hematology/Oncology
Bone Marrow Transplant Unit
University of Florida
Gainesville, FL 32610

John Graham Pole, M.D.
Professor and Associate Chief
Pediatric Hematology/Oncology
Bone Marrow Transplant Unit
University of Florida
Gainesville, FL 32610

Carlos E. Lee, M.T.
Bone Marrow Processing and
   Evaluation Laboratory
Bone Marrow Transplant Program
H. Lee Moffitt Cancer Center and
   Research Institute
University of South Florida
Tampa, FL

REFERENCES

1. Treleaven, J, et al: Removal of neuroblastoma cells from bone marrow with monoclonal antibodies conjugated to magnetic microspheres. Lancet 1:70, 1984.
2. Gee, AP, et al: Immunomagnetic purging and autologous transplantation in Stage D neuroblastoma. Bone Marrow Transplant 2(Suppl 2):89, 1987.
3. Freeman, RB: Method and apparatus for removal of cells from bone marrow, U.S. Patent No. 4,904,391. 1990.

COMBINATION PURGING

IMMUNOPHARMACOLOGIC PURGING OF MYELOMA CELLS

DESCRIPTION	The method for purging myeloma cells from bone marrow by using monoclonal antibodies and magnetic immunobeads is a sensitive and reproducible approach. However, its efficacy depends on the antigenic characteristics of myeloma cells such as the heterogeneity of surface antigen expression of myeloma cells and their progenitors. Therefore, the immunologic method alone might be insufficient to eliminate all clonogenic myeloma cells from bone marrow. While a number of nonimmunologic methods such as cytotoxic drugs, photoradiation, and hyperthermia are thought to be effective for purging contaminating tumor cells, combined methods using both immunoseparation and chemoseparation have been reported to be superior to either method alone. In this section, the immunopharmacologic method for purging myeloma cells from bone marrow is described.
TIME FOR PROCEDURE	Approximately 5 hours to process samples
SUMMARY OF PROCEDURE	1. Bone marrow mononuclear cells are incubated with 4-hydroperoxycyclophosphamide (4-HC).
	2. Bone marrow cells are then incubated with monoclonal antibodies.
	3. After washing, bone marrow cells are mixed with magnetic polystyrene beads coated with sheep antimouse IgG.
	4. Bead-cell complexes are removed by exposing the bone marrow suspension to the magnetic field.
	5. Purified bone marrow cells are mixed with cryoprotectant and stored in liquid nitrogen.
EQUIPMENT	1. Magnetic particle concentrator (MPC-BMP, No. 120.03) (Dynal A.S., Oslo, Norway)
	2. Standard variable speed peristaltic pump for flow rate 42 mL per minute (Masterflex PA-71)
	3. Multiplane tilting device (Heidroph 541 31 REAX 3)
	4. Plasma extractor (Terumo ACS-201)
	5. Blood bag heat sealer (Union Carbide)
	6. Plasma tube stripper (Delmed No. N5070 or equivalent)
	7. Centrifuge (Kubota Model 9810 or equivalent)
	8. Deep freezer ($-120°C$) or liquid nitrogen freezer
SUPPLIES AND REAGENTS	1. 4-HC (Shionogi and Co., Osaka, Japan)
	2. Monoclonal antibodies: PCA-1 (Coulter Immunology, Hialeah, FL), J-5 (CD10) (Coulter Immunology, Hialeah, FL), BL-3 (United Biomedical, Inc., Lake Success, NY)
	3. Dynabeads M-450 coated with sheep antimouse IgG-BMP (No. 310.02) Dynal A.S., Oslo, Norway

4. Cell culture medium (RPMI-1640)
5. Human serum albumin
6. Phosphate buffered saline
7. Blood bags: 150-, 600-, 2000-mL (Fenwal Nos. 4R2001, 4R2014, 4R4021)
8. Plasma transfer set (Travenol C2243)
9. Sterile, nonpyrogenic filter (Japan Millipore Ltd., Millex-GV, 0.22 μm)
10. Delmed blood freezing bag (style 20302)
11. Syringes: 3-, 5-, 10-, 20-, and 50-mL
12. Needles: 18- and 15-gauge
13. Sampling site couplers (Fenwal 4C2405)
14. Dimethyl sulfoxide (DMSO)
15. Hydroxyethyl starch (HES)

PROCEDURE

1. PURGING WITH 4-HC
   A. Obtain bone marrow buffy coat cells after removal of red blood cells by using HES or equivalent method (Chapter 6).
   B. Make cell suspension at a concentration of 20×10^6 cells per mL by adding medium. Check the volume of the blood bag.
   C. Dilute 4-HC with warmed phosphate buffered saline at the concentration of 400 μM, filtered in advance.
   D. Pour 4-HC solution (400 μM) at 1 volume to 9 volumes of cell suspension into the blood bag using a syringe (final concentration of 4-HC is 40 μM).
   E. Incubate cells at 37°C for 1 hour in the waterbath. Mix cells well every 15 minutes.
   F. After incubation, transfer cells into two to three 600-mL blood bags. Fill each blood bag with medium, followed by centrifugation ($200g$ for 10 minutes at 4°C).
   G. Place the bag on the plasma extractor.
   H. Express supernatant carefully so as not to lose cells. Then carefully express top layer of red blood cell buffy coat into 600-mL blood bag.
   I. Suspend the cells in medium at a concentration of approximately 50×10^6 cells per mL.

2. PURGING WITH MONOCLONAL ANTIBODIES AND MAGNETIC IMMUNOBEADS
   A. Cool the cell suspension on ice for 5 minutes.
   B. Add monoclonal antibodies: PCA-1, BL-3, and J-5 (5 μg of each per 10^6 cells).
   C. Incubate cells in a cold room at 4°C for 30 minutes with gentle tilt on the tilting device.
   D. Remove excess antibody by filling the bag with medium, followed by centrifugation ($200g$ for 10 minutes at 4°C). Remove supernatant and add new cold medium. Repeat the same procedure once.
   E. Suspend cells in cold medium at a concentration of 30×10^6 cells per mL. Maximum volume used in the bag is 350 mL (bag 4a) (Fig. 8–7).
   F. Wash desired number of magnetic beads (approximately 50 beads per target cell) three times with medium to remove sodium azide, resuspend in 20 mL of medium, aspirate into a syringe, and keep on ice.

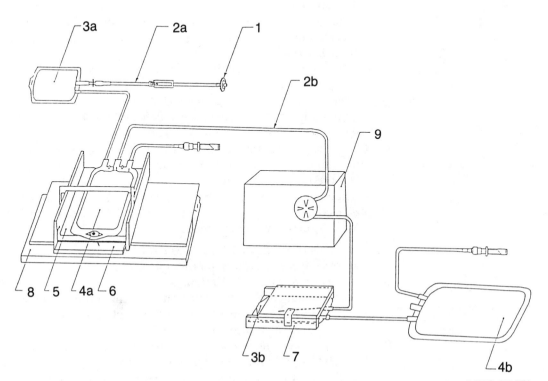

FIGURE 8–7   Dynal magnetic particle concentrator; bone marrow purging (MPC-BMP) and accessories. *1*, Sterile (0.2 μm) filter; *2a,b,* plasma transfer set; *3a,b,* 150-mL blood bags; *4a,b,* 600-mL blood bags; *5,* magnetic cassette; *6,* removable aluminum plate; *7,* magnetic filter; *8,* multiplane tilting device; *9,* peristaltic pump.

G. Insert the magnetic beads into blood bag 4a containing cell suspension and monoclonal antibodies as previously prepared.

H. Fasten blood bag 4a in the precooled cassette with the aluminum plate inserted and place on the tilting platform.

I. Put the plastic cover above blood bag 4a in the cassette to ensure even distribution of liquid.

J. Fix the 150-mL blood bag (3b) in the magnetic filter (7). Make sure that the cover is securely locked in place.

K. Incubate cells at 4°C for 30 minutes with gentle tilting.

L. Remove the aluminum plate and stop the tilting.

M. Lower the platform in stages with handle, taking 5 minutes each for stages 1 and 2, and 3 minutes each for stages 3 and 4.

N. Thereafter, immediately start the peristaltic pump (flow rate 42 mL per minute) and transfer the bone marrow suspension out of the blood bag, through the magnetic filter and into a new 600-mL Fenwal bag (4b).

O. Insert the aluminum plate into the cassette on the tilting platform. Transfer 50 mL medium into bag 4a from bag 3a. Remove the aluminum plate. Lower the platform to maximum magnetic strength for 2 minutes. Start the peristaltic pump and transfer the bone marrow cell suspension out of the blood bag through the magnetic filter into the 600-mL Fenwal bag (4b).

P. Before stopping the peristaltic pump, let air into the device by opening the drop controlling device on transfer set 2a, and transfer the remaining cell suspension from bags 4a and 3b.

Q. After purging, the cell suspension is concentrated by centrifuging the bag (4b) (500g for 15 minutes). Discard the supernatant.

R. Resuspend the cells in RPMI medium containing 40 percent human serum albumin to a final cell concentration of 2×10^8 cells per mL.

S. To ensure that the purified bone marrow cell suspension contains no magnetic beads, place bag 4b in the cassette again, compress with the plastic cover to give a thin layer of liquid, and then expose it for 2 minutes to the maximum field strength.

3. PROCEDURE FOR FREEZING CELL SUSPENSION
   A. Transfer cell suspension to another blood bag.
   B. Chill bag on wet ice for 15 minutes.
   C. Cryoprotectant containing 10 percent dimethyl sulfoxide (DMSO), 12 percent HES and 8 percent human albumin should also be chilled on ice for at least 30 minutes before use.
   D. Pour cryoprotectant at 1 volume to 1 volume of cell suspension into the blood bag using syringe. Make sure that as cryoprotectant is added a swirling motion is applied to bag to ensure immediate mixing.
   E. Return bag containing marrow-cryoprotectant mixture to the ice.
   F. Transfer the mixture to freezing bags. Each freezing bag should contain no more than 180 mL of mixture to minimize incidence of cracking bags upon thawing.
   G. Seal bags with heat sealer.
   H. Transfer bags to freezing tray, which is chilled in advance.
   I. Transfer trays to deep freezer at $-120°C$ in horizontal position for a minimum of 24 hours and then to liquid nitrogen for long-term storage.

ANTICIPATED RESULTS

The effect of immunomagnetic purging of myeloma cells depends on the surface antigen expression of these cells. Using the monoclonal antibody combination of PCA-1, BL-3, and J-5, more than 1.6 logs of fresh myeloma cells could be eliminated from bone marrow, while 4-HC decreases the clonogenic capacity of myeloma cells. The combination of these two methods is capable of removing more than 4 logs of cultured myeloma cells from bone marrow containing 10 percent myeloma cells.

NOTES

1. PURGING WITH 4-HC
   A. 4-HC is labile for heat and moisture, and should be stored in lyophilized form in the freezer. 4-HC is inactivated promptly after dissolving

with warmed phosphate buffered saline, and it should be used within 2 hours after dissolving.

B. Red blood cells contaminating in bone marrow buffy coat cells decrease the activity of 4-HC; therefore, it is important to minimize the contamination of red blood cells.

2. PURGING WITH MONOCLONAL ANTIBODIES AND MAGNETIC IMMUNOBEADS

A. The effect of immunomagnetic purging depends on the surface antigen expression of myeloma cells. Therefore, phenotypic analysis of myeloma cells in each case should be performed in advance.

B. In this section all operations should be carried out at 4°C to prevent antigenic modulation.

C. Evaluation of hematopoietic capacity in the marrow after purging should always be performed by standard colony-forming unit—granulocyte, macrophage (CFU-GM) or colony-forming unit—granulocyte, erythrocyte, macrophage, megakaryocyte (CFU-GEMM) assay before and after freezing.

AUTHORS

Chichiro Shimazaki, M.D.
Second Dept. of Medicine
Kyoto Prefectural University of
  Medicine
465 Kawaramachi-Hirokoji
Kamigyoku 602
Kyoto, Japan

Naohisa Fujita, M.D.
Second Dept. of Medicine
Kyoto Prefectural University of
  Medicine
465 Kawaramachi-Hirokoji
Kamigyoku 602
Kyoto, Japan

Tohru Inaba, M.D.
Second Dept. of Medicine
Kyoto Prefectural University of
  Medicine
465 Kawaramachi-Hirokoji
Kamigyoku 602
Kyoto, Japan

Masao Nakagawa, M.D.
Second Dept. of Medicine
Kyoto Prefectural University of
  Medicine
465 Kawaramachi-Hirokoji
Kamigyoku 602
Kyoto, Japan

Satoshi Murakami, M.D.
Second Dept. of Medicine
Kyoto Prefectural University of
  Medicine
465 Kawaramachi-Hirokoji
Kamigyoku 602
Kyoto, Japan

REFERENCES

1. Shimazaki, C, et al: Elimination of myeloma cells from bone marrow monoclonal antibodies and magnetic immunobeads. Blood 72:1248, 1988.

2. Shimazaki, C, et al: Ex vivo treatment of myeloma cells by 4-hydroperoxycyclophosphamide and VP-16-213. Acta Haematol 80:17, 1988.

3. Shimazaki, C, et al: Immunophenotypic analysis of lymphocytes and myeloma cells in patients with multiple myeloma. Acta Haematol 83:123, 1990.

4. Shimazaki, C, et al: Purging of myeloma cells from bone marrow using monoclonal antibodies and magnetic immunobeads in combination with 4-hydroperoxycyclophosphamide. In Gross, SR and Gee, A (eds): Bone Marrow Purging and Processing. Vol 333. Progress in Clinical and Biological Research. New York, Alan R. Liss, pp 311–319, 1990.

A COMBINATION PURGING PROCEDURE FOR BONE MARROW USING 4-HYDROPEROXYCYCLOPHOSPHAMIDE AND ANTIBODY-COATED MICROSPHERES

DESCRIPTION	In patients whose neoplastic disease involves the bone marrow, autologous marrow transplantation bears a risk of reinfusion of clonogenic tumor cells and potential development of diffuse metastases. To help obviate this complication, various purging techniques have been developed to kill or remove tumor from the marrow in vitro prior to cryopreservation. This procedure describes a combination purge of a mononuclear cell (MNC) fraction using two methods: pharmacologic with alkylating agent 4-hydroperoxycyclophosphamide (4-HC) and immunologic with monoclonal antibodies (MAb) and magnetic microspheres.
TIME FOR PROCEDURE	Approximately 4 to 7 hours, from obtainment of MNCs to preparation for cryopreservation

SUMMARY OF PROCEDURE

1. The MNC fraction is adjusted to a cell concentration of 2×10^7 white blood cells (WBC) per mL.

2. Dissolved 4-HC is added to the MNCs at a therapeutic concentration. After a 30-minute incubation in a 37°C waterbath, the MNCs are washed on the COBE 2991 processor with chilled saline.

3. Monoclonal antibodies specific to the tumor being treated are added to the MNCs. After a 60-minute incubation in an ice bath, the unbound antibody is removed by washing on the COBE processor.

4. Microscopic beads that contain a magnetite core and are coated with a secondary polyclonal antibody are added to the MNCs. A 60-minute incubation in a rotating ice bath follows.

5. The MNC suspension is placed on an array of neodymium magnets and gradually raised to a vertical position over a period of 8 minutes. The tumor-bead aggregates adhere to the wall of the bag on the magnet side and are left behind as the remaining suspension is pumped out of the bag.

6. The MNCs are centrifuged in the bag and then placed on a plasma expressor to reduce the volume prior to cryopreservation.

EQUIPMENT

1. COBE 2991 blood processor (COBE Laboratories, Lakewood, CO)
2. Plasma expressor (Baxter-Fenwal, Deerfield, IL)
3. RC-5B refrigerated centrifuge (du Pont, Wilmington, DE)
4. Magnetic purging apparatus (University Hospital, Denver, CO)
5. Sebra tube sealer (du Pont, Glenolden, PA)
6. AE-200 analytical balance (Mettler, Hightstown, NJ)
7. Waterbath (Lab-Line, Melrose Park, IL)
8. Heavy-duty rotator (Scientific Industries, Bohemia, NY)
9. Maxi-mix II mixer (Barnstead Thermolyne, Dubuque, IA)
10. Timer (Baxter, McGaw Park, IL)

11. Hemostats: Rochester-Pean (Fisher Scientific, Pittsburgh, PA)

12. Pipet-Aid pipettor (Drummond Scientific, Broomall, PA)

SUPPLIES AND REAGENTS

1. COBE 2991 single processing sets (Cobe, Lakewood, CO)

2. Two 1000-mL saline bags (hospital pharmacy): *chill at 4°C*

3. Autologous plasma, *irradiated with 2500 cGy*

4. TC-199 media (Gibco, Grand Island, NY)

5. 4-HC, 200 mg (Nova Pharmaceutical, Baltimore)

6. Monoclonal antibody panel (Monoclonal Core Laboratories, UCHSC, Denver)

7. Magnetic microspheres (Dynal Corp., Oslo, Norway)

8. Heparin, 10,000 U per mL (hospital pharmacy)

9. Transfer packs: 600- and 300-mL (Baxter-Fenwal, Deerfield, IL)

10. Transfer sets, with two couplers (Baxter-Fenwal, Deerfield, IL)

11. Transfer sets, with needle adaptor (Baxter-Fenwal, Deerfield, IL)

12. Sampling site couplers (Baxter-Fenwal, Deerfield, IL)

13. Syringes: 5-, 10-, and 60-mL, and 16-gauge needles (Becton Dickinson, Rutherford, NJ)

14. Syringe-top filter, 0.22 μm (Costar, Cambridge, MA)

15. Stopcocks (Baxter-Pharmaseal, Valencia, CA)

16. Serologic pipettes: 1-, 5-, 10-, and 25-mL (VWR Scientific, San Francisco)

17. Betadine solution (Purdue Fredrick, Norwalk, CT)

18. Povidone-iodine swabsticks (hospital supply)

PROCEDURE

1. Calculate the total number of cells by multiplying the cell count by the total MNC fraction volume.

2. Determine the volume of the incubation components as follows:

$$\text{Total volume} = \text{Total MNC per } 2.0 \times 10^7 \text{ cells per mL}$$
$$\text{Plasma volume (mL)} = \text{Total volume} \times 0.2$$
$$\text{Media volume (mL)} = \text{Total volume} - \text{cell volume} - \text{plasma volume}$$
$$\text{4-HC (mL)} = \text{Total volume} \times [\text{4-HC Rx] per } 10,000 \ \mu g/mL$$

3. Transfer the MNC suspension into a transfer bag of sufficient volume to contain the total volume calculated here.

4. Add the volume of *irradiated* plasma to the incubation bag.

5. Add the volume of TC-199 media to the incubation bag.

6. Reconstitute the 4-HC by adding 20 mL of sterile saline to the 200-mg vial. Shake until all particulate material has disappeared. This gives a stock concentration of 10 mg 4-HC per mL. Add the calculated volume of 4-HC to the bag via a syringe *through a 0.22-μm filter*. Mix by inverting.

7. Set a timer for 30 minutes and place the incubation bag in a 37°C water-bath. Tape the ports above the water line. Mix by inverting every 5 minutes.

8. During the incubation, install a new processing set on the COBE 2991 and make the instrument settings as below:

Centrifuge Speed	2000 rmp	Super-out Volume (mL)	500
Valve Selector	V-2	Spin Timer 1	3 minutes
Processing Switch	AUTO	Spin Timer 2	3 minutes
Super-out Rate (mL/min)	450		

9. Set the pinboard as diagrammed below:

10. When the timer rings, remove the incubation bag, spike to the RED line of the processing kit, and hang. Spike and hang the chilled saline bags to the GREEN and YELLOW lines.

11. Press BLOOD IN; allow the incubation bag to drain into the bowl.

12. Press STOP-RESET.

13. Clamp the CLEAR line just above the rotating seal.

14. Remove the incubation bag from the hanger bar. Press PREDILUTE. Allow about 100 mL of saline to flow into the incubation bag as a rinse, then press STOP-RESET.

15. Rehang the incubation bag, remove the clear clamp, and press BLOOD IN. Allow rinse to drain into bowl, then press STOP-RESET.

16. Press TUBE LOAD. Allow saline to fill bowl until flow stops, then press STOP-RESET.

17. Press BLOOD IN, then AIR OUT. When all air is out of the bowl, press BLOOD IN. When the fluid level is about 2 inches above the rotating seal, press STOP-RESET.

18. Press START-SPIN. The instrument will begin automated washing.

19. On the third (final) spin, change the super-out volume to the mark labeled "Final Spin." (This will leave between 40 and 70 mL in the bowl.)

20. When alarm sounds, press STOP-RESET. Seal the CLEAR tubing with the heat sealer or hand clips, then cut and remove the processing bag.

21. Insert a sampling site coupler into the port on the processing bag and remove the washed product to a 60-mL syringe. Remove 1 mL to a lavender-top tube for cell count and trypan blue viability. Record the remaining volume.

22. Using the disease-specific *Immunomagnetic Purge Worksheet*, calculate the total number of cells. Record on the worksheet.

23. Calculate and record the following parameters:

$$\text{Incubation volume} = \text{Total MNC} \div 2.0 \times 10^7 \text{ cells per ml}$$
$$\text{MAb } (\mu g) = \text{Incubation volume} \times [\text{MAb(Rx)}]$$
$$\text{MAb } (\mu L) = \text{MAb } (\mu g \div [\text{MAb(stock)}]$$

24. Attach a single stopcock to the syringe containing the MNC suspension. Make sure stopcock is closed to the syringe.

25. Attach a transfer bag (with needle adaptor) of sufficient size to contain the incubation volume to the stopcock port.

26. Clamp the syringe onto a ringstand.

27. Open the stopcock (valve directly downward) and push the MNC suspension into the transfer bag. Then clamp the line with hemostats.

28. Remove a sufficient number of antibody vials from the freezer. Allow them to thaw under the hood, then vortex each for 5 seconds at the lowest setting.

29. Close the stopcock valve to the transfer bag, then carefully remove the plunger from the syringe and stand it upright under the hood (or place on sterile gauze).

30. Close the stopcock valve downward.

31. Using the Pietman, add a volume (μL) of each monoclonal antibody equal to the amount calculated in step 23. Expel directly into the top of the open syringe.

32. When all antibodies have been added, remove the hemostats from the line. Add a sufficient amount of heparinized TC-199 media to reach the incubation volume (calculated in step 2).

33. Leaving a slight amount of air in the bag, seal the tubing with clamps. Cut off the excess tubing.

34. Place the transfer bag into a ziplock baggie, then place in an ice bath with povidone-iodine added, leaving the ports above the water line (tape if necessary).

35. Start a timer for the required MAb incubation period.

    NOTE: *The suspension* must be kept cold *from this point onward.*

36. When timer goes off, remove the bag from the ice bath.

37. Using the appropriate adaptor, place the bag in the large refrigerated centrifuge, set at 4°C, and spin at 1500 rpm for 10 minutes.

38. Place a waste collection beaker under the hood.

39. Place a stopcock onto a 60-mL syringe and clamp into the ringstand. Close the stopcock valve downward. Carefully remove the plunger and set aside.

40. Carefully remove the bucket from the centrifuge and place under the hood. Gently remove the bag from the bucket and place on the plasma expressor with the door locked open.

41. Close the roller clamp on a needle adaptor transfer set and spike into MNC bag.

42. Gently release the spring-loaded plasma expressor door.

43. Remove the sterile covering from the needle adaptor. Open the roller clamp and express the supernatant into the waste beaker until the cell layer begins to rise, then close the roller clamp.

44. Attach the needle adaptor to the stopcock port.

45. Open the roller clamp and add 200 mL of cold heparinized TC-199 media to the bag. Again clamp and cut the tubing. Gently agitate the bag to resuspend the cell layer.

46. Repeat steps 37 through 45 once more. *On the final wash, proceed directly from step 44 to step 47. Do **not** clamp tubing or remove from syringe.*

47. Calculate the volume of beads required using the following formulas:

$$\text{Tumor cells} = \text{Total MNC} \times \text{assumed tumor percentage}$$
$$\text{Number of beads} = \text{Tumor cells} \times \text{bead:tumor ratio}$$
$$\text{Volume of beads} = \text{Number of beads} \div 4 \times 10^8$$

48. Gently manually mix the stock bead vials, then remove the needed volume to conical centrifuge tube.

49. Top off the tube with TC-199 media and place on hand magnet. Allow beads to adhere to the wall of the tube nearest the magnet, then carefully decant the supernatant into the waste beaker. Repeat this step once more, then resuspend the beads in 10 mL of TC-199.

50. Add the beads to the bag via the syringe, then add sufficient volume of cold TC-199 to equal the incubation volume. Leave a slight amount of air in the bag, then seal and cut off excess tubing.

51. Place the bag in a resealable plastic bag, then place inside an ice bag with povidone-iodine on the rotator. Tilt rotator sideways, set at the slowest speed and start.

52. Set timer for the required bead incubation, and start.

53. Set the magnet array under the hood. Remove any nonfastened metal objects, then remove the magnet cover. Set the apparatus at the flat (horizontal) setting.

54. When timer sounds, gently remove incubation bag from the rotator and pat dry with paper towels. Place under hood and clean the unoccupied port with isopropanol. Then spike a 600-mL transfer into the port. Clamp the tubing with hemostats next to the port.

55. Place the incubation bag onto the magnetic array and secure the cover plate with the Velcro straps. Place the exit tubing into the secondary array, taking care not to kink it at the turns.

56. Start a timer. After 3 minutes, carefully raise the array one height level. Continue to raise one level per minute (three times total). Allow a full minute at the highest setting.

57. With the transfer bag lying on the hood deck, open the hemostats and allow the suspension to drain from the incubation bag. If flow stops, lower the transfer bag below deck level. When the transfer is complete, seal and cut the tubing.

58. Place the bag in the refrigerated centrifuge (4°C) and spin at 1500 rpm for 10 minutes.

59. Attach a stopcock to a 60-mL syringe. Do not remove the plunger. Make sure stopcock is closed downward.

60. When centrifuge stops, remove the MNC bag and place on the plasma expressor under the hood. Close the roller clamp on a needle adaptor transfer set and spike into the bag.

61. Remove the cover from the needle adaptor, then open the roller clamp and express the supernatant to a waste beaker. When the cell layer begins to

rise, close the roller clamp and attach the needle adaptor to the stopcock on the syringe. Agitate the bag to resuspend the cells.

62. Open the roller clamp, inject air into the bag, and then draw the MNC suspension into the syringe.

63. Record the purged MNC volume and proceed with cryopreservation.

| ANTICIPATED RESULTS | The average number of purged cells available for reinfusion following this procedure is 0.3×10^8 MNCs per kg patient weight. |

NOTES

1. Only unopened containers of media, saline, 4-HC, monoclonal antibodies, and magnetic beads are used. Lot numbers and expiration dates are recorded on the worksheet. Any unused 4-HC remaining in the vial is placed in a chemical waste container for subsequent pickup and incineration.

2. All sampling site ports are cleaned with povidone-iodine prior to needle entry.

3. Culture and sensitivity assays are sent to the central laboratory immediately following the procedure.

AUTHORS

Elizabeth J. Shpall, M.D.
Bone Marrow Transplant Program
University Hospital
Denver, CO 80262

Charles S. Johnston, M.T.(AMT)
Bone Marrow Transplant Program
University Hospital
Denver, CO 80262

REFERENCE

1. Shpall, EJ, et al: Immunopharmacologic bone marrow purging in metastatic breast cancer patients receiving high-dose chemotherapy with autologous marrow support. Proc Am Soc Clin Oncol 9:9, 1990.

TREATMENT OF DENSITY GRADIENT–SEPARATED CELLS WITH 4-HYDROPEROXYCYCLOPHOSPHAMIDE, VINCRISTINE, AND METHYLPREDNISOLONE

DESCRIPTION	Successful autologous marrow transplantation is limited by the presence of possible residual marrow tumor cells even though a clinical complete remission has been achieved. The use of 4-hydroperoxycyclophosphamide (4-HC) to purge tumor cells in marrows from patients with acute lymphocytic leukemia (ALL) has had minimal success. The purpose of this protocol is to explore the efficiency of in vitro incubation of the marrow graft with 4-HC, methylprednisolone (MP), and vincristine to remove tumor cells. The combination of these agents should enhance tumor cell kill and not significantly increase the toxicity to normal cells.
TIME FOR PROCEDURE	Approximately 2.5 hours for the incubations and washes of light-density cells (does not include time required for the collection of these cells)
SUMMARY OF PROCEDURE	1. Bone marrow is harvested. 2. Buffy coat cells are collected. 3. Backup cells are removed. 4. Cells are further purified using a density gradient. 5. Cells are incubated with 4-HC and vincristine for ½ hour. 6. Cells are washed. 7. Cells are incubated with MP for 1 hour. 8. Cells are washed, and then frozen.
EQUIPMENT	1. 37°C waterbath 2. COBE 2991 or other cell processor 3. Cell counter 4. Tube strippers 5. Tube sealer 6. Laminar flow hood
SUPPLIES AND REAGENTS	1. 2000-mL transfer pack (Fenwal 4R2041) 2. 1000-mL transfer pack (Fenwal 4R2031) 3. 600-mL transfer pack (Fenwal 4R2023) 4. 300-mL transfer pack (Fenwal 4R2014) 5. Sampling site couplers (Fenwal 4C2405) 6. Administration set (Cutter 20-5614) 7. Lifecell septum and cap (Fenwal 4C2471) 8. 4-HC (Nova Pharmaceutics) 9. Vincristine [Lilly (1 mg per mL concentration)] 10. MP sodium succinate [Abbott (1000 mg bottle = 125 mg per mL concentration)] 11. Deoxyribonuclease (DNAse) [Sigma (see Appendix)]

12. TC-199 (Gibco 320-1151)
13. Hank's Balanced Salt Solution (HBSS) (Gibco 320-4175 AG)
14. RPMI-1640 (4-L container) (Whittaker 12-167L)
15. Filters: 0.22-μm (Millipore 5LGS0250S)
16. 16-gauge needles
17. 60-mL luer-lock syringes
18. Alcohol wipes
19. Software for processing device

PROCEDURE

1. Prepare a buffy coat concentrate from the harvested marrow. Obtain a specimen for the following:
   A. Nucleated cell count
   B. Hematocrit (Hct)
   C. Progenitor cell assays
   D. Sterility

2. Determine the number of nucleated cells per kg patient weight present in the buffy coat concentrate. The primary fraction will be further purified by density gradient separation and treated. The secondary ("backup") fraction will be untreated.
   A. The recommended number of cells for the backup is at least 0.7×10^8 per kg.
   B. The remainder of the buffy coat cells (preferably more than 1.5×10^8 cells per kg) should be processed using a density gradient separation technique. Some patients may not have enough cells to allow for an untreated backup graft. The final decision is made by the medical director.

3. Determine the total number and volume of cells present in the primary and backup fractions. Transfer the appropriate volume (volume = cells per kg $\times$ patient weight $\div$ buffy coat cells per mL) of backup cells into properly labeled freeze bags and place them in the refrigerator. The cells that are to be further processed should be tranferred to a 600-mL transfer pack.

   NOTE: *All bags must be labeled with the patient's name, history number,* and *the type of treatment.*

4. After the light density cells are collected, they are washed with RPMI media and resuspended in a final volume of approximately 50 mL. Cell counts are performed to determine the number of cells to be treated. Specimens should be obtained for Hct and progenitor cell assays. Determine the volume of reagents using the following calculations:

$$\text{Total volume} = \text{Total number of cells} \div 2.0 \times 10^7 \text{ cells}$$
$$\text{mL plasma} = \text{Total volume} \times 0.2$$
$$\text{mg 4-HC} = \text{Total volume} \times 60\ \mu\text{g/mL} \div 1000\ \mu\text{g/mg}$$
$$\text{mL 4-HC} = \text{mg 4-HC} \div \text{4-HC stock concentration (mg/mL)}$$
$$\text{mL vincristine} = \text{Total volume} \times 3\ \mu\text{g/mL} \div 1000\ \mu\text{g/mL}$$
$$\text{mL media} = \text{Total volume} - \text{plasma volume} - \text{cell volume}$$
$$- \text{4-HC volume} - \text{vincristine volume}$$

5. Add the correct volume of autologous plasma to the incubation bag.

6. The appropriate number of TC-199 media bottles are stoppered using the Lifecell septums and caps.

7. Using an administration set and by weighing the bag on the balance, add the correct amount of TC-199 media. This may be syringed into the bag if the volume is small.

8. Place the bag in the 37°C waterbath and allow the cells to remain for 10 minutes before the addition of the 4-HC and vincristine.

9. The 4-HC (20 mg vial if available) should be reconstituted in 20 mL of room temperature TC-199 media. Refer to the package insert for details.

10. The dissolved 4-HC is added to the cells using a 0.22-μm filter attached to a syringe (to deliver small volumes of drug: filter the 4-HC into a sterile tube, remove the appropriate amount using 1-mL syringes and add the drug to the cells). Then add the appropriate amount of vincristine using a 1-mL syringe.

11. After the 4-HC and vincristine are added, mix the incubation bag and obtain a sample to determine the actual incubation cell count. Set a timer for 30 minutes. The ports of the bag should not be immersed in the water. They may be taped to the side of the water bath. Mix the bag every 5 minutes.

12. DURING THE INCUBATION PERIOD THE FOLLOWING SHOULD BE DONE:
    - Irradiate the plasma for use later in the procedure.
    - Remove one 10-mL bottle DNAse (5000 U/mL) from the freezer.
    - Prepare the appropriate amount of MP.

13. MP is obtained as a powder that is reconstituted with HBSS. Prior to the addition of the HBSS, the diluent must be removed from the MP container. The top of the container should be rinsed three times with HBSS. Then, using aseptic technique, add 8 mL of HBSS to the MP powder. The MP takes approximately 1 hour to dissolve. To calculate the amount of MP to prepare, take the total incubation volume from step 4 and multiply by 0.04.

14. After the 30-minute incubation, the cells should be washed on the COBE 2991 (or an equivalent device) with 1.5 L of *cold* RPMI media containing 2 percent autologous *irradiated* (more than 1500 rad) plasma.

15. THE COBE WASH PROCEDURE IS AS FOLLOWS: Attach the cells to the RED line and fill the bowl. The RPMI media should be attached to the GREEN line and the remainder of the bowl should be filled with media before beginning the program. The operator control panel should be set as follows:

Centrifuge Speed	Super-Out Rate	Minutes Agitate Time	Super-Out Volume (SOV)	Valve Selector
3000	450	80	450*	N/A

*At the start of the last cycle, change the super-out volume to 600.

Spin time 1: 2 minutes
Spin time 2: N/A
Auto/Manual: Auto

The board should be set as follows:

Timer	PC	Valve	SOV
X O	O	O X O	450
X O	O	O X O	450
X O	X	O O O	600

X = a peg in the slot
O = no peg in the slot

16. After the cells are washed, resuspend the product and obtain the final specimens as follows:
    A. Cell count
    B. Progenitor cell assays
    C. Differentials

17. MP INCUBATION: This step must begin within 1 hour after the completion of the 4-HC and vincristine incubation. Incubation volumes and reagent amounts are calculated according to the following formulas:

$$\text{Total incubation volume} = \text{Total number cells} \div 2 \times 10^7$$
$$\text{mL of DNAse} = \text{Total volume} \times 0.02$$
$$\text{mL of MP} = \text{Total volume} \times 5 \text{ mg/mL} \div 125$$
$$\text{mL of plasma} = \text{Total volume} \times 0.2$$
$$\text{mL of media} = \text{Total volume} - \text{volume of cells}$$
$$- \text{volume of DNAse}$$
$$- \text{volume of MP}$$
$$- \text{volume of plasma}$$

The addition of reagents will be in the following order: cells, irradiated plasma, media, DNAse, and MP. To ensure sterility, the DNAse and MP will be added through a 0.22-μm filter attached to a syringe.

18. Incubate the transfer pack containing the incubation mixture in a 37°C waterbath for 60 minutes with intermittent mixing. Secure the incubation bag such that the ports are not immersed.

19. Following the 60-minute incubation, wash the cells on the COBE 2991 as described in step 15. Use 1.5 L of media (RPMI or TC-199 containing 2 percent autologous irradiated plasma and 2.5 U/mL of beef lung heparin [1470 mL media, 30 mL plasma, and 0.38 mL heparin (10,000 U/mL)]. Transfer the cells to a freeze bag and obtain a final volume.

20. SAMPLES SHOULD BE OBTAINED FOR:
    A. Nucleated cell count
    B. Progenitor cell assays
    C. Sterility

21. Freeze the bone marrow according to the standard procedure.

ANTICIPATED RESULTS   This procedure should result in the recovery of more than 75 percent of the cells that were treated. The recovery of colony-forming unit—granulocyte, macrophages (CFU-GM) should be approximately 1 percent.

AUTHORS	Janice M. Davis, M.T.(ASCP), S.B.B. Cell Processing Laboratory The Johns Hopkins Oncology Center Baltimore, MD 21205	Scott D. Rowley, M.D., FACP Fred Hutchinson Cancer Research Center Seattle, WA 98104

REFERENCES

1. Rowley, SD, et al: Density-gradient separation of autologous bone marrow grafts before ex vivo purging with 4-hydroperoxycyclophosphamide. Bone Marrow Transplant (in press) 1991.
2. Rowley, SD, et al: Acute lymphoblastic leukemia (ALL): A phase I study of autologous bone marrow transplantation with combination drug purging (abst). Proc Am Soc Clin Oncol 9:202, 1990.

APPENDIX: DNASE PREPARATION

DESCRIPTION

DNAse is an enzyme that cleaves native DNA and is employed in assay systems subject to cell lysis to prevent gellation of the solution by free DNA. Experience has shown that 350 to 500 Kunitz units per mL of incubation solution may be adequate depending on conditions and the amount of cell lysis expected to occur. DNAse may also be used to dissolve clumps of cells. Even though no visible clumps remain, cell counts are not increased because the cells involved in this aggregation are presumably damaged and lost.

The DNAse is supplied as a lyophylized partially purified product that must be reconstituted prior to use in bone marrow processing. It is maximally soluble in salt containing solution, and HBSS has been arbitrarily selected for this purpose. The stock concentration will be 5000 U/mL and aliquots of 10 mL will be prepared. These will be frozen and stored.

Before clinical use, reconstituted DNAse must be determined to meet sterility and pyrogenicity standards as described by the United States Pharmacopoeia. Until the storage life span of reconstituted DNAse is determined, an empiric outdate of six months (at $-20°C$) from reconstitution will be maintained.

SUPPLIES AND REAGENTS

1. DNAse (Sigma Biochemical D5025)
2. HBSS (Gibco 310-417S, 100 mL)
3. Lifecell septum and cap (Fenwal 4C2471)
4. Serum bottles (Wheaton 223739, 10 mL)
5. Rubber stoppers (Wheaton 224124, 13 $\times$ 20 mm)
6. Aluminum seals (Wheaton 224183, 20 mm)
7. Filters (Millipore SLGS0250S, 0.22-μm)
8. Administration set (Cutter 20-5614)
9. 60-mL syringes
10. Three-way stopcock
11. Gloves
12. Labels

EQUIPMENT

1. Laminar flow hood
2. Autoclave
3. Bottle cap crimper

PROCEDURE

1. Wash glass vials and rubber stoppers, rinse with distilled water, and autoclave before use.

2. Store DNAse frozen and bring to room temperature before weighing. The entire bottle should be reconstituted at this time. The formula for reconstitution is as follows:

$$\text{Weight DNAse (mg)} \times \text{activity of stock (U per mg)} = \text{Total units}$$
$$\text{Total units} \div 5000 \text{ (U/mL)} = \text{Total reconstitution volume}$$

3. The DNAse is dissolved in the appropriate volume of HBSS. This should be done in a sterile 500-mL bottle.

4. Following reconstitution, membrane-filter sterilize the DNAse solution immediately. This step should be performed under the hood. Cap the bottle containing the dissolved DNAse using the Lifecell septum and cap. Spike the rubber stopper with an administration set. Place a three-way stopcock on the end of the administration set. Place a 60-mL syringe and a 0.22 μm filter on the two remaining ports on the stopcock. Place a 16-gauge needle onto the filter. Turn the three-way stopcock to fill the syringe with DNAse. Turn the three-way stopcock again to deliver 11 mL of reagent to each bottle. Sterilization occurs when the solution is pushed through the filter. The bottle is stoppered and the stoppers are fixed by crimping aluminum seals in place.

5. Appropriate labels will be affixed immediately after bottling. The following information must be included:

   - Product name
   - Lot number
   - Date expired
   - Store below $-20°C$
   - Activity
   - Volume

   The labels must also include the statement "For Investigational Use Only."

6. Freeze all vials at below $-20°C$ until immediately before use.

7. Sterility and pyrogenicity will be determined for sample vials as per the United States Pharmacopoeia. Appropriate records will be maintained, including lot numbers of supplies, date reconstituted, lot number of reconstituted DNAse, results of sterility and pyrogenicity testing, and outdate of reconstituted product.

9 | CRYOPRESERVATION AND STORAGE OF STEM CELLS

Commentary by N. C. GORIN

CONTROLLED-RATE FREEZING
Cryopreservation of Autografts Using
  Delmed Freezing Bags
Cryopreservation of Bone Marrow in Gambro
  Freezing Bags
Cryopreservation of Bone Marrow in
  Standardized Medium
Cryopreservation and Storage of Bone
  Marrow Cells in Fenwal Freezing Bags
Cryopreservation of T-Cell–Depleted Bone
  Marrow
MECHANICAL FREEZING
Cryopreservation of Bone Marrow Stem Cells
  in Dimethyl Sulfoxide and Hydroxyethyl
  Starch without Controlled-Rate Freezing
Cryopreservation of Bone Marrow with
  Hydroxyethyl Starch, Plasmalyte,
  Dextrose, and Dimethyl Sulfoxide Using a
  Mechanical Freezer

Refrigeration Storage of Bone Marrow
THAWING AND REINFUSION
Undiluted
  *Thawing and reinfusion of autografts
    using infusion set*
  *Infusion of thawed bone marrow using
    syringe*
Thawing and Dilution of Bone Marrow
CRYOPRESERVATION AND INFUSION OF
  PERIPHERAL BLOOD STEM CELLS
Cryopreservation of Peripheral Stem Cells
Cryopreservation of Peripheral Stem Cells
  Following Processing
Concentration and Cryopreservation of
  Peripheral Blood Mononuclear Cells
Cryopreservation of Hematopoietic
  Peripheral Blood Stem Cells in Gambro
  Freezing Bags
Infusion of Peripheral Blood Stem Cells

Studies on the effect of cold on viability of cells go back a very long time. Reaumur (1736) and Spalanzani (1787) opened the way with experiments on insects, sperm cells, and ova of various animal species. Despite numerous further attempts, no substantial improvement occurred until Polge, Smith, and Parkes[1] demonstrated revival of bull spermatozoa after vitrification and dehydration at low temperatures in the presence of glycerol, the first cryoprotective agent. In 1955, Barnes and Loutit,[2] using the Polge, Smith, and Parkes technique, demonstrated that bone marrow could be successfully preserved by freezing. From this period started the modern era of hematopoietic stem cell cryobiology. In addition to glycerol, other cryoprotective agents, such as dimethyl sulfoxide (DMSO)[3] and polyvinylpyrrolidone (PVP),[4] were introduced. Numerous animal models were established in rodents,[5,6] dogs,[7–10] and monkeys,[11–13] which clearly demonstrated that cryopreserved marrow retained the ability to reconstitute hematopoiesis following lethal irradiation. General principles for low-temperature preservation of bone marrow were progressively

*Bone Marrow Transplantation Unit, Formation Associée Claude-Bernard "Unité de Recherche sur les Greffes de Cellules Souches Hématopoiétiques" and Centre National de Transfusion Sanguine, Hôpital Saint-Antoine, Paris.

established[14-17] and later better adjusted with the availability of marrow culture techniques, the only in vitro tests at least partly relevant to assessment of viability following cryopreservation.[4,18-21] Recently, manipulations of marrow including stem cell concentration and in vitro treatment in various malignancies have brought additional information on increased sensitivity to cryoinjury either as a consequence of prefreezing treatment[22] or as a reflection of a specific intrinsic fragility such as for stem cells of chronic myelocytic leukemia (CML)[23] and for clonogenic progenitors (colony-forming units) of acute myelocytic leukemia (AML-CFU).[24]

The first attempts at autologous bone marrow transplantation (ABMT) between 1958 and 1965[25-28] produced questionable or disappointing results. Since 1975, however, several institutions have reported on clinical trials with ABMT clearly demonstrating the efficacy of cryopreserved marrow for hematopoietic recovery, and ABMT is nowadays performed on a large scale. Similarly, after first attempts in animals[29-32] and later first reports in humans with CML[33] and AML,[34-36] transplantation of autologous peripheral blood stem cells is now also widely used, for the treatment of both hematologic malignancies and solid tumors.

Three recent surveys show the importance of stem cell cryopreservation and autografting as so-called routine laboratory and clinical techniques. First, a report on facilities for cryopreservation and storage in the United States conducted in 1988 and 1989 identified a total of 47 centers of which 14 have cryopreserved fewer than 30 marrows per year; 15 have frozen 30 to 50, 12 have stored 50 to 100, and 6 have stored more than 100 marrows per year.[37] In 83 percent of the reporting centers a controlled-rate freezing program was used. In France alone, more than 1000 marrows have been cryopreserved in 1990.[38] Second, marrow can be successfully stored for long periods. A specific investigation on reinfusion of long-term cryopreserved marrow in Europe and at the Brigham and Women's Hospital in Boston has identified 33 patients who received marrow stored for more than 2 years and up to 11 years (median 2.8 years, range 2 to 11 years) of whom 30 of 32 engrafted successfully.[39] Finally, the last survey of the international registry on autologous bone marrow transplantation (ABMTR) has estimated the total number of autografts performed worldwide from 1987 to 1989 at 4000 per year,[40] a considerable increase over the two previously analyzed periods, 1985 to 1987[41] and before 1985.[42]

This chapter deals with cryopreservation and storage. Before detailing the various technical procedures, the principles of low-temperature preservation are reviewed and general guidelines proposed that should be considered by cryopreservation and transplant unit members.

THE CLASSIC PRINCIPLES OF LOW-TEMPERATURE PRESERVATION FOR NORMAL HEMATOPOIETIC STEM CELLS

Cooling of Cells to Temperatures above 0°C

Cooling above 0°C does not provide adequate storage for many practical purposes.[20]

1. Metabolism, although slowed down, does not cease at 0°C. In addition, all reactions are not quantitatively diminished to the same degree. Therefore, interrelated metabolic pathways are disturbed rather than put to rest.

2. Some consequences of cooling are directly harmful:
    *   Cooling switches off the Na pump and, as a result, cooled cells swell.
    *   Membrane lipids undergo phase changes that may in themselves be harmful and also modify reaction rates of membrane bound enzymes.[43]
    *   Poorly soluble materials may precipitate and dissociation constants change, resulting in changes in the composition and pH of solutions.[44]
3. Finally, for some unknown reason, rapid cooling can lead to cell death per se. This phenomenon, known as "thermal shock,"[45] is illustrated by the fact that, for instance, erythrocytes suspended in hypertonic salt solutions sufficient to produce only minimal hemolysis at 37°C are rapidly lysed if cooled to 0°C at a rate of -20°C/minute.

Therefore, the time for which cells can be preserved at temperatures above 0°C is limited, although in some instances, it may be sufficient for laboratory techniques and even clinical application. Several teams have successfully autografted marrows preserved at 4°C in the refrigerator for up to 56 hours.[46]

Freezing

The most dangerous events for the preservation of viability in a liquid system such as bone marrow occur during the freezing and thawing procedures. Critical periods during which a phase modification of the system takes place are transformation of liquid to a solid substance (ice crystal) and vice versa (Table 9–1).

DURING THE FREEZING PROCEDURE

Solution Effects Represent the Most Likely Source of Freezing Injury

The principal solute in biologic fluids is sodium chloride. When the isotonic sodium chloride (0.15 M) solution is cooled, it may supercool a few degrees, but if seeded, an ice crystal (containing exclusively water) forms and

Table 9–1 POTENTIAL DAMAGE OF CRYOPRESERVATION

Freezing Procedure
Solution effects
   Increased with slow cooling rates, reduced with the use of cryoprotective agents
Thermal shock
Phase transition time
Freezing rate after phase transition

Thawing
Recrystallization phenomenon
Dilution shock

---

starts growing. As cooling is continued, further water is incorporated into ice, sufficient at each temperature to concentrate the salt in the remaining liquid to produce a solution that has that freezing point. Thus the remaining solution is progressively diminished in volume and increased in molarity until at − 21.1°C the saline has reached a concentration of 5.2 M. At this temperature, the eutectic point, the remaining solution solidifies. When cells are suspended in isotonic saline and frozen, the ice crystal formation occurs first in the extracellular compartment because it is the largest one and therefore is more likely to contain a starting nucleus. This also occurs because thermal exchange is faster and an equilibrium more easily reached from the freezing chamber to the extracellular compartment than to the intracellular medium, which is somehow protected by the cell membrane. While freezing continues, cells are subjected to a 32-fold increase in sodium chloride concentration. Clearly, the most obvious effect of raised external osmolality is that cells shrink. The osmotic pressure may be increased to such a value that the cell membranes are damaged and become leaky to cations. A significant cell lysis occurs.

The solution effects are even more likely to affect cell survival when the cooling rate is slow. On the other hand, a very high cooling rate, which would avoid this risk, results in intracellular ice crystal formation and major intracellular structural disruption, also leading to cell lysis.

Cryoprotective agents make possible the use of slow cooling rates. Their mode of action is, however, complex and not perfectly understood.

- The best-known property of cryoprotectants is their ability to act as colligative agents.[47] They bind water molecules, which results in slowing down their incorporation into the growing ice crystal. This prevents a high increase in external osmotic pressure and reduces the solution effects. The rise in mole fraction of a NaCl solution initially isotonic, when cooling, is slowed down in the presence of increasing concentrations of glycerol. Therefore, a slow cooling rate that avoids intracellular freezing becomes possible (Fig. 9-1).
- The ability of the cryopreservative agent to penetrate the cell is certainly important. However, good cryopreservation has been obtained with agents that penetrate rapidly such as DMSO, slowly such as glycerol, or not at all such as PVP and hydroxyethyl starch (HES). When freezing rat pancreatic acinar cells with glycerol, best results yielding minimal ultrastructural alteration of the rough endoplasmic reticulum (RER) have been obtained by preincubation of cells with glycerol at 0°C—a temperature at which glycerol does not penetrate the cell.[48] Indeed, as discussed later, the diffusibility of the cryoprotective agent may be more critical at time of thawing when viability of cells can be decreased by the dilution shock phenomenon. Also these observations have led to speculation that the membrane may be one major site of action of some if not all cryoprotectants, which would interact directly or indirectly to stabilize the water-lipid-protein complex tertiary structure.[16]

The Phase Transition Time

The phase transition time has long been known to be a critical period. The phase transition occurs when the water in the liquid state releases its latent heat of fusion to transform to a solid phase. If the freezing program does not react at that time, the cooling rate, because of the liberation of the heat of fusion, diminishes—hence the freezing plateau (Fig. 9-2). The duration of the

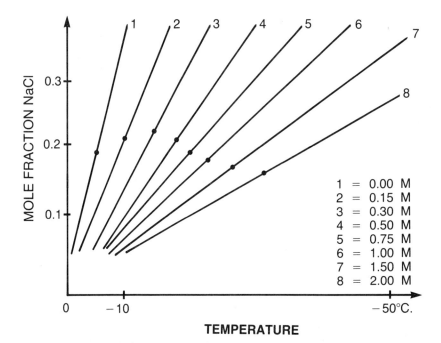

FIGURE 9–1 Graph showing the rise in mole fraction of NaCl in solutions initially containing the indicated molalities of glycerol and isotonic with respect to NaCl. (From Lovelock,[47] 1953, with permission.)

• Mole fraction NaCl giving 5 percent hemolysis.

phase transition is directly correlated to cell destruction.[49,50] For instance, by measuring viability through glycine-2-^{14}C incorporation, freezing bone marrow cells in the presence of 15 percent glycerol has resulted in 45 percent viability for a phase transition time less than 2 minutes and only 3 percent for a 15- to 25-minute phase transition duration. With 15 percent DMSO similar values of 52 percent and 2 percent, respectively, have been obtained.[16] In another experimental model, the recovery of mouse bone marrow cells decreased continuously as the freezing plateau was prolonged from 1 to 16 minutes.[50] The duration of the transition phase was also found to be an important factor of cell mortality when cooling canine kidneys and evaluating the damage from the release of lactic dehydrogenase (LDH) and glutamate-oxaloacetate transaminase (GOT) enzymes in the venous effluent.[51] Finally, Foreman and Pegg[52] found that the duration of the phase transition period did influence the survival of two tissue culture cell lines but did not influence survival of cryopreserved human lymphocytes. They suggested that with programmed cooling close to optimal, a longer freezing plateau was not damaging, as it allowed additional time for cell shrinkage and reduced the likelihood of intracellular freezing, while with suboptimal programmed cooling it would result in unnecessary exposure to solution effects when there was no danger of intracellular freezing. It seems logical to assume that the larger the bulk of a specimen being frozen, the greater the importance of control of the cooling process, including the phase transition period. With current freezing apparatus, it is conceivable that the release of the heat of fusion has more impact on cell viability when marrow is frozen in large volumes than in small aliquots.

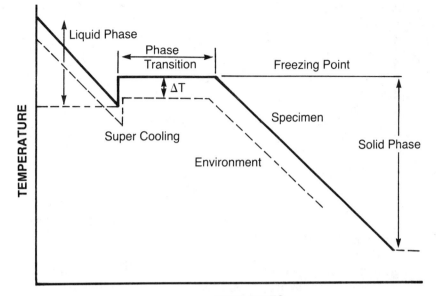

FIGURE 9–2   Cooling diagram illustrating the phases of transient heat transfer relationship between the biologic specimen and the cold environment. When measuring cooling rate, care should be exercised to obtain the temperature of the specimen and not that of the environment (freezing chamber). ΔT = the difference between the freezing chamber and the specimen. (From Rowe, AW,[16] 1966, with permission.)

Freezing Rate after the Heat of Fusion

While the cooling rate in the "pre–heat of fusion" liquid may vary within a certain range, in the "post–heat of fusion" phase a slow rate is considerably better than faster rates. Rowe[16] has reported for bone marrow cells viabilities of 78 and 45 percent, respectively, with slow (1°C per minute) and fast (8 to 9°C per minute) cooling rates after the heat of fusion. In our own experience,[53] on a total of 71 bags of frozen human marrow, we found recovery of CFU-GM to be 50 percent or more in 100 percent of cases when the freezing rate following heat of fusion was less than 5°C per minute, 45 percent for freezing rates between 5 and 10°C per minute, and 22 percent when the freezing rate exceeded 10°C per minute (n = 71; $P < .001$) (Fig. 9–3). We therefore cautioned against introducing too much nitrogen into the freezing chamber to annul the fusion heat, which could result in an overly marked increase in the subsequent freezing rate (the so called third slope of the freezing diagram). Figure 9–4 indicates the ideal bone marrow freezing rate obtained when the introduction of nitrogen vapor occurs at the time when the heat of fusion is generated, and is accurately calibrated both to counteract its effects and avoid subsequent brisk cooling (curve c).

STORAGE

If the freezing procedure is optimal and no cell damage has occurred, no further damage should be expected during the storage period provided that the

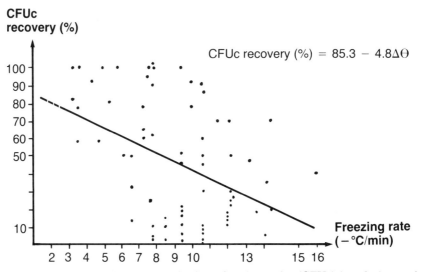

FIGURE 9–3   Percent recovery of colony-forming units (CFUc) in relation to freezing rates (°C/min) following release of heat of fusion. (From Gorin, NC,[53] 1983, with permission.)

temperature of preservation is low enough to block all the enzymatic pathways and the whole cell metabolism. The lower the storage temperature, the better.

Comparative in vitro studies of human marrow cryopreservation at $-79°C$ and $-196°C$[54,55] have shown far better recoveries in the latter situation. This has also been our experience when using the gas phase of liquid nitrogen for practical reasons (recorded temperature of $-194°C$ at the top of the gas phase). Nevertheless, liquid nitrogen, whenever possible, may be preferable, and a constant recording of the temperature in the storage chamber should be kept to trace any accidental warming occurring at any time of the storage. Ionizing events from background radiation have been shown not to interfere with effective long-term storage,[56] despite the blockade of the DNA repair enzymatic system. In fact, until recently little was known about the possible effect or lack of effect of duration of storage on in vivo stem cell viability in humans. Several teams have performed ABMT with marrows preserved for several years leading to hematopoietic recoveries within normal intervals.[39]

We recently reviewed retrospectively the engraftment data of 33 patients from the European Cooperative Group for bone marrow transplantation (EBMT) and the Brigham and Women's Hospital in Boston,[39] who received stem cells cryopreserved for more than 2 years from 1981 to 1989. The source of stem cells was bone marrow in 32 patients and peripheral blood in 1 patient. Nineteen patients had acute lymphoblastic leukemia, 11 acute myelogenous leukemia, and 3 chronic myelogenous leukemia. Median age at time of transplant was 22 years (range 7 to 57 years). The bone marrow was treated with mafosfamide in 14 patients and with monoclonal antibody in 3 patients; it was left untreated in the remaining 19 patients. Data on cryopreservation methods were available in 16 of 33 patients. The rate of freezing and the final storage temperature varied from institution to institution. However, in all cases stem cells were frozen in liquid nitrogen with a programmed freezer and stored at

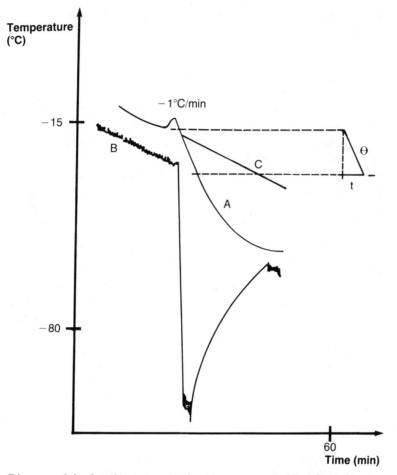

FIGURE 9–4 Diagram of the freezing curves in the marrow sample (A or C) and in the freezing chamber (B). Curve C is the ideal curve, while curve A shows an increase in the rate of cooling on the so-called third slope, which results from an overcompensation to annul the heat of fusion. Freezing following curve A induced poor stem cell recovery. (From Gorin, NC,[53] 1983, with permission.)

temperatures at or below −140°C. The median duration of cryopreservation was 2.8 years (range 2 to 11 years).

All patients received ablative doses of chemotherapy with or without irradiation. One patient died of sepsis on day 5 and was inevaluable for engraftment. Thirty of thirty-two evaluable patients (94 percent) achieved granulocyte counts of more than 500 per μL (median 23 days; range 10 to 119 days); 26 of 32 (74 percent) achieved platelets more than 50,000 per μL (median 30 days; range 19 to 128 days), and 22 of 32 patients (69 percent) achieved platelets more than 100,000 per μL (median 45 days; range 20 to 328 days). The numbers of colony-forming unit—granulocyte, macrophage (CFU-GM) were measured before stem cell infusion in 15 patients. The median CFU-GM dose infused was 1.1×10^4 per kg (range 0 to 17×10^4 per kg). The three patients infused with less than 1000 CFU-GM per kg achieved polymorphonuclears (PMNs) greater than 500 per μL. This demonstrates that human stem cells cryopreserved for up to 11 years are capable of engrafting.

THAWING

Severe effects may occur during the last step of cryopreservation, the thawing procedure. Several studies have shown that rapid thawing is desirable. For instance, Leibo and colleagues[4] have reported a major increase ($\times$ 2) in marrow cell viability with a 90°C per minute warming rate, as compared with 2°C per minute. However, when studying CFU cryopreservation in mice, they showed that rapid thawing was better only in a situation when the freezing rate used had been nonoptimal. Kubota and associates[51] similarly showed better results in canine kidney preservation when using rapid rates of thawing (70 to 110°C). It has been proposed that rapid thawing may avoid the recrystallization phenomenon during which ice crystal reorganization favoring inclusion of small crystals into bigger ones may destroy cells mechanically. During thawing, cells are submitted to the "dilution shock," as the course of events is the reverse of what occurred during freezing. The ice crystal melts, which generates free water, and the extracellular fluid becomes progressively hypotonic. The cells swell. There is a greater sensitivity of cells to swelling than to shrinkage. Cell lysis will occur, especially when using a cryoprotective agent that penetrates intracellularly or diffuses poorly, or both, and therefore remains located inside the cell membranes after thawing. For this reason, there may be an advantage to select agents that either do not penetrate cells or have a very high diffusibility, such as DMSO.

ADDITIONAL FACTORS INTERVENING IN THE EFFICACY OF CRYOPRESERVATION OF HUMAN MARROW

Optimal Freezing Rate

The best cooling rate for marrow stem cells evaluated by CFUs or CFU-GM recovery, has been shown to range between 1 and 3°C per minute both with glycerol and DMSO.[4,57] When cryopreserving marrow, one must bear in mind that the cooling rates used are very effective for preservation of bacteria and yeast, while inducing red cell hemolysis.

Concentration of Cryopreservation Agents

DMSO has been shown to be superior to glycerol for human marrow stem cell cryopreservation and the recommended final concentration is 10 percent.[58,59]

Contact of Stem Cells With DMSO

DMSO at the concentration of 10 percent is highly toxic to stem cells. We have shown that the recovery of CFU-GM following contact times with DMSO of 15 and 60 minutes at 4°C falls to 49 percent and 23 percent, respectively.[60] Therefore, freezing of marrow should be started very quickly as soon as DMSO has been introduced. Likewise, infusion of the marrow should be done immediately after thawing through a central venous line, ideally within 10 to 15 minutes.

The Role of Serum

Macromolecules such as serum proteins protect cells during freezing, as well as protecting them against handling injury after thawing. Human serum is much superior to fetal calf serum.[61] Usual final concentrations used are 5 to 10 percent.

Influence of Cell Concentration

When freezing red blood cells, high cellular concentrations result in cell loss.[62] For this reason, and also to avoid cell clumping after thawing, we have used concentrations below 20×10^6 per mL in the final medium. However, if preparations include only mononuclear cells, the final concentration can probably be increased.

Freezing in Ampoules or Bags

Cryopreservation in ampoules and bags for larger volumes are both satisfactory. However, as mentioned before, freezing in bags necessitates a more careful monitoring, especially at the time of release of the heat of fusion. Common lipophilic plasticizers are toxic for the cell membrane and should not be used.[63]

Polyolefin and Teflon-Kapton bags have been used successfully. From our experience in 500 frozen marrows, Teflon-Kapton bags (Gambro Dyalisatoren, West Germany) are more resistant to breakage and therefore safer. Test tubes should not be used as probes to control the efficacy of cryopreservation when marrow is frozen in bags for further clinical use. Indeed, we have studied the recovery of hematopoietic progenitor cells (CFU-GM, burst-forming units—erythroid [BFU-E]) in 52 ampoules and compared it with the recovery in 83 standard bags. Our data showed significantly deficient CFU-GM and BFU-E recoveries (47 ± 31 percent and 31 ± 30 percent, respectively) in ampoules when compared to bags (72 ± 22 percent and 64 ± 19 percent, respectively; $P < .001$). Moreover, a good progenitor cell recovery (more than 50 percent) was observed in only 46 percent of frozen ampoules versus 100 percent in frozen bags ($P < .05$). We were able to relate this nonoptimal recovery to an excessively rapid freezing rate of $-9°C$ per minute following the release of fusion heat which occurred in ampoules, while the freezing rate was constantly maintained at $-2°C$ per minute in the corresponding bags (Fig. 9–5). We concluded that the cooling conditions have to be carefully controlled to ensure that the bags and ampoules are both cooled under the same conditions. Otherwise, ampoules would not be a reliable indicator of the true progenitor cells' cryopreservation efficiency in bags.

Therefore, when using bags, there is no better way to test the cryopreservation efficiency than to use a bag of marrow as a probe.[64]

Influence of Red Cells or Red Blood Cell Hemolysate on Cryopreservation

By uptake of tritiated thymidine, Pyle and Boyer[65] showed a rejuvenating effect of fresh red blood cells when added to thawed marrow. Red blood cell hemolysate also increases CFU-GM growth.[66,67] Therefore, it is conceivable that, when freezing total nonfractionated marrow, the presence of red blood cells is favorable.

Table 9–2 summarizes the requirements for effective cryopreservation of human bone marrow.

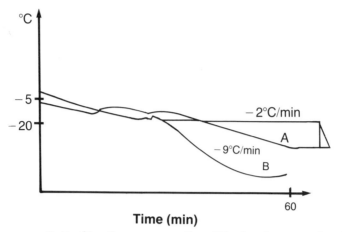

FIGURE 9–5 Simultaneous recording of the freezing curves in a bag of marrow (*A*) and in the corresponding ampoule (*B*). The cooling rate after the release of fusion heat ($\Delta\theta = \theta/t$) was calculated in the space defined by a horizontal line through the point where the release of fusion heat begins and a second horizontal line 13.5°C lower. (From Douay, L,[64] 1986, with permission.)

ATTEMPTS TO SIMPLIFY FREEZING OF NORMAL STEM CELLS: MECHANICAL FREEZING

Despite the numerous preclinical experiments in favor of controlled-rate freezing, several teams have investigated the possibility of freezing marrow without costly programmed equipment, and some have apparently been suc-

Table 9–2 REQUIREMENTS FOR EFFECTIVE CRYOPRESERVATION OF HUMAN BONE MARROW

Freezing Procedure
Low cellular concentration
Cryoprotective agent to reduce the solution effects
Slow cooling rate (−1 to −3°C per minute), constant before and after the transition phase
No lag in the cooling curve (increased nitrogen release to compensate for the heat of fusion) and no acceleration in the freezing rate after the heat of fusion
Use of bags containing no lipophilic plasticizer: polyolefin or Teflon-Kapton
Each bag should be squeezed between two flat aluminum plates so that a thin monolayer preparation is obtained and uniform freezing occurs
Tubes should not be used as probes to test freezing and cryopreservation efficiency in bags

Storage
Storage should be done at the lowest and steadiest available temperature with a constant recording to detect any accidental warming.

Thawing
Very rapid warming should be used to avoid growth of small ice crystals by the process of recrystallization (above −50°C)
The slow stepwise dilution technique is not essential, prior to autografting
Thawed cells are fragile and should not be manipulated prior to infusion
Thawed cells should be infused through a central venous line within less than 15 minutes to avoid toxicity from DMSO.

cessful. Stiff and colleagues have used a mixture of DMSO, HES, and human albumin at final concentrations of 5, 6, and 4 percent, respectively, to freeze marrow by immersion into a $-80°C$ freezer until the time of reinfusion. These authors have reported percentage recoveries as high as 82 and 90 percent, respectively, for CFU-GM and BFU-E, further confirmed by successful engraftment in a series of 60 patients undergoing 72 transplants.[68] This technique has been further adapted with success by others[69] and, more specifically, the comparison of several freezing media combining DMSO and HES has been in favor of the 5 percent DMSO plus 6 percent HES (final) suggested initially by Makino and associates.[70] When recording temperature in the samples of marrow subjected to mechanical freezing, both the freezing rates in the pretransition and in the post-transition periods remain in the range of the rates usually achieved by controlled freezers. Also, with a few exceptions (which mainly concern large samples of marrow in bags) the duration of the transition phase is reduced to a minimum.[71] Therefore, whereas an interesting consequence of mechanical freezing may be to avoid the use of possibly unnecessarily costly devices, it does not negate the general principles of cryopreservation outlined earlier—namely, and essentially, the need for cryoprotective agents, slow freezing rates, and short transition phases (although this last point is still under investigation).

INCREASED CRYOSENSITIVITY OF CLONOGENIC LEUKEMIC CELLS

Although the problem has been ignored for many years, it now appears that CML stem cells and CFU-GM on the one hand and AML-CFU both in the brown Norway rat leukemia model[72] and in human AML on the other hand express an increased sensitivity to cryopreservation when optimal techniques for normal hematopoietic stem cells, as described earlier, are used.

For chronic myelocytic leukemia, our attention was initially attracted by two observations. First, in our series of more than 100 ABMTs, most failures of engraftment, either partial or total, occurred, with a high rate (7 of 14), in patients with CML receiving marrow stem cells.[73] Second, in a patient in acute transformation treated by high-dose chemotherapy and total body irradiation followed by ABMT with marrow stem cells collected at a time when a mosaicism was detected (50 percent Ph chromosome), not only did the cytogenetic marker of the transformation disappear but so did the Ph chromosome. We hypothesized that CML stem cells bearing the Ph chromosome were more sensitive to cryoinjury favoring engraftment of Ph$^-$ stem cells.[74] We studied 41 bags of frozen marrows from 25 patients with CML and indeed found an overall cryopreservation recovery deficiency[23] with a mean of CFU-GM recovery of 55 $\pm$ 38 percent only, versus 73 $\pm$ 19 percent in a control group of patients with other malignancies ($P < .01$). Our data also showed an inverse linear relationship (n $= -.40$; $P < .05$) between CFU-GM concentration and recovery after freezing. A good CFU-GM recovery (at least 50 percent) was observed in 70 percent of cases when the concentrations were less than 6500 CFU-GM per mL as compared with 30 percent only when the concentration was more than 6500 CFU-GM per mL ($P < .01$).

We failed to improve the recovery by diluting marrows when necessary to reduce the concentration below this threshold. There was no relation between the freezing recovery and the nucleated cell concentration. These results suggest a particular fragility of CML stem cells to freezing, probably related to their excessive amplification. Our clinical and laboratory observations are consistent with the experiences of others.

Finally, relevant to the specific problem of CML stem cells is that busulfan is highly toxic for cells in G_o, which are more sensitive to freezing.[75,76] Norman and associates[77] have shown a decreased level of CFU-GM in the peripheral blood and a lowered rate of recovery after freezing when the patients were treated with high cumulative doses of busulfan (greater than 768 mg) and the marrow collected too soon after discontinuation of the drug (fewer than 42 days).

We recently investigated cryopreservation efficiency for human AML-CFU.[24] We selected six freezing techniques that vary with respect to different parameters in order to compare the cryopreservation rate of normal progenitors (CFU-GM and BFU-E) and leukemic clonogenic cells (AML-CFU). Eleven patients with AML were studied at diagnosis to settle the AML-CFU colony assay conditions. Five of these patients entered the study for AML-CFU recovery after cryopreservation. Normal hematopoietic progenitor cell recovery (CFU-GM and BFU-E) was evaluated in five normal donors for allogeneic bone marrow transplantation. Six freezing techniques from five different institutions were used. Freezing vials were cryopreserved directly at $-80°C$ or by a programmed freezing technique (Nicool ST 20 or Minicool LCD 40) with a cooling rate of $-2°C$ per minute. Each specimen was rapidly thawed in a waterbath at $37°C$ and instantly diluted in nine volumes of the corresponding thawing solution, to reduce to 1 percent the concentration of DMSO, thus avoiding cell toxicity. Samples were washed once and resuspended in 10 percent FCS-containing medium. Cells were immediately prepared for in vitro cultures: CFU-GM, BFU-E, or AML-CFU. Recoveries from frozen samples (CFU-GM, BFU-E, AML-CFU) were compared with fresh sample growth and expressed in terms of percentage. The median CFU-GM and BFU-E recoveries using the six different techniques were 47 percent (27 to 76 percent) and 40 percent (34 to 50 percent), respectively. In spite of a good cell viability after thawing, the median absolute recovery of AML-CFU was only 0.5 percent (0.02 to 2.6 percent). On the whole, the AML-CFU recovery was significantly lower than that of normal progenitors CFU-GM and BFU-E ($P < .05$).

These results suggest an intrinsic defect of leukemic progenitors, with increased sensitivity to cryoinjury. These data are similar to those we reported earlier on failure of bone marrow cryopreservation in patients with chronic myelogenous leukemia, but in this study any influence of previous therapy was excluded, as all experiments were performed before therapy. This particular sensitivity of leukemic cells suggests a possible purging effect of cryopreservation in those with AML in complete remission, even in the absence of any in vitro purging method per se.

CONCLUSIONS AND GUIDELINES

Stem cell cryopreservation is a very widely used technique; because of this, it is somehow considered as routine. Furthermore, recent attempts at simplification, mainly by omitting programmed freezing, may place even greater and more dangerous limits on quality control. We propose, in conclusion, our own guidelines used in our department at Hôpital Saint-Antoine, Paris, which can be summarized as follows:

1. Inappropriate freezing of stem cells can lead directly or indirectly to cell death.

2. There may be a minimum dose of stem cells to infuse for successful engraftment. Evaluated prior to freezing and in the absence of purging, this dose is approximately 10^4 CFU-GM per kg for marrow and 10^5 CFU-GM per kg for peripheral blood stem cells.

3. Each freezing procedure must be directly supervised by a trained technician. In particular, we always record the temperature both in the marrow sample and in the freezing chamber.

4. With or without a programmed freezer, the background rules for freezing, storage, and thawing are the same.

5. A cryopreservation test may be useful in making the decision to autograft. Recovery of CFU-GM in cryopreserved marrow reflects the quality of the stem cell pool and may predict engraftment. A CFU-GM percentage recovery of at least 50 percent reflects good quality control. Recoveries of less than 50 percent may indicate the necessity for a second marrow collection and cryopreservation. Test tubes may not be adequate indicators for bags.

6. There is an individual sensitivity to cryopreservation, as indicated by the correlation between several CFU-GM cryopreservation efficiency determinations in the same individual. This may also be related in part to the underlying disease or the chemotherapy regimens previously given, or both.

7. Purging with mafosfamide or 4-hydroperoxycyclophosphamide (4-HC) increases the cryosensitivity.

8. Cryosensitivity of CFU-GM is higher for AML than for ALL, lymphomas, and solid tumors.

9. The maximum risk of failure or delay of engraftment exists with AML and marrow purged with mafosfamide or 4-HC, for which quality control criteria must be carefully evaluated. These may include short-term liquid cultures to assess the repopulating potential of purged marrow.

10. A permanent recording of the temperature in the storage chamber is mandatory to detect any unexpected transient warming that could destroy the stem cells.

11. Thawed bone marrow should be infused rapidly within 10 minutes through a central venous line.

REFERENCES

1. Polge, C, Smith, AU, and Parkes, AS: Revival of spermatozoa after vitrification and dehydration at low temperatures. Nature 164:666, 1949.
2. Barnes, DWH and Loutit, JF: The radiation recovery factor: Preservation by the Polge-Smith-Parkes technique. J Nat Cancer Inst 15:901, 1955.
3. Lovelock, JE and Bishop, MWH: Prevention of freezing damage to living cells by Dimethyl-sulfoxide. Nature 183:1394, 1959.

4. Leibo, SP, et al: Effects of freezing on marrow stem cell suspensions: Interactions of cooling and warming rates in the presence of PVP, sucrose or glycerol. Cryobiology 6:315, 1970.

5. Ashwood-Smith, MJ: Preservation of mouse bone marrow at −79°C with Dimethyl-sulfoxide. Nature 190:1204, 1961.

6. Smith, LH and Phan, TT: Long term preservation of bone marrow. Nature 205:503, 1965.

7. Cavins, JA, et al: Recovery of lethally irradiated dogs following infusion of autologous marrow stored at low temperature in Dimethyl-sulfoxide. Blood 20:730, 1962.

8. Gorin, NC, et al: Long term preservation of bone marrow and stem cell pool in dogs. Blood 51:257, 1978.

9. Appelbaum, FR, et al: Study of cell dose and storage time on engraftment of cryopreserved autologous bone marrow in a canine model. Transplantation 26:245, 1978.

10. Storb, R, et al: Transplantation of allogeneic canine bone marrow stored at −80°C in Dimethyl-sulfoxide. Blood 33:918, 1969.

11. Buckner, CD, et al: Low temperature preservation of monkey marrow in Dimethyl-sulfoxide. Cryobiology 7:136, 1970.

12. Schaefer, UW, Dicke, KA, and Van Bekkum, DW: Recovery of haemopoiesis in lethally irradiated monkeys by frozen allogeneic bone marrow grafts. Revue Europeenne d'Etudes Cliniques et Biologiques 17:483, 1972.

13. Merritt, CB, et al: Rescue of rhesus monkeys from acute lethal graft versus host disease using Cyclophosphamide and frozen autologous bone marrow. Transplantation 15:154, 1973.

14. Meryman, HT: Mechanics of freezing in living cells and tissues. Science 124:515, 1956.

15. Meryman, HT: Preservation of living cells. Fed Proc 22:81, 1963.

16. Rowe, AW: Biochemical aspect of cryoprotective agents in freezing and thawing. Cryobiology 3:12, 1966.

17. Meryman, HT: Cryoprotective agents. Cryobiology 8:173, 1971.

18. Abrahams, S, et al: Assessment of viability of frozen bone marrow cells using a cell culture method. Cell Tissue Kinet 1:255, 1968.

19. Gray, JL and Robinson, WA: In vitro colony formation by human bone marrow cells after freezing. J Lab Clin Med 31:317, 1973.

20. Pegg, DE: Long term preservation of cells and tissues: A review. J Clin Pathol 29:271, 1976.

21. Douay, L, Gorin, NC, and Lemarie, E: Recovery of CFUGM in cryopreserved marrow and in vivo evaluation after autologous bone marrow transplantation are predictive of engraftment. Exp Hematol 14:358, 1986.

22. Douay, L, et al: Asta Z 7557 (INN Mafosfamide) for the in vitro treatment of human leukemia bone marrow. Invest New Drugs 2:187, 1984.

23. Douay, L, Gorin, NC, and Lopez, M: Failure of bone marrow cryopreservation in chronic granulocytic leukaemia: Relation to excessive granulo-macrophagic progenitor pool. Int J Cell Cloning 4:250, 1986.

24. Allieri, MA, et al: Establishment of an AML-CFU colony assay to evaluate the sensitivity of leukemic progenitors to cryopreservation: Incidence for bone marrow transplantation. Exp Hematol Today, Springer-Verlag, New-York, 1989, pp 69–71.

25. Kurnick, NB, et al: Preliminary observations and the treatment of post irradition haematopoietic depression in man by the infusion of stored autogenous bone marrow. Ann Intern Med 49:969, 1958.

26. Newton, KA, et al: Total thoracic supervoltage irradiation followed by the intravenous infusion of stored autogenous marrow. Br Med J 1:531, 1959.

27. McFarland, WF, Granville, NB, and Dameshek, W: Autologous bone marrow infusion as an adjunct in therapy of malignant disease. Blood 14:503, 1959.

28. McGovern, JJ, et al: Treatment of terminal leukemic relapse by total body irradiation and intravenous infusion of stored autologous bone marrow obtained during remission. New Engl J Med 260:675, 1959.

29. Malinin, TI, et al: Peripheral leukocyte infusion into lethally irradiated guinea pigs. Blood 25:693, 1965.

30. Debelak-Fehir, KM and Epstein, RB: Restoration of hematopoiesis in dogs by infusion of cryopreserved autologous peripheral white cells following Busulfan-Cyclophosphamide treatment. Transplantation 20:63, 1975.

31. Calvo, W, et al: Regeneration of blood forming organs after autologous leukocyte transfusion in lethally irradiated dogs. II. Distribution and cellularity of the marrow in irradiated and transfused animals. Blood 47:593, 1976.

32. Storb, R, et al: Demonstration of hemopoietic stem cells in the peripheral blood of baboons by cross circulation. Blood 50:537, 1977.

33. Goldman, JM, et al: Haematological reconstitution after autografting for chronic granulocytic leukaemia in transformation. The influence of previous splenectomy. Br J Haematol 45:223, 1980.

34. Juttner, CA, et al: Circulating autologous stem cells collected in very early remission from acute nonlymphoblastic leukaemia produce prompt but incomplete haemopoietic reconstitution after high dose Melphalan or supralethal chemoradiotherapy. Br J Haematol 61:739, 1985.

35. Reiffers, J, et al: Hematopoietic reconstitution after autologous blood stem cell transplantation: A report of 46 cases. Plasma Therapy and Transfusion Technology 8:360, 1987.

36. Laporte, JP, et al: A relapse after autografting with peripheral blood stem cells [letter]. Lancet 2:1393, 1987.

37. Areman, EM, Sacher, RA, and Deeg, HJ: Processing and storage of human bone marrow: A survey of current practices. Bone Marrow Transplant 6:203, 1990.

38. Rapport annuel France Autogreffe. In preparation.

39. Aird, W, et al: Long term cryopreservation of human bone marrow. Blood 76 (Suppl 1):525a, 1990.

40. Armitage, J and Gorin, NC: Trends in autologous bone marrow transplantation: Results of the 2nd survey of ABMTR. In preparation.

41. Gorin, NC, Gale, RP, and Armitage, J: Autologous bone marrow transplants: Different indications in Europe and North America. Lancet 2:317, 1989.

42. Bone marrow autotransplantation in man: Report of an international cooperative study. Lancet 2:960, 1986.

43. Lyons, JM: Phase transitions and control of cellular metabolism at low temperatures. Cryobiology 9:341, 1972.

44. Van Den Berg, L and Rose, D: Effect of freezing on the pH and composition of sodium and potassium phosphate solutions. Arch Biochem 81:319, 1959.

45. Lovelock, JE: Haemolysis by thermal shock. Br J Haematol 1:117, 1955.

46. Burnett, AK, et al: Haematological reconstitution following high dose supralethal chemoradiotherapy using stored non cryopreserved autologous bone marrow. Br J Hematol 54:309, 1982.

47. Lovelock, JE: The mechanism of the protective action of glycerol against haemolysis by freezing and thawing. Biochem Biophys Acta 2:28, 1953.

48. Sherman, JK and Liu, KC: Relation of ice formation to ultrastructural cryoinjury and cryoprotection of rough endoplasmic reticulum. Cryobiology 13:599, 1976.

49. Rowe, AW and Rinfret, AP: Controlled rate freezing of bone marrow. Blood 20:636, 1962.

50. Lewis, JP, Passovoy, M, and Trobaugh, FE: The effect of cooling regimens on the transplantation potential of marrow. Transfusion 7:17, 1967.

51. Kubota, S, et al: The effect of freeze rate, duration of phase transition and warming rate on survival of frozen canine kidneys. Cryobiology 13:455, 1976.

52. Foreman, J and Pegg, DE: Cell preservation in a programmed cooling machine: The effect of variations in supercooling. Cryobiology 16:315, 1979.

53. Gorin, NC, et al: Delayed kinetics of recovery of haematopoiesis following autologous bone marrow transplantation. The role of excessively rapid marrow freezing rates after the release of fusion heat. Eur J Cancer Clin Oncol 19:485, 1983.

54. Malinin, TI, et al: Long term storage of bone marrow cells liquid nitrogen and dry ice temperature. Cryobiology 7:65, 1970.

55. O'Grady, LF and Lewis, JP: The long term preservation of bone marrow. Transfusion 12:312, 1972.

56. Ashwood-Smith, MJ and Friedman, GB: Lethal and chromosomal effects of freezing, thawing, storage time, and X irradiation on mammilian cells preserved at $-196°C$ in DMSO. Cryobiology 16:132, 1979.

57. Mazur, P: Theoretical and experimental effects of cooling and warming velocity on the survival of frozen and thawed cells. Cryobiology 2:181, 1966.

58. Ashwood-Smith, MJ: The preservation of bone marrow. Cryobiology 1:61, 1964.

59. Ragab, AH, Gilkerson, E, and Choi, SC: The cryopreservation of colony forming cells from the bone marrow of children with acute lymphocytic leukaemia. Cancer Res 34:942, 1974.

60. Douay, L, et al: Study of granulocyte-macrophage progenitor (CFUc) preservation after slow freezing of bone marrow in the gas phase of liquid nitrogen. Exp Hematol 10:360, 1982.

61. Grill, G, Porcellini, A, and Lucarelli, G: Role of serum cryopreservation and subsequent viability of mouse bone marrow hemopoietic stem cells. Cryobiology 17:516, 1980.

62. Nei, T: Effect of initial cell concentration on the post thaw hemolysis of frozen erythrocytes. Cryobiology 13:651, 1976.

63. Kim, BK and Baldini, MG: Preservation of viable platelets by freezing. Effect of plastic containers. Proc Exp Biol Med 142:845, 1973.

64. Douay, L, Lopez, M, and Gorin, NC: A technical bias: Differences in cooling rates prevent ampoules from being a reliable index of stem cell cryopreservation in large volumes. Cryobiology 23:296, 1986.

65. Pyle, HM and Boyer, HF: Factors influencing the post storage viability of human bone marrow. Ann NY Acad Sci 114:686, 1964.

66. Bradley, TR, Telfer, PA, and Fry, P: The effect of erythrocytes on mouse bone marrow colony development in vitro. Blood 38:353, 1971.

67. Rothmann, J, Hertogs, CF, and Pluznik, DH: Growth enhancement and serum replacement in cloning of murine mastocytoma and granulocyte-macrophage precursor cells: Two distinct activities present in hemolysates. Exp Hematol 7:352, 1979.

68. Stiff, J, et al: Autologous bone marrow transplantation using unfractionated cells cryopreserved in dimethylsulfoxide and hydroxyethylstarch without controlled rat freezing. Blood 70:974, 1987.

69. Gulati, S, et al: Cryopreserving stem cells without controlled rate freezing the fifth international symposium on autologous bone marrow transplantation (abstr). Omaha, NE, August 1990.

70. Makino, S, et al: A simplified method for cryopreservation of peripheral blood stem cells at $-80°C$ without rate controlled freezing. Bone Marrow Transplant 8:239, 1991.

71. Clark, J, Pati, A, and McCarthy, D: Successful cryopreservation of human bone marrow does not require a controlled rate freezer. Bone Marrow Transplant 7:121, 1991.

72. Hagenbeek, A and Martens, ACM: Cryopreservation of autologous marrow grafts in acute leukemia: Survival of in vivo clonogenic leukemic cells and normal hemopoietic stem cells. Leukemia 3:535, 1989.

73. Lemonnier, MP, et al: Autologous marrow transplantation for patients with chronic myeloid leukemia in accelerated or blastic phase: Report of 14 cases. Exp Haematol 14:654, 1986.

74. Gorin, NC, et al: Disappearance of Philadelphia chromosome after autologous bone marrows transplantation for treatment of chronic myeloid leukaemia in acute crisis (letter). Lancet 1:44, 1982.

75. Dunn, CDR: The chemical and biological properties of Busulfan. Exp Hematol 2:101, 1974.

76. Frim, J, et al: Survival of unprotected mammalian plateau phase cells following freezing in liquid nitrogen. Cryobiology 13:475, 1976.

77. Norman, JE, et al: Collection and cryopreservation of peripheral blood progenitor cells in chronic granulocytic leukemia. A comparison of treated and untreated patients. Pathology 13:609, 1981.

CONTROLLED-RATE FREEZING

CRYOPRESERVATION OF AUTOGRAFTS USING DELMED FREEZING BAGS

DESCRIPTION	Patients with cancer, who are at high risk of relapse or who have failed conventional chemotherapy regimens, may have the option of an autologous bone marrow harvest if their marrow is free of disease or if the marrow can be purged in vitro with drugs or monoclonal antibodies to eliminate residual tumor cells. The harvested marrow is cryopreserved and stored.
TIME FOR PROCEDURE	2 hours (steps 4 through 8 of summary)
SUMMARY OF PROCEDURE	1. Harvested bone marrow is delivered to the laboratory in one transfer bag. Samples are taken for a nucleated count, hematocrit (Hct), and microbiologic cultures.
	2. Volume is reduced and red cells are depleted in one of two ways (method is determined by Hct and total marrow volume): concentration protocol or Ficoll-Hypaque protocol of the Haemonetics model V-50.
	3. Platelets are depleted by centrifuging at 900 rpm for 10 minutes with no brake. The platelet-rich supernatants are discarded.
	4. The bone marrow pellets are combined and dispensed into a bone marrow freezing bag. A sample of this bulk bone marrow is taken to put over Ficoll-Hypaque.
	5. Freezing solutions are made and cooled on ice.
	6. Freezing solution is added to bulk bone marrow and to the Ficoll-Hypaqued sample.
	7. Marrow is cryopreserved in a programmable freezer at a controlled freezing rate.
	8. Cryopreserved marrow is placed in a cryostorage tank.
	9. Colony-forming assays are performed on the bulk and post–Ficoll-Hypaque samples.
EQUIPMENT	1. Laminar air flow hood
	2. Planar biomed programmable freezer (Kryo 10) or equivalent
	3. Taylor Wharton 27K cryostorage system with M300 controller or equivalent
SUPPLIES AND REAGENTS	1. Two Delmed blood freezing bags (style 2030-2)
	2. 2 boxes (4 sets) of Fenwal plasma transfer sets with coupler and needle adapter (4C2240)
	3. 60- and 35-mL syringes
	4. 2 three-way stopcocks
	5. Two 20-gauge $\times$ 1½-inch needles
	6. 250-mL conical centrifuge tube

7. Two 50-mL conical centrifuge tubes

8. 1-, 5-, and 10-mL pipettes

9. Freezing cassettes (usually two)

10. Hank's balanced salt solution (HBSS) without bicarbonate, calcium, or magnesium salts (Hank's 1×)

11. Dimethyl sulfoxide (DMSO)—CryoServ from Research Industries (Rimso 100)

12. Type-specific fresh frozen plasma (FFP) (blood bank)

13. Preservative-free heparin (5 U per mL final concentration)

PROCEDURE

1. After red cell and platelet depletion transfer marrow into a 250-mL conical centrifuge tube. Sterilely dispense marrow into a freezing bag as follows:

   A. Attach the coupler end of a plasma transfer set to a freezing bag. Attach a three-way stopcock to the needle adapter end of the plasma transfer set along with a 60-mL syringe and a needle (see Fig. 9–6). Remove the barrel of the syringe and close the valve on the plasma transfer tube.

   B. Pour the marrow into the syringe and measure the volume. Open the three-way stopcock to the bag and let the marrow flow into the bag. Take a marrow sample for a cell count and determine the total number of cells to be frozen and the number of cells per kilogram of patient's weight. Take 3×10^6 cells for CFU-GM assay. The normal volume of marrow for an adult is 120 mL; the minimum for a child is 50 mL. The marrow volume is adjusted with HBSS plus heparin (5 U per mL). Place marrow bag in ice.

   C. Take 10 mL of marrow from bag and separate over Ficoll-Hypaque. These cells are to be frozen as mononuclear cells and to set up CFU-GM assays.

2. PREPARE FREEZING SOLUTION AS FOLLOWS

   A. For the bulk marrow, obtain the patient's type-specific FFP, or autologous plasma if available, from the blood bank. In a 250-mL conical centrifuge tube, mix a solution of 50 percent FFP, 20 percent DMSO, and 30 percent HBSS without Ca^{2+} or Mg^{2+} plus heparin (i.e., for 120-mL volume, use 60 mL FFP, 24 mL DMSO, 36 mL HBSS and heparin). Add FFP and HBSS and heparin to the conical tube, and put on ice until it is cold. Add DMSO over 5 minutes to the ice-cold 50 percent FFP plus 30 percent HBSS and heparin. Keep conical tube on ice until ready for use.

   B. For the post–Ficoll-Hypaque cells, make 10 mL of a 20 percent DMSO solution (2 mL of DMSO plus 8 mL HBSS and heparin). Add DMSO dropwise to cold HBSS and heparin. Keep on ice until ready to use.

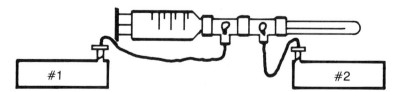

FIGURE 9–6 Diagram showing sterile dispensing of marrow into freezing bag from syringe.

3. START THE PROGRAMMABLE FREEZER
    A. Close the freezer lid.
    B. Open the safety release valve on the delivery pump (heating coil); attach the heating coil to the dewar filled with liquid nitrogen. Close the safety release valve.
    C. Turn on main power switch (make sure the auto/manual switch is on auto).
    D. Pressurize the dewar by turning on the switch on the roller platform under the dewar. The light on the roller platform goes out when the tank is fully pressurized (between 0.25 and 0.050 lb).
    E. Turn the keyswitch to READ to check the program, which is as follows:
- Ramp 1: The temperature decreases at $-1°C$ per minute until a temperature of $+4°C$ is reached.
- Ramp 2: The temperature rate is held at 0.00 (so temperature in chamber remains at $+4°C$) for 30 minutes (program temperature $+0.30°C$).
- Ramp 3: The temperature rate decreases at $-1°C$ per minute until a temperature of $-40°C$ is reached (program temperature $-40°C$).
- Ramp 4: The temperature rate decreases at $-12°C$ per minute to a temperature of $-120°C$ (program temperature $-120°C$).
- Ramp 5: Recycle.

    F. Turn on power to chart recorder and chart paper.
    G. Turn keyswitch to RUN; program number 1 flashes; press SELECT TO TEMPERATURE function and enter $4°C$ by pressing digit button to $+4°C$.
    H. Press START button; program will go to ramp 2; temperature in chamber will go to $+4°C$ and hold there for 30 minutes. (Press SELECT button to TIME function to see how much time is left; you can speed up or hold using FAST RUN switch).

4. After the post–Ficoll-Hypaque cells are washed and counted, add the freezing solutions to the bone marrow. This is best accomplished by two technicians.
    A. Everything is ice cold and the freezing solutions must be added to the cells while the cells are on ice.
    B. One technician adds the freezing solution to the bulk marrow in the freezing bag over 10 minutes' time (if 120 mL is to be added, add 12 mL per minute). Use the 60-mL syringe graduations to measure.
    C. The other technician adds an equal volume of 20 percent DMSO to the post–Ficoll-Hypaque cells. This is done over 10 minutes also.
       (1) Dispense the post–Ficoll-Hypaque cells into sterile freezing vials 1 mL per vial.
       (2) Cap the vials and keep on ice or in the planar freezer at $4°C$ until the bulk marrow bags are ready.

5. Bulk marrow is dispensed into two freezing bags:
    A. Attach a plasma transfer tube and a three-way stopcock to the second freezing bag. Attach in tandem with the freezing bag containing the bulk marrow as follows:
    B. Transfer one-half the volume of bulk marrow–DMSO to the second freezing bag by pulling up with a syringe and manipulating the stopcocks (see Fig. 9–6).

    C. Take 4 to 5 mL from one of the bulk marrow freezing bags and add this to some freezing vials (1 mL per vial).

    D. Remove the plasma transfer tubing from the freezing bags. Reattach two new plasma transfer tubes to the bags using the smaller ends (the end without the wide spikes).

    E. Express air from the freezing bags and tie or clamp off so bag is sealed. Dry the bags and put into cold freezing cassettes.

6. Put the vials and cassettes into the programmable freezer being held at 4°C. Press the select button to time function to see how much time is left in 30-minute hold. Three to 4 minutes should be left to let chamber cool down to 4°C again.

7. Program then automatically goes to ramp 3 and the temperature in the freezing chamber decreases at −1°C per minute to −40°C. Program then automatically goes to ramp 4 and the temperature decreases at −12°C per minute to −120°C, at which point an alarm sounds. Program will hold at this temperature for as long as there is a nitrogen supply.

8. Turn off the main power and remove the frozen cassettes and vials. Place frozen marrow immediately into a liquid nitrogen storage tank (we use vapor phase).

9. Turn on main power; replace lid and turn on manual heat to warm up chamber; turn keyswitch to READ.

10. Open safety release valve on heating coil in dewar and let the pressure fall to 0 before removing the heating coil. Store heating coil upright so condensation will drop away from coil head.

11. When chamber temperature reaches +20°C, turn keyswitch to OFF; return manual heat switch to AUTO position. Turn off chart recorder and main power.

12. Set up colony-forming assays on bulk and post–Ficoll-Hypaque marrow samples.

ANTICIPATED RESULTS

We find it is optimal to freeze marrow at a final concentration (in bag or vials) of 2×10^7 to 1×10^8 per mL. We like to have a minimum of 1×10^8 bone marrow cells per kg to freeze.

NOTES

We freeze patient marrow in at least two freezing bags with a minimum volume of 50 mL per bag, and not more than 125 mL per bag. If more than two freezing bags are needed, just attach more stopcocks and bags in sequence. The heat of fusion (while marrow is being frozen) should occur below 0°C.

AUTHORS

Roy S. Weiner, M.D.
University of Florida
Gainesville, FL 32610

Mary Ann Gross, M.T.(ASCP)
Shands Hospital
University of Florida
Gainesville, FL 32610

REFERENCES

1. Weiner, RS, Tobias, JS, and Yankee, RA: The processing of human bone marrow for cryo preservation and infusion. Biomedicine 24:226, 1976.
2. Weiner, RS: Cryopreservation of lymphocytes for use in in vitro assays of cellular immunity. J Immunol Methods 10:49, 1976.
3. Weiner, RS, Richman, CM, and Yankee, RA: Dilution techniques for optimum recovery of cryopreserved bone marrow cells. Exp Hematol 7:1, 1979.
4. Parker, LM, et al: Prolonged cryopreservation of human bone marrow. Transplantation 31:454, 1981.

CRYOPRESERVATION OF BONE MARROW IN GAMBRO FREEZING BAGS

DESCRIPTION	Cryopreserved autologous bone marrow buffy coat can be used for reinfusion to repopulate hematopoietic cells following conditioning therapy for bone marrow transplantation. The buffy coat concentrate is cryopreserved in a programmable controlled-rate freezing unit, in order to obtain maximum viability.
TIME FOR PROCEDURE	Approximately 90 minutes for 250 mL of buffy coat

SUMMARY OF PROCEDURE

1. Bone marrow buffy coat is obtained from harvested bone marrow.
2. Freezing cell count is adjusted with autologous plasma.
3. Freezing solution is prepared with 60 percent tissue culture media, 20 percent dimethyl sulfoxide (DMSO), and 20 percent autologous plasma.
4. Buffy coat and freezing solution are combined in a 1:1 ratio.
5. Cryoprocessor is set up for user-defined program 7.
6. Cryobags are transferred to storage cassettes and stored in a liquid nitrogen freezer at vapor phase.

EQUIPMENT

1. CryoMed 1010A programmable freezing unit
2. Sterilgard hood (Baker Company) or equivalent
3. CryoMed freezer CMS-450A
4. Gambro welding device No. WD2 (Gambro-Hospa Ingstrom)
5. Gambro storage cassettes No. DF200 (CryoMed)
6. Copper plates: 2 plates per set with one cut out for transfusion port of bag; size 22.5 mm $\times$ 15.5 mm $\times$ 1.0 mm
7. 30-mL sterile glass syringe
8. Large binder clips
9. COBE 2991 cell washer (Cobe Laboratories, Lakewood, CO)

SUPPLIES AND REAGENTS

1. Gambro Hemofreeze bag DF200: 1 bag per 25 mL of buffy coat
2. Plasma transfer set with coupler
3. 500-mL sterile evacuated container: 1 bottle per 500 mL (or less) of buffy coat
4. 35-mL sterile syringe
5. Two 60-mL sterile syringes
6. 16-gauge $\times$ 1½-inch needles; 1 needle per Hemofreeze bag
7. Sampling site coupler (Fenwal No. 4C2405); 1 coupler per Hemofreeze bag
8. Three-way stopcock
9. Double female luer-lock adapter
10. Double male luer-lock adapter
11. 12-inch transfer tubing with spike (adapted from Fenwal transfer pack, sterilized in house)
12. Two 2.0-mL cryovials

13. Alcohol swabs
14. 0.22-μm Millipore filter
15. Hi-Low Temperature Labels (Shamrock Specialty Labels)
16. DMSO—sterile, nonpyrogenic (CryoServ Multi-Sample Vial)
17. Tissue culture medium (TC-199) (Gibco No. 320-1151)
18. Autologous plasma
19. Ice bath
20. 70 percent methanol solution

PROCEDURE

1. FREEZING CELL COUNT ADJUSTMENT
   A. The buffy coat cell count is adjusted to $8.0 \pm 2.0 \times 10^7$ cells per mL with autologous plasma.
   B. Calculate the approximate volume of buffy coat to be frozen:

   $$\text{Final volume} = \frac{\text{Total nucleated cell count per total volume}}{8.0 \times 10^7 \text{ cells per mL}}$$

   Round down to the nearest multiple of 25 plus 1 mL.
   C. Add the appropriate volume of plasma.

   $$\text{Volume of plasma} = \text{Final volume} - \text{buffy coat}$$

2. FREEZING SOLUTION PREPARATION
   A. Prepare the volume of freezing solution to the nearest 50 mL in excess of the calculated final volume.
   B. The freezing solution contains:
      60 percent tissue culture media (TC-199)
      20 percent DMSO
      20 percent autologous plasma
   C. In a laminar air flow (LAF) hood, filter the exact amount of TC-199 tissue culture media required through a 0.22-μm Millipore filter.
   D. Add the appropriate volume of autologous plasma to the sterile tissue culture media to make up a 20 percent solution.
   E. Remove the seal from the multisample bottle of sterile DMSO and swab the top with alcohol. Using a glass syringe, transfer the necessary DMSO to make up a 20 percent solution to the sterile tissue culture mixture.
   F. Immediately transfer the freezing solution to the sterile glass evacuated bottle.
      (1) Remove the metal seal from the evacuated bottle and wipe off with alcohol.
      (2) Close the roller clamp on the plasma transfer set and insert into the evacuated bottle, saving the spiked end cover.
      (3) Remove the cover from the coupler end of the plasma transfer set and aseptically insert into the freezing solution.
      (4) Open the roller clamp and allow the freezing solution to be transferred to the glass evacuated bottle. Cap the coupler end and place solution in ice.
   G. Place one set of copper plates into the refrigerator for each bag being frozen.

3. PROCESSING OF BUFFY COAT FOR FREEZING

  A. Turn on the WD2 welding device and the CryoMed 1010A, and adjust the chart baselines accordingly.

  B. Label the Hemofreeze bags and the high-low temperature labels on the storage cassettes.

  C. In a laminar flow hood, aseptically attach a three-way stopcock to the buffy coat bag, using the spiked end connected to a 1-inch segment of rubber tubing.

  D. Attach a 35-mL syringe to the next port.

  E. Attach the spiked transfer tubing to a double male luer-lock adaptor, then to the last port.

  F. Attach the first Hemofreeze bag to the end of the Fenwal tubing attached to the right port.

  G. Gently mix the buffy coat bag, open the stopcock, and aspirate 25 mL of buffy coat. (For the first bag, compensate for the marrow occupying the dead space of the tubing.)

  H. Change the stopcock position and express the buffy coat into the Hemofreeze bag.

   I. Remove the tubing from the Hemofreeze bag, express out the air, and replace the tubing with a sampling site coupler.

   J. Attach the transfer tubing to the next Hemofreeze bag. (Using a scalpel to make an incision into the port will allow you to insert the spike more easily.)

  K. After all the buffy coat is aliquoted, transfer the remaining 1.0 mL of buffy coat to 2 to 2.0 mL cryovials, 0.5 mL of marrow into each.

  L. Remove the freezing solution from the ice bath, rinse bottle off with 70 percent methanol, and hang on the overhead rod in hood.

  M. Attach a double female luer-lock adaptor to the coupler end of the plasma transfer set attached to the freezing solution.

  N. To the female adapter attach a 60-mL syringe.

  O. Release the roller clamp and aspirate 25 mL of the freezing solution, remove syringe, and attach another 60-mL syringe.

  P. Attach a 16-gauge needle to the syringe with the freezing solution.

  Q. Swab the sample site coupler of the first Hemofreeze bag, insert the syringe, and push the freezing solution into the bag while gently swirling the buffy coat.

  R. Double weld the top port and cut off the used port.

  S. Remove two copper plates and four binder clips for each bag.

  T. Dry bag and place between one set of copper plates, secure with the binder clips, and return plates to the refrigerator.

  U. After all the bags are filled, add 0.5 mL of freezing solution to each cryovial; then cap, gently mix, and place in rack in chamber.

  V. After half the bags are loaded into the freezing chamber, insert the plate thermocouple to the center of the next bag.

  W. Select user-defined program 7 and press RUN to initiate the program. When the chamber temperature reaches 0°C, press RUN to advance to the next section of the freezing program (see Table 9–3 for details).

  X. At the end of the last section the alarm will sound; press ALARM RESET.

  Y. When the sample temperature reaches −80°C, press RUN to terminate

Table 9–3 USER-DEFINED
PROGRAM FOR CryoMed 1010A
PROGRAM 7

Section	Rate	Desired Temperature*	Location
1	Wait	0°C	Chamber
2	1°C/min	−6°C	Sample
3	25°C/min	−50°C	Chamber
4	15°C/min	−20°C	Chamber
5	1°C/min	−45°C	Chamber
6	10°C/min	−90°C	Chamber
7	End		

*Transfer bags to liquid nitrogen freezer when the sample
temperature reaches −80°C.

the program. Immediately remove bags, insert into prediluted storage cassettes, and transfer to a liquid nitrogen freezer for storage.
Z. Document storage information on the patient's worksheet.

ANTICIPATED RESULTS	1. Heat of fusion should be released between −6 and −11°C.
	2. Freezing program should take between 1 and 1½ hours to be processed.

NOTES	1. In double sealing the Gambro bag, to ensure a bubble-free seam, reseal over the original seam and hold clamp down for 10 seconds to allow seam to cool and seal.
	2. If cryofreeze bags are moist, when pressed between the copper plates, the bags will stick to the plates when you try to remove them for storage.

AUTHORS	Lorraine Y. Soken, M.T. (ASCP) St. Francis Medical Center Dept. of Pathology Tissue Bank Honolulu, HI 96817

CRYOPRESERVATION OF BONE MARROW IN STANDARDIZED MEDIUM

DESCRIPTION	Bone marrow cells are suspended in a *standardized* medium designed to enhance cell membrane integrity at low temperatures (medium-199 plus 10 percent Plasma-Plex plus 10 percent dimethyl sulfoxide [DMSO]). The cell suspension is frozen at a controlled rate of temperature decline, which compensates for eutectic point transitions (changes in the molecular structure of ice that occur with decreasing temperatures below $-35°C$).
TIME FOR PROCEDURE	Approximately 2 to 3 hours from completion of wash process to completion of freezing procedure
SUMMARY OF PROCEDURE	Processed bone marrow cells are placed in a standardized medium containing medium-199, 10 percent Plasma-Plex, and 10 percent DMSO before being partitioned into four bags each of roughly equal volume. The marrow in these four bags is then frozen in a preprogrammed low-temperature freezer.
SUPPLIES AND REAGENTS	1. DMSO (CryoServ, Research Industries Co., Salt Lake City, UT)
	2. Medium-199 without phenol red (Formula No. 79-04158K, Grand Island Biological Company, Grand Island, NY)
	3. Purified Protein Fraction (PPF) of human plasma (Plasma-Plex, Armour Pharmaceutical Co., Kankakee, IL)
	4. Liquid nitrogen (in low-pressure supply cylinder)
	5. Freezing bags (Fenwal No. 4R2116)
	6. Sterile towels or gauze squares
	7. Sample vials for cryostorage
EQUIPMENT	1. Programmable freezer (CryoMed model 1010, New Baltimore, MI)
	2. Liquid nitrogen storage bank (CryoMed CPII, New Baltimore, MI)
PROCEDURE	1. Prepare a mixture of 10 percent plasma protein fraction in medium-199 (199+PPF).
	2. If the marrow cells are not already suspended in 199+PPF, replace existing medium with 199+PPF. *Use of an automated blood cell washer for this step is recommended.*
	3. Adjust volume of suspended marrow cells to approximately 247 mL.
	4. Remove 1.5 mL of suspended cells and send in an Isolator tube to the microbiology laboratory for culturing. Remove 2 mL of suspended cells and set aside for hematopoietic cell assays. Remove 0.5 mL of suspended cells for counting and differential analysis.
	5. Withdraw an additional 3 mL of marrow cell suspension and aliquot into two cryostorage vials (1.5 mL each). These vials will have DMSO added and will be frozen for any contingency testing that may be required.
	6. Using 60-mL syringes, divide the remaining marrow suspension (about 240 mL) into four equal parts, and inject into freezing bags.
	7. Using waterproof felt-tip marker, clearly label each freezing bag with (a) patient name; (b) patient medical record number; and (c) date marrow

is being frozen. Record the same information on the outside of the metal freezing frames.

8. Place marrow bags, and an extra bag with 199 + PPF (for thermocouple), into an ice bath. Ensure that all bags are well covered with ice. Chill for at least 30 minutes to ensure that the temperature of the cells and surrounding medium has completely dropped to about 0°C.

9. Draw CryoServ into 20-mL syringes equal to 10 percent of bag volume (approximately 6 mL).

10. While allowing marrow to chill, start programmed freezer, and allow chamber temperature to come down to +4°C. To do this:
    A. Turn on freezer.
    B. Using up and down buttons on freezer control panel, set freezer to step 1. 1 (not the same as 1 1, complete program described farther on).
    C. Press SCAN button on freezer control panel.
    D. Press RUN button on freezer control panel.

11. With freezing bags containing marrow still packed in ice, attach syringe with CryoServ to each one. Draw back syringe plunger, removing air from bag, until marrow enters syringe. Push back plunger until fluid-air interface has almost reached bag, and heat seal inlet tube. Repeat for each bag.
    Add 0.15 mL of CryoServ to each of the two vials that have been set aside.

12. Cut all inlet tubes at heat seals.

13. Remove bags from ice, wipe off excess water with sterile towel or gauze. Place bags in metal freezing frames, and place in rack in freezer. Bag with medium only should have thermocouple forced through one of spike ports, and place in special frame in freezer. Place cryostorage vials into freezer.

14. Close freezer, and initiate freezing program by pressing RUN button:

    Freezing program is as follows:

From	To	Rate	Comments
4°C	−10°C	2.0°C/min	Chamber temp, hold for 10 minutes
−10°C	−50°C	25°C/min	Chamber temp, absorbs heat of fusion which is released at approximately −12°C
−50°C	−14°C	15°C/min	Chamber temp, return to approximate sample temp
−14°C	−60°C	1.0°C/min	Sample temp
−60°C	−90°C	5.0°C/min	Sample temp, END of program

15. Transfer frozen cannister, bags, and marrow quickly from programmed freezer into liquid nitrogen storage bank. *Be sure that all cannisters are fully submerged in the liquid nitrogen.*

ANTICIPATED RESULTS   Upon thawing, frozen marrow cells should have a 70 to 90 percent viability. Heat of fusion release should occur at −10°C to −20°C in the freezing process.

NOTES   1. *Because of the adverse effects of DMSO on cells at temperatures above 0°C, steps 11 through 14 must be undertaken with deliberation and speed.*

2. *Extreme care should be exercised when handling the liquid nitrogen. If spilled on skin, liquid nitrogen can cause severe burns.*

3. Following freezing operation, the door to the programmed freezer should be left open to allow the unit to dry. Otherwise, water condensation will collect and eventually cause corrosion or contamination or both.

QUALITY CONTROL

1. A sample of the marrow is held aside before beginning the procedure. From this sample, viable cell counts are performed (trypan blue exclusion test), an eight-part differential analysis is made, and hematopoietic progenitor colony assays are set up. When the marrow is thawed, a sample of the thawed material should be obtained, and comparison with prefreezing established.

2. If microbiologic assays have not been set up before freezing procedure, then both aerobic and anaerobic microbiologic assay vials should be seeded with marrow sample before starting freezing.

3. The programmed freezer generates a strip chart record of chamber temperatures and temperature of the mock sample in the thermocouple bag. This chart should be labeled with the patient identifying information and retained.

AUTHORS

William E. Janssen, Ph.D.
Bone Marrow Processing and
 Evaluation Laboratory
Bone Marrow Transplant Program
H. Lee Moffitt Cancer Center and
 Research Institute
University of South Florida
12902 Magnolia Dr.
Tampa, FL 33612-9497

Carlos E. Lee, M.T.
Bone Marrow Processing and
 Evaluation Laboratory
Bone Marrow Transplant Program
H. Lee Moffitt Cancer Center and
 Research Institute
University of South Florida
12902 Magnolia Dr.
Tampa, FL 33612-9497

REFERENCES

1. Lewis, JP, et al: The effect of cooling regimens on the transplantation potential of marrow. Transfusion 7:17, 1967.
2. Wells, JR, et al: Isolation, cryopreservation, and autotransplantation of human stem cells. Exp Hematol 7(Suppl 5):12, 1979.
3. Ashwood-Smith, HJ: Lack of genetic damage in mammalian cells after cryopreservation at −196°C. Exp Hematol 7(Suppl 5):21, 1979.
4. Robinson, WA, et al: Recovery of CFU-C after freezing of normal and leukemic human bone marrow. Exp Hematol 7(Suppl 5):27, 1979.
5. Hill, RS, et al: The survival of cryopreserved human bone marrow stem cells. Pathology 11:361, 1979.
6. Körbling, M, et al: Description of a closed plastic bag system for the collection and cryopreservation of leukapheresis-derived blood mononuclear leukocytes and CFUc from human donors. Transfusion 20:293, 1980.

CRYOPRESERVATION AND STORAGE OF BONE MARROW CELLS IN FENWAL FREEZING BAGS

DESCRIPTION	Cryopreservation of bone marrow cells is performed using a controlled-rate cell freezer and storage in liquid nitrogen. Separated buffy coat cells, suspended in RPMI-1640 (without phenol red) containing autologous plasma and a cryoprotectant (dimethyl sulfoxide [DMSO]), are cryopreserved in liquid nitrogen at 1°C per minute in a controlled-rate, programmable cell freezer. The frozen bone marrow is stored in a designated location in the liquid nitrogen freezer.
TIME FOR PROCEDURE	2 to 3 hours
SUMMARY OF PROCEDURE	Controlled cooling of bone marrow cells permits preservation and long-term storage of hematopoietic stem cells in the liquid phase of liquid nitrogen (−196°C) without significant loss of viability. Bone marrow cells are mixed with a cryoprotective media that protects the cells from harmful ice formation during the freezing process.
EQUIPMENT	1. Biologic laminar flow hood 2. CryoMed model 990C cell freezer or equivalent 3. CryoMed model 1010 microcomputer programmable cell processor and chart recorder or equivalent 4. Blood bag sealer or metal clips and hand sealer
SUPPLIES AND REAGENTS	1. 60-mL sterile syringes 2. Intralock sterile three-way stopcocks 3. Plasma transfer set, with coupler and needle adapter (Fenwal 4C2240) 4. Fenwal freezing bags (250-mL or 300-mL) 5. Metal-rimmed tags for labeling freezing bags 6. Removable 2- × 2-inch white stickers for labeling 7. Metal freezing plates and large binder clips 8. Liquid nitrogen 9. RPMI-1640 media with L-glutamine, without phenol red 10. DMSO (Research Industries Co., Salt Lake City, UT) 11. Autologous human plasma
PROCEDURE	1. Label four white metal-rimmed tags with the patient's name, collection number, and date. 2. Attach one tag to the bottom of each of four freezing bags. 3. Label each bag with a permanent marking pen with the patient's name, medical record number, date, and collection number. 4. Close all ports of the freezing bags, and remove all caps. 5. Prepare the freezing solution containing 10 percent DMSO and 10 percent patient plasma, as follows: add 20 mL of DMSO to 60 mL of RPMI, mix well and cool, then add 20 mL of patient plasma collected during processing

procedure. Keep mixture cold. This freezing solution may be prepared in advance and kept refrigerated until ready to use.

NOTE: *If the patient's bone marrow cell count exceeds 200,000 per μL, the bone marrow must be diluted accordingly, and more freezing solution will be needed.*

6. Spike the transfer pack containing buffy coat with a plasma transfer set.

7. Attach a three-way stopcock to the needle adapter end of the transfer tubing and attach a 60-mL syringe and extension set to the other two ends of the stopcock.

8. Transfer the freezing solution into the bag of marrow and mix.

9. Replace the extension set site on the three-way stopcock with one of the freezing bags and transfer 50 mL of the marrow mixture into the bag. Repeat this step for the remaining freezing bags.

10. Heat seal the bags as close to the port as possible. Seal twice and cut the remaining tubing off. (Metal clips can be used in place of the heat seal: Using the hand sealer, seal the tubing with the metal clips as close to the port as possible; cut off the remaining tubing.)

11. Each bag should be placed between two metal freezing plates. Use the binder clips to clamp the plates. The side of the bag with the ports should be facing out and at the top of the plates. The clamps should be placed so the bag is uniformly flattened.

12. One bag should have the sample thermocouple of the CryoMed controlled-rate freezer securely taped against the side of the bag before being placed between the freezing plates.

13. Place the plates into the freezer, making sure that the tubing of the ports is not bent. (Bent tubing can cause cracking, resulting in bag failure after freezing.)

14. Close and secure the freezer door.

15. Remove the cap from the pen on the printer and turn the microcomputer on. Push the CHAM key on the TC SCANNER panel and adjust the pen to −180°C on the paper. Push the SAMP key and adjust to 0°C. Repeat pushing the CHAM and SAMP keys until they are aligned properly. With the recorder calibration complete, press the SCAN key and turn the chart drive switch ON.

16. Select either the semiautomated (program 8) or the automated (program 7) freezing program. The programs run in an automated mode, except where noted in the semiautomated program.

17. SEMIAUTOMATED PROGRAM
     The following freezing sequence is used for the semiautomated program:

Prog. No./ Sect. No.	Funct.	Temp./Time	Target Temp.	Probe Mode	Add. Keys
8.1	Wait	0°C	−10°C	Chamber	
8.2	Ramp	1°C/min	−40°C	Sample	COOL+
8.3	Ramp	5°C/min	−60°C	Sample	COOL+
8.4	Ramp	10°C/min	−90°C	Sample	COOL+
8.5	End				

A. Press RUN key and let chamber and sample cool to 0°C. With the WAIT function, the freezer will cool the chamber to the desired target temperature and hold the target temperature indefinitely, unless instructed otherwise.

B. When 0°C is reached, press the RUN key again to advance to section 8.2. Allow cells to reach heat of fusion (temperature at which liquid becomes solid) and press COOL+ key in 20-second bursts to boost the cells through the heat of fusion. Once the sample returns to the heat of fusion temperature, the program will continue in an automatic mode to the end of the program.

18. AUTOMATIC PROGRAM
The following freezing sequence is used for the automatic program:

Prog. No./ Sect. No.	Funct.	Temp./Time	Target Temp.	Probe Mode	Add. Keys
7.1	Ramp	3°C/min	+2°C	Sample	COOL+
7.2	Hold	1 min	+0°C	Chamber	
7.3	Ramp	1.5°C/min	−10°C	Sample	COOL+
7.4	Hold	3 min	−50°C	Chamber	COOL+
7.5	Hold	2 min	−30°C	Chamber	
7.6	Ramp	5°C/min	−60°C	Sample	COOL+
7.8	End				

A. To activate program, press RUN key and the program will enter program section 7.1 and continue until it finishes the program.

19. The alarm will sound, signaling the end of the program. Press the PROG key to shut the freezer off, open the door and take the frozen bone marrow out carefully. Unclamp the plates and remove the thermocouple gently.

20. Place the bone marrow in the appropriate frame and canisters and replace the frame in the liquid nitrogen storage freezer.

21. In this institution, patient labels (name, medical record number, date, collection number) are placed in duplicate freezer inventory/patient log notebooks and on the freezing chart record. The labels are placed in the freezer inventory/patient log notebooks in the position corresponding to the bone marrow position in the liquid nitrogen freezer. The freezing chart is stapled to the back of a completed bone marrow processing report form and becomes a permanent part of patient's record. In addition, the following information is also entered on the Rolodex file card for each patient: freezer number, frame and canister number(s), the total number of bone marrow (BM) nucleated cells, number BM nucleated cells per kg, and number BM nucleated cells per kg per bag.

NOTE: *When the cell count requires further dilution of the buffy coat, additional freezing bags may be required. Do not place more than 100 mL of cell suspension into each freezing bag. Always maintain the appropriate proportions of RPMI, DMSO, and autologous plasma when making the freezing solution. Always mix equal amounts of freezing solution and buffy coat cell suspension.*

NOTES	The patient's bone marrow is stored until needed for transplant. The frozen bone marrow bag is stored in metal canisters to protect against damage to the plastic bag, which becomes brittle at liquid nitrogen temperatures. From the freezing curve, the heat of fusion and the freezing rate can be determined.

QUALITY CONTROL	**CELL FREEZING** A strip chart recording is prepared simultaneously with the freezing of the sample. This recording provides a permanent record of the cell freezing process and is attached to the bone marrow processing record. **CELL STORAGE–LIQUID NITROGEN** The liquid nitrogen storage freezer has an automatic fill for maintaining appropriate levels of liquid nitrogen. If the level of liquid nitrogen falls below its indicated level, or if the storage unit is shut off, a remote alarm should be connected to the blood bank or another location which is staffed 24 hours a day so that the appropriate personnel can be notified at once of a malfunction. Daily records are kept in the bone marrow transplant laboratory of the level of liquid nitrogen in the storage freezer.

AUTHORS	Richard C. Meagher, M.D. James Graham Brown Cancer Center University of Louisville Louisville, KY 40292 Roger H. Herzig, M.D. James Graham Brown Cancer Center University of Louisville Louisville, KY 40292	G. P. Herzig, M.D. Washington University School of Medicine St. Louis, MO 63110

REFERENCES	1. Lovelock, JE and Bishop, MWH: Prevention of freezing damage to living cells by dimethylsulfoxide. Nature 183:1394, 1959. 2. Appelbaum, FR, et al: Study of cell dose and storage time on engraftment of cryopreserved autologous bone marrow in a canine model. Transplantation 26:245, 1978. 3. Ashwood-Smith, MJ: The preservation of bone marrow. Cryobiology 1:61, 1964.

CRYOPRESERVATION OF T-CELL–DEPLETED BONE MARROW

DESCRIPTION	This procedure describes the cryopreservation of bone marrow that has been purged with monoclonal antibodies and complement to reduce the number of mature donor T lymphocytes. T-cell–depleted marrow is resuspended in 5 percent human albumin and then frozen with dimethyl sulfoxide (DMSO) at a final concentration of 10 percent in a programmable freezing chamber at the rate of 1 to 2°C per minute. Marrow is stored in the liquid phase of liquid nitrogen. This procedure is useful to store purged marrow for prolonged periods.
TIME FOR PROCEDURE	Approximately 3 hours
SUMMARY OF PROCEDURE	1. Bone marrow, purged with monoclonal antibodies and complement, is resuspended in 5 percent human albumin to a nucleated cell count of less than 200×10^6 per mL. 2. The purged marrow is transferred to freezing bags. DMSO is added to the marrow for a final concentration of 10 percent. 3. The marrow is frozen in a programmable freezing chamber at 1°C per minute to $-60°C$, then 3°C per minute to $-100°C$. 4. The marrow is stored in the liquid phase of liquid nitrogen.
EQUIPMENT	1. Laminar flow hood 2. Heat sealer 3. Controlled-rate freezer 4. Liquid nitrogen storage container 5. Pipette aid, vacuum pressure 6. Syringe rack (made by University's machine shop)
SUPPLIES AND REAGENTS	1. Minimal essential media (MEM) with Hanks' balanced salt solution and L-glutamine 2. Human serum albumin, 25 percent 3. DMSO 4. Liquid nitrogen 5. Sampling site coupler 6. Plastic pipettes, sterile 7. Syringes: 60-mL 8. Thermocouple bag (Stericon) 9. Freezing bags 10. Freezing canister 11. Sterile flask 12. Ice bucket 13. Cryoprotectant gloves
PROCEDURE	1. PREPARE 5 PERCENT HUMAN ALBUMIN MEDIA: To each of two 100-mL bottles of MEM add 25 mL of 25 percent human albumin. Mix well.

2. RESUSPEND T-CELL–DEPLETED MARROW CELLS IN 5 PERCENT HUMAN ALBUMIN

   A. Harvested bone marrow collected in the operating room using standard procedure is processed by a method using monoclonal antibodies and complement to reduce the number of mature donor T lymphocytes (see Chapter 7). At the completion of the purging procedure the marrow cells are resuspended in 5 percent human albumin media to a volume of 50 mL.

   B. Remove a sample for postprocessing tests: nucleated cell count, differential, and microbiology cultures.

   C. The nucleated cell count should be less than 200×10^6 per mL to freeze. If the nucleated cell count is greater than or equal to 200×10^6 per mL, dilute the T-cell–depleted marrow cells with the 5 percent human albumin media.

3. PREPARE CRYOPROTECTANT (20 PERCENT DMSO SOLUTION)

   A. The volume needed is the total sum of the following:
      (1) The volume of T-cell–depleted marrow
      (2) Half the volume of the thermocouple bag
      (3) Sample for microbiology cultures

   B. The cryoprotectant solution is 60 percent MEM media, 20 percent DMSO, and 20 percent of 5 percent human albumin.
      (1) Place a sterile flask in an ice bath and add the following consecutively:
         (a) MEM media
         (b) DMSO (mix and allow mixture to cool on ice 5 minutes)
         (c) 5 percent human albumin media (mix and keep mixture on ice)

4. PREPARE CONTROLLED-RATE FREEZER

   A. Set controlled-rate freezer program to a starting temperature of 0°C. Freeze at a rate of 1°C per minute to −60°C, then 3°C per minute to −100°C. The phase change begins at −8°C with a phase change chamber temperature drop to −52°C. These settings are approximate and may vary slightly with each freezer.

   B. Turn the controlled-rate freezer on and cool the freezing chamber to 0°C.

5. PREPARE THE THERMOCOUPLE BAG

   A. The final volume of this monitoring bag should be the same as that for the marrow bags being frozen.

   B. Insert sampling site coupler into port. Add half volume of 5 percent human albumin media and half volume of 20 percent DMSO solution.

   C. Heat seal bag just below the fill port. Cut off port. Insert sample thermocoupler into bag. Place bag into canister and set aside.

6. TRANSFER T-CELL–DEPLETED MARROW AND CRYOPROTECTANT TO FREEZING BAGS

   A. Determine the volume of marrow to add to each freezing bag, taking into consideration the following:
      (1) The ratio of marrow to cryoprotectant for each bag will be 1:1.
      (2) The total volume of each bag (marrow plus cryoprotectant) should be 50 mL or less. This allows for the marrow to be thawed in manageable aliquots for easier infusion to recipient.

(3) Allow a small percentage of marrow to be stored in small aliquots to be thawed separately for postcryopreservation tests if desired.

B. Remove plunger from sterile 60-mL syringe. Attach syringe to adaptor of freezing bag. Place inverted syringe on syringe rack to be used as a siphon for marrow and cryoprotectant.

C. Using one 25-mL pipette, transfer marrow to the syringes. Allow marrow to run into the bags.

D. Using a 25-mL pipette, transfer the appropriate amount of cooled 20 percent DMSO solution to two bags at a time. Heat seal bags just below the fill port. Cut off port and tubing. Place bags in canisters. Place canisters into the freezing chamber. Once the DMSO is added to the marrow, the bags must be placed into the freezing chamber quickly. The final concentration of DMSO (10 percent) is toxic to the marrow cells at room temperature. The marrow-DMSO mixture must be lowered to 4°C or less within 15 minutes.

7. FREEZE MARROW

A. Place thermocouple bag into freezing chamber. Adjust controls to scan both chamber and sample temperatures.

B. When the sample and freezing chamber temperatures have stabilized and are approximately equal, adjust controls to start the controlled-rate freezing.

C. Monitor the freezing curve closely. If necessary, the freezing rate may need to be controlled manually.

D. When the sample temperature reaches −100°C, transfer the marrow canisters to storage frames and immerse in liquid nitrogen.

NOTES

1. The marrow is processed and placed into bags using sterile techniques in a laminar flow hood.

2. T-cell–depleted marrow cells tend to clump when resuspended in autologous plasma. The use of 5 percent human albumin for resuspension of T-cell–depleted marrow cells may prevent this phenomenon.

AUTHORS

Marita G. Hill, M.T.(ASCP), S.B.B.
Blood Bank Immunohematologist
University of Kentucky Medical
  Center
Lexington, KY 40536

Vickie M. Robertson, M.T.(ASCP),
  S.B.B.
Blood Bank Bone Marrow
  Coordinator
University of Kentucky Medical
  Center
Lexington, KY 40536

Larry G. Dickson, M.D.
Director, Blood Bank
Clinical Laboratory
University of Kentucky Medical
  Center
Lexington, KY 40536

REFERENCES

1. Thomas, SR: Technique for human marrow grafting. Blood 36:507, 1970.
2. Appelbaum, F, et al: Successful engraftment of cryopreserved autologous bone marrow in patients with malignant lymphoma. Blood 52:85, 1978.

MECHANICAL FREEZING

CRYOPRESERVATION OF BONE MARROW STEM CELLS IN DIMETHYL SULFOXIDE AND HYDROXYETHYL STARCH WITHOUT CONTROLLED-RATE FREEZING

DESCRIPTION	The cryoprotectant combination of dimethyl sulfoxide (DMSO) and hydroxyethyl starch (HES) provides a simplified, inexpensive, rapid, and effective method of bone marrow stem cell cryopreservation. The technique eliminates the time and cost involved with controlled-rate freezing and liquid nitrogen storage.
TIME FOR PROCEDURE	Approximately 60 minutes to process and freeze a typical bone marrow harvest of 1000 mL.
SUMMARY OF PROCEDURE	1. Preparation of cryoprotectant 2. Transfer of RPMI-1640 into evacuated bottle 3. Dilution of buffy coat 4. Cryoprotectant and buffy coat simultaneously added into freezing bags 5. Thawing and reinfusion
EQUIPMENT	1. COBE 2991 cell washer 2. Blood bank freezer at $-80°C$ 3. Blood freezing bag heat sealer
SUPPLIES AND REAGENTS	1. Sterile 500-mL bottle with rubber septum screw cap 2. CharterMed 4403-2 blood freezing bags (triplicate set) 3. Sterile 500-mL bottle of RPMI-1640 without L-glutamine 4. 140 mL sterile Normosol-R in D_5W (Abbott Laboratories) 5. 42 g low molecular weight HES (DuPont Critical Care), average molecular weight, 150,700; requires investigational new drug (IND) from Food and Drug Administration (FDA) 6. 100 mL sterile 25 percent human serum albumin 7. 70 mL 50 percent DMSO (Rimso-50, Research Industries Corp.) 8. 250 mL evacuated bottle (Abbott Laboratories) 9. Sampling site coupler (Fenwal) 10. Four 16-gauge $\times$ 1½-inch hypodermic needles 11. Venting needle 12. 19-gauge $\times$ ⅞-inch butterfly infusion set 13. Three 60-mL disposable syringes 14. Plasma transfer set (Fenwal) 15. 2 CryoMed aluminum freezing frames, 10 $\times$ 11 $\times$ ½ inch (No. BP-2P, CryoMed Inc.)

PROCEDURE

1. PREPARATION OF CRYOPROTECTANT
    A. In a sterile 500-mL bottle with a rubber septum cap, add the following:
        (1) 42 g low molecular weight HES (Pentastarch)
        (2) 140 mL sterile Normosol in D_5W
    B. Shake this mixture to mix, and steam autoclave for 20 minutes; then seal the bottle and cool to room temperature.
    C. To the room temperature mixture, using a 50-mL syringe, add:
        (1) 100 mL sterile 25 percent human serum albumin
        (2) 70 mL 50 percent DMSO (Rimso-50)
        The final volume is approximately 350 mL.
    D. Put the cryoprotectant on ice until ready for use.

2. TRANSFER OF RPMI-1640 INTO A 250-mL EVACUATED BOTTLE
    A. Attach a 19-gauge $\times$ ⅞ butterfly infusion set to a 60-mL disposable syringe.
    B. Remove the plunger from the syringe and discard.
    C. Pour sterile RPMI-1640 directly into the open syringe. When the syringe is full, plunge the butterfly needle into a 250-mL evacuated bottle.
    D. The bottle will begin to fill. As it does, replenish the supply of RPMI-1640 in the 60-mL syringe. Continue to add RPMI to the syringe until the volume in the bottle is approximately 250 mL.
    E. Remove and discard the butterfly and syringe.
    F. Vent the bottle with a venting needle.
    G. Insert the spiked end of a Fenwal plasma transfer set into the bottle.
    H. Attach a 16-gauge needle to the needle adaptor end of the plasma transfer set.
    I. The bottle of RPMI-1640 is now ready to dilute the buffy coat.

3. DILUTION OF THE BUFFY COAT
    A. Collect the buffy coat from the cell separator (volume approximately 150 mL) into a 600-mL plasma transfer bag. Once collected, seal the bag and insert a sampling site coupler.
    B. Insert the needle from the prepared bottle of RPMI into the sampling site coupler. Allow the RPMI to flow into the bag and bring the collected buffy coat cells to a final volume of 300 mL (determined by weight).
    C. Mix thoroughly.

4. TRANSFER OF CRYOPROTECTANT AND BUFFY COAT INTO FREEZING BAGS
    A. All processing is done on wet ice (2°C).
    B. Simultaneously add 300 mL of the cryoprotectant and the 300 mL of buffy coat cells to one of the bags of the CharterMed 4403-2 triplicate set.
    C. Once the addition is complete, mix the final volume (approximately 600 mL) thoroughly and distribute equally into two of the freezing bags of the triplicate set. Discard the third bag.
    D. After samples are removed, seal the two bags and weigh them to determine the final volume.
    E. Put the bags back on ice for 2 to 3 minutes before transfer into freezer.

5. TRANSFER OF BAGS INTO FREEZER
   A. Place each freezing bag into a prechilled labeled aluminum freezing frame. The frames can be cooled by being put on ice or into a $-20°C$ freezer.
   B. Place the aluminum freezing frames containing the bags horizontally into a $-80°C$ blood bank freezer. The freezer must be equipped with an active alarm system.

6. THAW AND REINFUSION
   A. At the time of reinfusion, rapidly thaw the bags in a 37°C waterbath.
   B. Reinfuse the marrow in 300-mL aliquots (one bag) over a 30-minute period via an infusion pump.

ANTICIPATED RESULTS	
	1. Post-thaw recovery of nucleated cells is about 95 percent, with trypan blue viability at 80 to 90 percent.
	2. Post-thaw colony-forming unit—granulocyte, macrophage (CFU-GM) recovery is 80 to 90 percent of the prefreeze value, and burst-forming unit—erythroid (BFU-E) recovery is 85 to 95 percent.

NOTES

1. No volume adjustment is made for cell count. The final mixture has an average cell count of 30 to 50 $\times$ 10^6 cells per mL.
2. There is no evidence of clumping or gel formation of unfractionated cells in this technique.
3. Cell viability remains unchanged for at least 2 years of storage.

AUTHORS

David H. Oldenburg
Section of Hematology/Oncology
Loyola University Medical Center
Maywood, IL 60153

Patrick J. Stiff, M.D.
Section of Hematology/Oncology
Loyola University Medical Center
Maywood, IL 60153

REFERENCES

1. Stiff, PJ, et al: Unfractionated human marrow cell cryopreservation using dimethylsulfoxide and hydroxyethyl starch. Cryobiology 20:17, 1983.
2. Stiff, PJ, et al: Autologous bone marrow transplantation using unfractionated cells cryopreserved in dimethylsulfoxide and hydroxyethyl starch without controlled rate freezing. Blood 70:974, 1987.

CRYOPRESERVATION OF BONE MARROW WITH HYDROXYETHYL STARCH, PLASMALYTE, DEXTROSE, AND DIMETHYL SULFOXIDE USING A MECHANICAL FREEZER

DESCRIPTION	Bone marrow frozen in cryoprotectant consisting of dimethyl sulfoxide (DMSO)/hydroxyethyl starch (HES) may be frozen at $-80°C$ for years. The rate of freezing in a mechanical freezer is approximately $3°C$ per minute. Viability and engraftment have been documented to be adequate when bone marrow is frozen in this way.
TIME FOR PROCEDURE	Preparation of cryoprotectant takes approximately 2 hours and may be done in advance of the actual cryopreservation procedure; cryopreservation of bone marrow requires approximately 40 minutes.
SUMMARY OF PROCEDURE	Bone marrow cells to be frozen should be adjusted to a cell concentration of not greater than 1×10^8 cells per mL. Bone marrow is slowly mixed with cryoprotectant in a freezing bag while being gently agitated, submerged in crushed ice. The bone marrow bag is sealed and placed in a metal canister and transferred to a $-80°C$ freezer to be frozen overnight in a horizontal position. The canister may then be stored vertically in a designated freezer.
EQUIPMENT	1. Laminar flow hood
	2. Bio-freezer ($-80°C$)
	3. Autoclave
	4. Eberbacker shaker
	5. Heat sealer
	6. Heated stir plate
SUPPLIES AND REAGENTS	1. Freezing bags (Fenwal 4R2422)
	2. Metal freezing canisters (Stericon RCM-3D)
	3. Plastic tub large enough to hold freezing bags and crushed ice
	4. 500-mL screw-top bottles (hospital supply)
	5. 250-mL vacuum bottles (hospital supply)
	6. Ultrapore filter (Millipore Co.)
	7. Plasma-Lyte (240 mL) (Baxter Laboratories 2B2544)
	8. Dextrose (anhydrous) 0.54 g (Fisher Scientific Co.)
	9. 200 mL human serum albumin (25 percent) (New York Blood Center)
	10. 50 mL CryoServ DMSO (not less than 99 percent) (Tera Pharmaceutical Inc.)
	11. 60 g HES (molecular weight 250,000) (American Critical Care)
PROCEDURE	1. PREPARATION OF CRYOPROTECTANT
	A. Add Plasma-lyte, dextrose, and HES to a 500-mL bottle and mix well by stirring on a heated stirplate for 30 minutes. Autoclave. This mixture may be stored at $4°C$ for up to 1 month.
	B. Immediately prior to use, bring volume up to 450-mL with 25 percent human serum albumin.

C. Mix well. Add 50 mL filtered DMSO slowly. If any precipitant appears, continue to mix until completely dissolved. Transfer cryoprotectant to 250- or 500-mL vacuum bottles. The final concentration of DMSO is 10 percent. The final concentration of HES is 12.5 percent.

NOTE: *Steps 1B and 1C are carried out sterilely in a laminar flow hood. Unused, unopened cryoprotectant may be stored at 4°C for not more than 1 week. Preparer should initial and date each bottle.*

2. BONE MARROW CRYOPRESERVATION

A. Bone marrow should be diluted, if necessary, with RPMI to yield a cell concentration of not greater than 1×10^8 cells per mL.

B. Close both clamps on bifurcating tubing of freezing bag. Connect end of one tubing to the bag containing bone marrow and the second tubing to the bottle containing cryoprotectant. The volume of cryoprotectant used should be equal to the volume of bone marrow to be frozen.

C. Place freezing bag into a tub on a bed of crushed ice, covering with additional crushed ice. Place tub on shaker and start at three cycles per second.

D. Unclamp tubing from cryoprotectant bottle, allowing the cryoprotectant to flow into the freezing bag.

E. Once cryoprotectant has reached the freezing bag, unclamp tubing from bone marrow bag and allow both cryoprotectant and bone marrow to flow into the freezing bag at approximately the same rate (process should be complete within 10 minutes). Allow a small amount of cryoprotectant to remain in bottle after the bone marrow bag has emptied. Clamp tubing to freezing bag and run the remaining cryoprotectant into the bone marrow bag to wash out any remaining bone marrow. Allow a small amount of bone marrow to remain in tubing to be sent for microbiologic culture.

F. Heat-seal tubing at point as close as possible to the freezing bag. Weigh all bags, transfer into metal canisters, and place horizontally in mechanical freezer. Record processing information and location of bags in bone marrow processing record. Multiple bags should be frozen in separate freezers. They may be changed from horizontal to vertical storage after 12 hours.

ANTICIPATED RESULTS	The final volume of frozen bone marrow is typically 400 to 500 mL, with a total cell count of 1 to 4×10^{10} cells.
NOTES	If the total concentration of cells allows, bone marrow should be frozen in at least two aliquots so that each canister may be placed in a separate freezer as a safety precaution.
AUTHORS	Oksana Rosina, M.T.(ASCP) Mount Sinai Medical Center New York, NY 10029 Robert Jiang, M.T.(ASCP) Mount Sinai Medical Center New York, NY 10029

AUTHORS   Oksana Rosina, M.T.(ASCP)   Robert Jiang, M.T.(ASCP)
Mount Sinai Medical Center   Mount Sinai Medical Center
New York, NY 10029   New York, NY 10029

REFERENCES

1. Stiff, PJ, et al: Autologous bone marrow transplantation using unfractionated cells cryopreserved in dimethylsulfoxide and hydroxyethyl starch without controlled rate freezing. Blood 70:974, 1987.

2. Bone Marrow Processing Manual, Bone Marrow Processing Laboratory, Mount Sinai Hospital Blood Bank, 1991.

REFRIGERATION STORAGE OF BONE MARROW

DESCRIPTION

Refrigeration storage of bone marrow is effective in reconstituting hematopoiesis.[1–3] The minimum storage interval between the collection and reinfusion of marrow depends on the time required to administer the therapeutic regimen and the half-life of the drugs used. By contrast, cryopreservation of marrow requires specialized equipment and technical expertise, which limits its availability.[4]

In a series of experiments (Preti, R, unpublished data) refrigerated marrow colony-forming unit—granulocyte, macrophage (CFU-GM) colonies and nucleated cell viability were comparable to cryopreserved marrow for up to 10 days. In fact, CFU-GM colonies increased almost threefold at 4°C. Other investigators have also confirmed the validity of refrigerated marrow storage.[5–10]

The average cost of refrigeration storage at Westchester County Medical Center was \$50.00 compared with \$970.00 for cryopreservation. Controlled-rate freezing and liquid nitrogen were not used in the method detailed in this study and would have added to the cost of cryopreservation.

Marrow can be refrigerated after red cells have been removed. The cell viability is comparable to whole marrow. Marrow stored in this fashion could be used for ex vivo treatment at the end of the storage period.

TIME FOR PROCEDURE

Approximately 20 minutes

SUMMARY OF PROCEDURE

1. Marrow is aspirated under general or spinal anesthesia.
2. Marrow is mixed with 200 mL of tissue culture medium TC-199 (Gibco, Grand Island, NY) and 120×10^3 units of commercially available preservative-containing sodium heparin (so-called preservative-free heparin solution also contains preservatives). Alternatively 100 mL of ACD-A solution, 100 mL TC-199, and 60×10^3 units of sodium heparin may be used. At least 2.0×10^8 cells per kg body weight are aspirated.
3. Marrow is filtered through coarse and fine wire meshes and then collected in 1000-mL nonbreathing plastic bags.
4. Marrow is placed in a standard blood bank refrigerator and maintained at 4°C (range 1 to 6°C) for up to 6 days. Marrow is shaken manually for 2 minutes twice daily.

EQUIPMENT/ SUPPLIES AND REAGENTS

1. Tissue culture medium TC-199 (Gibco Laboratories, Grand Island, NY)
2. Nonbreathing plastic bags (T-1000) (Terumo Laboratories, Piscataway, NJ)
3. Refrigerator (Jewett T-100-1, Buffalo, NY, or equivalent)

ANTICIPATED RESULTS

In a previous analysis,[1] patients undergoing refrigerated marrow storage were compared with patients whose marrow was cryopreserved with regard to the number of days until white blood cell (WBC) and platelet count recovery and number of days to red blood cell (RBC) transfusion independence. The median time to recovery of WBCs was 17 days (range 11 to 43 days) after refrigerated bone marrow infusion and 23 days (range 9 to 50 days) for cryopreserved bone marrows. A self-sustaining platelet count of more than 20×10^9 per L was achieved at a median of 24 days (range 10 to 125 days) following the infusion of refrigerated marrow and 51 days (range 18 to 90 days) after cryopreserved bone marrow infusion (p = ns). Independence from RBC transfusions occurred after a median of 21 days (range 0 to 77 days) for refrigerated marrow and 61 days (range 0 to 110) for cryopreserved marrow, which was statistically significant ($P < .038$). The frequency of delayed recovery of platelets was 11 percent in the refrigeration group versus 27 percent in the cryopreservation group (p = ns). Prolonged RBC transfusion dependence occurred in 3 percent of the refrigeration storage group versus 27 percent for cryopreservation group ($P < .008$).

A variety of high-dose chemotherapy-radiotherapy regimens has been used in conjunction with refrigerated autologous marrow, including (a) etoposide 1500 to 2000 mg per m^2, cyclophosphamide 5000 mg per m^2, carmustine 400–600 mg per m^2; (b) cyclophosphamide 5000 mg per m^2; total body irradiation 1200 rad; with or without etoposide 2000 mg per m^2; (c) Thiotepa 750 to 900 mg per m^2; (d) Thiotepa 900 mg per m^2, vinblastine 0.4 to 0.6 mg per kg, with or without cytarabine 3 to 6 g per m^2.

Refrigeration storage of marrow is simple and effective and should be considered for patients undergoing marrow transplantation within a few days of harvesting.

NOTES

1. Bleeding may occur at harvest sites when heparinized refrigerated marrow is used. This can be prevented by using 500 mg of protamine sulfate infusion over 20 minutes.

2. Marrow should be infused without using any filters. In the event that RBCs clump, the marrow may need to be drawn up in syringes and pushed manually.

AUTHORS

Tauseef Ahmed, M.D.
Director of Bone Marrow
   Transplantation Services
New York Medical College
Valhalla, NY

David Wuest, M.D.
Associate Director
Hudson Valley Blood Services
Valhalla, NY

Robert Preti, Ph.D.
Associate Investigator
Hudson Valley Blood Services
Valhalla, NY

REFERENCES

1. Ahmed, T, et al: Marrow storage techniques: A clinical comparison of refrigeration versus cryopreservation. Acta Hematol (in press).

2. Carella, AM, et al: High dose chemotherapy and non frozen autologous bone marrow transplantation in relapsed advanced lymphoma or those resistant to conventional chemotherapy. Cancer 54:2836, 1984.

3. Burnett, AK, et al: Hematological reconstitution following high dose and supralethal chemoradiotherapy using stored non-cryopreserved autologous bone marrow. Br J Haematol 54:309, 1983.

4. Stiff, PJ, et al: Autologous bone marrow transplantation using unfractionated cells cryopreserved in dimethyl sulfoxide and hydroxyethyl starch without controlled rate freezing. Blood 70:974, 1987.

5. Billen, D: Recovery of lethally irradiated mice by treatment with bone marrow cells maintained in vitro. Nature 179:574, 1957.

6. Urso, IS and Congdon, CC: Short term preservation of mouse bone marrow at refrigerator and room temperature for irradiation experiments. J Appl Physiol 10:314, 1957.

7. Kohsaki, M, et al: Non-frozen preservation of committed hematopoietic stem cells from normal human bone marrow. Cells 1:111, 1981.

8. Lasky, LC, McCullough, J, and Zanjani, ED: Liquid storage of unseparated human bone marrow: Evaluation of hematopoietic progenitors by clonal assay. Transfusion 26:331, 1986.

9. Takahashi, M and Singer, JW: Effects of marrow storage at 4°C on the subsequent generation of long term cultures. Exp Hematol 13:691, 1985.

10. Delforge, A, et al: Granulocyte-macrophage progenitor cell preservation at 4°C.

THAWING AND REINFUSION

Undiluted

THAWING AND REINFUSION OF AUTOGRAFTS USING INFUSION SETS

DESCRIPTION	Cryopreserved bone marrow can be thawed quickly in a waterbath and reinfused immediately, without washing out the dimethyl sulfoxide (DMSO) and without significant cell loss.
TIME FOR PROCEDURE	Approximately 2 hours (for two freezing bags)

SUMMARY OF PROCEDURE

1. Appropriate time for reinfusion is determined with the doctor or nurses in the unit.
2. Waterbath and other necessary laboratory supplies are prepared and location of cassettes in cryostorage determined.
3. In the bone marrow transplant unit (BMTU), marrow is thawed at bedside. Samples are taken for counts and cultures.
4. In the laboratory cell counts, viabilities and colony-forming unit assays are performed.

EQUIPMENT

1. Waterbath
2. Baker laminar flow hood

SUPPLIES AND REAGENTS

1. Two 35×75 snap-cap test tubes (or 1 tube per marrow bag)
2. Blood components recipient set (Fenwal 4C2100)
3. Container to transport bone marrow cassettes that can hold liquid nitrogen
4. Cryogloves
5. Trypan blue solution 0.4 percent
6. Minimal essential media (MEM) alpha plus 6 percent fetal calf serum plus heparin (5 U per mL)
7. Ethanol
8. Plastic centrifuge bags

PROCEDURE

1. On the morning of the reinfusion, talk with the nurses and/or doctors concerning the best time to reinfuse the marrow. Inform them at this time of the number of marrow bags frozen and the total volume in them to be reinfused.
2. In the laboratory clean the waterbath and disinfect with 70 or 95 percent ethanol. Fill the waterbath to a convenient depth (approximately half full) with water (sterile water can be used). Turn on the waterbath and bring it to a temperature of 40°C. Place ice and the 35×75 mL tubes (one for each bag to thaw) in an ice bucket. Put some liquid nitrogen in a container large enough to keep the marrow cassettes frozen during transport to the BMTU

and preparation for reinfusion. Place the bone marrow cassettes in the liquid nitrogen. Assemble all of this on a cart to transport to the patient's bedside.

3. Remove the marrow cassettes from the cryostorage tank and place in the carrying container with liquid nitrogen in it.

4. At the agreed upon time, take cart to the patient's bedside. Plug in the waterbath.

5. When the nurse is ready (after preparatory medications are given and vital signs taken), thaw the first bag. Remove frozen marrow bag from metal cassette. Place the bag of marrow into a centrifuge bag and place in 40°C bath. Do not allow water to enter outer bag. As the marrow bag thaws, gently massage the bag to break up clumps of ice. When the marrow has thawed to a slushy consistency, remove from waterbath.

6. Attach the blood component recipient set to the thawed bag. Close the clamp on the set and fill the filter and line. Hang the marrow using sterile technique. The marrow is allowed to flow as fast as the patients can tolerate it. A small amount (3 to 5 mL) is left in the line. Use 1 to 2 mL for the aerobic and anaerobic culture bottles and dispense the rest sterilely into the 35- $\times$ 75-mm tube. The tube is placed on ice.

7. The remaining bags are thawed in a similar fashion. Completely finish the reinfusion of one bag before thawing the next. The bags can be cultured aerobically and anaerobically either individually or together.

8. In the laboratory, perform nucleated cell counts and viabilities. The total cell dose and the total viable cell dose are determined.

9. Samples from each bag are washed, either individually or together, one time with MEM alpha plus 6 percent fetal calf serum plus heparin, counted, and plated for the colony-forming assays.

ANTICIPATED RESULTS

Our average total cell recovery after cryopreservation is 74 percent $\pm$ 17 percent. The average percentage of viable cells is 66.5 percent $\pm$ 16 percent. Both of these numbers are "worst case scenarios" because the cell count is done on the last portion left in the line, which may not be representative of the whole bag as the bag is not mixed after it is hung. The viability is not determined until after we return to the laboratory (about 1 hour after first bag is reinfused).

NOTES

1. Have enough volume in the waterbath so the temperature of the water is approximately 40°C after thawing the marrow.

2. Sometimes small strings or clumps of cells are seen in the thawed bag. This may be due to the fact that cells are frozen at a concentration as high as 1×10^8 per mL. The more concentrated the cells, the more they tend to clump. Excess platelets or granulocytes may also contribute to clumping. If the filter clogs to the extent that marrow is hardly dripping, the marrow can be put into a syringe (with a three-way stopcock) and "pushed." Care must be taken not to injure patient's Hickman catheter.

3. Marrow should be allowed to drip as fast as possible to increase the number of viable cells reinfused (the longer DMSO is with cells at room temperature, the more damage is done to the cells) and to decrease cell clumping.

AUTHORS   Roy S. Weiner, M.D.   Mary Ann Gross, M.T.(ASCP)
           University of Florida   Shands Hospital
           Gainesville, FL 32610   University of Florida
                                           Gainesville, FL 32610

REFERENCE   1. Weiner, RS, Richman, CM, and Yankee, RA: Dilution techniques for optimum recovery of cryo-
              preserved bone marrow cells. Exp Hematol 7:16, 1979.

INFUSION OF THAWED BONE MARROW USING SYRINGE

DESCRIPTION	Cryopreserved marrow that has been frozen in aliquots of 50 mL or less is thawed rapidly in a 40°C saline bath. The thawed marrow is transferred from freezing bag to syringe and given by intravenous infusion.
TIME FOR PROCEDURE	Approximately 10 minutes per bag thawed
SUMMARY OF PROCEDURE	1. Bone marrow, frozen in aliquots of 50 mL or less and stored in individual canisters, is transferred to a styrofoam box filled with liquid nitrogen for transport to the area designated for thawing marrow.
	2. Sterile supplies used to thaw marrow are placed in a laminar flow hood.
	3. The marrow, thawed rapidly in a 40°C saline bath in a laminar flow hood, is transferred from bag to syringe and given by intravenous (IV) infusion within 5 minutes from time of thaw.
EQUIPMENT	1. Laminar flow hood
	2. Waterbath
SUPPLIES AND REAGENTS	1. 1-L bottles of saline, sterile: 3 per bag thawed
	2. Sterile basin: 1 per bag thawed
	3. Sterile syringes: 60-mL
	4. Needles: 16-gauge × 1½-inch
	5. Sterile hemostats
	6. Sterile scissors
	7. Sterile towels
	8. Sterile gauze
	9. Alcohol swabs
	10. Sampling site coupler
	11. Stopwatch
	12. Cryogloves
	13. Styrofoam box
PROCEDURE	1. PREPARATION FOR THAWING OF MARROW
	A. Place bottles of saline in waterbath and warm to 40°C.
	B. Place the following supplies in the laminar flow hood.
	(1) Sterile towels spread to cover working area
	(2) Sterile basin for saline
	(3) Sterile gauze
	(4) Sterile hemostats and scissors
	(5) Sampling site coupler
	(6) 60-mL syringe with 16-gauge needle
	(7) Alcohol swabs
	C. Remove the designated canisters to be thawed from storage and place in a styrofoam box filled with liquid nitrogen. Transport to room with hood.

  D. Check the identification of each canister of marrow to be thawed with the patient's physician before beginning the actual thawing process.

2. THAWING AND INFUSION OF MARROW
  A. When the physician, nurse, and patient are ready, thaw the marrow, one bag at a time as follows:
  (1) Pour three bottles of the 40°C saline into the basin in the hood.
  (2) Quickly remove one canister from liquid nitrogen and submerge it in the 40°C saline.
  (3) As soon as the canister warms enough, quickly but carefully open canister. Remove bag and resubmerge bag in the warm saline.
  (4) When the marrow is partially thawed, briefly remove bag from saline. Wipe bag with white gauze to look for possible crack in the bag. If a crack is observed, secure bag with a sterile hemostat.
  (5) Resubmerge partially thawed marrow bag into the warm saline. Gently knead bag until marrow is completely thawed.
  (6) When marrow is completely thawed, start stopwatch.
  (7) Remove plastic cover from bag port. Wipe port with alcohol swab and insert sampling site coupler.
  (8) Transfer marrow from bag to a 60-mL syringe with a 16-gauge needle.
  (9) Place patient identification label on syringe and quickly transport to patient's bedside. When infusion is completed by the patient's physician, stop stopwatch.

  NOTE: *The marrow should be infused within 5 minutes from the time of thawing in order to decrease exposure of thawed marrow cells to concentrated DMSO.*

  B. If more than one bag of marrow is to be infused, repeat step 2A for each bag.

AUTHORS

Marita G. Hill, M.T.(ASCP), S.B.B.
Blood Bank Immunohematologist
University of Kentucky Medical Center
Lexington, KY 40536

Vickie M. Robertson, M.T.(ASCP), S.B.B.
Blood Bank Bone Marrow Coordinator
University of Kentucky Medical Center
Lexington, KY 40536

Larry G. Dickson, M.D.
Director, Blood Bank
Clinical Laboratory
University of Kentucky Medical Center
Lexington, KY 40536

REFERENCE

1. Appelbaum, F, et al: Successful engraftment of cryopreserved autologous bone marrow in patients with malignant lymphoma. Blood 52:85, 1978.

Thawing and Dilution of Bone Marrow

DESCRIPTION	Bone marrow cells frozen at a high concentration may clump at the time of thawing. Addition of citrate phosphate dextrose acid (CPDA), followed by dilution with hydroxyethyl starch (HES) and human serum albumin, can eliminate cell aggregates. Bone marrow may then be reconstituted to a desired smaller volume. These steps achieve avoidance of clumping, removal of DMSO, and control of the final infused volume. This method has been developed for use with bone marrow cryopreserved with DMSO/HES.
TIME FOR PROCEDURE	Approximately 1 hour and 30 minutes from the time the bone marrow is removed from the freezer until it is ready for infusion into the patient

SUMMARY OF PROCEDURE

1. The bag containing frozen bone marrow is removed from the freezer, the name of the patient confirmed, and the bone marrow bag examined for any damage.
2. The bone marrow is partially thawed by submersion into a 37°C waterbath followed by the addition of CPDA.
3. After the bone marrow is completely thawed, a previously prepared "wash solution" of HES/albumin is added.
4. The bone marrow is centrifuged and the supernatant removed.
5. The remaining cell pellet is then reconstituted to a desired volume with the HES/albumin solution.
6. The final product is agitated for a few minutes at room temperature and checked for the presence of any cell aggregates.
7. The volume of the product is measured and a sample is taken for cell count. The bone marrow is now ready to be infused.

EQUIPMENT

1. Sorvall RC-3B centrifuge or equivalent
2. Plasma extracter
3. Laminar flow hood
4. Heat sealer
5. Tube strippers
6. 37°C waterbath

SUPPLIES AND REAGENTS

1. 600-mL transfer pack (Fenwal 4R2023)
2. Plasma transfer set with needle adaptor (Fenwal 4C2240)
3. Plasma transfer set with two couplers (Fenwal 4C2243)
4. 60-mL syringes (hospital supply)
5. 16-gauge needles (hospital supply)
6. 500 mL Hespan (6 percent HES in 0.9 percent NaCl for injection) (DuPont Critical Care)
7. 100 mL human serum albumin (25 percent)
8. 70 mL CPDA-1 (Fenwal)

PROCEDURE

1. Remove freezing bag containing bone marrow from metal canister and place in 37°C waterbath for 1 to 2 minutes, until bone marrow is partially thawed (do not submerge ports of bone marrow bag).

2. Remove bag from waterbath after the bone marrow is partially thawed and insert the sampling site coupler into the port of the marrow bag.

3. Inject 20 mL CPDA-1 anticoagulant into the marrow bag, mix gently, and resubmerge into the waterbath making sure not to submerge the bag ports. Incubate until the bone marrow is completely thawed. Remove bag from waterbath.

4. Inject an additional 50 mL CPDA-1 into the completely thawed bone marrow. Mix gently.

5. Inject the "wash solution" of HES/albumin in a volume equal to the initial volume of bone marrow. Gently agitate the marrow bag as the wash solution is added.

6. Transfer the bone marrow/wash mixture into a 600-mL transfer pack and expel the excess air from the bag. Connect a second transfer pack to the bag now containing bone marrow (to collect the supernatant).

7. Centrifuge the bone marrow/wash mixture for 10 minutes at 2000 rpm at 4°C.

8. Using the plasma expressor apparatus, expel the supernatant from the marrow bag and resuspend the remaining cell pellet by adding additional wash solution to a minimum volume of 150 mL.

9. Inspect the final product for the presence of aggregates.

10. Weigh bag to determine final volume. Obtain specimens for cell count, stem cell culture, and microbiologic culture. Calculate the number of nucleated cells infused and record data in the bone marrow processing record.

ANTICIPATED RESULTS

This procedure typically yields a bone marrow product in a volume of 150 to 200 mL with a cell count of 5 to 10×10^7 nucleated cells per mL. This method of thawing enables the removal of supernatant containing free hemoglobin and DMSO and allows the concentration of bone marrow into a small volume.

NOTES

1. Thawed bone marrow should be infused as quickly as possible via a central IV catheter without any filter.

2. The patient should be informed of potential side effects associated with reinfusion of marrow including nausea, vomiting, palpitations, fever, dyspnea, rash, chest, and back pain.

3. Urine may turn red but should clear within 12 hours.

AUTHORS

Oksana Rosina, M.T.(ASCP)
Mount Sinai Medical Center
New York, NY 10029

Donna Tabrizi, M.D.
Mount Sinai Medical Center
New York, NY 10029

Shengly Zhou, M.D.
Mount Sinai Medical Center
New York, NY 10029

Eileen Scigliano, M.D.
Mount Sinai Medical Center
New York, NY 10029

REFERENCES

1. Leiderman, IZ and Zaroulis, CG: A simple method to prevent clumping of previously frozen hematopoietic progenitor cells. Personal communication, 1991.

CRYOPRESERVATION AND INFUSION OF PERIPHERAL BLOOD STEM CELLS

CRYOPRESERVATION OF PERIPHERAL STEM CELLS

DESCRIPTION	Autologous stem cell rescue (ASCR) is used to restore hematopoietic function following high-dose chemotherapy-radiotherapy. For patients with metastatic malignant disease involving the bone marrow, the alternative to marrow stem cells is circulating stem cells found in peripheral blood. Autologous mononuclear cells in peripheral blood are collected using a continuous flow cell separator (Fenwal CS3000). During the interval between cell collection and reinfusion, the cells' metabolic "clock" must completely halt. Successful freezing or cryopreservation of mononuclear cells prohibits further metabolism while maximizing viability. The key aspects include use of a cryoprotective agent such as dimethyl sulfoxide (DMSO) and a controlled rate of cooling.
TIME FOR PROCEDURE	Between 2 and 3 hours for 50 to 200 mL.

SUMMARY OF PROCEDURE

1. Prepare DMSO-medium solution.
2. Label cryobags, cryovials, and holders with patient's name, hospital number, and date. Chill.
3. Divide specimen evenly between cryobags, label volume on cryobags and holders. Chill.
4. Aspirate equal volumes of DMSO-medium in syringes. Chill.
5. Just before the freeze, prepare cryovials. Chill in ice.
6. Inject each cryobag with DMSO-medium, seal, cut off tubing, fit in holder. Put cryovials in box.
7. Cryopreserve cryobags and cryovials according to protocol.
8. Store.

EQUIPMENT

1. The CryoMed system contains the following three pieces: Model 1010 A micro computer, model 990 freezing chamber with capacity for either ribbon thermocouple (indirect specimen contact) or probe thermocouple (direct specimen contact), and Linseis model 6100 flat bed recorder.
2. Dielectric tube sealer
3. Laminar flow hood

SUPPLIES AND REAGENTS	See under each heading.

PROCEDURE

1. PREPARING THE DMSO-MEDIUM SOLUTION

   NOTE: *The DMSO-medium solution should be made on the same day as the cryopreservation.*

   A. The final concentration of DMSO when DMSO-medium is mixed with cells in a 1:1 proportion is 10 percent. Hence, the initial concentration of DMSO in medium must be twice that, or 20 percent. To determine

Table 9–4 DMSO-MEDIUM
VALUES FOR EXACT
MEASUREMENTS OF 20 PERCENT
DMSO IN MEDIUM

Total (mL)	=	DMSO	+	Medium
5		1		4
10		2		8
15		3		12
20		4		16
25		5		20
30		6		24
35		7		28
40		8		32
45		9		36
50		10		40
55		11		44
60		12		48
65		13		52
70		14		56
75		15		60
80		16		64
85		17		68
90		18		72
95		19		76
100		20		80
105		21		84
110		22		88
115		23		92
120		24		96
125		25		100
130		26		104
135		27		108
140		28		112
145		29		116
150		30		120
160		32		128
170		34		136
180		36		144
190		38		152
200		40		160
250		50		200
300		60		240

the total amount of DMSO and medium needed, weigh the specimen. The weight approximates the specimen's volume for which an equal volume of DMSO-medium solution is required. In addition, a few extra milliliters for cryovials are needed (Table 9–4).

Under a laminar flow hood place:

- Tissue culture medium (Gibco TC-199 with Hank's balanced salt solution and L-glutamine, cat. no. 320-1151AG)
- DMSO (Cryoserv multidose, Research Industries Corp.)
- 2 sterile 50-mL tubes
- Sterile 30-mL or 20-mL syringe

- 16-gauge 1.5-inch hypodermic needle
- Sterile alcohol preparation pads
- Styrofoam tube holder
- Pipet-Aid
- Sterile 25-mL pipette
- Cryovials: 1.8 mL (Nunc 377267)

    (1) Remove plastic wrap from bottle of medium and loosen cap.
    (2) Pour medium carefully into each of two 50-mL tubes (any sterile container is appropriate).
    (3) Pipette appropriate volume back into glass bottle.
    (4) Recap loosely.

B. Attach 16-gauge 1.5-inch needle to 30-mL syringe (20-mL for final volumes of 100 mL or less) and set aside.

    (1) Remove metal cap from CryoServ with an alcohol preparation pad.
    (2) Wipe rubber injection site with alcohol.
    (3) Insert needle and aspirate DMSO.

C. Squirt DMSO into medium, cap tightly, shake well (outside of hood), and chill in refrigerator (4°C).

2. THE SPECIMEN OF PERIPHERAL STEM CELLS

NOTE: *Your cryobags and their metal holders should be labeled with name, specimen type (peripheral stem cell [PSC] total volume), date, and any other pertinent information such as hospital number. Do not write directly on the cryobag plastic through which you will see specimen because the ink might diffuse into the cryobag; instead write on upper left and right corners of cryobags. To ensure the same freeze rate, each bag should contain approximately the same volume (i.e., 3 bags of 80 is preferable to 2 of 100 plus 1 of 40). Chill the cryobags and holders for an hour or longer while awaiting the specimen.*

A. Use Fenwal medium-sized Cryocyte freezing containers with plastic PL269, code 4R5462. Total volume in each cryobag should not exceed 110 mL because the bag will be too large to enclose in metal holders. Each cryobag has two female leads for transferring DMSO-medium and specimen. The plastic tubing adjacent to the bag seals easily in a SEBRA hand-held tube sealer. Two sterile ports remain at the top center of the bag for use after thawing. A Fenwal blood component infusion set (bcis), code 4C2223, produces a closed system, thereby acting as an added measure against contamination. In addition, it contains a filter (pore size of 170 to 210 μm). The Fenwal cryobags fit imperfectly but adequately in the Stericon metal holders, catalogue no. RCM-91D, which, in turn, fit into Stericon frames, catalogue no. RCM-91-FR-4 for storage in liquid nitrogen.

Under the hood place with your specimen:

- Cryobags
- Blood component infusion set (bcis)
- 60-mL syringe
- Sterile tube(s)
- Styrofoam tube holder
- 16-gauge 1.5-inch needle

(1) Close all clamps on cryobags.

(2) Remove bcis from box and close all clamps.

(3) Remove cover from the specimen bag outlet port and carefully (without touching port) set aside.

(4) Insert bcis coupler into outlet port of specimen bag.

(5) Open syringe and set aside.

(6) Remove cover from bcis female luer connector and attach syringe.

(7) Remove luer adaptor cover from one cryobag lead and attach bcis coupler.

(8) Open clamp to specimen bag.

(9) Using syringe, withdraw specimen (the amount should be half the total calculated volume for each cryobag; for example, 50 mL total volume = 25 mL specimen + 25 mL DMSO-medium).

NOTE: *Remember to save a few mL for cryovials.*

(10) Close clamp to specimen bag, then open clamps on cryobag-bcis and inject specimen.

(11) Pull about 5 mL of air back into syringe and inject it to push through the specimen caught in the tubing.

(12) Close all clamps on cryobag-bcis (close clamp on cryobag near the luer connector).

(13) Attach next cryobag to bcis and repeat procedure.

B. When all cryobags have been filled, withdraw from specimen bag 2 to 3 mL for at least four cryovials.

(1) Attach a 16-gauge 1.5-inch needle to syringe and put specimen in tube(s).

(2) Put tube(s) in refrigerator.

C. Using SEBRA tube sealer, seal cryobag tubing (below clamp) that was used for injecting specimen, pull or cut off, and discard.

D. Finish labeling cryobags and holders with volumes. Chill.

3. PREPARING THE SYRINGES OF DMSO-MEDIUM

A. Under the hood place:

- 16-gauge 1.5-inch needle(s)
- DMSO-medium (shaken)
- Tray for holding syringes at more than a 30-degree angle (if necessary)

(1) Loosen cap on DMSO-medium.

(2) Open syringe and set aside.

(3) Attach needle to syringe (do not touch the tapered end of the syringe as it may rest on the sterile tube or bottle of DMSO-medium).

(4) For each volume of specimen, withdraw an equal volume of DMSO-medium.

(5) Label if necessary.

(6) Chill in refrigerator for 45 minutes.

4. THE CRYOVIALS

A. This step is performed 10 to 15 minutes before commencing cryopreservation. Cryovials should already be labeled with patient's name, specimen type, hospital number, and date. Like the cryobags, there is a one-to-one correspondence of specimen to DMSO-medium for a total of 1 mL in each cryovial. Because of their smaller volume, cryovials of specimen do not have the same eutectic point as their cryobag counterparts. Ideally, the cryovials should be cryopreserved separately from the bags; but if they are cryopreserved together, the cryovials should be placed first in a styrofoam blood tube box to stagger the rate at which they freeze. In any event, cryovials should not be used to measure viability, as they are typically unreliable indicators of cryobag viability.

Under the hood place:

- Labeled cryovials
- Sterile 1-mL pipettes
- Cryovial rack
- Specimen and DMSO-medium in 0°C ice

(1) Just prior to putting them in ice under the hood, shake the DMSO-medium and vortex the specimen tube.
(2) Put the specimen tube and DMSO-medium in ice under the hood and loosen the caps on each.
(3) Loosen two cryovial caps.
(4) Pipette 1 mL of specimen and put 0.5 mL specimen in each of two cryovials. Dispose of pipette.
(5) Pipette 1 mL of DMSO-medium and put 0.5 mL in each of the aforementioned two cryovials. Dispose of pipette.
(6) Tighten cryovial caps, agitate, and submerge in ice.

   B. Repeat for remaining cryovials; then remove from hood and place near freezer.

5. UNIVERSITY OF CHICAGO MEDICAL CENTER CRYOMED FREEZER PROGRAM

   A. This program is intended for cryobag volumes between 40 and 110 mL, inclusive. Heat of fusion occurs between -8 and $-20°C$. Typically, heat of fusion occurs between -12 and $-16°C$, inclusive. Ideally, at heat of fusion the specimen heats minimally (between 2 and 8°C), warming to a temperature that is not warmer than $-6°C$, and returns to the temperature at which heat of fusion occurred within 4 minutes, certainly no more than 8 minutes, and thereafter cools at -1 to $-2°C$ per minute. Precisely at heat of fusion and thereafter until the specimen's rate of cooling is stable, cooling and warming of the chamber is controlled manually. The program is run in "unlimited access mode," which over-rides the function that would not otherwise facilitate manual intervention. Also, the program includes several WAIT functions, which allow a one-button push to pause, advance, or reverse the program steps. Those timely seconds saved by unlimited access mode and the WAIT function features are critical at the heat of fusion when decisions must be made every 10 seconds or less. WAIT functions serve to drop the specimen or chamber to a designated temperature until the operator advances (or reverses) the program. S refers to specimen; CH to chamber. The numbers 1.1 and so on indicate program number 1 and steps 1 through 9. With the exception of heat of fusion, the specimen is typically about 10°C warmer than the chamber.

1.1	WAIT ------------>	+0 CH (S IS ABOUT +12–14 DEGREES)	COOL+
1.2	−1 d/m ---------->	−10 S	COOL+
1.3	WAIT ------------>	−20 CH; heat of fusion ? S	COOL+
1.4	WAIT ------------>	−75 CH	COOL+
1.5	WAIT ------------>	−60 CH	COOL+
1.6	+35 d/m -------->	−26 CH	HEAT
1.7	−1 d/m ---------->	−45 S	COOL+
1.8	−10 d/m -------->	−90 S	COOL+
1.9	END		

d/m = degree C per minute.

    B. Before adding DMSO-medium to the cryobags, close the chamber door.
- (1) Turn on the computer.
- (2) Raise the visor on the flat bed recorder, remove the protective rubber cap on the pen, and place it on the chart drive metal button (or a place where you will not lose it—the pen can dry out overnight).
- (3) Looking again at the computer, push the buttons PROG (program), 1, 2, 3, ENT (enter), 1, 1, in that exact sequence. If 1.1 already appears in the program number and section number boxes, it is not necessary to push the last two buttons of the above sequence: 1, 1.
- (4) Returning to the recorder, turn on the machine, lower the pen, and push CHART DRIVE, a white button, using the green button to 0 the machine as necessary.
- (5) Raise the pen.
- (6) On the computer, push SCAN. The red light will fluctuate between SAMP (sample) and CHAM (chamber). Check that the following red lights are on: PWR (power), COOL, COOL+, and CHAMBER.
- (7) Ascertain that the PROG red light is flashing. If not, turn off and on the computer and repeat the previous sequence.
- (8) Under system status WAIT should appear highlighted in red.
- (9) Under program display in red are 1.1 and +0.

6. MIXING THE DMSO-MEDIUM AND SPECIMEN

    A. Perform this step immediately before cryopreserving the specimen in order to limit the degree to which the DMSO, which may be lethal to cells at room temperature, warms. The mixing should be done as quickly as possible without compromising sterile technique.

NOTE: *All labeling must be done prior to mixing.*

A bag containing an average volume of those being cryopreserved should be chosen as the reference bag. If the controlled-rate freezer is not next to the hood where the mixing is done, then the cryobags should travel to the freezer on a bed of ice (0°C) to prevent as much warming as possible. The bed of ice should be on a cart with wheels. If the liquid nitrogen storage refrigerator is not located next to the freezer, then a styrofoam box of approximate dimensions 16 × 16 × 16 inch should be partially filled with liquid nitrogen prior to the end of the freeze cycle, then used to transport the frozen specimen to the liquid nitrogen refrigerator. During transportation, the specimen should not rest in the liquid but just above it in the gas phase. A metal shelf placed in the bottom of the styrofoam box is adequate for elevating the frozen specimen. The following instructions assume that the hood is next to the freezer with a refrigerator (4°C) directly beneath the bench on which the freezer chamber rests.

Next to the hood have available:

- Plasma extractor
- SEBRA hand-held tube sealer, Model 1100 (turned on)
- Scissors
- Styrofoam blood tube box (for cryovials)

(1) Quickly, choose a bag of specimen and a syringe of equal volume.

(2) Put them under the hood, remove the protective cover from the cryobag lead, remove the needle from the syringe, and attach the syringe to the bag.

(3) Remove from hood the coupled bag-syringe, open clamp, and inject DMSO-medium in cryobag—*do not detach syringe!*—mix, and place in plasma extractor.

(4) Extract excess air into syringe plus a little specimen.

(5) Inject specimen, close clamp, and put under hood.

CAUTION: *Ascertain that the bag does not have excess air. If there is more than 60-mL of air pulled into the syringe, you can put the coupled cryobag-syringe back under the hood, disconnect the syringe, eject some of the air from the syringe, reconnect it, and place it in the plasma extractor to continue withdrawing air from the bag.*

(6) Seal tubing; cut and discard tubing with coupled syringe.

(7) Put cryobag in holder and put in refrigerator.

B. Repeat for each cryobag *until one remains.*

7. CRYOPRESERVATION

A. At computer, push RUN (the red light will turn off under PROG and flash under RUN) and quickly turn on the liquid nitrogen.

B. Inject the last bag as the chamber cools to 0°C.

(1) Push PROG (its red light is flashing).

(2) Open the chamber door and place the ribbon thermocouple on the center of the reference bag. Close the holder (*carefully* on the thermocouple).

(3) Insert the holder with port upright in the rack.

(4) Quickly insert the other holders, and close the door.

(5) Computer—hit RUN (flashing light).

(6) Recorder—lower pen, and turn CHART DRIVE metal button on.

(7) Put the cryovials in a small styrofoam box, hit PROG, insert the box upright in the chamber, and hit RUN.

(8) Computer—Under display, push PROG/ACT and CHAM/SAMP to see the actual sample temperature according to the computer.

(9) As soon as the chamber is 0°C or cooler, push RUN once to advance the program to −1°C per minute (step 1.2). The red light will continue to flash throughout the freeze process.

C. The specimen temperature should now drop at an appropriate rate and does not need to be monitored until it is about −8°C.

D. Just before and definitely after step 1.3 engages (1.3 WAIT → −20 CH; HEAT OF FUSION ? S), watch the recorder pen very carefully in order to detect specimen warming. Have your finger poised on the RUN button and push it as soon as heat of fusion occurs. If the chamber warms to within 6°C of the temperature of the specimen, give short BLASTS by toggling between PROG and RUN to maintain a rate of −1°C per minute.

E. After heat of fusion occurs, quickly return the specimen temperature to the same temperature at which heat of fusion occurred without incurring too rapid a cooling rate thereafter. As a rule, extreme cooling of the chamber (steps 1.4 and 1.5) should not be engaged for more than 4 minutes. If the specimen starts to cool quickly ("hairpin curve"), engage the chamber warming step (step 1.6), but if the specimen then cools at less than −1°C per minute or plateaus, advance to −1°C per minute cooling (step 1.7) and toggle between warming (step 1.6) and steady cooling (step 1.7).

CAUTION: *Any step engaged for too long can cause excessive warming or cooling.*

F. After the specimen has returned to the point of heat of fusion, monitor it for about 10 minutes to verify that it cools at not more than −2°C per minute. Although step 1.7 is programmed to decrease at −1°C per minute, it will generally decrease at −2°C per minute for several minutes, and then reduce its rate to −1°C per minute. The rate at which the temperature decreases is determined by the length of the extreme cooling (steps 1.4 and 1.5).

G. The program is reliable hereafter and need not be monitored. It is inadvisable to leave the room, however.

H. The computer will alarm audibly when the freeze is finished.
   (1) Push PROG, turn off liquid nitrogen.
   (2) Put on cryogloves.
   (3) Open the chamber door and put all of the holders except the reference bag into the styrofoam box.

   NOTE: *Be gentle but quick. Do not drop them!*

   (4) Remove the thermocouple from the reference bag, lift the pen, reclose the holder on the reference bag, and put bag in transport box along with box of cryovials.
   (5) Transport to storage in liquid nitrogen refrigerator.
   (6) Mark a frame with patient's name, date, and other pertinent information.
   (7) Put holders in frame, ports facing in, and submerge in liquid nitrogen refrigerator.

ANTICIPATED RESULTS	The viability, based on a trypan blue test using a sample taken from a reinfused cryobag, should be between 80 and 95 percent, inclusive.
NOTES	If peripheral stem cells and bone marrow specimen could follow the ideal freeze curve, they would cool at −1°C per minute until reaching −45°C, thereafter cooling at −10°C per minute until reaching −90°C. However, heat of fusion intervenes, and must be overcome without destroying the cells by freezing them too fast or too slow. Specimens vary greatly in volume, cell count, and number

of bags, thus giving a variable heat of fusion point. A lot of flexibility in the program is required and the technician's discretion is called upon in order to manually control the specimen's freeze curve through the heat of fusion point. The most difficult aspect of the freeze is judging whether the specimen temperature is decreasing properly after heat of fusion and when to advance to the next step. One learns to recognize visual cues without being able to verbalize the exact measurements. Here are a few hints:

1. Be ready to cool the chamber as soon as the graph recorder pen indicates heat of fusion—the pen will shoot 90° directly to the right.

A GOOD FREEZE

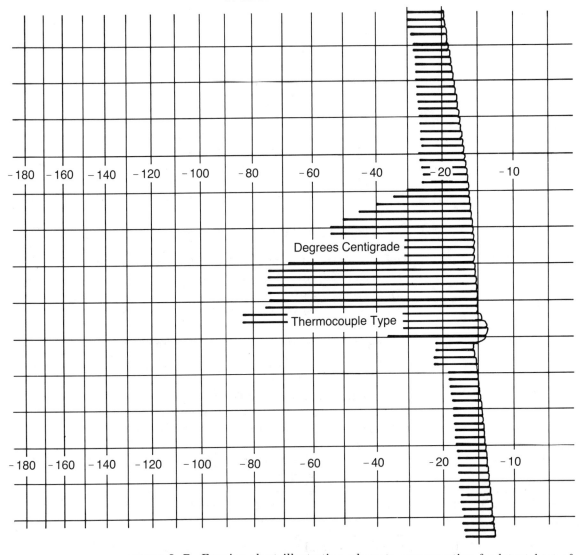

FIGURE 9–7 Freezing chart illustrating adequate compensation for latent heat of fusion released by specimen during freezing. Each horizontal line represents chamber (lower) and sample (higher) temperatures (°C). Each box represents 10°C horizontally and 1 minute vertically.

2. If a specimen at heat of fusion reverses its warming trend immediately after the WAIT function to cool the chamber to $-75°C$ is initiated (step 1.4), then advance to the next step, cooling the chamber to only $-60°C$ (press RUN just once—do not accidently press it twice or you will be in *limited* access mode; if you do accidently press RUN twice, press your code to restore *unlimited* access mode—ours is PROG, 1, 2, 3, ENTER).

3. If the chamber temperature reaches its maximum cold temperature and the specimen starts to warm, even slightly, or seems to plateau, press PROG, advance to $-1°C$ per minute cooling (step 1.7), and allow the specimen to start cooling until the warming trend is reversed.

4. Experience dictates that the lower heat of fusion occurs, $-15°C$ or lower, the greater the tendency for the specimen to warm—as much as $8°C$. For higher heat of fusion temperature, between -8 and $-12°C$, there is the opposite tendency. In other words, a heat of fusion that occurs at $-15°C$ is likely to warm to $-9°C$ $(6°C)$ and take approximately 5 or 6 minutes to return to $-15°C$ (provided that the chamber temperature is properly controlled and not overcooled), whereas heat of fusion that occurs at $-10°C$ might only warm $2°C$ to $-8°C$ and return to $-10°C$ in 2 minutes or less. For the latter, decisions concerning warming or cooling have to made much more quickly.

5. "Eyeball" the rate: each pen marking of the specimen represents 10 seconds, whereas the recording of the chamber—the "spike"—represents 2 seconds. Five of these "boxes," therefore, equal a minute. Ideally, your specimen temperature will take five boxes to lower 1 (or 2) $°C$.

6. Toggle between steady cooling (step 1.7) and warming (step 1.6), nursing the specimen back to the heat of fusion temperature while also endeavoring to ensure a rate of $-1°C$ (or $-2°C$) thereafter. This takes practice. The danger in adhering too closely to the aforementioned formula (minimizing the warming of specimen temperature and number of minutes to return to heat of fusion) is that the chamber will cool too much or for too long, thereby engendering a specimen cooling rate of much greater than $-1°C$ per minute thereafter. Rates of more than $-5°C$ per minute are detrimental to the specimen (Fig. 9–7).

AUTHOR   Kristi Hollingsworth, M.A.
University of Chicago Medical
  Center
Chicago, IL 60637

REFERENCES   1. Gorin, NC: Collection, manipulation, and freezing of haemopoietic stem cells. Clin Haematol 15:19, 1986.
2. Douay, L, Lopez, M, and Gorin, N: A technical bias: Differences in cooling rates prevent ampoules from being a reliable index of stem cell cryopreservation in large volumes. Cryobiology 23:296, 1986.
3. Gorin, N, et al: Delayed kinetics of recovery of haemopoiesis following autologous bone marrow transplantation. The role of excessively rapid marrow freezing rates after the release of fusion heat. Eur J Cancer Clin Oncol 19:485, 1983.

CRYOPRESERVATION OF PERIPHERAL STEM CELLS FOLLOWING PROCESSING

DESCRIPTION	Peripheral blood stem cells are cryopreserved for use in transplantation. A mononuclear cell suspension is prepared from peripheral blood harvested by apheresis. Dimethyl sulfoxide (DMSO) is added as a cryoprotectant and the cells are controlled-rate frozen to $-80°C$ and stored at $-196°C$ in liquid nitrogen.
TIME FOR PROCEDURE	Approximately 1.5 hours

SUMMARY OF PROCEDURE

1. A suspension of mononuclear cells and plasma prepared from the apheresis product are cooled on ice prior to the cryopreservation procedure.
2. Cryoprotectant is added to the cell suspension.
3. The cell suspension is dispensed into containers for freezing.
4. The cell suspension is frozen to $-80°C$ at a controlled rate of approximately $-1°C$ per minute.
5. The frozen cell product is stored in liquid nitrogen.

EQUIPMENT

1. Kryo 10 Model 10-20 programmable controlled-rate freezer (Planer Biomed, United Kingdom)
2. Sebra tube sealer (Tuta, Australia)
3. Class II biologic safety cabinet (BH series, Gelman Sciences, MI)

SUPPLIES AND REAGENTS

1. Hank's balanced salt solution (HBSS) supplied as powder (Flow Laboratories, Australia, or equivalent)
2. DMSO (BDH Chemicals, Australia, or equivalent)
3. Fenwal cryocyte freezing containers 500-mL or 250-mL capacity (Baxter Healthcare Catalog Nos. 4R5462 and 4R5461, Deerfield, IL)
4. Nunc 1.8-mL cryotubes (Intermed Catalog No. 368632, Sweden)
5. Sterile, individually wrapped, mixing cannulas (Indoplas Catalog No. 500.11.012, Australia)
6. Sterile disposable 30-mL syringes

PROCEDURE

1. Perform all processing of the cell suspension for cryopreservation aseptically in a biologic safety cabinet.
2. Prepare the mononuclear cell suspension and plasma as described in "Processing of Blood Stem Cells" (Chapter 5). The plasma in two 50-mL sterile disposable centrifuge tubes is cooled on ice. The mononuclear cell suspension is placed in a 250-mL sterile Erlenmeyer flask on ice in preparation for the cryopreservation procedure.
3. Perform a white cell count on the cell suspension. The total number of cells is calculated by multiplying cell volume (measured as described in "Processing of Blood Stem Cells" [Chapter 5]) by cell concentration.
4. Cells should be frozen within the concentration range 20 to 40×10^6 per mL. The volume in which the cells are stored is thus approximated by dividing total cell number by the median concentration. Final storage vol-

ume can be adjusted to suit storage containers, as long as cell concentration is within the desired range.

5. After calculating the required volume the amount of each constituent of the freeze mixture can be calculated from the ratio:

10%	DMSO
40%	Autologous plasma (effectively 20% as plasma is diluted 1:2 during cell separation
50%	Cells + HBSS

6. The plasma, HBSS, and DMSO are measured into a 250-mL sterile disposable centrifuge tube and left on ice to cool for several minutes.

7. The DMSO-plasma mixture is then added to the cell suspension. This is done dropwise with constant swirling for the first 30 mL; thereafter, it can be added at a faster rate, still ensuring constant mixing. Throughout this procedure, and until the cell suspension is frozen, the reaction mixture should be kept on ice.

8. When cells and freeze mixture have been completely mixed, approximately 6 mL of the suspension is removed using a 30-mL syringe and mixing cannula; this is dispensed aseptically in 1-mL aliquots into each of six 2-mL cryotubes, which are then kept on ice (see Note 5).

9. The remaining mixture is dispensed into a Fenwal cryocyte freezing container using a 30-mL syringe and mixing cannula, ensuring that sterility is maintained. Once the entire cell suspension has been transferred, excess air must be aspirated from the bag using a syringe.

10. The access port is double-sealed as close as possible to the container using a dielectric tube sealer.

11. The freezing container is removed from ice and wiped dry. It is then placed in a Kryo 10 freezing cassette. The cryotubes are placed in a rack. These are then placed in the freezing chamber of the Kryo 10 freezer.

12. The actual freezing program that produces controlled-rate freezing of $-1°C$ per minute depends on the type of freezing machine used. The program we use on the Kryo 10 is listed in the accompanying notes.

13. The freezing cassette and rack are removed from the freezing chamber and the cryocyte container and cryotubes removed and placed in storage cassettes in liquid phase in a liquid nitrogen vessel.

ANTICIPATED RESULT	On completion of cryopreservation the cell suspension should be completely frozen and at $-80°C$.

NOTES	1.	The cryopreservation procedure must be started as soon as the mononuclear cell suspension is prepared.
	2.	Preparation of the cryoprotectant freeze mixture and its addition to the cell suspension must be carried out on ice.
	3.	When using a 500-mL freezing container, a minimum of 80 mL and a maximum of 140 mL of cell suspension should be stored. Similarly, when using a 250-mL freezing container, a minimum of 40 mL and a maximum of 80 mL should be stored.

4. Cells must be stored at the recommended concentration range. This minimizes damage to cells during cryopreservation by ensuring that cells are adequately exposed to cryoprotectant and medium.

5. The six 1-mL aliquots of frozen cells are available to thaw for colony-forming unit—granulocyte, macrophage (CFU-GM) cultures to quantitate the number of stem cells present in the storage sample.

6. For maximal recovery of stem cells after cryopreservation, the cells must be frozen to $-80°C$ at a slow, controlled rate. We have also shown that cells should be stored at temperatures much lower than $-70°C$ for optimal recovery of stem cells as measured in the (CFU-GM) culture.

7. The cryopreservation program on the Kryo 10 is as follows:

Ramp No.	Starting Temp	Cooling Rate	Temp at End of Ramp
1	$+5°C$	$1°C$/min	$-12°C$
2	$-12°C$	$4°C$/min	$-20°C$
3	$-20°C$	$0°C$/min for 5 min	$-20°C$
4	$-20°C$	$1°C$/min	$-40°C$
5	$-40°C$	$3°C$/min	$-80°C$

AUTHORS

Pamela G. Dyson, B.Sc.(Hons)
Leukaemia Research Unit
Institute of Medical and Veterinary
    Science
Adelaide, South Australia 5000

David N. Haylock, B.App.Sc.
Leukaemia Research Unit
Institute of Medical and Veterinary
    Science
Adelaide, South Australia 5000

Luen Bik To, M.D., M.B.B.S.
Leukaemia Research Unit
Division of Haematology
Institute of Medical and Veterinary
    Science
Adelaide, South Australia 5000

and

Royal Adelaide Hospital
Adelaide, South Australia 5000

REFERENCES

1. Ellis, WM, Aitken, W, and Dobrostanski, B: The effect of cryopreservation of committed stem cells (CFU-c's) in humans. Cryobiology 18:238, 1981.
2. Hill, RS, et al: A new controlled-rate cooling apparatus for freezing hematopoietic cells at $-196°C$. Cryobiology 10:1, 1973.
3. Haylock, DN, To, LB, and Juttner, CJ: A simplified bone marrow cryopreservation method. Blood 72:1102, 1988.

CONCENTRATION AND CRYOPRESERVATION OF PERIPHERAL BLOOD MONONUCLEAR CELLS

DESCRIPTION	Peripheral blood stem cell (PBSC) concentrate, after autologous apheresis procedure, is consolidated and cryopreserved in the laboratory.
TIME FOR PROCEDURE	Approximately 2 hours from receiving the product to storing it in the freezer
SUMMARY OF PROCEDURE	1. The PBSC product is spun down in blood bag cup, and extra clear plasma is removed by a plasma extractor.
	2. The cell pellet is resuspended in autologous plasma and cryopreserved in a final concentration of 10 percent dimethyl sulfoxide (DMSO)
EQUIPMENT	1. Blood bag centrifuge
	2. Plasma extractor
	3. 60-mL disposable sterile syringes
	4. 14-gauge cannulas
	5. 600-mL transfer packs
	6. 50-mL sterile tubes
	7. Freezing bags (Fenwal Cryocyte 4R5462 or equivalent)
	8. Hemostats
	9. Cryovial
	10. 16-gauge needles
SUPPLIES AND REAGENTS	1. Heparin sodium, preservative-free; 1000 U per mL, 5-mL bottle
	2. DMSO (CryoServ, Research Industries)
	3. Medium-199 (TC-199)
PROCEDURE	1. Prepare TC-199-DMSO solution beforehand, and store on ice or in the refrigerator. For each 100-mL freezer bag, one 50-mL tube is prepared with: A. 20.4 mL TC-199 B. 10.2 mL DMSO Use 30 mL of this mixture at the freezing step.
	2. PBSC concentrate should have had at least 5000 U of heparin added in the bag before collection. Mix the product and take 0.1 mL specimen with a tuberculin syringe from the coupler for cell count.
	3. Transfer product into new 600-mL transfer pack. Sampling site couplers or spikes should not be placed in bag that will be centrifuged, to prevent possible damage to the product bag.
	4. Place the product in a centrifuge bag and fit into a blood bag cup, with the top seam parallel to the cup flats.
	5. Balance the loaded cup with a dummy bag and cup.
	6. Centrifuge at 400g for 15 minutes with no brake at room temperature.
	7. Carefully remove the product from the cup, and hook the bag onto the plasma extractor.
	8. Gently release the plasma extractor handle.

9. Swab the coupler site with povidine-iodine and connect a 600-mL transfer pack with a 16-gauge needle.

10. Plasma will start flowing into the transfer pack. With a hemostat, stop the flow when approximately 50 mL are left.

11. Resuspend cells in remaining autologous plasma; examine any clumps by gently massaging the bag.

12. Under the sterile hood, aspirate the product with a 60-mL syringe and a cannula. Transfer into a freezer bag.

13. Release the hemostat and allow a small amount of plasma to enter the product bag to rinse out the residual cells.

14. Measure with the syringe to make a total of 70-mL cell suspension in the freezer bag. Mix well, and take samples aseptically for cell count, percent mononuclear cells (MNCs), and viability test.

15. Leave the freezer bag on wet ice or in the refrigerator for 10 minutes.

16. Precool the freezer chamber to 4°C.

17. Add 30 mL TC-199-DMSO mixture to each bag with agitation. Reserve 0.5 mL for one reference vial for post-thaw colony-forming unit—granulocyte, macrophage (CFU-GM) culture.

18. Start freezing with no delay. (See previous procedures for examples of freezing programs.)

ANTICIPATED RESULT	Each 100-mL freezer bag can safely cryopreserve 10×10^9 nucleated cells.

NOTES:

Before adding TC-199-DMSO solution, make sure everything is ready in order to minimize time delay for freezing:

1. A bag holder cassette is properly labeled, prechilled in the refrigerator.

2. One reference vial is labeled, sitting on ice bath with cap open, under the sterile hood.

3. When prefreezer specimen is heavily contaminated with mature granulocytes, 20 units of DNAse can be added before freezing.

AUTHOR   Jean T. Yao, M.S., S.B.B.(ASCP)
Research and Development
  Associate
Blood Bank
Methodist Medical Center
221 N.E. Glen Oak Ave.
Peoria, IL 61636

CRYOPRESERVATION OF HEMATOPOIETIC PERIPHERAL BLOOD STEM CELLS IN GAMBRO FREEZING BAGS

DESCRIPTION	Immediately after the apheresis run, the cells are placed in a cryoprotective solution to be frozen in a controlled-rate freezer and stored in liquid nitrogen.
TIME FOR PROCEDURE	• Preparation of the cryoprotective solution: 15 minutes • Preparation of the cell concentrate: 15 minutes • Addition of the cryoprotective solution: 30 minutes • Freezing: 60 minutes
SUMMARY OF PROCEDURE	1. Prepare cryoprotective solution. 2. Concentrate stem cell suspension. 3. Add plasma and cryoprotectant. 4. Freeze in programmable freezer. 5. Store in liquid nitrogen.
EQUIPMENT	1. Laminar flow hood 2. Sorvall centrifuge (or equivalent) 3. Plasma extractor 4. Gambro bag welder 5. NICOOL ST 20 programmable freezer (or equivalent)
SUPPLIES AND REAGENTS	1. Hank's Balanced Salt Solution (HBSS) 2. Dimethyl sulfoxide (DMSO) 3. 0.22-μm Yvex filter (or equivalent) 4. 600-mL transfer pack 5. Gambro freezing bags 6. Cryopreservation vials

PROCEDURE	1. All manipulations are carried out in a laminar flow hood.
	2. Cryoprotective solution: Sterile Hank's balanced salt solution (HBSS) containing 20 percent dimethyl sulfoxide (DMSO) is filtered through a 0.22-μm Yvex filter into a transfer pack.
	3. The cell concentrate is centrifuged in a Sorvall programmable centrifuge with the integrator set at 7.5×10^6 and the brake at setting 3, which is the equivalent of 1000 rpm for 10 minutes.
	4. Collect the platelet-rich plasma and centrifuge it at 4000 rpm for 10 minutes. Draw the plasma into a transfer pack.
	5. Store at 4°C for at least 1 hour:
	  • The cryoprotective solution
	  • The stem cell concentrate
	  • The autologous plasma

ON A COLD PACK OR ON WET ICE:

6. Transfer the cell pellet by syringe to a Teflon-Kapton DF700 Gambro freezing bag. Measure the cell pellet during the transfer. Fill to 125 mL

with the autologous plasma and then rinse the initial bag containing the stem cells with a few milliliters of plasma.

7. Slowly add 125 mL of the cryoprotective solution while gently agitating the bag containing the stem cells. The concentration of DMSO should now be at 10 percent in the final solution.

8. Aliquot the contents of the bag into two Gambro freezer bags. Remove the air from the bags and correctly identify them.

9. Aspirate 10 mL of the solution containing the stem cells and DMSO for a cell count and differential. Cryopreservation tubes containing the stem cells are frozen at the same time as the bags and serve to control the quality of the apheresis prior to transplantation.

10. Freezing must commence as soon as possible after the addition of the cryoprotective solution.

11. Controlled-rate freezing is carried out with the NICOOL ST 20 programmable freezer. The freezer must be stabilized at 6°C before starting the freezing program. The temperature falls at a rate of 2°C per minute until the temperature reaches −40°C, whereby the rate increases to 5°C per minute until the temperature attains −140°C. A probe to control the temperature is put into a DF700 Gambro freezer bag containing 60 mL plasma and 60 mL of the cryoprotective solution.

12. Store in liquid nitrogen.

ANTICIPATED RESULTS	
1.	The final freezing volume is 240 mL with a hematocrit (Hct) of 20 percent and an average cell concentration of 4×10^7 per mL.
2.	The average cell recovery after freezing is 80 percent.

AUTHORS

Ridha Bouzgarou, M.D.
Centre Régional de Transfusion
  Sanguine de Bordeaux
Bordeaux, France

Gérald Cristol, M.D.
Centre Régional de Transfusion
  Sanguine de Bordeaux
Bordeaux, France

Françoise Hau, M.D.
Centre Régional de Transfusion
  Sanguine de Bordeaux
Bordeaux, France

Gérard Vezon, M.D.
Centre Régional de Transfusion
  Sanguine de Bordeaux
Bordeaux, France

Josy Reiffers, M.D.
Bone Marrow Transplant Unit
Centre Hospitalier Régional
Bordeaux, France

REFERENCES

1. Reiffers, J, et al: Stem cell apheresis in patients with acute nonlymphocytic leukemia. Plasma Ther Transfus Technol 9:115, 1988.
2. Reiffers, J, et al: Collection et congelation des cellules souches sanguines au cours des leucemies alques non lymphoblastiques. Rev Fr Transfus Immunohematol 29:193, 1986.
3. Reiffers, J, et al: Autogreffe de cellules souches sanguines. Bull Cancer 76:931, 1989.
4. Reiffers, J, et al: Haematopoietic reconstitution after autologous blood stem cell transplantation. In Bone Marrow Transplantation: Current controversies, Alan R. Liss, New York, 1989, p 313.

5. Reiffers, J, et al: Hematopoietic reconstitution after autologous blood stem cell transplantation: A report of 46 cases. Plasma Ther Transfus Technol 8:360, 1987.
6. Reiffers, J, et al: Collection of circulating granulocyte-macrophage precursors in patients with acute nonlymphocytic leukemia. Plasma Ther Transfus Technol 7:93, 1986.
7. Reiffers, J, et al: Collection de cellules souches sanguines et applications therapeutiques. Ann Med Interne, 139(suppl.1):3, 1988.

INFUSION OF PERIPHERAL BLOOD STEM CELLS

DESCRIPTION	This technique concerns autologous transplantation of peripheral blood stem cells. We will refer only to cells cryopreserved in bags (the only technique actually in use). Stem cells frozen and stored in cryotubes represent only a small number of transplants carried out before January 1987.

TIME FOR PROCEDURE

1. Preparation of material at the bedside: 20 minutes
2. Stem cell infusion: approximately 20 minutes per bag; therefore, 2 hours and 30 minutes for 12 bags, without taking into account any interruptions in the procedure related to the condition of the patient.

EQUIPMENT

1. Container of liquid nitrogen
2. Sterile waterbath
3. Large pair of tweezers (gynecologic)
4. 10-L container of sterile distilled water
5. 3 bags of antiseptic solution
6. Five 10-mL syringes with 19-gauge needles
7. 4 sample site couplers AE9
8. Three 16-gauge $\times$ 1¼-inch needles
9. 1 L sterile physiologic saline
10. Transfusion set with three branches (Travenol C2210)
11. 250 mL of 4 percent albumin (125 mL per freezer bag)
12. Airways No. 5

SUPPLIES AND REAGENTS

1. Alcohol, iodinated alcohol
2. Gauze, cotton, adhesive tape
3. Transfusion stand
4. Furosemide, chlorpromazine, hydrocortisone, intravenous (IV)
5. Sterile gown, hat, mask, boots

PROCEDURE

1. Transport the cryopreserved stem cells in a container of liquid nitrogen, to the bedside of the patient. There are 8 to 14 bags for a peripheral blood stem cell transplant (two bags per apheresis session).
   A. Preparation of the waterbath
      (1) Fill the waterbath with the 10 L of sterile distilled water and the antiseptic solution. Heat the water bath to 37°C.
   B. Preparation of the transfusion set
      (1) Connect the three-branched transfusion set to the physiologic saline.
      (2) Purge the injection tubing.
      (3) Attach the flask of albumin to one of the branches of the three-way transfusion set.
   C. Venous access
      (1) Use a 16-gauge needle or a 19-gauge butterfly.
      (2) Introduce the needle into a peripheral vein (at the elbow if possible).

      (3) Keep the vein clear with a saline drip.

      (4) Alternatively, the cells may be infused through a central venous catheter.

D. Premedication, when required, should be administered before thawing of cells is begun.

E. Thawing the cytaphereses products

      (1) Remove a bag from the liquid nitrogen with a pair of tweezers (start with the bags that are to be tested in the laboratory).

      (2) Plunge the bag into the 37°C waterbath for 1 minute; gently swirl the bag but do not attempt to dissociate the ice.

      (3) Take the bag out of the waterbath when the ice in the center of the bag is about 2.5 cm in diameter. (Do not wait too long as DMSO is toxic to cells at temperatures above 10°C.)

      (4) Attach a sample site coupler AE9 to the bag (if a sample is to be taken), and aspirate 5 mL of cells from the bag and inject them into the prepared sterile culture tube.

      (5) Attach the bag to the third branch of the transfusion set.

      (6) Stop the physiologic saline; start the albumin and the stem cells.

      (7) Fill the bag with 125 mL of albumin by placing the bag containing the stem cells lower than the bag with the albumin and gently mix.

2. PBSC INFUSION

A. Stop the albumin and hang the bag containing the stem cells and albumin on the transfusion stand.

B. Control the flow rate, so that the bag takes approximately 10 minutes to run through (not too fast, so as to avoid the cold sensations at the start of infusion, but speeding up the flow rate toward the end).

C. When the bag is empty, flush the line with a saline drip to keep the vein clear.

D. Start the next bag (if the patient's condition allows it).

3. SURVEILLANCE

A. Check the arterial pressure after the infusion of every three bags.

B. Follow the diuresis (do not exceed 750-mL volume overload, the equivalent of three bags, and inject 20 to 40 mg ampoules of furosemide if necessary).

C. In the case of nausea and vomiting, which generally occur toward the infusion of the 10th bag and are due to the cumulative effect of the DMSO, slow down the flow rate and administer 1 ampoule of chlorpromazine.

4. END OF THE STEM CELL INFUSION PROCEDURE

A. If the patient's clinical condition is satisfactory, remove the drip and make sure to compress the vein manually for at least 5 minutes before applying the bandage.

B. Empty the waterbath in the bathroom.

C. Put all disposables in a rubbish bag and the needles in an appropriate container.

D. Return the waterbath to be sterilized.

E. Write up the patient's file, detailing the transplant and the follow-up required.

AUTHORS

Ridha Bouzgarou, M.D.
Centre Régional de Transfusion
   Sanguine de Bordeaux
Bordeaux, France

Gérald Cristol, M.D.
Centre Régional de Transfusion
   Sanguine de Bordeaux
Bordeaux, France

Françoise Hau, M.D.
Centre Régional de Transfusion
   Sanguine de Bordeaux
Bordeaux, France

Gérard Vezon
Centre Régional de Transfusion
   Sanguine de Bordeaux
Bordeaux, France

Josy Reiffers, M.D.
Bone Marrow Transplant Unit
Centre Hospitalier Régional
Bordeaux, France

REFERENCES

1. Reiffers, J, et al: Stem cell apheresis in patients with acute nonlymphocytic leukemia. Plasma Ther Transfus Technol 9:115, 1988.
2. Reiffers, J, et al: Collection et congelation des cellules souches sanguines au cours des leucemies alques non lymphoblastiques. Rev Fr Transfus Immunohematol 29:193, 1986.
3. Reiffers, J, et al: Autogreffe de cellules souches sanguines. Bull Cancer 76:931, 1989.
4. Reiffers, J, et al: Haematopoietic reconstitution after autologous blood stem cell transplantation. Bone Marrow Transplantation: Current controversies. Alan R. Liss, New York, 1989, p 313.
5. Reiffers, J, et al: Hematopoietic reconstitution after autologous blood stem cell transplantation: A report of 46 cases. Plasma Ther Transfus Technol 8:360, 1987.
6. Reiffers, J, et al: Collection of circulating granulocyte-macrophage precursors in patients with acute nonlymphocytic leukemia. Plasma Ther Transfus Technol 7:93, 1986.
7. Reiffers, J, et al: Collection de cellules souches sanguines et applications therapeutiques. Ann Med Interne 139(suppl 1):3, 1988.

PEDIATRIC BONE MARROW TRANSPLANTATION AND PROCESSING | 10

Commentary by K. W. CHAN and L. D. WADSWORTH

BUFFY COAT COLLECTION FROM SMALL- VOLUME ABO-INCOMPATIBLE BONE MARROW	BUFFY COAT WITH THE FENWAL CS3000 PLUS
AUTOMATED DENSITY GRADIENT SEPARATION OF SMALL-VOLUME BONE MARROW OR BONE MARROW	COLLECTION AND PROCESSING OF CORD BLOOD FOR PRESERVATION AND HEMATOPOIETIC TRANSPLANTATION

Bone marrow transplantation (BMT) is an established treatment modality in children with diseases involving the hematopoietic stem cells (HSCs). Although the procedure itself is identical in adults and children, there are differences relating primarily to clinical indication, source of HSCs, donor care, and some aspects of marrow processing.

CLINICAL INDICATIONS FOR BONE MARROW TRANSPLANTATION IN CHILDREN

As with adult patients, acute lymphoblastic and myeloblastic leukemia and aplastic anemia are the main indications for BMT in childhood. The prognosis for childhood acute lymphoblastic leukemia, however, in many risk groups is so good that BMT is reserved for patients whose disease has recurred during or shortly following chemotherapy and some other high-risk situations. In contrast, chronic granulocytic leukemia and myelodysplastic syndromes, although rarely seen in childhood, both require BMT for curative therapy. Hodgkin's disease and non-Hodgkin's lymphomas relapsing after primary chemotherapy are indications for intensive chemotherapy followed by allogeneic BMT, or autologous BMT if there is no evidence of bone marrow disease. The majority of solid tumors in childhood are sensitive to chemotherapy and radiation therapy. These disorders are models, therefore, for intensive therapy followed by allogeneic or autologous BMT. Advanced neuroblastoma, for example, has been treated by this approach, and 25 to 43 percent disease-free survival has been achieved.[14,20] Neoplasms currently being treated experimen-

363

Table 10–1   INDICATIONS FOR BMT IN CHILDREN

A. Malignant disorders
   1. Involving hematopoietic precursor cells[6]
      (a) Acute lymphoblastic leukemia*
      (b) Acute myeloblastic leukemia*
      (c) Chronic granulocytic leukemia
      (d) Myelodysplastic syndromes
      (e) Langerhans' cell histiocytosis
   2. Others[6,14,20]
      (a) Hodgkin's disease†
      (b) Non-Hodgkin's lymphoma†
      (c) Neuroblastoma†
      (d) Ewing's sarcoma†
      (e) Rhabdomyosarcoma†
      (f) Wilms' tumor†
      (g) Germ cell tumor†
      (h) Brain tumors†
B. Inherited disorders of immunity[9,19]
   1. Severe combined immunodeficiency and variants
   2. Wiskott-Aldrich syndrome
   3. Bare lymphocyte syndrome
   4. Lymphokine and interleukin receptor deficiency
   5. Other nonfunctional T- and B-cell disorders
C. Lysosomal storage disorders and disorders of myeloid-monocyte stem cells[9,15]
   1. Gaucher's disease
   2. Niemann-Pick disease
   3. Mucopolysaccharidosis (types I, III, IV, VI)
   4. Fabry's disease
   5. Wolman's disease
   6. Metachromatic leukodystrophy
   7. Chronic granulomatous disease
   8. Chédiak-Higashi syndrome
   9. Osteopetrosis
   10. Kostmann's syndrome
D. Bone marrow failure syndromes, inherited cytopenias, and other disorders[6,13]
   1. Severe aplastic anemia
   2. Fanconi's anemia
   3. Diamond-Blackfan syndrome
   4. Congenital amegakaryocytic thrombocytopenia
   5. β-thalassemia major
   6. Sickle-cell anemia
   7. Glanzmann's disease
   8. Paroxysmal nocturnal hemoglobinuria

*Sometimes using purged autologous BMT.
†Often autologous BMT.

tally by this type of protocol also include high-risk or recurrent astrocytoma, rhabdomyosarcoma, Ewing's sarcoma, germ cell tumor, and others.[20] A list of these disorders is shown in Table 10–1(A). There are case reports of other tumors that have been managed by autologous BMT in childhood, including Wilms' tumor, osteosarcoma, and retinoblastoma, but further prospective studies are required to validate BMT as an option for these entities.[20]

   A number of inborn errors involving the HSCs are diagnosed in childhood. When it became clear that bone marrow contained competent immune stem cells, the management of inherited immunodeficiencies by allogeneic BMT provided a curative modality for what had previously been severe disorders with profound morbidity and considerable mortality. Disorders of lymphoid stem cells that can be successfully managed by BMT are listed in Table 10–1(B). It is particularly interesting that HLA-mismatched grafts can sometimes be performed in these patients, without ablative therapy or subsequent immunosuppression—particularly in those with decreased T-cell function.[12]

Many inherited disorders are due to problems of lysosomal storage, secondary to abnormalities of catabolic enzymes. Because BMT will replace abnormally functioning macrophages with normal cells from the bone marrow donor, curative therapy for a variety of macrophage and storage disorders became possible. A full list of these disorders is given in Table 10–1(C), together with other disorders of the myeloid-monocyte stem cells that have been shown to respond favorably to BMT. In order for BMT to be successful in these circumstances "displacement" of the recipient's marrow, using cyclophosphamide and busulfan, is required.[9]

A variety of hemoglobinopathies and bone marrow failure syndromes that constitute severe management problems for the pediatric hematologist can now be cured by BMT; these are listed in Table 10–1(D). Ethical considerations relating to BMT in patients with β-thalassemia and sickle-cell anemia, both nonfatal disorders, are still being debated.

Clinical recovery after BMT in inherited disorders is variable and depends on preexisting organ damage.[11] Because BMT does not necessarily reverse secondary complication such as hepatic fibrosis or esophageal varices, which may complicate some of the inherited disorders, the earlier the BMT is performed in the patient's clinical course, the better the final outcome.[13] Early transplantation is also important because the better the overall health of the recipient, the more favorable the outcome. If engraftment is successful, patients with thalassemia major rapidly become transfusion-independent; transfusion-induced iron overload resolves more slowly. Patients with osteopetrosis and Gaucher's disease recover slowly and it may be several months before tissue macrophages of donor origin are found and a year before Gaucher's cells disappear from the bone marrow.[13,15] In transplanted patients with mucopolysaccharidosis, significant improvement in the non–central nervous system (CNS) disease manifestations occurs within 6 months after BMT. It is controversial whether CNS manifestations will reverse because doubts exist regarding the extent to which donor bone marrow–derived cells or their products gain access to the recipient's CNS.[11,13]

In the transplantation of inborn errors of metabolism, it is important, therefore, that the donor bone marrow cells contain the missing enzyme and that this enzyme is accessible to tissue in which metabolite accumulations have occurred. For these reasons, BMT in Pompe's disease and Lesch-Nyhan syndrome has not been successful and is not recommended.[13]

SOURCE OF HEMATOPOIETIC STEM CELLS

As for adults, HSCs can be collected for children from syngeneic, allogeneic, or autologous sources. Because of the age of the pediatric patient, a larger range of donors (including siblings, cousins, parents, uncles, and aunts) is generally available for testing for potential bone marrow donation than is usual for the adult patient.

Some unique sources of stem cells for pediatric patients merit special discussion. Liver cells obtained from 12- to 16-week fetuses have been successfully transplanted into infants with severe combined immunodeficiency syndromes, leading to full reconstitution of the immune system.[2] A similar technique has been used in treatment of patients with Fabry's disease and Niemann-Pick disease.[15,17] More recently, umbilical cord blood from healthy newborn siblings has been used in transplantation of patients with Fanconi's anemia, resulting in correction of the hematologic abnormalities.[7] The disadvantage of these approaches is the increased risk for microbial contamination of the infused HSCs; however, meticulous attention to aseptic technique should allow both these options to become readily available, although rarely used, procedures for stem cell transplantation in children. Owing to the small dose of recoverable cells, these techniques will probably be limited to young children. The advantage of umbilical blood as a potential source of HSCs is the much higher concentration of stem cells per unit volume found in cord blood.[1] Factors affecting cell recovery and purification for this attractive source of normal HSCs are being investigated.

The suggested method used for harvesting umbilical cord and placental blood is described herein (see "Collection and Processing of Cord Blood for Preservation and Hematopoietic Transplantation"). HSCs harvested in this way are usually cryopreserved and can be infused into the recipient at a more convenient time. It is important to note that attempts so far to concentrate the HSCs in harvested umbilical blood have been unsuccessful. It is advisable, therefore, to freeze the umbilical cord blood intact and not to filter or wash prior to cryopreservation.

The use of peripheral blood stem cells harvested by apheresis is well recognized as an alternative to bone marrow HSC for autotransplantation in adults.[10,16,18] This approach is particularly favored in patients in whom the bone marrow is fibrotic, necrotic, or infiltrated with metastatic neoplasm, or if the respective areas were previously irradiated. The use of this technique is still experimental in children and, owing to difficulties in venous access and flow rate, will probably be limited initially to children over 4 years of age. The disadvantages of peripheral blood stem cell harvesting in small children relate to the extracorporeal blood volume required by the apheresis hardware, together with the technical problems of restraining small infants during a protracted procedure. Developments in apheresis hardware and software may increase the scope of this harvesting technique, making it a safe option for small children.

CARE OF THE PEDIATRIC MARROW DONOR

The care of the sibling marrow donor for the pediatric BMT recipient warrants special mention. Iron supplementation is given empirically for at least 2 weeks before donation. The donor must avoid contact with other children known to have infectious diseases. Prolonged fasting prior to anesthesia on the day of marrow harvesting is not recommended. Small aliquots of marrow (2 to 5 mL) are aspirated with each puncture from the posterior iliac crest; the use of the anterior iliac crest to obtain additional marrow is encouraged. For donors under age 10, a 16-gauge needle is used, somewhat depending on the size of the donor. Donor morbidity is extremely low and a hospital stay of only 1 to 3 days is usually needed.[3] Postoperative pain can usually be managed with oral analgesics such as acetaminophen. Most children can ambulate the day after bone marrow donation. Oral iron therapy should be continued for 2 months after marrow harvest.

In situations when the donor is much smaller than the recipient, the risks to the donor of hypovolemia and excessive blood loss must be considered. To avoid these complications and to avoid needless transfusion of random donor blood to the sibling marrow donor, various steps can be taken. It is our practice to collect routinely an autologous unit of blood from the bone marrow donor 2 to 3 weeks before the date of transplantation. An autologous donation consisting of 10 percent of the donor's total blood volume is taken. This can be easily performed in children over 8 years of age with a regular adult blood donor pack; sometimes the anticoagulant volume must be reduced if the anticipated donation is less than 250 to 300 mL. For smaller children with small veins, special blood packs may have to be used, and experiments anastomosing smaller needles to regular donor packs using a sterile connecting device are underway. For small infant and newborn bone marrow donors, pre-transplantation autologous blood donation is not an option. It is our policy to avoid homologous transfusion, and in more than 60 BMTs performed at British Columbia Children's Hospital (BCCH), no allogeneic bone marrow donor has ever been transfused with homologous donor blood. Other steps to avoid homologous transfusion are discussed subsequently. In the very rare event when nonautologous blood must be administered to the donor during marrow procurement, such blood must be irradiated to prevent the engraftment of non–HLA-identical immunocompetent cells in the recipient.

TECHNICAL ASPECTS OF BONE MARROW PROCESSING FOR CHILDREN

As a rule, more varied and complex manipulations of donor bone marrow are required for the pediatric patient, thereby increasing the risk of microbial contamination of the harvested marrow. The consequence of such contamination may be severe. Great care must therefore be exercised during marrow manipulation. It is important to employ personnel such as blood bank technologists who are skilled in the handling and manipulation of blood products for the pediatric patient to process marrow for pediatric BMT recipients.

In contrast to the adult situation, bone marrow manipulation is often performed for the benefit of the donor as well as for the recipient. In order to minimize the effects of marrow donation for the donor who is small, sometimes only a quarter of the recipient's weight and blood volume, the marrow may be collected in aliquots that are sequentially centrifuged to harvest donor red cells, which are immediately returned to the donor while a further aliquot of marrow is being aspirated. This technique has been successfully used to achieve a full engraftment of a 20-kg patient with aplastic anemia while avoiding transfusion or morbidity in a 9.4-kg donor.[5] Attention to aseptic technique is particularly important with this type of manipulation, as two recipients are involved.

Problems with ABO-incompatible marrow are potentially very serious for infants and children. Conventional methods such as plasmapheresis, to reduce isoagglutinin levels in the recipient and thereby minimize the risk of infusion of ABO-incompatible erythrocytes, are logistically impossible for small patients. Centrifugation techniques with or without added rouleaux-inducing agents are very difficult when the harvested marrow has a small volume. In our experience, marrow manipulation, such as washing or erythrocyte removal, using the COBE 2991 requires a marrow harvest volume of at least 500 mL. If the marrow donor and recipient are small, however, such a large marrow harvest volume may be contraindicated. In these circumstances, manipulation to avoid infusion of large volumes of ABO-incompatible erythrocytes can be successfully achieved by using a "shelf" of erythrocytes from a fully tested, cytomegalovirus (CMV)–seronegative, washed and irradiated unit of group O, Rh-compatible packed red cells from a third-party donor (see "Buffy Coat Collection from Small-Volume ABO-Incompatible Bone Marrow"). After the marrow has been spun in a conventional refrigerated centrifuge and packed red cells have been removed for return to the marrow donor, the remaining marrow is pumped into the COBE 2991 processing unit on top of the third-party red cells. The addition of this shelf of packed cells helps fill the processing pack and allows manipulation of small volumes of marrow using the COBE intrument. There is also a dilution of any residual ABO-incompatible erythrocytes with compatible group O erythrocytes. In our experience, this technique has been used successfully to obtain full engraftment in nine patients, aged 6 months to 11.5 years (mean 5 years). The marrow harvest volume for these patients was 145 to 625 mL (mean 363 mL), with a nucleated cell recovery after processing of 65 to 85 percent (mean 75 percent). The final product contained 1.1 to 7 mL (mean 5 mL) of ABO-incompatible erythrocytes. During marrow infusion the recipients were managed as described farther on, and no morbidity was encountered.[8]

An automated technique has been described when small-volume bone marrow harvests (10 to 80 mL packed cell volume) require reduction of erythrocyte or granulocyte content prior to infusion, purging, or cryopreservation. This method involves the use of a Ficoll-Hypaque density gradient and a Fenwal CS3000 apheresis instrument and is based on a procedure for automated density gradient separation of mononuclear cells.[4] Yields of approximately 50 percent of marrow mononuclear cells with a significant reduction in erythrocytes and granulocytes should be obtained (see "Automated Density Gradient Separation of Small-Volume Bone Marrow or Bone Marrow Buffy Coat with the Fenwal CS3000 Plus").

CARE OF THE PATIENT DURING MARROW INFUSION

Infusion of Allogeneic Marrow

Bone marrow should be infused, without a filter, through a central venous catheter as soon as possible after procurement. The infusion should be completed, if possible, in less than 2 hours. For ABO-incompatible transplants, the recipients should be prehydrated, with or without mannitol diuresis, for several hours before marrow infusion. Oxygen and antianaphylaxis treatment should be available at the bedside. The first several milliliters of marrow should be infused very slowly, while observing carefully for evidence of transfusion reaction. The rate of infusion may then be increased if no problem has been encountered. Transient hemoglobinuria may occur for up to 12 hours after marrow infusion, but acute reactions are rare.

Infusion of Cryopreserved Marrow

Children should be sedated with dimenhydrinate (Gravol) at 1 mg per kg prior to infusion. In the setting of autologous transplantation, the marrow aliquots are thawed at the bedside and are given consecutively by intravenous (IV) push. The bone marrow aliquots should be warmed by the attendant's hands or by using warm towels, to avoid hypothermia. The rate of infusion should be reduced if bradycardia or vomiting occurs. Marrow infusion should be discontinued if the heart rate is less than 80 beats per minute because further decreases in heart rate may occur.

Conclusions

The scope of BMT in childhood has expanded rapidly in the last decade. The indications for the procedure are many and include a large number of non-neoplastic, inborn errors. An increasing variety of sources of HSCs are available to the pediatric patient. Specific problems occur owing to the small size of the recipient, and in many cases of the donor. Various processing techniques are available to reduce the risks of marrow harvesting and infusion for the donor and recipient, respectively.

REFERENCES

1. Broxmeyer, HE, et al: Human umbilical cord blood as a potential source of transplantable hematopoietic stem/progenitor cells. Proc Natl Acad Sci USA 86:3828, 1989.
2. Buckley, RH, et al: Correction of severe combined immunodeficiency by fetal liver cells. N Engl J Med 234:1076, 1976.
3. Cairo, MS, et al: Clinical and laboratory experience in marrow harvesting in children for autologous bone marrow transplantation. Bone Marrow Transplant 4:305, 1989.
4. Carter, CS, et al: Use of a continuous-flow cell separator in density gradient isolation of lymphocytes. Transfusion 27:362, 1987.
5. Chan, KW, Stanley, C, and Wadsworth, LD: Bone marrow harvesting avoiding allogeneic blood transfusion in an infant. Transfusion 27:441, 1987.
6. Chao, NJ and Blume, KG: Bone marrow transplantation. Part I. Allogeneic. West J Med 151:638, 1989.
7. Gluckman, E: Hematopoietic reconstitution in a patient with Fanconi's anemia by means of umbilical-cord blood from an HLA-identical sibling. N Engl J Med 321:1174, 1989.
8. Herd, S, et al: Unpublished observations, 1990.
9. Hobbs, JR: Displacement bone marrow transplantation and immunoprophylaxis for genetic diseases. Adv Inter Med 33:81, 1988.
10. Kessinger, A, et al: Autologous peripheral hematopoietic stem cells transplantation restores hematopoietic function following marrow ablative therapy. Blood 71:723, 1988.

11. Krivit, W, et al: Lysosomal storage diseases treated by bone marrow transplantation: Review of 21 patients. In Johnson, FL and Pochedly, C (eds): Bone Marrow Transplantation in Children. Raven Press, Lancaster, CA, 1990, p 261.

12. Moen, RC, et al: Immunologic reconstitution after haploidentical bone marrow transplantation for immune deficiency disorders, treatment of bone marrow cells with monoclonal antibody CT_2 and complement. Blood 70:664, 1987.

13. Parkman, R: Future perspective for bone marrow transplantation in pediatrics. In Sacher, RA and Strauss, R (eds): Contemporary Issues in Pediatric Transfusion Medicine. American Association of Blood Banks, Arlington, VA, 1989.

14. Pinkerton, R, et al: Autologous bone marrow transplantation in pediatric solid tumours. Clin Hematol 15(1):1987, 1986.

15. Ringden, O, et al: Bone marrow transplantation for metabolic disorders of Huddinge Hospital. Transplant Proc 22:198, 1990.

16. To, LD, et al: The optimization of collection of peripheral blood stem cells for autotransplantation in acute myeloid leukemia. Bone Marrow Transplant 4:41, 1989.

17. Touraine, JL and Malik, MC: Fetal liver transplantation in Fabry disease (abstr). Blut 41(Suppl 3):190, 1980.

18. Watanabe, T, et al: Peripheral blood stem cell autotransplantation in treatment of childhood cancer. Bone Marrow Transplant 4:261, 1989.

19. Weinberg, K and Parkman, R: Severe combined immunodeficiency due to a specific defect in the production of interleukin-2. N Engl J Med 322:1718, 1990.

20. Yaniv, I, et al: Autologous bone marrow transplantation in pediatric solid tumours. Pediatr Hematol 7:35, 1990.

BUFFY COAT COLLECTION FROM SMALL-VOLUME ABO-INCOMPATIBLE BONE MARROW

DESCRIPTION	A bone marrow transplant involves major ABO incompatibility if the recipient possesses ABO isoagglutinins, which may cause hemolysis of the donor erythrocytes contained in the transplanted bone marrow. The problem can be circumvented by reducing antibody titers in the recipient using plasma exchange or by removing red blood cells (RBCs) from the bone marrow before infusion. Small-volume bone marrow can be difficult to process using automated techniques. The method described here provides a simple technique for automated processing of small-volume, ABO-incompatible bone marrow without the use of gravity sedimentation or density gradient separation.[1]

TIME FOR PROCEDURE	Approximately 2 hours to process 500 mL of bone marrow

SUMMARY OF PROCEDURE	1. Harvested bone marrow is delivered as soon as possible to the processing laboratory.
	2. Marrow is centrifuged in an inverted position for 10 minutes at $600g$ at 22°C. Using a syringe, 60 to 70 percent of RBCs are removed.
	3. A marrow buffy coat collection is done on the COBE 2991 blood cell washer using crossmatch compatible irradiated leukocyte-depleted washed Group O Rh-compatible RBCs (anti-cytomegalovirus [CMV]-nonreactive if appropriate) as a "shelf" on which the buffy coat layer collects.
	4. Agglutination studies are done to determine the volume of ABO-incompatible RBCs in the final marrow preparation.

EQUIPMENT	1. COBE 2991 Blood Cell Processor, preferably with fifth pinch valve option, COBE Laboratories
	2. Laminar flow hood

SUPPLIES AND REAGENTS	1. 2 COBE 2991 blood cell processor processing sets
	2. 300-mL transfer pack
	3. 2 sampling site couplers
	4. Three 16-gauge × ¾-inch needles
	5. Leukocyte-depletion filters
	6. 60-mL syringes
	7. 500-mL bag sterile saline
	8. 1000-mL bag sterile saline

PROCEDURE	1. CENTRIFUGATION OF MARROW
	A. If necessary, transfer the marrow to an appropriately sized transfer pack to allow good separation of the RBCs and supernatant.
	B. Centrifuge the marrow in an inverted position for 10 minutes at $600g$ at 22°C.
	2. INITIAL REMOVAL OF RED BLOOD CELLS
	A. After centrifugation, hang the marrow bag in an inverted position inside a laminar flow hood.
	B. Insert a sampling site coupler into one port of the transfer pack.

C. Withdraw into a syringe 65 to 70 percent of the RBCs in the bone marrow. Cap the needle. The RBCs can be reinfused to the donor if required. See method "Reinfusion of Bone Marrow Red Blood Cells to the Pediatric Marrow Donor" (Chapter 12).

3. PREPARATION OF LEUKOCYTE-DEPLETED WASHED RED CELL "SHELF"
   A. Install the COBE processing set according to the instructions in the operator's guide.
   B. Set up the pinboard and control panel as follows:

WASHED RED BLOOD CELL PINBOARD DIAGRAM

	Timer 1 2	Stop PC	Valve 1 2 3	Stop RC	RCO
1	● ○	○	○ ● ○	○	●
2	○ ●	○	○ ● ○	○	●
3	○ ●	●	○ ○ ○	○	●

Centrifuge Speed	Super-Out Rate	Minimum Agitate Time	Super-Out Volume
3000 rpm	450 mL/min	50 sec	600 mL

Spin timer 1: 2.75 min
Spin timer 2: 1.5 min
AUTO/MANUAL to AUTO
RCO* time: 2.0 seconds

*RCO = red cell override.

C. Connect the GREEN line to 1000 mL bag of saline.
D. Connect the RED line to a unit of crossmatch-compatible irradiated packed cells (anti-CMV nonreactive if appropriate). Leave the bag lying in front of the centrifuge cover.
E. Place a hemostat on the CLEAR line just below the red cell detector.
F. Press PREDILUTE. The V1 and V2 valves will open and saline will flow into the packed cell bag. Mix the cells thoroughly during this time.
G. When approximately 200 mL of saline has been added, press STOP/RESET.
H. Ensure the diluted RBCs are well mixed and hang the bag from the left post. Remove the hemostat from the CLEAR line.
I. Press BLOOD IN. Blood will run into the processing bag.
J. When the flow of blood has stopped, press AIR OUT. The centrifuge will start and excess air will be expressed back into the original bag.
K. When all of the air is out of the RED line, press the BLOOD IN button and the remainder of the blood will flow into the processing set. Press STOP/RESET.
L. Turn the VALVE SELECTOR dial to V2. Press TUBE LOAD and let saline run into the processing bag until it is full. Press STOP/RESET.
M. Press START/SPIN. The machine will proceed through the programmed wash cycles. Press STOP/RESET to silence the alarm.
N. Seal off the CLEAR line.
O. Remove the processing bag containing the washed RBCs from the centrifuge.
P. Filter the washed RBCs using a leukocyte-depletion filter.
Q. Irradiate the washed RBCs with 2000 to 3000 cGy of gamma radiation.

4. BUFFY COAT COLLECTION
   A. Installation of processing set and initial setup
      (1) Load the COBE processing set onto COBE 2991 according to the instructions in the operator's guide.
      (2) Remove the CLEAR line from the RBC detector.
      (3) Set the AUTO/MANUAL switch to MANUAL.
      (4) Set the SUPER-OUT rate to 100 mL per minute.
      (5) Connect the GREEN line to a 500-mL bag of sterile saline.
      (6) Connect the BLUE line to a 300-mL transfer pack. Place the transfer pack on a scale and tare to collect the desired volume of buffy coat. This volume will vary depending on the volume of marrow processed. The volume of ABO-incompatible RBCs that can be tolerated will vary with the size of the recipient.
   B. Addition of washed RBC shelf
      (1) Connect the RED line to the washed RBCs.
      (2) Press BLOOD IN to allow the washed RBCs to flow into the processing bag.
      (3) When the flow has stopped, press AIR OUT.
      (4) When all the air is out of the RED line, press BLOOD IN and allow the remaining RBCs to flow into processing bag. Press STOP/RESET.
   C. Addition of bone marrow
      (1) Remove the empty washed RBC bag from the RED line and attach the bone marrow bag.
      (2) Press BLOOD IN to allow the bone marrow to flow into the processing bag.
      (3) When the flow has stopped, press AIR OUT.
      (4) When all the air is out of the RED line, press BLOOD IN to allow the remaining bone marrow to drain into the processing bag. Press STOP/RESET.
      (5) Place a hemostat on the CLEAR line just below the RBC detector.
      (6) Press PREDILUTE and allow 25 to 30 mL saline to flow into the empty marrow bag. Press STOP/RESET.
      (7) Gently rotate the marrow bag to rinse it.
      (8) Remove the hemostat from the CLEAR line. Press BLOOD IN to allow the saline rinse to flow into the processing bag. Press STOP/RESET.
      (9) Set the valve indicator to V2. Press TUBE LOAD to allow saline to flow into the processing bag until the bag is full. Press STOP/RESET.
   D. Collection of buffy coat
      (1) Press START/SPIN. Centrifuge for 5 minutes at 3000 rpm.
      (2) Press SUPER-OUT. Allow the supernatant to flow out of the processing bag until the supernatant red cell interface is 0.5 cm from the edge of the metal plate on the centrifuge cover. Turn the SUPER-OUT rate to 0 for 5 minutes.
      (3) Slowly turn the SUPER-OUT rate up to 60 mL per minute and allow the supernatant to flow into the waste bag.
      (4) When the buffy coat is visible below the junction block, flip the COLLECT/SOV switch to the COLLECT position.

(5) Collect the required volume of buffy coat. Press STOP/RESET.
(6) Seal the BLUE line and remove the transfer pack. Gently mix the buffy coat.

5. AGGLUTINATION STUDIES
   A. Preparation of cell suspensions
      (1) Prepare RBCs suspensions of varying concentrations of the appropriate group A, B, or AB in group O cells (e.g., if the donor is group A and the recipient is group O, prepare 5, 10, 15, 20, 25, 30 percent A/O cells).
   B. Slide testing
      (1) Perform slide testing with appropriate ABO antisera. Compare the concentration of ABO-incompatible RBCs in the buffy coat preparation to the known suspensions by comparing the agglutination reaction strengths.
      (2) Calculate the volume of ABO-incompatible RBCs in the buffy coat preparation.

6. CALCULATION OF ABO-INCOMPATIBLE RED BLOOD CELL VOLUME
   A. The volume of ABO-incompatible RBCs can be calculated using the formula described by Rosenfeld and colleagues[2]:

   $$\text{Volume-incompatible cells} = B \times \frac{A}{A + C}$$

   where   A = volume RBCs in bone marrow
           B = volume RBCs in buffy coat
           C = volume RBCs in packed RBC shelf

ANTICIPATED RESULT

This procedure should yield a buffy coat preparation containing less than or equal to 20 percent (less than or equal to 10 mL) ABO-incompatible RBCs in a marrow buffy coat preparation of 35 mL.

NOTE

Sampling for nucleated cell counts, cell cultures, or sterilities will vary with each processing laboratory. In this procedure it is important to calculate the total nucleated cells contained in the red cells that were removed prior to processing on the COBE 2991.

AUTHORS

Carol Stanely, A.R.T.
British Columbia Children's Hospital
Vancouver, British Columbia Canada

Sharon Herd, A.R.T.
British Columbia Children's Hospital
Vancouver, British Columbia Canada

L. D. Wadsworth, M.B., FRCP(C), FRCPath
Hematopathology/ Immunohematology
British Columbia Children's Hospital
Vancouver, British Columbia Canada

REFERENCES

1. Chan, KW, et al: ABO-incompatible pediatric bone marrow transplantation: A simple method to remove red blood cells from small volume marrow grafts. Bone Marrow Transplant (in press).
2. Rosenfeld, CS, et al: A double buffy coat method for red cell removal from ABO incompatible marrow. Transfusion 29:415, 1989.

AUTOMATED DENSITY GRADIENT SEPARATION OF SMALL-VOLUME BONE MARROW OR BONE MARROW BUFFY COAT WITH THE FENWAL CS3000 PLUS

DESCRIPTION	This procedure is based on the procedure by Carter and colleagues[1] for automated density gradient separation of mononuclear cells. It is designed for small-volume autologous or allogeneic bone marrows or bone marrow buffy coats that require reduction of red blood cell (RBC) and granulocyte content prior to infusion, secondary processing (purging), or cryopreservation. The total packed cell volume of the marrow or buffy coat should be at least 10 mL but should not exceed 80 mL.
TIME FOR PROCEDURE	2 hours

SUMMARY OF PROCEDURE

1. Harvested bone marrow is delivered to the processing laboratory in a transfer pack. Volume, nucleated cell count, and hematocrit (Hct) of the marrow are measured, and the packed cell volume of the marrow is estimated by multiplying the Hct (percent) by the marrow volume. If the packed cell volume is between 10 and 80 mL, this procedure is appropriate. For marrows with somewhat higher packed cell volume (80 to 140 mL), a manual buffy coat procedure should be carried out before proceeding. For marrows with packed cell volumes greater than 140 mL that require density gradient separation, we usually carry out an initial mononuclear cell concentration procedure prior to the density gradient separation procedure in the granulocyte chamber.

2. FAT REMOVAL: Bone marrow with substantial fat content should be centrifuged in a DuPont Sorvall RC3 or comparable centrifuge with the transfer pack in an inverted position for 11.5 minutes at 4000 rpm at 20°C. The packed cells and some of the plasma are drained into another transfer pack, leaving the fat layer behind.

3. DEVICE SETUP: A standard Fenwal open system apheresis kit is installed on the CS3000 Plus and primed with normal saline.

4. LOAD MARROW INTO CHAMBER: The bone marrow cell suspension is diluted with normal saline and loaded into the A35 collection chamber.

5. DENSITY GRADIENT SEPARATION: Ficoll-Hypaque density gradient medium is pumped into the A35 collection chamber to underlay the marrow cells. Centrifugation causes the red blood cells and granulocytes to sediment through the Ficoll-Hypaque density gradient, leaving the marrow mononuclear cells in a layer that can be pumped up from the A35 chamber into a bag.

6. WASH: The marrow cells are loaded into the granulocyte separation chamber and washed free of the Ficoll-Hypaque density gradient medium, and resuspended in an appropriate medium for infusion, further processing, or cryopreservation.

EQUIPMENT

1. Fenwal CS3000 Plus blood cell separator (4R4530) with granulocyte separation chamber and A35 collection chamber (Fenwal Division, Baxter Healthcare)

2. Scale and balance bags

3. Heat sealer

4. Sterile connection device (DuPont/Haemonetics)

SUPPLIES AND REAGENTS

1. Fenwal open system apheresis kit for CS3000

2. 2 three-lead blood recipient sets (Fenwal 4C2210), with all roller clamps closed before using

3. Blood component recipient set (Fenwal 4C2100)

4. 2 Y connectors (Cutter 812-70)

5. Two 600-mL transfer packs (Fenwal 4R2024)

6. 2000-mL transfer pack (Fenwal 4R2041)

7. Three 1000-mL bags normal saline (Kendall-McGaw Y94-001-769)

8. 19-gauge sterile needles (Monoject)

9. Ficoll-Hypaque (LSM, Whittaker Bioproducts, Walkersville, MD), 300 mL, sterile, in a plastic transfer pack

10. 1000-mL bag sterile tissue culture medium or Hank's balanced salt solution (HBSS without Ca, Mg, and phenol red, Whittaker Bioproducts), supplemented as desired (this will be the final resuspension fluid)

11. Plastic tape

12. Hemostats

PROCEDURE

1. SET UP APHERESIS KIT AND PRIME

   A. Set up the CS3000 Plus using the open system apheresis kit as directed by the manufacturer, with the following modifications (Fig. 10–1):

   (1) To the plasma collect line, attach the straight portion of a Y connector, and then two 600-mL transfer packs to the arms of the Y connector. Then connect the 2000-mL transfer pack to one of the 600-mL transfer packs. Place a hemostat on the tubing below one of the 600-mL transfer packs, and hang the hemostat on one of the hooks above the device (this bag will be the cell collection bag, while the other two will be waste bags).

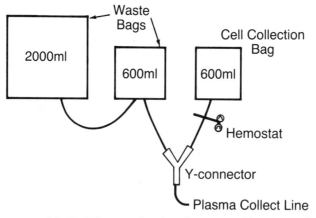

FIGURE 10–1 Diagram showing the connection of transfer bags for automated processing of small-volume marrow using the Fenwal CS3000 Plus.

(2) Leave the anticoagulant (AC) line alone, but connect a bag of saline to the saline and vent lines.

(3) Open the roller clamps on the saline, vent, and plasma collect lines (the clamps on the AC, whole blood (WB), and return lines should be closed). Make sure that the position of the roller clamps allows enough tubing between the clamp and the end of the line for future sterile connections.

(4) Label packed red blood cell (PRBC) and component ride plasma (CRP) lines with tape for easy identification.

(5) Reprogram procedure end-point volume as follows: Press DISPLAY/EDIT. Use arrows at top left of panel to select END POINT. Press ENTER. Use arrows to increase volume to 9000 mL. Press ENTER. Press DISPLAY/EDIT.

B. Perform an auto prime (prime cycle takes about 10 minutes):

(1) Press MODE.

(2) Press START/RESUME.

(3) Lift platen over whole blood pump to release air; then close.

(4) Press START/RESUME.

(5) Invert the air trap until it is filled with saline prime.

2. PREPARE BONE MARROW SUSPENSION AND SOLUTIONS

A. If necessary, transfer the marrow cells to a 300-mL transfer pack with an available port.

B. Weigh and sample the marrow as needed for cell counts and so on before beginning procedure.

C. All solutions should be in transfer packs that have at least one unused port.

3. PRERUN EXCLUDE AIR

A. Set the PROCEDURE SELECT switch to 5.

B. Place the RUN switch to MANUAL.

C. Press MODE; then press START/RESUME twice.

D. Set pump flow rates (PLASMA and BLOOD) to 0 mL per minute.

E. Press buttons to OPEN clamps to SALINE (2), PLASMA RETURN (5), and VENT (6).

F. Start BLOOD pump and set rate at maximum (88 mL per minute).

G. Start PLASMA pump and set rate at 45 mL per minute.

H. Press START/RESUME.

I. Flick air out of tubing sampling sites.

4. PRIME WITH FICOLL-HYPAQUE AND SALINE

A. Attach the Ficoll-Hypaque bag to a blood component recipient set (4C2100), and attach this and a three-lead set to the arms of a Y connector. Attach the straight portion of the Y connector to a 19-gauge needle, and place the needle aseptically into the CRP injection port (Fig. 10–2).

B. To the leads of the three-lead set, attach the marrow bag to one, a 1000-mL bag of normal saline to another, and nothing to the third (Fig. 10–2).

C. Fill the bubble trap on the component recipient set with Ficoll-Hypaque.

D. Stop the plasma pump and place a hemostat on the CRP line below the injection site.

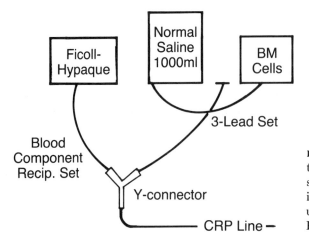

FIGURE **10–2** Flow diagram to show Ficoll-Hypaque and saline prime used for processing small-volume marrow using the Fenwal CS3000 Plus.

    E. Prime the Ficoll-Hypaque line by opening its roller clamp and also opening the roller clamps on the three-lead set and on the unused line of the three-lead set. Close the clamps once the line has been primed. Ficoll-Hypaque should go just beyond the Y.

    F. Prime the three-lead line with saline by removing the hemostat and opening the roller clamp on the three-lead line and the unused line. (Saline will flow up through the line and into the bottom of the air trap and filter.) Once the lower chamber (air trap) has filled, close the three-lead line and unused line roller clamps.

    G. To prime the upper chamber of the three-lead set and rinse the cells from the marrow bag, lower the marrow cell bag, open its roller clamp, and open the roller clamp of the saline. Allow about 100 mL saline to go into marrow bag. Close the roller clamps on both bags.

    H. Start the plasma pump (45 mL per minute). (This prevents air bubbles from entering the system.)

  5. INPUT OF MARROW INTO A35 COLLECTION CHAMBER

    A. Start the centrifuge, and allow it to come to full speed (1600 rpm) before proceeding.

    B. Stop the plasma pump.

    C. Place a hemostat on the CRP line below the injection site.

    D. Open the roller clamps to the marrow bag and on the three-lead line. Check that the other clamps on the three-lead line are closed.

    E. Close PLASMA RETURN (5). Open PLASMA COLLECT (7).

    F. Start the plasma pump forward to 45 mL per minute.

    G. Cells are now being pumped into the A35 collection chamber.

    H. Once the marrow cell bag has emptied, simultaneously open the saline line and close the cell line. Allow approximately 40 to 50 mL of saline to flow through the filter. Rinse the marrow cell bag with saline by lowering the product bag and opening its roller clamp, letting 25 to 50 mL of saline into the bag and then closing the roller clamp. Shake the bag and place it into an upright position; then simultaneously close the saline line while opening the marrow cell line. After the cells drain into the system, allow saline to flow through the system so that all the cells are rinsed into the collection chamber.

I. During the saline rinse step just described, open the hemostat below the CRP injection site for 2 to 3 seconds to flush cells that may have sedimented in this space toward the collection chamber.

6. SIPHONING OF EXCESS SALINE AND PLASMA FROM THE A35 CHAMBER
    A. Stop the plasma pump. Close the roller clamp to the three-lead set. Open the roller clamp to the Ficoll-Hypaque bag.
    B. Squeeze air from the 2-L bag into the attached 600-mL bag. Then place a hemostat at the outlet of the 2-L bag.
    C. Lower the primary waste bag (600-mL) to the floor.
    D. Check that the PLASMA COLLECT clamp is open.
    E. Stop the centrifuge. The cell-free effluent will now siphon out of the chamber and flow into the 600-mL waste bag.
    F. While the siphon step is in progress, you may remove the used three-lead set by heat sealing.
    G. When about 40 to 80 mL of fluid have been siphoned into the transfer pack (measure by visual estimation or use scale), or when cellular components appear in the line that exits the collection chamber, close PLASMA COLLECT. Note and record the plasma volume from the panel.
    H. Stop the blood pump.
    I. Close VENT and SALINE clamps. Place a hemostat on the PRBC line below the blue box. Move any lines or supplies from the top of the centrifuge. Open the centrifuge door (mute the alarm). Resuspend the cells in the A35 chamber by shaking bag. Place the bag back in the chamber, and close the centrifuge door.
    J. Press RESUME. Decrease plasma pump to 0. Open PLASMA RETURN.
    K. Start plasma pump, and set at 10 mL per minute. Cells will now be underlayed with Ficoll-Hypaque until the code 52 alarm signals, indicating that the A35 chamber is full (200 mL total volume in chamber). When alarm signals, STOP the plasma pump, close PLASMA RETURN, and press START/RESUME. Plasma return clamp should then close. Remove hemostat from PRBC line. If the code 52 is still present, press START/RESUME once more.
    L. Note and record plasma volume on panel. Subtract volume recorded in step 6G from this volume to calculate the amount of Ficoll-Hypaque that was pumped into the A35 chamber (should be 40 to 80 mL).

7. DENSITY GRADIENT SEPARATION
    A. Open SALINE and VENT. Start the whole blood pump forward to maximum speed.
    B. Start the centrifuge (1600 rpm). While the centrifuge increases its speed, open PLASMA COLLECT (7) for 1 to 2 seconds; then close PLASMA COLLECT (7) to allow cells in the line above the chamber to be drawn back into the chamber. Next, open the plasma pump platen for several seconds; then close (this allows Ficoll-Hypaque to fill the chamber as it expands during centrifugation).
    C. Open PLASMA COLLECT. Start plasma pump, and set rate to 4 to 5 mL per minute. A faster flow rate may lead to RBC contamination of the final product.
    D. Place a hemostat directly below the Y on the plasma return line (short portion), to prevent any sedimentation of cells into this line.
    E. After about 4 minutes, about 20 mL of Ficoll-Hypaque have been

pumped into the collection chamber, as can be noted on the plasma pump volume on the panel. At this point, switch the hemostat from the line to the clean 600-mL cell collection bag to the 600-mL waste bag.

F. As the density gradient separation continues, you will see plasma, medium, mononuclear cells, and finally Ficoll-Hypaque coming up into the clean 600-mL bag. The separation and collection should continue until you see a distinct clear layer (the Ficoll-Hypaque) below the mononuclear cell layer in the bag. This will take about 30 minutes.

G. While waiting for the separation to be completed, you will have time to set up the bags and solutions for the wash procedure (described subsequently).

H. When separation is complete, stop the plasma pump. Close the roller clamp to the density gradient solution, and heat seal its line. Remove the needle in the injection site and discard. Remove the hemostat just below the CRP injection site. Remember, PLASMA COLLECT is left open.

I. Heat seal the collection bag containing the cells as close to the bag as possible. Detach the bag, and gently mix the cells.

8. WASH AND RESUSPEND THE CELLS

A. Aseptically attach the long tubing end of a three-lead set to the PRBC injection port with a 19-gauge needle. Position the needle so that the bevel faces the other arm of the Y (i.e., toward the separation chamber). Figure 10–3 shows correct needle placement. Prime the line by opening the roller clamp to the three-lead set and on one of the unused lines of the three-lead set. Saline will flow up through the line into the air trap. After the air trap fills, close the open roller clamps.

B. Regarding the three leads of the three-lead set, attach the marrow cell

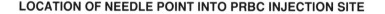

LOCATION OF NEEDLE POINT INTO PRBC INJECTION SITE

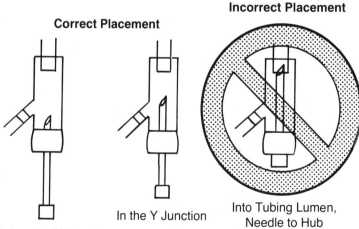

FIGURE 10–3   Figure showing correct placement of needle in packed RBC injection site when using the Fenwal CS3000 Plus for density gradient separation of small volumes of marrow.

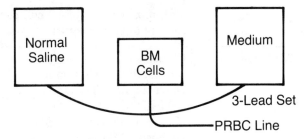

FIGURE 10–4   Flow diagram showing sg7-up for resuspension of bone marrow cells in saline and tissue culture medium following density gradient separation.

product bag to one, a 1-L bag of saline to one, and a 1-L bag of tissue culture medium or HBSS to one (Fig. 10–4).

C. Dilute the cells with 300 to 400 mL of saline by lowering the cell bag and opening the roller clamps to the bag and to the saline. Close the roller clamps.

D. Stop the whole blood pump. Close SALINE and VENT. Place a hemostat on the PRBC line above the injection site (just below the blue box).

E. Open the roller clamps to the three-lead line and cell line. Check that the PLASMA COLLECT is in the open position, and remove the hemostat on the waste bag(s), both the 600-mL transfer packs, and the 2-L transfer pack.

F. Start the plasma pump, and set rate to 60 mL per minute. Cells are now being pumped into the granulocyte separation chamber.

NOTE: *Do not allow bag and its tubing to empty to the point where air is allowed into the system. If this occurs, you will need to remove the product from the chamber and carry out a manual wash.*

G. Once the cell bag has emptied, close the roller clamp to the bag and open the saline line. Allow 40 to 60 mL of saline to enter the filter. Rinse the cell bag with saline by lowering the cell bag and opening its roller clamp, allowing 50 to 75 mL of saline into the bag and then closing the roller clamp. Shake the bag and place upright. Simultaneously close the saline line and open the cell line.

H. After the cell bag has emptied, simultaneously open the saline line and close the cell line. Allow saline to flow through the system so that all the cells are rinsed into the collection chamber. Simultaneously close the saline line and open the roller clamp to the tissue culture medium.

I. After the bag of tissue culture medium (or HBSS) is almost empty, stop the plasma pump. Close PLASMA COLLECT. Stop the centrifuge, and close the three-lead clamp.

J. Remove the cell bag from the chamber, heat-seal (above the level where cells have sedimented in the lines), and remove from the device. Discard all disposables.

K. Use the sterile connection device to transfer the cells to an appropriate bag. Weigh and sample the cells.

ANTICIPATED RESULTS   This procedure should yield about 50 percent of marrow mononuclear cells from the marrow cell suspension or buffy coat, in a volume of about 140 mL, with minimal red blood cell contamination, and significant reduction in the content of granulocytes.

AUTHORS

Charles S. Carter
Special Services Laboratory
Department of Transfusion
  Medicine
National institutes of Health
Bethesda, MD 20892

Holly Goetzman
Special Services Laboratory
Department of Transfusion
  Medicine
National Institutes of Health
Bethesda, MD 20892

Elizabeth J. Read, M.D.
Department of Pathology
University of Utah Medical Center
Salt Lake City, UT

REFERENCE

1. Carter, CS, et al: Use of a continuous-flow cell separator in density gradient isolation of lymphocytes. Transfusion 27:362,1987.

COLLECTION AND PROCESSING OF CORD BLOOD FOR PRESERVATION AND HEMATOPOIETIC TRANSPLANTATION

DESCRIPTION	Based on recent observations by Broxmeyer and colleagues that human umbilical cord blood is a rich source of hematopoietic precursors, we developed a procedure for processing cord blood for cryopreservation for subsequent transplantation.[1,2] Because the volume of cord blood obtained after normal delivery is limited, a procedure was developed to maximize recovery of fetal blood from the umbilical veins and placenta. Furthermore, the umbilical cord blood processing method was devised with the goal of retaining quantitative (100 percent) recovery of the processed hematopoietic cells. The technique is simple to perform and results in samples that retain high viability as judged both by in vitro (colony-forming unit [CFU]) assays and by their consistent ability to repopulate marrow ablated allogeneic recipients.

TIME FOR PROCEDURE	• For harvesting cord blood: 60 to 120 minutes • For processing cord blood: 30 minutes • For freezing processed blood: 120 minutes

EQUIPMENT	1. CryoMed (or equivalent) programmed-rate freezer 2. Ice bath 3. Sterile basin for placenta; sterile table for work area

SUPPLIES AND REAGENTS	1. 1-L bag isotonic sodium chloride for injection/infusion 2. 2 Charter Med 2030-2 cryogenic blood component freezing bags 3. 2 plasma transfer sets with coupler and needle adaptors 4. 50-mL sterile, pyrogen-free dimethyl sulfoxide (DMSO) 5. 30-mL syringes (10 to 15) containing 5 mL of acid citrate dextrose (ACD) for cord blood aspiration 6. Four 200-mL sterile plastic screw cap beakers (Corning), each containing 15 mL of ACD 7. 10 to 20 assorted-gauge needles (16- to 25-gauge), including ten 20-gauge needles 8. 1,000,000 U penicillin G for injection (Squibb) 9. 1 g streptomycin sulfate (Lilly), dissolved in water, for injection 10. Two 10-mL vials of sterile water, for injection 11. Two 10-mL syringes

PROCEDURE	1. COLLECTION OF CORD BLOOD A. After the baby is delivered by cesarean section or by vaginal delivery, double-clamp the cord within 3 inches of the umbilicus and sever between the clamps. The cord is clamped immediately because backflow from cord to fetus begins within seconds, reducing the volume available for collection. The distal end of the clamped cord is introduced into the collection beaker containing 15 mL of ACD. The clamp is released and the cord blood allowed to flow into the beaker. Collection is continued as long as there is flow; the cord is milked gently and continuously by hand. Care should be taken to avoid contamination of

the collection by maternal blood. When the collection is finished, penicillin (10,000 U) and streptomycin (10 mg) are added to the contents of each 100-mL beaker. The beaker is then closed. The placenta is then placed into the sterile basin and handed to the technician responsible for collection. The placenta is placed on the sterile table and turned shiny side up. At the root of the cord, a dilation area is present from which several large vessels branch out. These vessels are engorged with fetal blood, which is aspirated with the 20-mL syringes (containing 5 mL ACD) through 20-gauge needles. Various needle sizes are used for aspiration of fetal blood from other vessels in the placenta, depending on the size of the vessel. Fetal blood aspiration from these vessels has to be performed very carefully because the vessel walls are thin and collapse easily. Blood from the placenta is placed in another beaker; antibiotics are then added and the top tightened. Samples of cord blood are sent for white cell and CFU analysis. The volume of the remainder is determined and sent to the processing laboratory for preservation.

2. CORD BLOOD PROCESSING

   A. Early attempts to remove and concentrate hematopoietic leukocytes from cord blood by enhanced sedimentation, density gradient centrifugation, erythrocyte lysis, or other techniques failed for technical reasons. The decision was therefore made to process cord blood intact, without prior separation of blood components. Because no fatty material or marrow particles are present, the need for washing and filtering before processing was obviated. The cord blood is processed by chilling it to 4°C in the freezing bags. Also, a 20 percent solution of DMSO in saline is brought to 4°C in ice baths. Each bag contains 50 mL or less of unseparated cord blood. After cooling, an equal volume of chilled 20 percent DMSO is quickly added with vigorous agitation. The bags are sealed and cryopreserved by standard methods at a heat loss rate of 1 to 2°C per minute.[3] Frozen cord blood is kept in the liquid phase of a liquid nitrogen freezer until transplantation.

3. INFUSION INTO PATIENTS: The frozen cord blood is brought in a styrofoam container in liquid nitrogen to the patient's room along with a waterbath at 40°C. The cord blood is rapidly thawed in the waterbath and quickly infused intravenously.

NOTES

1. Cord blood provides a valuable source of hematopoietic cells for transplantation.

2. Engraftment has been achieved after 1.0×10^8 cryopreserved cord blood mononuclear leukocytes were thawed and infused into young, allogeneic recipients.

3. The use of this technique, both for autologous and for allogeneic transplantation, will expand in the near future.

AUTHORS

Denis English, Ph.D.
Director, Bone Marrow Transplant
   Laboratory
Methodist Hospital of Indiana
1701 N. Senate
MPC, Rm 1417
Indianapolis, IN 46202

Scott Cooper, B.S.
Walther Oncology Center
Indiana University School of
   Medicine
Indianapolis, IN 46202

Gordon Douglas, M.D.
Department of Obstetrics and
  Gynecology
New York University Medical Center
New York, NY 10016

Hal E. Broxmeyer, Ph.D.
Walther Oncology Center
Indiana University School of
  Medicine
Indianapolis, IN 46202

REFERENCES

1. Broxmeyer, HE, et al: Human umbilical cord blood is a source of transplantable hematopoietic stem/progenitor cells. Proc Natl Acad Sci USA 86:3828, 1989.
2. Gluckman, E, et al: Hematopoietic reconstitution in a patient with Fanconi's anemia by means of umbilical cord blood from an HLA-identical sibling. N Engl J Med 321:1174, 1989.
3. English, D, et al: Semiautomatic processing of bone marrow grafts for transplantation. Transfusion 29:12, 1989.

11 QUALITY ASSURANCE IN MARROW PROCESSING

Commentary by LARRY C. LASKY and NANCY L. JOHNSON

An ever-increasing number of laboratories is becoming involved in processing autologous and allogeneic bone marrow for transplantation. Although there are currently no federal regulations concerning these activities, the American Association of Blood Banks (AABB) has recently introduced standards regarding bone marrow processing.[1,2] With or without published requirements, quality assurance measures are an integral part of good laboratory practice and should be applied to marrow processing. The purpose of this chapter is to provide a guideline for developing such a quality assurance program. The published requirements for blood banks and transfusion services can be used as a model when setting up a program: Code of Federal Regulations (CFR), AABB standards, Joint Commission on Accreditation of Healthcare Organizations (JCAHO).[3-5] The AABB Technical Manual and Accreditation Requirements Manual are also good reference materials.[6,7]

GENERAL CONSIDERATIONS

An essential component of any quality assurance program is a manual of standard operating procedures. This manual should detail all methods and procedures in use in the laboratory. All personnel must follow the procedures as described in the manual. Because some techniques and equipment may not be familiar to the staff, adequate training is important.

Technical personnel from a variety of backgrounds have been used to staff marrow processing laboratories. Those with blood bank experience may have some familiarity with the equipment and quality control procedures and appreciate the importance of documentation and patient identification. To facilitate training, a mock marrow can be prepared by mixing red blood cells, plasma, buffy coats prepared from fresh whole blood units, and heparinized tissue culture media into an appropriately sized transfer pack. This allows the staff to practice handling marrow, preparing a buffy coat either by manual or by automated methods, using the laminar flow hood and sterile technique and to gain confidence in the use of reagents, supplies, and equipment. Documentation should be kept of training and the competence of staff to perform procedures.

Proper documentation and record-keeping is another important aspect of quality assurance. This begins with the informed consent of the patient for the entire procedure including processing. Obtaining consent is usually the responsibility of the patient's physician. Some institutions also require consent for storage of marrow, delineating time limits for storage, criteria for disposal, and any fees for extended storage. Alternatively, a written release may be required before removing marrow from storage.

The processing laboratory should have in its records a prescription by a physician to process marrow, usually a request form. Complete documentation of the processing procedure itself must be kept. This is usually performed by completing a flow sheet or other standardized form. The form should include patient information, date and time of marrow collection and processing, results of measurements taken or test results (volume, nucleated cell counts, hematocrit), calculations, and reagent lot numbers and expiration dates. Storage information such as location in freezer and records of the disposition of the marrow should be kept. Documentation of the freezing process, if done, would include the chart recording of the freeze and lot numbers and manufacturer of the freezing bags. If marrow has been shipped or received, date and time shipped/received, personnel identification, and temperature records should be kept. The infusion of the marrow and post-transplant events also require appropriate documentation. The record of the infusion should include date, time, number of bags and volume infused, number of nucleated cells and dose given, personnel involved in patient identification and infusion, problems encountered (e.g., cracked bags), and patient reaction. Clinical data on the recipient should be collected to evaluate the post-transplant course such as time to hematopoietic recovery, transfusion requirements, transplant-related complications (graft-versus-host [GVH] disease), and disease recurrence.

Of paramount importance in marrow processing is, of course, donor and patient identification. Every record, form, or label must provide for the recording of this information. All containers (bags, syringes, and the like) used for marrow or plasma for transfusion or analysis should be labeled to facilitate identification. The AABB Standards for Blood Banks and Transfusion Services and Technical Manual can be consulted in regard to requirements for patient identification, labels, and forms, as well as patient, donor, and quality control records.[3,7]

EQUIPMENT

Equipment should be calibrated and maintained following standard laboratory practice and the manufacturer's instructions. Suggestions for equipment monitoring have been taken from several sources, including the CFR, AABB reference materials, and the National Committee for Clinical Laboratory Standards (NCCLS) for Temperature Monitoring and Recording in Blood Bank.[3,5-8] For temperature-dependent or heat-regulated equipment, the temperature should be monitored at least on the day of use (refrigerators, freezers, waterbaths, incubators, refrigerated centrifuge). Refrigerators and mechanical freezers that store reagents, blood components, or marrow should have a continuous-recording thermometer or temperature-monitoring system and an alarm system with audible signals as well as a remote alarm connection to an area staffed 24 hours a day. Carbon dioxide (CO_2) incubators (stem cell cultures) should have CO_2 levels measured periodically and relative humidity monitored in addition to temperature. Centrifuges should have speed (rpm) and timer checked at least every 6 months. Laminar flow biologic safety cabinets should be recertified to factory standards at installation, annually, and after moving or repair. Liquid nitrogen (LN_2) storage freezers should be equipped with an audible alarm system to detect low or unsafe levels of LN_2 and ideally with an automatic-fill mechanism. If it is not monitored 24 hours a day, remote or central alarm monitoring devices are available. Alarm systems on temperature-dependent equipment should be checked periodically for function. The freezer should have locking capability for security. LN_2 levels should be monitored daily. If an automated blood processor is used for preparation of a buffy coat, mononuclear cell separation, or washing the marrow, the manufacturer's instructions should be followed for routine use and maintenance. Appropriate parameters of the marrow can be monitored to check equipment function such as before and after processing nucleated cell counts, percent recovery and yield, and differentials. Quality control of cell counters includes counting known controls as dictated by standard laboratory practice. Blood cell irradiators should be monitored for radiation leakage and to ensure that the designated dose is delivered, usually on installation and at 6-month intervals. The procedure manual should contain procedures for equipment quality control and maintenance. Laboratory records should contain documentation of the aforementioned.

SUPPLIES AND REAGENTS

Many of the reagents used in marrow processing are not approved by the Food and Drug Administration (FDA) for use in humans. Consequently, when selecting reagents, consideration should be given to whether they conform to regulations governing infusables (sterility, pyrogenicity, isotonicity, and so on). Certain reagents used in the treatment of marrow (such as purging) may require approval under the Investigational New Drug Exemption. Documentation is usually required of the use of these reagents. Some reagents prepared by a facility may need quality control testing before being put into use. For instance, when changing lot numbers of prepared reagents used in hematopoietic progenitor cultures, duplicate cultures can be set up using reagents from the old lot and the new lot. The concentration of a reagent also may need to be determined before use. In progenitor cultures, the appropriate amount of a growth factor to be added is determined by setting up a series of cultures with varying concentrations of the growth factor. It should be kept in mind that these cultures can be affected by a variety of factors. For instance, the distilled water used in the preparation of some reagents should be endotoxin-free.

It is important to maintain the sterility of the reagents used in marrow processing and progenitor cultures. This can be facilitated by using a closed system or a laminar flow hood if a closed system is not possible. A sterile docking device is available for maintenance of a closed system. Filtering devices such as a 0.22- or 0.45-μm syringe filter can be used if sterility of reagents is in doubt.

Reviewing quality control results may point to a problem with a reagent. In one reported case, a series of positive routine marrow bacterial culture results led to the finding of a lot of preservative-free heparin used for marrow anticoagulation at harvest to be infected with *Pseudomonas putida*.[9] Consequently, a method of marrow anticoagulation was developed that did not require preservative-free heparin. Reagent lot number and expiration date should be documented for each marrow processed. Laboratory records should note date received.

Many of the supplies used must be sterile and may be purchased as sterile disposables. Those supplies that must be reused should be sterilized and the appropriate quality control testing documented. Lot numbers of some disposables such as freezing bags and commercially purchased harvest kits should be recorded, as are those of reagents. Problems with breakage and leaks in the freezing bags have occurred usually in particular lot numbers of bags.

QUALITY ASSURANCE OF THE STEM CELL PREPARATION

In addition to standard laboratory quality control procedures for monitoring equipment function and reagent quality, the processing procedures and the marrow function and viability are monitored through various laboratory measurements and observations. This is much like the quality control testing of blood components prepared by the blood bank. Included in the parameters monitored are hematologic measurements, sterility, and hematopoietic progenitor assays. When additional processing is done, other assays can be used to monitor specific effects of the processing, such as determining T-cell numbers or the presence of residual neoplastic cells.

Total and Differential Counts

Several basic hematologic parameters are measured at various stages in marrow processing. Nucleated cell counts may be done in the operating room to determine the amount of marrow to be harvested, after buffy coat preparation or density gradient separation, or both, after purging or other specific processing, and before freezing. Nucleated cell counts can be done by manual methods or by automated cell counters (see Chapter 4). These numbers are also used in calculations to determine dose (nucleated cells per kilogram of recipient weight) and percent recovery. The percent recovery figure is useful in monitoring methods or equipment, or both, used in buffy coat or density gradient separation.

Microscopic examination of marrow films and smears can be helpful. Slides can be made directly from the marrow (buffy coat, treated, or otherwise processed marrow), or via the cytospin method, from a suspension of cells. After appropriate staining the slides can be examined to determine hematopoietic cell types or the presence or absence of recognizable neoplastic cells. This can be also useful in monitoring methods of mononuclear cell separation. Large numbers of granulocytes found after separation can indicate a problem in that isolation step. Slides should be made in duplicate with one set unstained. All slides are kept for future reference.

Packed Cell Volume

The packed red cell volume (hematocrit) is measured during and after processing to monitor red cell content. Because the cryopreservation regimen for marrow does not preserve red cells but allows them to lyse, the amount of red cells in the marrow is important information for the clinician as the breakdown products of red cells can have harmful effects on the patient after infusion. Red cell content also may be critical for some purging procedures. For example, when using 4-hydroperoxycyclophosphamide (4-HC) to purge marrow of tumor cells, excess red cells may contribute to drug inactivation.[10]

Sterility

Maintenance of sterility is an important consideration in marrow processing. Rowley and colleagues[11] reported a total contamination rate of 22 percent in a study of 63 patients receiving allogeneic transplants and 37 receiving autologous transplants, whose marrow was collected in open containers. The organisms identified were flora normally found on skin and did not cause clinically obvious infections in the recipients. Contamination can occur during collection of the marrow and at several stages in the processing procedure. The availability of semiclosed harvest kits and automated processing equipment may reduce the opportunity for contamination; however, sterility should be monitored with bacterial and fungal cultures. Samples are taken for culture from marrow collected in the operating room, from the buffy coat or light density fraction or both, after further treatment such as purging, and from marrow when it is thawed for infusion. Routine blood culture techniques can be used. Organism identification and sensitivities should be done on cultures that test positive. Although the major purpose of this testing is the protection of the patient, it also provides useful epidemiologic information about the laboratory and transplant activities in general.

Cryopreservation

The observation and recording of the freezing curve can be an indication of the success of the cryopreservation process and indirectly of cell viability. For instance, too rapid cooling just after phase change can result in delayed hematopoietic recovery after infusion.[12]

Viability and Progenitor Content

The ideal quality control test for ensuring the quality of the marrow graft and monitoring the processing and cryopreservation procedures would be to assess the viability of the pluripotent stem cell in the marrow and its ability to differentiate into committed hematopoietic progenitors and eventually into mature blood cells. Unfortunately, no assay procedure for the pluripotent stem cell, other than that which demonstrates engraftment after marrow infusion, is currently available. There are, however, other procedures that can be used to measure marrow viability. The trypan blue viability test is based on the ability of viable cells to exclude the dye (trypan blue). Nonviable cells stain blue when viewed under a microscope. This test can be done on a sample of marrow taken at the time of infusion, as in the procedure described in this chapter, and also on a sample of the fresh marrow prior to freezing and another sample thawed after cryopreservation. The dye exclusion test is usually carried out on the mononuclear cell fraction prepared from these samples. Unfortunately, this is a measure of the integrity of the cell membrane of each of the nucleated cells in the sample, and not specifically of the progenitor cells, which are usually present in very small quantities.

A potentially valuable in vitro method of assessing marrow viability is hematopoietic progenitor clonogenic assays. Most transplant centers use some form of these cultures to document the viability and reconstitutive potential of the marrow. Committed hematopoietic progenitors can be detected in vitro by the colonies of mature or maturing blood cells that arise when they are put into culture in the proper conditions. The types of progenitors that can be detected in human cell preparations include the committed colony-forming unit—granulocyte, monocyte (CFU-GM), the more and less committed colony-forming unit—erythroid (CFU-E) and burst-forming unit—erythroid (BFU-E), the multipotential progenitor CFU-MIX or colony-forming unit—granulocyte, erythrocyte, monocyte, megakaryocyte (CFU-GEMM), and the committed colony-forming unit—megakaryocyte (CFU-meg or CFU-MK). Although there is some controversy about the extent to which these in vitro assays of committed progenitors predict post-transplant hematopoietic recovery, some researchers have found at least some correlation between numbers of progenitors infused and speed of recovery.[13–15] The number of progenitors (as measured by clonogenic assay) needed for recovery is controversial for both allogeneic and autologous marrow and autologous peripheral blood stem cell transplantation.[13]

A reliable assay for the cell responsible for engraftment in human marrow transplantation is not currently available. Rather than assaying for this primordial undifferentiated and self-renewing cell, current assays measure the presence of CFUs of a more or less committed nature. The controversy arises in large part from the nature of the assays themselves. The assays, including the most-used CFU-GM, can be performed in many ways, and different institutions use different techniques or variations of the same technique. The assays can be affected by such factors as source of colony-stimulating activity (e.g., lymphocyte feeder layer, phytohemagglutinin-stimulated leukocyte conditioned medium [PHA-LCM], recombinant granulocyte-monocyte- [GM-] or granulocyte- [G-] or monocyte–colony-stimulating factor [M-CSF], Mo-cell conditioned medium), incubation conditions (e.g., 20 or 5 percent O_2; 4, 5, or 7.5 percent CO_2), other nonprogenitor cells in the population being plated (e.g., monocytes can be either inhibitory or stimulatory if not removed before plating, depending on culture conditions), and other culture ingredients (e.g., lot number of fetal calf serum; presence, type, and amount of steroids and reducing agents used). In published studies, these factors are often not explicitly stated, and, when they are, they vary considerably. Moreover, only rarely are reference ranges provided so that the reader can evaluate the numbers given in light of some standard.

Spitzer and associates[13] were the first to suggest that the number of committed hematopoietic progenitors infused during an autologous marrow transplant helped determine the speed of hematopoietic recovery. They showed that patients receiving a large number of day 7 CFU-GM experienced a more rapid circulating granulocyte recovery. Douay and colleagues[16] found similar results for day 10 CFU-GM. On the other hand, several investigators[17–19] have found no or little correlation between the numbers of CFU-GM infused and recovery. Rowley and coworkers[14] have shown that the number of CFU-GM infused (as detected by growth in the presence of small amounts of prednisolone) correlates with postinfusion hematopoietic recovery following 4-HC–treated autologous marrow.

The lack of consensus regarding the utility and predictive nature of committed progenitor culture in autologous marrow transplantation situations is also observed in the literature regarding allogeneic transplantation. Atkinson and associates[20] found no correlation with marrow recovery compared with the number of CFU-GM or CFU-E infused. Jansen and colleagues[21] found a weak but significant correlation between the CFU-GM numbers infused and neutrophil and reticulocyte recovery after allogeneic transplant. Arnold and coworkers[22] found a correlation between several parameters of engraftment, and CFU-GM, BFU-E, and CFU-E numbers infused. Messner and others[15] found a correlation between pretransplant CFU-meg (referred to as CFU-M in their paper) and hematopoietic recovery after allogeneic transplant.

However, for peripheral blood stem cells, within one institution, if a consistent culture technique is used, the results of clonogenic assays may be useful. One group has proposed a level of CFU-GM infused below which recovery is delayed or temporary in their institution: 50×10^4 CFU-GM per kg. They have examined the use of the less-committed CFU-GEMM or CFU-MIX, but have found that it rises in concert with the CFU-GM level during cyclic chemotherapy rebound and hence is no better a predictor of hematopoietic recovery.[23,24] In a study of the available literature, these investigators found that a dose higher than 30×10^4 CFU-GM per kg afforded rapid and prolonged engraftment. Another group has proposed 15×10^4 CFU-GM per kg as the cutoff, based on 72 peripheral blood stem cell (PBSC) rescues performed in France.[25] However, several groups[26,27] have reported successful enduring hematopoietic recoveries using considerably lower doses of CFU-GM—as much as 1 to 2 orders of magnitude lower. To and associates[23] have speculated that because the number of CFU-GEMM or CFU-MIX contained in these PBSCs correlated with the number of CFU-GM, the former were no more predictive than the latter.

Additional culture techniques that more closely represent the repopulating cell may be possible in the future. Leary and Ogawa's group[28] has described an assay for marrow progenitors that produce self-renewing and differentiating blastlike cells in vitro. From their in vitro characteristics, these cells appear much closer in the differentiation pathway to the primordial marrow repopulating cell than progenitors measured in the assays described earlier. The problem with the current application of this assay in evaluation of marrow or PBSCs is that these cells are extremely rare, and they have yet to be cultured from peripheral blood other than cord blood.

In addition to these clonogenic assays, various culture systems are used in evaluating new progenitor-processing techniques. Long-term Dexter-type cultures have been used, for instance, to evaluate the marrow repopulating ability of 4-HC–treated marrow.[29] Douay and others[30] have used this technique to examine the regenerative characteristics of blood-derived progenitors. They found they could establish long-term CFU-GM production using PBSCs in the absence of an adherent marrow stromal cell layer. This technique may be used in the future to evaluate PBSC preparations for their marrow restoration potential. Smith and Broxmeyer[31] have used liquid suspension culture to observe the growth of progenitors isolated from human cord blood under different conditions.

Several practical considerations are necessary when considering setting up and using these culture techniques. "Cake-mix" kits for hematopoietic progenitor assays are available commercially. When evaluating the effect of the cryopreservation process, usually samples in small bags or tubes are frozen at the same time as the primary marrow inoculum. These samples can be thawed after freezing and sufficiently long enough before infusion to allow outgrowth of colonies in culture. Because the geometry of tubes and small bags is different from the most-used larger freezing bags, the rate at which these samples freeze may be different.[32] However, gross errors in the freezing process, such as accidentally using another reagent instead of dimethyl sulfoxide (DMSO) as a cryoprotectant or encountering major freezing problems, will be detected.

The human hematopoietic progenitor antigen CD34 has been used experimentally to positively select progenitor cells for use in autologous marrow transplantation.[33,34] It is possible that the number of CD34-positive cells in a given cellular support inoculum may be indicative of its potential ability to restore hematopoiesis. This has yet to be established.

Purging and T-Cell Removal

Another parameter to follow is the number of residual unwanted cells. If T cells or malignant cells are physically removed (as in elutriation or with antibody and complement), then immunologic marking techniques such as immunofluorescence using microscopy or flow cytometry can be performed. Some methods of purging leave the antigenic structure of unwanted cells intact, at least initially. Purging with the toxin ricin and with the chemotoxic compound 4-HC are examples of such methods.[35] In the case of T cells, functional assays can be performed, including lectin stimulation and limiting dilution analysis.[36]

In some malignancies, clonogenic assays of malignant progenitors may be possible.[37,38] Chromium release assays using labeled malignant cell lines can be carried out in parallel to the actual purging to check the efficiency of the purging process. Chromosomal markers or clonal gene rearrangements can also be followed. Polymerase chain reaction techniques may allow detection of malignant cells with a resolution as high as 1 in 100,000.[39]

Infusion and Clinical Effect

The effect of the infusion of the marrow inoculum can indicate several things about the quality of the processing. Fever, chills, hemoglobinuria, and other untoward symptoms and signs may occur with some frequency even if no problems with the processing have occurred.[40] On the other hand, these can be associated with unintentional contamination with undesirable cells, pathogens, or chemicals, and thus should be followed closely as part of marrow processing quality assurance.

An important measure of the safety of the marrow manipulation process is the clinical outcome. If the desired hematopoietic progenitors in the marrow have been substantially damaged, hematopoietic recovery may be considerably delayed or may fail to occur in one or more cell lines. The time in which the patient's white count exceeds 1000 per μL or absolute neutrophil count exceeds 500 per μL may range from 2 weeks to 3 months. Platelet recovery may and usually does take longer than white cell or neutrophil recovery.

Other clinical factors may be related to the effectiveness of marrow processing. In allogeneic transplants, the incidence and degree of GVH disease may be related to the degree of T-cell depletion. On the other hand, T-cell depletion may be associated with graft failure and an increase in the incidence of disease recurrence (the latter due to abrogation of the graft-vs-leukemia effect). Although disease recurrence following autologous transplant is often thought to be due to residual disease in the patient,[41] inadequate in vitro purging may also be a factor. For these reasons, the clinical outcome of the patient with respect to hematopoietic recovery, disease recurrence, and GVH disease should be followed closely by those responsible for marrow processing, as well as the patient's clinical physicians.

REFERENCES

1. Rowley, SD and Davis, JM: Standards for bone marrow processing laboratories. Transfusion 30:571, 1990.
2. Areman, EM, Sacher, RA, and Deeg, HJ: Bone marrow storage and processing: Is it time to set standards? Transfusion 30:574, 1990.
3. Standards for Blood Banks and Transfusion Services, ed 13. American Association of Blood Banks, Arlington, VA, 1989.
4. Van Schoonhoven, P, Berkman, EM, and Lehmann, R: Medical Staff Monitoring Functions: Blood Usage Review. Joint Commission on Accreditation of Hospitals, Chicago, 1987.
5. Code of Federal Regulations: Title 21, Parts 600 to 799. US Government Printing Office, Washington, DC, 1990.
6. Accreditation Requirements Manual, ed 3. American Association of Blood Banks, Arlington, Virginia, 1990.

7. Technical Manual, ed 10. American Association of Blood Banks, Arlington, VA, 1990.

8. Temperature Monitoring and Recording in Blood Banks. Tentative Guidelines. NCCLS Document I 16-T. National Committee for Clinical Laboratory Standards, Villanova, PA, 1986.

9. Cameron, S, et al: Reported contamination of heparin sodium with pseudomonas putida. MMWR 35:123, 1986.

10. Jones, RJ, et al: Variability in 4-hydroperoxycyclophosphamide activity during clinical purging for autologous bone marrow transplantation. Blood 70:1490, 1987.

11. Rowley, SD, et al: Bacterial contamination of bone marrow grafts intended for autologous and allogeneic bone marrow transplantation. Transfusion 28:109, 1988.

12. Abrams, RA, et al: Haemopoietic recovery in Ewing's sarcoma after intensive combination therapy and autologous marrow infusion. Lancet 2:385, 1980.

13. Spitzer, G, et al: The myeloid progenitor cell—its value in predicting hematopoietic recovery after autologous bone marrow transplantation. Blood 55:317, 1980.

14. Rowley, SD, et al: CFU-GM content of bone marrow graft correlates with time to hematologic reconstitution following autologous bone marrow transplantation with 4-hydroperoxycyclophosphamide–purged bone marrow. Blood 70:271, 1987.

15. Messner, HA, et al: Clonogenic hemopoietic precursors in bone marrow transplantation. Blood 70:1425, 1987.

16. Douay, L, et al: Recovery of CFU-GM from cryopreserved marrow and in vivo evaluation after autologous bone marrow transplantation are predictive of engraftment. Exp Hematol 14:358, 1986.

17. Gilmore, MJML, et al: A technique for the concentration of nucleated bone marrow cells for in vitro manipulation or cryopreservation using the IBM2991 blood cell processor. Vox Sang 45:294, 1983.

18. Beaujean, F, et al: Successful infusion of 40 cryopreserved autologous bone-marrows. In vitro studies of the freezing procedure. Biomed Pharmacother 38:348, 1984.

19. Hartmann, O, et al: Hematopoietic recovery following autologous bone marrow transplantation: Role of cryopreservation, number of cells infused and nature of high-dose chemotherapy. Eur J Cancer Clin Oncol 21:53, 1985.

20. Atkinson, K, et al: Lack of correlation between nucleated bone marrow CFU-GM dose or marrow CFU-E dose and the rate of HLA-identical sibling marrow engraftment. Br J Haematol 60:245, 1985.

21. Jansen, J, et al: The impact of the composition of the bone marrow on engraftment and graft-versus-host disease. Exp Hematol 11:967, 1983.

22. Arnold, R, et al: Hemopoietic reconstitution after bone marrow transplantation. Exp Hematol 14:271, 1986.

23. To, LB, et al: CFU-mix are no better than CFU-GM in predicting hematopoietic reconstitutive capacity of peripheral blood stem cells collected in the very early remission phase of acute non-lymphoblastic leukemia. Exp Hematol 15:351, 1987.

24. To, LB, Dyson, PG, and Juttner, CA: Cell-dose effect in circulating stem-cell autografting (letter). Lancet 2:404, 1986.

25. Reiffers, J, et al: Autologous blood stem cell transplantation in patients with haematological malignancies. Bone Marrow Transplant 3(Suppl 1):167, 1988.

26. Lasky, LC, et al: Clinical collection and use of peripheral blood stem cells in pediatric patients. Transplantation 47:613, 1989.

27. Körbling, M, et al: Autologous blood stem cell transplantation (ABSCT) in 34 patients: Its methodological advantage and limitation. Blood Marrow Transplant 3(Suppl 1):51, 1988.

28. Leary, AG and Ogawa, M: Blast cell colony assay for umbilical cord blood and adult bone marrow progenitors. Blood 69:953, 1987.

29. Winton, EF and Colenda, KW: Use of long-term human marrow cultures to demonstrate progenitor cell precursors in marrow treated with 4-hydroperoxycyclophosphamide. Exp Hematol 15:710, 1987.

30. Douay, L, et al: Long-term human blood cultures: Application to circulating progenitor cell autografting. Bone Marrow Transplant 2:67, 1987.

31. Smith, S and Broxmeyer, HE: The influence of oxygen tension on the long-term growth in vitro of haematopoietic progenitor cells from human cord blood. Br J Haematol 63:29, 1986.

32. Douay, L, Lopez, M, and Gorin, NC: A technical bias: Differences in cooling rates prevent ampules from being a reliable index of stem cell cryopreservation in large volumes. Cryobiology 23:296, 1986.

33. Berenson, RJ, et al. Stem cell selection—clinical experience. Prog Clin Biol Res 333:403, 1990.

34. Bensinger, WI, et al: Positive selection of hematopoietic progenitors from marrow and peripheral blood for transplantation. J Clin Apheresis 5:74, 1990.

35. Vallera, DA, et al: Bone marrow purification. In Edwards-Moulds, J and Masouredis, S (eds): Monoclonal Antibodies. American Association of Blood Banks, Arlington, VA, 1989, p 181.

36. Filipovich, AH, et al: T cell depletion with anti-CD5 immunotoxin in histocompatible bone marrow transplantation. The correlation between residual CD5 negative T cells and subsequent graft-versus-host disease. Transplantation 50:410, 1990.

37. Uckun, FM, et al: Marrow purging in autologous bone marrow transplantation for T-lineage acute lymphoblastic leukemia: Efficacy of ex vivo treatment with immunotoxins and 4-hydroperoxycyclophosphamide against fresh leukemic marrow progenitor cells. Blood 69:361, 1987.

38. Uckun, FM, et al: Use of fluorescence activated cell sorting (FACS) in combination with leukemic progenitor cell (LPC) assays for quantitative analysis of residual disease in bone marrow (BM) samples from high risk remission b-lineage who undergo autologous bone marrow transplantation (BMT) (abstract). Blood 74(Suppl 1):281a, 1989.

39. Hansen-Hagge, TE, Yokota, S, and Bartram, CR: Detection of minimal residual disease in acute lymphoblastic leukemia by in vitro amplification of rearranged T-cell receptor delta chain sequences. Blood 74:1762, 1989.

40. Yeager, AM, et al: Autologous bone marrow transplantation in patient with acute nonlymphocytic leukemia, using ex vivo marrow treatment with 4-hydroperoxycyclophosphamide. N Engl J Med 315:141, 1986.

41. Kersey, JH, et al: Comparison of autologous and allogeneic bone marrow transplantation for treatment of high-risk refractory acute lymphoblastic leukemia. N Engl J Med 317:461, 1987.

THAWING MARROW FOR ASSAYS

THAWING OF CRYOPRESERVED BONE MARROW SAMPLES FOR ASSAYS

DESCRIPTION	This procedure describes the thawing and washing of a 10-mL aliquot of concentrated bone marrow buffy coat cryopreserved with dimethyl sulfoxide (DMSO) at a final concentration of 10 percent. This technique is useful in recovering cryopreserved bone marrow for microbiology cultures and hematopoietic progenitor colony assays and to evaluate the percentage of cells recovered after thawing.
TIME FOR PROCEDURE	Approximately 2 hours

SUMMARY OF PROCEDURE

1. A 10-mL sample bag of cryopreserved bone marrow is thawed rapidly in a 37°C waterbath.
2. The thawed marrow is diluted with media to lower the DMSO concentration to 1 percent or less and then is centrifuged to concentrate cells.
3. The recovered marrow cells are layered over a gradient of Ficoll-Hypaque to isolate the mononuclear cells.
4. The mononuclear cells are washed with media to remove Ficoll-Hypaque and to concentrate marrow cells for desired tests.

EQUIPMENT

1. Laminar flow hood
2. Centrifuge and tube holders for 50- and 15-mL conical tubes
3. Pipette aid, vacuum-pressure
4. Hemostats

SUPPLIES AND REAGENTS

1. 200-mL Minimum Essential Medium (MEM) with Hank's salts and L-glutamine
2. 2.5 mL of micrococcal nuclease from *Staphylococcus aureus* (20.0 units per mL)
3. 50 mL human serum albumin, 25 percent
4. 1 mL heparin sodium 10,000 USP U per mL
5. 15 mL Ficoll-Hypaque gradient
6. Alcohol and iodine swabs
7. Sampling site coupler
8. Plastic pipettes, sterile: 25-mL, 10-mL, 2-mL, 1-mL
9. Syringes: 60-mL, 20-mL, 3-mL
10. Needles: 16-gauge × 1½ inch
11. Sterile polypropolyene conical tubes with caps: 50-mL, 15-mL

PROCEDURE

1. PREPARATION OF DILUTING MEDIA
   A. To each of two 100-mL bottles of MEM, add the following:
      (1) 25 mL of albumin

        (2) 0.5 mL of heparin
        (3) 1.25 mL of a 20 U per mL solution of nuclease for a final concentration of 0.2 U per mL
  B. Mix media well using a 25-mL pipette
  C. Add prepared media to sterile conical tubes as follows:
        (1) 10 mL of media to one 50-mL tube
        (2) 9 mL of media to one 50-mL tube

> **NOTE:** *If volume of marrow sample bag is greater than 10 mL, calculate the amount of diluting media needed for each marrow aliquot using the following calculations and then adjust procedure accordingly. The cryopreserved marrow sample must be diluted 1:10 (1 part marrow to 9 parts media) in order to reduce the DMSO concentration to 1 percent or less.*

Total volume frozen marrow (10 mL) $\times$ 10 = 100 mL total volume of marrow plus media

100 mL − 10 mL marrow = 90 mL of media required to dilute 10 mL of 10 percent DMSO to 1 percent DMSO

2. THAWING AND DILUTION OF MARROW ALIQUOTS

  A. Fill a 1000-mL beaker with 37°C water.
  B. Submerge the frozen marrow aliquot into the 37°C water. Gently massage bag until marrow is thawed.
  C. Wipe bag with gauze and then break off protective cover from port on marrow bag. Insert a sampling site coupler.
  D. Wipe coupler with an alcohol swab. Using a 20-mL syringe with a 16-gauge needle, inject 5 cc of air into the sample bag. Withdraw marrow into syringe.
  E. Transfer marrow from syringe into a sterile 50-mL conical tube. Using a 10-mL sterile pipette quickly measure the volume of the thawed marrow and record volume.
  F. Using the same pipette as in step 2E, transfer 1 mL of thawed marrow to a tube containing 9 mL of media to be used as a 1:10 dilution for a nucleated cell count, differential, and dye viability test. Pipette the remaining marrow to the 50-mL tube containing 10 mL of media. Allow mixture to equilibrate for 1 minute and then transfer equal aliquots of this mixture to two 50-mL tubes. Further dilute mixture by slowly adding 40 mL of media to each aliquot in a stepwise manner within 5 minutes.
  G. Allow diluted marrow to stand at 18 to 22°C for 10 minutes and then centrifuge at 400*g* for 10 minutes at 18 to 22°C.
  H. After centrifugation of diluted marrow, discard supernatant. Resuspend and pool cell buttons into a 15-mL tube. Add media to bring volume to 15 mL.

3. MONONUCLEAR CELL SEPARATION

  A. With a 30-mL syringe and needle, remove 15 mL of Ficoll-Hypaque from bottle and transfer 5 mL of gradient to each of three 15-mL sterile conical tubes.

B. Gently overlayer each 5 mL of Ficoll-Hypaque with 5 mL of thawed marrow.

C. Before starting centrifuge, turn centrifuge brake to OFF position. When starting centrifugation, gradually increase rpms from 0 to the appropriate setting. Centrifuge at $400g$ for 30 minutes at 18 to 22°C.

4. WASHING OF MONONUCLEAR CELLS

A. Using a 10-mL pipette, carefully remove the mononuclear cell layer and pool in a 50-mL sterile conical tube.

B. Add media to bring the cell volume up to 50 mL. Centrifuge at $400g$ for 10 minutes at 18 to 22°C.

C. Remove supernatant. Wash cells again by resuspending the cell button and adding media to bring volume up to 50 mL. Mix well. Centrifuge at $400g$ for 10 minutes at 18 to 22°C.

D. Repeat step 4C for a third wash. After the third wash, resuspend the cell button and add media to bring volume to 2 mL.

5. POST-THAWING TESTS

A. Remove 0.1 mL of cells and add to 0.9 mL of media (1:10 dilution) for post-thawing tests: nucleated cell counts, differential, and dye viability.

B. The remaining 1.9 mL of cells may be used for additional assays such as hematopoietic progenitor colony assays.

C. Calculate the percent recovery of frozen thawed marrow using the immediate post-thaw nucleated cell count and the volume of marrow measured in step 2E.

6. MICROBIOLOGY CULTURES

A. Prepare sample from 10-mL marrow bag for microbiology cultures. Wipe sampling site coupler with alcohol and iodine swabs. Allow to dry. Using a 3-mL syringe and needle inject 2-mL of media into the 10-mL sample bag. Leaving needle inserted in bag, mix and transfer fluid back into the syringe. Transfer fluid to a sterile tube for microbiology cultures.

ANTICIPATED RESULTS	1. Greater than 99 percent dye viability of frozen-thawed mononuclear cells
	2. Greater than 80 percent recovery of frozen-thawed mononuclear cells
	3. Minimum mononuclear cell count of 1.0×10^6 of washed cells (final product volume 1.9 mL) for hematopoietic progenitor colony assays
NOTE	All work for the procedure is performed in a laminar flow hood using sterile technique to prepare marrow for microbiology cultures and hematopoietic progenitor colony assays.

AUTHORS

Marita G. Hill, M.T.(ASCP), S.B.B.
Blood Bank Immunohematologist
University of Kentucky Medical
    Center
Lexington, KY 40536

Vickie M. Robertson, M.T.(ASCP),
    S.B.B.
Blood Bank Bone Marrow
    Transplant Coordinator
University of Kentucky Medical
    Center
Lexington, KY 40536

Larry G. Dickson, M.D.
Director, Blood Bank
Clinical Laboratory
University of Kentucky Medical
    Center
Lexington, KY 40536

REFERENCE   1. Visani, G, et al: Recovery of CFU-GM after freezing of normal human bone marrow: Effect of
                    three dilution techniques after thawing. Cryobiology 20:587, 1983.

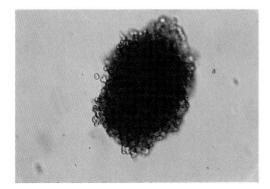

Figure 11–1   BFU-E (×75)

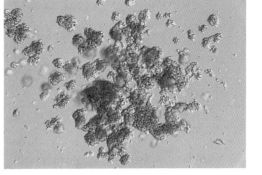

Figure 11–2   BFU-E (×37.5)

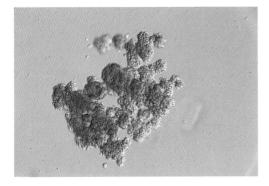

Figure 11–3   BFU-E (×37.5)

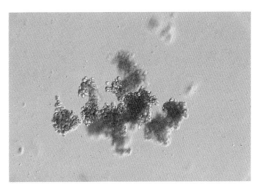

Figure 11–4   BFU-E (×37.5)

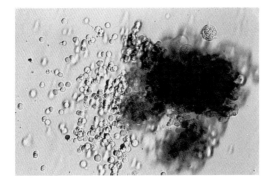

Figure 11–5   CFU-GEMM (×75)

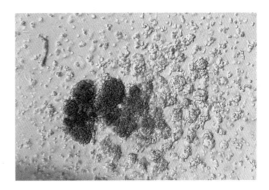

Figure 11–6   CFU-GEMM (×37.5)

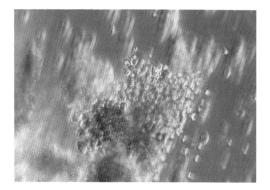

Figure 11–7   CFU-GEMM (×150)

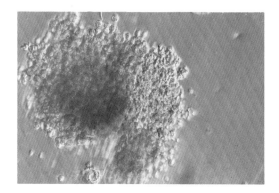

Figure 11–8   CFU-GEMM (×150)

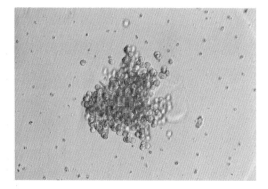

Figure 11–9   CFU-GM (×75)

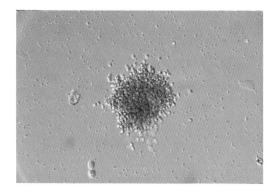

Figure 11–10   CFU-GM (×37.5)

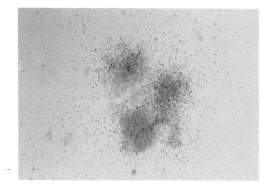

Figure 11–11   CFU-GM (×15)

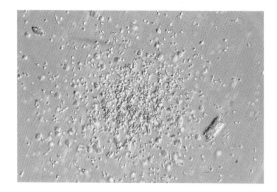

Figure 11–12   CFU-GM (×37.5)

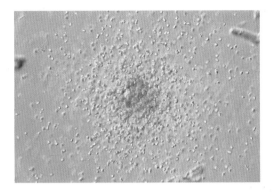

Figure 11–13 CFU-GM (×37.5)

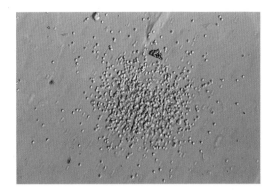

Figure 11–14 CFU-GM (×37.5)

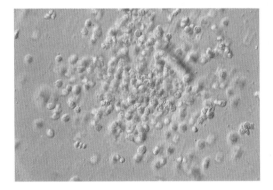

Figure 11–15 CFU-GM (macrophage) (×37.5)

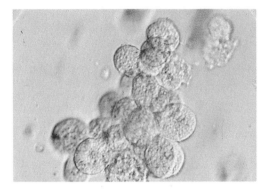

Figure 11–16 CFU-GM (macrophage) (×150)

Figures 11–1 to 11–4. BFU-E-derived colonies. The colony depicted in Figure 11–1 did not grow with subclusters, but the large size and time of appearance in culture (all colonies were photographed after 14 to 16 days in culture) distinguish this colony from the much smaller and earlier CFU-E-derived colonies. **Figure 11–2.** The other extreme of a BFU-E giving rise to a large number of subclusters is illustrated. The color (amount of hemoglobin) and size of the subclusters are very consistent within the colonies depicted in these figures.

Figures 11–5 to 11–8. Mixed erythroid/myeloid colonies (CFU-GEMM, CFU-GEM, or CFU-mix are common terms for the progenitor cell giving rise to this type of colony). The colonies in Figures 11–5 and possibly 11–6 could be read as overlap colonies as well, showing the need to develop one's own criteria for defining this colony type. Figures 11–7 and 11–8 are high-magnification photomicrographs showing the intimate admixture of cells usually found in this colony type. Colonies of mixed myeloid cells (neutrophils with macrophages or eosinophils, for example) contain cells from the same lineage, and therefore are not classified as CFU-GEMM-derived.

Figures 11–9 to 11–16. Myeloid colonies. Some colonies, especially eosinophil colonies (Figure 11–9) may form in tight balls. Others may form in multiple subclusters similar to erythroid colonies (Figure 11–11). Figures 11–12 to 11–14 show more typical myeloid colonies of the "fried-egg" appearance of a dense center and a periphery of migrating neutrophils. Macrophages, large cells with "foamy" cytoplasm, can be seen in Figures 11–15 and 11–16.

HEMATOPOIETIC CELL COLONIES
Scott D. Rowley, M.D., FACP
(See procedure: HEMATOPOIETIC PROGENITOR CELL ASSAY)

Culture of hematopoietic progenitor cells requires interpretation of the colonies found in the culture dishes. Therefore, it is important to define what features constitute a colony. In general, colonies are groupings of greater than 40 cells, in contrast to clusters, which are smaller groupings. CFU-E- and CFU-megakaryocyte-derived colonies are smaller and may be defined in some assays as groupings of only four to eight cells. BFU-E-derived colonies are sometimes defined as requiring three or more subclusters. Terminology may also differ among different laboratories—we believe that colonies arise from single cells called *colony-forming units*. It always should be understood that the colony found in the culture dish is not a CFU, but rather a CFU-derived colony. (In actuality, the hematopoietic cell probably should be termed a CFC [colony-forming *cell*] instead of a CFU [colony-forming *unit*].) Only in the most precise experimental hematology research will the progenitor cells be classified by the actual composition of resulting colonies (e.g., CFU-eosinophil, CFU-neutrophil, CFU-basophil, CFU-neutrophil/eosinophil, etc.). Instead, colonies are usually grouped as arising from progenitor cells of fairly similar potential (i.e., all of the above can be classified as CFU-GM). Our laboratory generally classifies all colonies into one of three groupings: CFU-GM-, BFU-E-, or CFU-GEMM-derived. Not all CFU-GM-derived colonies contain macrophages, and some are composed only of neutrophils or macrophages or eosinophils. Likewise, we have never looked for megakaryocytes in our CFU-GEMM-derived colonies, accepting instead that this progenitor cell, capable of giving rise to both erythroid and myeloid cells in our cultures, is probably the same progenitor cell that other investigators have shown can give rise to megakaryocytes.[1] The cells of BFU-E-derived colonies always contain hemoglobin and can be identified by the red color in situ. CFU-GEMM-derived colonies contain a mixture of erythroid and myeloid cells. Immature red cells without red pigment should not be mistaken for myeloid cells: high-magnification examination may be necessary to determine cell type. Colonies can also be aspirated from the culture dishes, diluted into media, and cytospun onto glass slides for staining and examination of composition. CFU-GM has generally replaced the term CFU-C (colony-forming unit, culture) found in earlier hematology reports.

Cell culture is as much an art as a science. We are frequently asked which technique is best for quality control of a bone marrow processing facility. Every laboratory has its own biases about the proper techniques and reagents for culturing hematopoietic progenitor cells. What matters, however, is the utility of the data obtained. If the culture results do not relate to the question asked, then alternate techniques should be tested. We found, for example, that one technique could be used to predict engraftment after autografting with 4-HC purged marrows, while a second technique provided no relevant data.[2] Obviously, we no longer use the irrelevant assay as quality control in our laboratory. The major differences between these two assays were the concentration of fetal-bovine serum, and the growth stimulant used. Successful cell culture laboratories continuously monitor the quality of their reagents, and will not even change plastic-ware manufacturers without comparing the new lots to the old. Quality control is as important in the cell culture laboratory as it is in the bone marrow processing laboratory.

Scoring of culture dishes requires interpretation that is not easily depicted in photomicrographs. In obtaining these pictures, we had the benefit of seeing the entire culture dish and could isolate individual colonies at the lower magnification used for scoring. In crowded culture dishes, overlap of colonies will occur, leading to artificially lower counts. To distinguish overlap colonies, we look for concentricity. (For instance, does it appear that there are two distinct centers?) Cultures are three-dimensional, so spatial separation may also be vertical. Cell lineages (are there also two distinct cell types such as eosinophils and neutrophils?) and maturity (are the red blood cells in one grouping more hemoglobinized than they are in the other?) also enter into the interpretation of concentricity.

REFERENCES

1. Fauser, AA and Messner, HA: Identification of megakaryocytes, macrophages, and eosinophils in colonies of human bone marrow containing neutrophilic granulocytes and erythroblasts. Blood 53:1023, 1979.
2. Rowley, SD, et al: CFU-GM content of bone marrow graft correlates with time to hematologic reconstitution following autologous bone marrow transplantation with 4-hydroperoxycyclophosphamide-purged bone marrow. Blood 70:271, 1987.

COLLECTION AND QUALITY ASSURANCE OF SAMPLES FROM BONE MARROW THAWED FOR INFUSION

DESCRIPTION	Bone marrow, frozen in bags and stored in liquid nitrogen ($-196°C$) is rapidly thawed at 37°C and immediately infused into the recipient, diluting the dimethyl sulfoxide (DMSO) cryopreservative before substantial hematopoietic cell damage may occur. Sampling of the bone marrow is necessary for quality control assessment (microbiology and cell viability and quantitations).
TIME FOR PROCEDURE	Approximately 1 to 3 hours from thawing of first bag and its reinfusion to thawing and reinfusing the last bag, varying with the number of bags (usually four) and patient's reaction(s).
SUMMARY OF PROCEDURE	1. Marrow bags are thawed one at a time. 2. Each marrow bag is sampled for quality control.
EQUIPMENT	1. Waterbath, circulating type (should be on a movable cart) 2. Hemacytometer 3. Microscope
SUPPLIES AND REAGENTS	1. 3-mL syringes (1 per bag of marrow thawed) 2. Microbiologic assay vials 3. Culture tube containing 3.5 mL TC-199 plus 5.0 mL fetal bovine serum (FBS) plus 0.5 mL heparin 4. Microscope slides 5. Trypan blue dye 6. Wright-Giemsa stain 7. Alcohol swipes
PROCEDURE	1. Immediately after marrow flow has begun, hand 3-mL syringe to nurse, who will draw a 2.5-mL sample of marrow through sterile stopcock in infusion line. 2. Fit syringe with needle, wipe top of microbiologic assay vial with alcohol wipe, and inject 1.5 mL into vial. 3. Inject remaining 1 mL into culture tube containing 3.5 mL of TC-199 plus 5.0 mL FBS plus 0.5 mL heparin (to dilute DMSO and prevent further degradation of cells before counting and assay). From this sample, smear or cytospin preparations can be made for differential analysis, hematopoietic progenitor cell colony assays can be set up, and cell viability can be assessed by trypan blue exclusion.
ANTICIPATED RESULTS	1. The thawing procedure should yield a viable cell fraction equal to 65 to 95 percent. 2. A recovery of 40 to 70 percent of the original cell number frozen is expected.
NOTES	1. *USE EXTREME CAUTION WHEN HANDLING LIQUID NITROGEN. IF SPILLED ON SKIN, SERIOUS BURNS MAY RESULT.* 2. Because of the adverse effects of DMSO on cells above 0°C, samples should be chilled (0 to 4°C) after collection and should be tested as soon as possible.

AUTHORS

Carlos E. Lee, M.T.
Bone Marrow Processing and
   Evaluation Laboratory
Bone Marrow Transplant Program
H. Lee Moffitt Cancer Center and
   Research Institute
University of South Florida
12902 Magnolia Dr.
Tampa, FL 33612-9497

William E. Janssen, Ph.D.
Bone Marrow Processing and
   Evaluation Laboratory
Bone Marrow Transplant Program
H. Lee Moffitt Cancer Center and
   Research Institute
University of South Florida
12902 Magnolia Dr.
Tampa, FL 33612-9497

REFERENCES

1. Weiner, RS, Richman, CM, and Yankee, RA: Dilution techniques for optimum recovery of cryopreserved bone marrow cells. Exp Hematol 7(Suppl 5):1, 1979.
2. Warkentin, PI, Ramsay, NK, and McCullough, J: Effect of procedural variations on *in vitro* viability of cryopreserved bone marrow (abstr.). Transfusion 20:640, 1980.

DYE EXCLUSION TEST FOR BONE MARROW VIABILITY

DESCRIPTION	The trypan blue viability test is based on the ability of the cell membrane of live (viable) cells to exclude the dye. The nonviable cells are blue when viewed with a microscope.

TIME FOR PROCEDURE	Approximately 15 to 20 minutes

SUMMARY OF PROCEDURE	1. At the time of the bone marrow infusion, a volume of bone marrow is removed and placed into cold medium for transport to the laboratory.
	2. The specimen is centrifuged, the supernatant removed, and the remaining cells slowly diluted with medium until the desired concentration is achieved.
	3. The trypan blue dye is added to the cells and after a brief period the cells are loaded onto a hemacytometer and examined with a microscope. The viable cells are enumerated and the percent viability reported.

EQUIPMENT	1. Centrifuge
	2. Hemacytometer
	3. Microscope

SUPPLIES AND REAGENTS	1. TC-199 with Earle's salts and L-glutamine
	2. 0.4 percent trypan blue (Gibco No. 630-5250)
	3. Fetal bovine serum (FBS)
	4. Tissue culture tubes: 50-mL and 15-mL
	5. Pipettes

PROCEDURE	1. SPECIMEN PREPARATION
	A. Make a 15 percent FBS solution using TC-199 as the diluent: To a 50-mL tube add 7.5 mL of FBS to 42.5 mL of TC-199. Mix well and add 12 mL of the TC-199/FBS solution to a 15-mL tube and refrigerate until used.
	B. Add 0.5 mL of bone marrow to the 12 mL of TC-199/FBS and mix thoroughly.
	2. CENTRIFUGATION AND INCUBATION
	A. Centrifuge the TC-199/FBS containing the marrow specimen for 7 minutes at $400g$ at 12°C.
	B. Aspirate and discard the supernatant.
	C. To the cell button, slowly add TC-199/FBS solution mixing well after each addition, until the volume is approximately 12 mL.
	D. Centrifuge 7 minutes at $400g$ at 12°C.
	E. Aspirate and discard the supernatant.
	F. To the cell button slowly add TC-199/FBS until a suitable cell concentration is achieved.
	G. To 0.2 mL of the diluted cell suspension, add 0.05 mL of 0.4 percent trypan blue solution.

    H. After 5 minutes load the trypan blue suspension onto a hemacytometer. Count the number of viable white blood cells (not blue) per 100 total white blood cells (viable and nonviable). Report as percent viable cells.

ANTICIPATED RESULTS	Viabilities will range from 70 to 90 percent using this trypan blue exclusion method.
NOTES	1. This procedure dilutes the dimethyl sulfoxide (DMSO) to a concentration low enough that it should not be harmful to the cells. The marrow sample can be procured at the time of infusion and transported to the laboratory for completion of testing.
	2. The trypan blue should not incubate longer than 5 minutes with the cell suspension because viable cells will begin to take up the dye and cause low viability results.
	3. Between 200 and 300 total white blood cells should be counted and the viabilities averaged.
AUTHOR	Barbara A. Reeb, M.T.(ASCP)
	Brooke Army Medical Center
	Dept. of Clinical Investigation
	Fort Sam Houston, TX 78234-6200
REFERENCE	1. Merchant, D, Kahn, R, and Murphy, W: Handbook of Cell and Organ Culture. Burgess Publishing, Broken Arrow, OK, 1964, p 157.

STERILITY CHECKS DURING BONE MARROW PROCESSING

DESCRIPTION	A closed system cannot be maintained during all phases of in vitro bone marrow processing and purging. Bacterial cultures should be performed when marrow is delivered to the laboratory, following marrow manipulation, and at the end of processing.
TIME FOR PROCEDURE	2 minutes per set of cultures
SUMMARY OF PROCEDURE	1. Marrow is sampled when received in the laboratory and at various stages of processing. 2. Marrow sample is inoculated into aerobic and anaerobic blood culture bottles.
EQUIPMENT	None
SUPPLIES AND REAGENTS	1. Aerobic and anaerobic blood culture bottles (1 of each for each sample to be cultured) 2. 5- or 10-mL syringes 3. 16-gauge hypodermic needles 4. Alcohol preparation swabs 5. Providone-iodine swabs 6. Sampling site couplers
PROCEDURE	1. Obtain one aerobic and one anaerobic blood culture bottle for each culture event. Label bottles. 2. Insert a sampling site coupler into marrow pack. 3. Clean sampling site coupler with Povidone iodine. 4. Remove tops from blood culture bottles and clean diaphragms with alcohol preparation swabs. 5. Using a 5- or 10-mL syringe and 16-gauge needle, draw required volume of marrow. 6. Inoculate each of the culture bottles with required volume of marrow.
ANTICIPATED RESULTS	Confirmation of sterility of product at all stages of processing.
AUTHOR	Sarah F. Donnelly, M.T.(ASCP), S.B.B. University of Virginia Health Sciences Center Blood Bank and Transfusion Services Charlottesville, VA 22908

BONE MARROW CELL CULTURE

HEMATOPOIETIC PROGENITOR CELL ASSAY

DESCRIPTION	Bone marrow samples can be cultured for 14 days and the progenitor cells in that sample quantitated. Using this information, one can follow the progenitor cells through the processing of the marrow to provide quality assurance throughout the technique. Also, one may be able to use this information to predict the kinetics of engraftment (e.g., the number of days to 500 granulocytes per microliter) for the recipients of hydroperoxycyclophosphamide (4-HC)–purged grafts.
TIME FOR PROCEDURE	2 hours
SUMMARY OF PROCEDURE	1. Light density cells (specific gravity less than 1.078 g per mL) are isolated. 2. Cells are placed in culture with growth-stimulating media. 3. Colonies are enumerated after 14 days of incubation.
EQUIPMENT	1. Centrifuge 2. Cell counter 3. Laminar flow hood 4. Automatic pipettor 5. Adjustable pipettors (1 to 10, 10 to 100, and 100 to 1000 μL) 6. Incubator (37°C and 5 percent [CO_2]) 7. Inverted microscope
SUPPLIES AND REAGENTS	1. 35- $\times$ 10-mm tissue culture plates (Lux 5221-R)* 2. 15- $\times$ 100-mm tissue culture plates (VWR Scientific 25384-070) 3. 5- and 10-mL syringes 4. Blunt 15-gauge needles (Sherwood Medical) 5. 50-mL conical tubes (Corning 25330-50) 6. Serologic pipettes (1, 2, 5, and 10), sterile 7. Sterile distilled water 8. Ficoll-Hypaque (specific gravity less than 1.078) (Organon Teknika 36427) 9. Methylcellulose media (MC); see Appendix A 10. Fetal bovine serum (FBS) (Sigma F4010) 11. Conditioned medium (PHA-LCM); see Appendix B 12. Bovine serum albumin (BSA) (Boehringer Mannheim 652237) 13. 2-Mercaptoethanol (BME) (Bio Rad 161-0710) 14. Methylprednisolone (MP) (Abbott NDC0074-5631-08) 15. Alpha minimum essential medium (MEM) (Gibco 320-2561)

---

*Sources are suggestions only, and equivalent substitutes may be used.

16. Erythropoietin (TCepo) (Amgen Biologicals 08500)

17. 18-gauge spinal needle, 3½-inch

Aliquot and store all reagents according to usage.

NOTE: *Do not reconstitute MP with diluent provided: it contains preservatives.*

NOTE: *Growth of bone marrow progenitor cells is very dependent on reagents and supplies. Changes in source or even lot number can enhance or suppress colony formation; therefore test each lot.*

PROCEDURE

1. Isolate bone marrow nononuclear cells from the bone marrow with Ficoll-Hypaque, using no more than 8×10^7 cells per gradient.* Dilute cells in MEM as needed up to 16 mL in a 50-mL tube. Carefully layer 8 mL of Ficoll-Hypaque under the cell volume using a spinal needle. Spin the gradient for 30 minutes at $400g$. Harvest the interface of the Ficoll-Hypaque suspension that contains the mononuclear cells and wash these three times using MEM. Measure the volume and count the remaining cells to calculate total cell numbers and percent recovery.

2. Mix the ingredients for the plating mixture in 50-mL conical tubes. Quantities that follow are for a 5-mL total mixture. All reagents should be at room temperature.
    A. MC—2.2 mL of a 3 percent solution (using a syringe with blunt needle)
    B. FBS—1.5 mL
    C. PHA—0.25 mL
    D. BSA—0.5 mL of a 10 percent solution
    E. BME—0.05 mL of a 10^{-2}-M stock solution
    F. MP—0.05 mL of a 10^{-4}-M stock solution
    G. TCepo—0.05 mL of a 100 U per mL stock
    H. Cells and media—0.40 mL

    To calculate volume of cells used for each tube to produce four plates per tube:

    $$\frac{\text{Desired concentration of cells} \times 5\dagger}{\text{Cell count (cells per mL) of sample}}$$

3. Plating densities (cells per mL) are as follows:
    A. Pre sample: 5×10^4
    B. Buffy coat sample: 5×10^4
    C. Machine Ficoll-Hypaque sample: $5 \times 10^4\ddagger$
    D. 4-HC–treated sample: 5×10^5 and 1×10^6§

4. Record patient information and sample concentration. Label four 35- $\times$ 10-mm tissue culture dishes per sample with the appropriate information.

---

*If the marrow has already been density gradient separated, a second Ficoll-Hypaque separation is not required. However, additional washing of 4-HC–treated cells is recommended to ensure that no 4-HC is unintentionally carried into the culture medium.

†Recipe is multiplied by 5 in order to achieve enough volume for four plates (because almost a full milliliter cannot be recovered from the 50-mL tube). Add the appropriate volume of cells to each tube and enough remaining volume with MEM to reach 0.40 mL (5 mL final volume). Gently mix the tubes.

‡When cells are density gradient separated using automated cell separators.

§Concentration per plate will be changed in accordance with the treatment of the bone marrow. Untreated samples should not be cultured above 5×10^4.

Make hydration dishes using one 35- $\times$ 10-mm open dish containing sterile distilled water seated inside the larger 15- $\times$ 100-mm tissue culture dish. One of these is needed for every two 35- $\times$ 10-mm dishes.

5. Draw up 4 mL of the cell mixture from each 50-mL conical tube into a 5-mL syringe using a blunt needle, after expelling air from the syringe. Place 1 mL into each 35- $\times$ 10-mm dish. Culture dishes are then placed into the incubation dishes (two per incubation dish) and placed into a 37°C, 5 percent CO_2, fully humidified incubator.

   NOTE: *Do not allow CO_2 to fall below 5 percent. Preferably, maintain CO_2 slightly above 5 percent (5.2 to 5.5 percent). The incubator should be checked at least weekly.*

6. Cell colonies should be quantitated after 14 days of incubation. Colonies to be counted are burst-forming units—erythroid (BFU-E), colony-forming units—granulocyte, macrophage (CFU-GM), and CFU-Mix colonies. The number of colonies per dish is recorded, and then averaged for further calculations. (See color slides 11–1 to 11–16.)

APPENDIX A: METHYLCELLULOSE MEDIA

SUPPLIES	1.	Methylcellulose powder, 1500 centipoise (cp) (Sigma M-0387)*
	2.	Double-strength alpha-MEM (Gibco 410-2000EB)
	3.	Sterile distilled water
	4.	Sodium bicarbonate (Gibco 895-1810)
EQUIPMENT	1.	2-L Erlenmeyer flask
	2.	Magnetic stirrer
	3.	Large sterile stirbar
	4.	100-mL sterile bottles
	5.	Hotplate
	6.	Laminar flow hood
PROCEDURE	1.	Into a sterile 2-L Erlenmeyer flask, add 500 mL of sterile distilled water and replace the foil cap. Boil for a few minutes.
	2.	Add 30 g of methylcellulose, cover, and swirl until wet.
	3.	Heat again until boiling (do not let foam). Remove from the heat and swirl.
	4.	Cool to 40 to 50°C under cool running water.
	5.	Add 500 mL double-strength media (add antibiotic if desired at this point).
	6.	Add a large sterile stirbar, cover securely, and stir at least 4 hours (or overnight) in the cold (4°C).
	7.	Pour into sterile bottles and label. Store in a −20°C freezer. This will keep for at least 6 months in the freezer or from 4 to 6 weeks when stored at 4°C.
	8.	Test each lot for sterility and growth activity.

*Sources are suggestions only.

APPENDIX B: PHYTOHEMAGGLUTININ-STIMULATED LYMPHOCYTE-CONDITIONED MEDIUM

SUPPLIES	1. Alpha minimum essential medium (MEM) (Gibco 320-2561)*
	2. Fetal bovine serum (Sigma F4010)
	3. Phytohemagglutinin (PHA) (Sigma L-9132)
	4. Ficoll-Hypaque (specific gravity less than 1.078) (Organon Teknika 36427)
	5. Fresh, healthy donor blood
	6. Tissue culture flasks, 75 cm^2 (Corning 25116-75)
	7. Sterile 5-mL disposable tubes (Falcon 2054)
	8. 0.22-μm filter (Millipore SLGS0250S)

EQUIPMENT	1. Carbon dioxide (CO_2) incubator
	2. Centrifuge
	3. Freezer ($-70°C$)

PROCEDURE	1. Separate whole blood from a healthy donor with Ficoll-Hypaque to obtain the lymphocyte fraction.
	2. Prepare PHA-P with sterile water at 1000 μg per mL.
	3. To a tissue culture flask, add:
	A. 1×10^6 cells per mL in media
	B. 20 percent fetal bovine serum
	C. 1 percent PHA-P
	Volume is determined by the number of lymphocytes available. Maximum volume per flask is 50 mL.
	4. Incubate at 37°C in 5 percent CO_2 humidified atmosphere for 7 days undisturbed.
	5. Centrifuge media. Recover the supernatant and filter with a 0.22-μm filter.
	6. Aliquot, label, and freeze at $-70°C$.
	7. Test each lot for sterility and growth activity.

ANTICIPATED RESULTS	Healthy donor bone marrow should give rise to 70 to 120 BFU-E and CFU-GM–derived colonies and 3 to 5 CFU-Mix–derived colonies per 5×10^4 cells plated. Patient marrow samples will have fewer progenitor cells because of previous treatment. Chemical-purged (4-HC) marrows may have very few progenitors. Culture of progenitor cells is largely dependent on good reagents.

AUTHOR	Scott D. Rowley, M.D., FACP The Fred Hutchinson Cancer Research Center Seattle, WA 98104

REFERENCE	1. Rowley, SD, et al: CFU-GM content of bone marrow graft correlates with time to hematologic reconstitution following autologous bone marrow transplantation with 4-hydroperoxycyclophosphamide–purged bone marrow. Blood 70:271, 1987.

*Sources are suggestions only.

BONE MARROW STEM CELL DIFFERENTIATION IN SEMISOLID MEDIUM

DESCRIPTION	In the past, bone marrow stromal layers consisting of reticular cells, fibroblasts, macrophages, and adipocytes have been used for the in vitro growth and differentiation of bone marrow stem cells.[1,2] The stromal cells have been thought to exert their effects by production of the extracellular matrix and the secretion of humoral factors in vivo.[3,4] Owing to the troublesome nature of this method a methylcellulose-based system has been developed that mimics the supportive environment of the extracellular matrix.[5,6] This culture system will support the growth and differentiation of granulocytic, erythroid, macrophage, megakaryocytic, and eosinophilic progenitors as recognized by the formation of characteristic colony-forming units (CFUs). These CFUs are the burst-forming unit—erythroid (BFU-E), the CFU in culture (CFU-C), which is synonymous with the CFU-GM colony-forming unit—granulocyte, macrophage (CFU-GM), and the mixed colony, loosely defined here as the colony-forming unit—granulocyte, erythrocyte, monocyte, megakaryocyte (CFU-GEMM).
	The methylcellulose colony assay can be used to elucidate a number of problems that have faced researchers for some time. For example, using this culture system, it is possible to investigate the complex interactions of factors that affect cell-cell communications influencing hematopoiesis, in order to provide insight into the regulatory control mechanisms that are responsible for commitment toward specific lineages.[7] Determination of the synergistic effects that specific factors have on blood cell differentiation may also aid studies of diseases of the bone marrow involving atypical blood cell production, such as leukemia and aplastic anemia.[8] In addition, the toxic effects of various antitumor therapeutic agents on bone marrow differentiation may be explored using this assay.

TIME FOR PROCEDURE	1.	45 minutes to separate mononuclear cells and make appropriate dilution
	2.	15 minutes to set up cultures
	3.	2 weeks' incubation
	4.	1 hour to count colonies

SUMMARY OF PROCEDURE	1.	Whole bone marrow is separated on a Ficoll-Hypaque gradient, and the mononuclear cells are collected.
	2.	After the cells are diluted to the appropriate concentration, they are added to tubes containing growth medium.
	3.	Tubes are vortexed vigorously, bubbles are allowed to rise, and tube contents are aliquoted into culture plates.
	4.	Colonies are scored 2 weeks later.

SUPPLIES AND REAGENTS	1.	Fenwal stem cell CFU Kit No. 4R5526
	2.	Ficoll-Hypaque (Pharmacia No. 17-0840-02)
	3.	Sterile water
	4.	Hank's balanced salt solution (HBSS) containing phenol red
	5.	12- $\times$ 75-mm sterile polystyrene tubes with push caps
	6.	1-mL syringes

7. Sterile 15-mL centrifuge tubes

8. Sterile pipettes

PROCEDURE This procedure is a modification of the methylcellulose assay,[5] as initially described by Iscove.[6]

1. SEPARATION OF MONONUCLEAR CELLS
   A. Dilute fresh bone marrow by adding an equal volume of HBSS.
   B. Carefully layer 5 mL diluted bone marrow on top of 3 mL Ficoll-Hypaque in a 15-mL sterile centrifuge tube, being careful not to disturb the Ficoll-Hypaque layer.
   C. Centrifuge at $400g$ for 30 to 40 minutes at room temperature.
   D. Collect the mononuclear cells at the interface and transfer them to a sterile 15-mL centrifuge tube containing 10 mL HBSS. Centrifuge at $1500g$ for 5 minutes. Wash the pellet twice with 10 mL HBSS.
   E. Resuspend pellet and adjust the isolated bone marrow mononuclear cells to 0.5×10^6 cells per mL with dilution medium. These mononuclear cells can be stored at 4°C overnight at this point, if needed.

2. SETTING UP CULTURES: Additional growth factors may be added to increase the number and size of certain colonies, if desired.
   A. For each sample, add the following together in a 12- $\times$ 75-mm sterile polystyrene tube
      (1) 0.5 mL bone marrow mononuclear cells at 0.5×10^6 per mL
      (2) 1.5 mL CFU culture medium (supplied in the stem cell CFU kit), added via a 1-mL syringe
      (3) If external factors are to be tested, they should be added in small volumes of 5 to 10 μL
   B. Vortex the tube vigorously (highest setting) until the contents of the tube are well mixed.
   C. Let the tube stand for approximately 10 minutes to allow the large bubbles to rise.
   D. Aliquot the contents of the tube into three wells of a four-well culture plate (supplied in the stem cell CFU kit) using a 1-mL syringe (about 0.5 mL per well).
   E. Fill the remaining empty well with 0.5 mL sterile water in order to provide for an adequately humidified atmosphere.
   F. Incubate the plate for 10 to 14 days in a humidified incubator at 37°C and 5 to 10 percent carbon dioxide (CO_2) (10 percent is recommended but not essential). It is advisable to place the plate in an area that will not be disturbed for the duration of incubation.

3. SCORING COLONIES: The various hematopoietic colonies can be easily recognized by their distinct colors and morphologies via an inverted microscope. A colony consists of at least 40 cells. The following are the criteria used to evaluate colony formation.
   A. The granulocyte macrophage colony (CFU-C or CFU-GM) is typically a flat, nonhemoglobinized colony that consists of only translucent cells. These colonies are sometimes very dense and at other times appear to be more spread out, possibly containing a more dense centralized region.
   B. The erythroid burst colony (BFU-E) is a densely packed colony of

orange to dark red (hemoglobinized) cells containing no translucent cells.

    C. The pluripotent mixed colony (CFU-GEMM) has a "fried-egg" appearance with a compact hemoglobinized area that may be central to, or to one side of, a peripheral flat lawn of nonhemoglobinized translucent cells that may be either large or small. This colony is basically a mixture of the CFU-C and BFU-E colonies.

ANTICIPATED RESULTS

1. The numbers of CFU-C colonies that can be expected using this procedure may range from 30 to 90 colonies per well (approximately 8.3×10^4 cells). BFU-E colony numbers should be in the range of 80 to 120 colonies per well, and CFU-GEMM colonies in the range of 5 to 30 colonies per well.

2. These numbers are based on studies using normal human bone marrow, and may vary somewhat if the marrow has been compromised in any way.

NOTES

1. It is always necessary to use a syringe when working with methylcellulose because it is extremely viscous and sticks to most surfaces. Normal pipette suction will not suffice as an alternative.

2. Ficoll-Hypaque is a registered trademark of Pharmacia-LKB.

AUTHOR

Suzanne Beckner, Ph.D.   Bonny Bass, B.S.
Life Technologies, Inc.   Life Technologies, Inc.
8717 Grovemont Cir.   8717 Grovemont Cir.
Gaithersburg, MD 20877   Gaithersburg, MD 20877

REFERENCES

1. Dexter, TM, Allen, TD, and Lajtha, LG: Conditions controlling the proliferation of hemopoietic stem cells in vitro. J Cell Physiol 91:335, 1976.
2. Dexter, TM: Stromal cell associated haemopoiesis. J Cell Physiol (Suppl) 1:87, 1982.
3. Gordon, MY, et al; Compartmentalization of a haematopoietic growth factor (GM-CSF) by glycosaminoglycans in the bone marrow microenvironment. Nature 326:403, 1987.
4. Dexter, TM: Growth factors involved in haemopoiesis. J Cell Sci 88:1, 1987.
5. Fauser, AA and Messner, HA: Identification of megakaryocytes, macrophages, and eosinophils in colonies of human bone marrow containing neutrophilic granulocytes and erythrocytes. Blood 53:1023, 1979.
6. Iscove, NN: Colony formation by normal and leukemic marrow cells in culture: Effect of conditioned medium from human leukocytes. Blood 37:1, 1971.
7. Iscove, NN, et al: Molecules stimulating early red cell, granulocyte, macrophage and megakaryocyte precursors in culture: Similarity in size, hydrophobicity and charge. J Cell Physiol (Suppl) 1:65, 1982.
8. Boettiger, D, Andersen, S, and Dexter, TM: Effect of src infection on long-term marrow cultures: Increased self-renewal of hemopoietic progenitor cells without leukemia. Cell 36:763, 1984.

COLONY-FORMING UNIT ASSAY—AGAR METHOD

DESCRIPTION	The colony-forming unit—in culture (CFU-C) assay is an in vitro assay using a solid agar base, enriched with McCoy's medium, various amino acids, fetal calf serum, and colony-stimulating factors. By counting the CFU-C in the agar–McCoy's 5A medium, proliferation of pluripotent hematopoietic stem cells can be determined.
TIME FOR PROCEDURE	60 minutes

SUMMARY OF PROCEDURE

1. ++ McCoy's 5A medium plus additives is prepared from double-strength ($\times\times$); McCoy's 5A medium is prepared.
2. Dense and light agar are prepared.
3. ++ McCoy's 5A is combined with agar in a 3:2 proportion.
4. Colony-stimulating factor is placed in dense agar underlayer and stem cells are placed in light agar overlayers.
5. Plates with cells are incubated for 2 weeks at 37°C in 7 percent carbon dioxide (CO_2).
6. Colonies containing greater than 40 cells are scored.

EQUIPMENT

1. 37°C and 44°C waterbath (Precision Scientific Group dual-chamber waterbath No. 66552-25 or equivalent).
2. 37°C incubator (7 percent CO_2, 99 percent humidity)
3. Dissecting microscope (Olympus VM $1\times$–$4\times$).
4. Laminar air flow hood
5. Stirring plate (Corning No. PC-351)
6. Analytic balance (Mettler model PM460)

SUPPLIES AND REAGENTS

1. McCoy's 5A medium (modified) powder with L-glutamine, without sodium bicarbonate (Gibco No. 430-1500EB)
2. $NaHCO_3$ (Gibco No. 895-1810)
3. Penicillin-streptomycin, 10,000 U per mL and 10,000 mg per mL (Gibco No. 600-5140 PE)
4. Fetal calf serum (Hyclone No. A1111D), heat inactivated. (To heat inactivate, place a bottle of fetal calf serum [at room temperature] in 56°C bath for 30 minutes; store indefinitely at 2 to 8°C.)
5. 100 mM sodium pyruvate (Gibco No. 320-1360AG)
6. 50$\times$ essential amino acids (MEM) (Gibco No. 320-1135A6)
7. 100$\times$ vitamins (MEM) (Gibco No. 320-1120AG)
8. 100$\times$ nonessential amino acids, 10 mM (Gibco No. 320-1140AG)
9. 100$\times$ L-glutamine, 200 mM (Gibco No. 320-5030AE)
10. L-serine (Gibco No. 810-1101IL), (add 0.525 g to 25 mL sterile distilled water; filter; freeze in 1-mL aliquots. Stable 6 months at -20°C)
11. L-asparagine (Gibco No. 810-1013IL), (add 0.25 g to 25 mL sterile distilled water; filter 0.22 μm and freeze in 1-mL aliquots. Stable 6 months at -20°C)

12. Bacto-Agar (Difco No. 0140-01), 25°C
    - *Dense agar:* 0.72 g agar in 60 mL sterile distilled water, boil 4 minutes, store in 44°C bath until ready to use; store at 25°C when not in use. Reheat over flame until just melted to reuse; stable 1 week or three melts.
    - *Light agar:* 0.44 g agar in 60 mL sterile distilled water; stability and treatment same as previously described.

13. Distilled water

14. 35- × 10-mm petri dishes (Falcon No. 3001)

15. McCoy's 5A medium, modified, 1× liquid with L-glutamine (Gibco No. 320-6600AG)

16. Colony-stimulating factor (Moore T-cell supernatant), concentration determined by growth response curve (American Type Culture Collection [ATCC], 800-638-6597)

17. Human bone marrow stem cells, 4 M per mL and 2 M per mL

18. Hemacytometer

19. Counting grid

20. 0.22- and 0.45-μm filters (Nalgene Nos. 130-4045 and 120-0020)

PROCEDURE

1. PREPARATION OF MEDIA
    A. Double-strength McCoy's (××):
        (1) Ingredients
            (a) 12.1 g McCoy's 5A salts
            (b) 2.2 g sodium bicarbonate ($NaHCO_3$)
            (c) 20 mL penicillin-streptomycin
            (d) 480 mL sterile distilled water
        (2) Combine materials in a beaker.
        (3) Cover with parafilm and stir until dissolved.
        (4) Under a sterile hood, filter ×× stock through a 0.45-μm filter into sterile container.
        (5) Store 5 days at 2 to 8°C.
    B. ×× stock plus additives:
        (1) Into a 100-mL sterile bottle add:

        - 66.5 mL ×× stock
        - 1.68 mL sodium pyruvate 100 mM
        - 1.35 mL 50× essential amino acids
        - 0.68 mL 100× vitamins
        - 0.68 mL 100× nonessential amino acids
        - 0.68 mL 100× L-glutamine
        - 0.068 mL L-serine
        - 0.28 mL L-asparagine

        2. Mix and filter through a 0.22-μm filter into sterile container.
        3. Add 25 mL heat-inactivated fetal calf serum and mix.
        4. Store 5 days at 2 to 8°C.
        5. Warm 20 minutes at 37°C before use.
    C. Diluting media for cell suspension (100 mL volume)
        (1) 80 percent McCoy's 5A medium

(2) 20 percent heat-inactivated fetal calf serum

(3) 1 percent penicillin-streptomycin

D. Store 2 to 8°C for 5 days.

2. PREPARATION OF CULTURE PLATES

   A. Prepare underlayers for plates

     (1) Place 0.2 mL colony-stimulating factor in plates.

     (2) Add 1.0 mL of + + and dense agar mixture, previously prepared in a tube at a 3:2 ratio at 37°C. For six plates, use 6 mL + + and 4 mL agar.

     (3) Swirl to mix. Let stand 5 minutes.

     (4) May be stored at 2 to 8°C up to 5 days or used immediately.

   B. Prepare overlayers for plates

     (1) In a tube at 37°C, make a 3:2 ratio of + + and light agar. Subtract cell suspension volume to be used from + + volume. For three plates, use 2.5 mL + + and 2 mL agar.

     (2) Add calculated cell suspension volume to overlayer mixture. For three plates, use 0.5 mL of 4 m per mL and 2 m per mL, respectively.

     (3) Place 1.0 mL of overlayer cell-assay mixture on each previously prepared underlayer.

   C. Incubate at 37°C, 7 percent CO_2 for 2 weeks.

3. DETERMINE NUMBER OF CFU-C PER 1×10^5 CELLS AND TOTAL CFU-C PER MARROW

   A. Count colonies per plate. Colony equals more than 40 cells.

   B. To obtain CFU-C per 1×10^5 cells, divide number of colonies on plate by cell concentration placed on plate.

   C. To obtain total CFU-C per bone marrow, multiply CFU-C per 1×10^5 cells by total cells in bone marrow.

ANTICIPATED RESULTS — 100 colonies per 1×10^5 bone marrow cells

NOTES

1. Large cell volumes to be plated should be warmed to 37°C.

2. Plate quickly before agar hardens in tube. A beaker with water kept at 37°C can be used in hood to prevent solidification.

3. Large numbers of plates should be prepared in groups, not at once.

4. IL-3 (500 μm per mL) and GM-CSF (600 μm per mL) may be used as alternative stimulators.

AUTHORS

Mitsi Wood, B.S.
University of Virginia Health Sciences Center
Charlottesville, VA 22908

Gerda Pirsch, M.S.
University of Virginia Health Sciences Center
Charlottesville, VA 22908

REFERENCE

1. Kurland, JI: Granulocyte-monocyte progenitor cells. In Golde, D (ed): Methods in Hematology, Hematopoiesis. New York, Churchill Livingstone, 1984, p 87.

QUANTITATION OF PERIPHERAL BLOOD STEM CELLS PRIOR TO CRYOPRESERVATION

DESCRIPTION	The progenitor cell number has been shown to be a better indicator of the hematopoietic reconstituting capacity of a blood stem cell storage specimen than the nucleated cell number. Progenitor cells are measured in the colony-forming unit—granulocyte, macrophage (CFU-GM) culture. Quantitation of CFU-GM assesses the suitability of a blood stem cell storage specimen for hematopoietic rescue following cytotoxic therapy.
TIME FOR PROCEDURE	Approximately 0.5 hours
SUMMARY OF PROCEDURE	1. A known number of mononuclear cells is added to a suspension medium containing nutrients.
	2. This cell suspension is dispensed in 1-mL aliquots into 35-mm tissue culture plates to which a source of colony-stimulating activity has been added.
	3. The plates are incubated at 37°C with 5 percent carbon dioxide (CO_2) in a humidified atmosphere for 14 days.
	4. After 14 days aggregates of at least 40 cells are scored as colonies using a dissecting microscope.
	5. A differential cell count performed on a cytospin preparation of the mononuclear cell sample is performed so that CFU-GM values can be expressed per milliliter of blood.
EQUIPMENT	1. Contherm M190 CO_2 controlled incubator (Contherm Scientific, New Zealand, or equivalent)
	2. Class II biologic safety cabinet or equivalent
	3. Dissecting microscope (Model SZH, Olympus, Tokyo, or equivalent)
	4. Shandon cytocentrifuge (Cytospin II, Shandon, United Kingdom, or equivalent)
SUPPLIES AND REAGENTS	1. Iscove's modified Dulbecco's medium (IMDM) with L-glutamine, without bicarbonate, supplied as powder (Gibco Laboratories, Grand Island, New York)
	2. DEAE-Dextran (Pharmacia No. 170350-01, Sweden)
	3. L-asparagine (Sigma)
	4. 2-Mercaptoethanol (Sigma)
	5. Bacto-Agar (Difco, Detroit)
	6. Fetal calf serum (FCS) (CSL, Australia)
	7. 35- × 10-mm sterile tissue culture dishes (Corning, Ontario)
	8. Human placental conditioned medium (HPCM) (see Notes)
	9. Penicillin (CSL, Australia)
	10. Streptomycin (CSL, Australia)
	11. Sodium bicarbonate (AR, BDH, Australia)

12. Jenner Giemsa stain

13. Esterase stain

PROCEDURE

1. Prepare CFU-GM cultures aseptically in a biologic safety cabinet.

2. Use an aliquot of the mononuclear cell suspension of known concentration prepared as described in "Processing of Peripheral Blood Stem Cells" (Chapter 5) for CFU-GM culture.

3. Perform peripheral blood CFU-GM cultures at three cell concentrations—usually 3, 1, and 0.5×10^5 per mL.

4. Label culture dishes according to cell concentration and stimulus. For each cell concentration, five culture dishes are prepared—one with no added stimulus, four with HPCM added.

5. Add HPCM to labeled dishes. The amount of HPCM for optimal stimulation should be determined when batch testing is carried out (see Note 3) but should not exceed 0.1 mL per dish.

6. Prepare culture suspensions by mixing 0.66 percent agar with double-strength IMDM with 50 percent FCS. 0.66 percent agar should constitute half the required volume, the remainder consisting of double-strength IMDM with FCS and the cell sample (the resulting suspension medium will be 0.33 percent agar in single-strength IMDM with 25 percent FCS). The volume of cell sample added should not exceed 10 percent of the final volume. The volume of the culture suspension should exceed the volume required for plating by at least 1 mL.

7. Label three 10-mL sterile centrifuge tubes for the three cell concentrations used. Calculate amount of cell sample and volumes of reagents for each cell concentration. Add the required volume of double-strength IMDM with FCS to the 10-mL tubes.

8. Bring 0.66 percent agar to a boil and keep at 45°C until required. Cultures should be set up one concentration at a time to prevent premature gelling of suspensions. For each concentration, add required volume of agar to the dispensed medium, add cell sample, and dispense with gentle swirling in 1 mL volumes into labeled tissue culture dishes.

9. Place culture dishes in a clean plastic box on a wire grid over sterile distilled water. Partially cover box and place in humidified, CO_2 incubator (5 percent CO_2 in air) at 37°C for 14 days.

10. Prepare two cytospin slides from the initial cell suspension consisting of 1×10^5 cells per slide. One should be stained with Jenner Giemsa stain and one with esterase stain.

11. After 14 days, use a dissecting microscope to enumerate colonies (greater than 40 cells).

12. Perform differential count on cytospin preparations.

13. Express culture results as the number of CFU-GM per mL, which is calculated using the following formula:

$$\text{CFU-GM per mL} = (\text{CP/C6}) \times (\%\text{MNB}/\%\text{MNC}) \times \text{WCC}$$

where: CP = Average number of colonies scored per plate
        C6 = Number of cells plated in units of 10^6

> %MNC = Percent mononuclear cells from cytospin (i.e., cells cultured)
>
> WCC = White cell count in units of 10^6 per mL blood
>
> %MNB = Percent mononuclear cells in peripheral blood determined by differential count

The highest result calculated from the three concentrations plated is reported.

ANTICIPATED RESULTS

In our laboratory the reference range values for blood CFU-GM values are 46 to 855 per mL for normal males and 14 to 411 per mL for normal females.

NOTES

1. IMDM medium is prepared according to the formula communicated by Dr. G. Johnson, Walter and Eliza Hall Institute, Melbourne, Australia (personal communication):
   - 1 L pack IMDM
   - 390 mL distilled water
   - 60 mg penicillin
   - 100 mg streptomycin
   - 1.5 mL (50 mg per mL) DEAE-Dextran
   - 0.2 g L-asparagine

   Mix and aliquot in 50-mL lots. When required, to one aliquot add 50 mL FCS, 0.01 mL 1N 2-mercaptoethanol, and 0.6 g $NaHCO_2$. Sterilize by filtration.

2. Rigorous quality control for all reagents is essential. At least five batches of fetal calf serum from different suppliers are tested in our laboratory before purchase to ensure an optimal batch. New batches of prepared media should be tested against those currently in use.

3. Human placental conditioned medium is prepared according to the method of Schlunk.[3] Several 5-L batches are prepared and screened individually for colony-stimulating activity in the CFU-GM culture. A pool is then prepared from suitable batches and titrated to determine the volume required for optimal colony stimulation. Pooled HPCM is stored in 100-mL aliquots at −70°C.

4. 0.66 percent agar is prepared by adding 0.66 g agar powder to 100 mL distilled water in a 100-mL reagent bottle. Autoclave at 15 psig for 15 minutes. Remove from autoclave as soon as possible.

5. Optimal growth of peripheral blood CFU-GM occurs when mononuclear cells are cultured at concentrations that optimize the stimulatory influence of monocytes within the culture system. As there are sample-to-sample variations in the numbers of monocytes present, and in their stimulatory or inhibitory effect on CFU-GM, it is essential to perform the culture at a range of cell concentrations.

6. As the CFU-GM culture is complex and can be influenced by numerous media components, interlaboratory standardization remains difficult. There are considerable differences in the growth-supporting ability between batches of media and fetal calf serum. There is still no commonly agreed-on standard for the colony-stimulating factor in the culture. At present the best option is for each laboratory to establish a reference range based on normal subjects so that some degree of relativity among CFU-GM data from different laboratories can be achieved.

7. Pure recombinant growth factors that are now commercially available present an option for standardizing the CFU-GM colony-stimulating activity. However, recombinant growth factors alone do not stimulate maximal numbers of colonies, and further work is needed to define the combination of recombinant growth factors that will optimally stimulate colony proliferation and differentiation.

8. Sources of supplies and reagents are suggested. Comparable equivalents may be substituted.

AUTHORS

Pamela G. Dyson, B.Sc.(Hons)
Leukaemia Research Unit
Institute of Medical and Veterinary
    Science
Adelaide, South Australia 5000

David N. Haylock, B.App.Sc.
Leukaemia Research Unit
Department of Haematology
Institute of Medical and Veterinary
    Science
Adelaide, South Australia 5000

REFERENCES

1. To, LB, et al: The effect of monocytes in the peripheral blood CFU-GM assay system. Blood 61:112, 1983.
2. Burgess, AW, Wilson, EMA, and Metcalf, D: Stimulation by human placental conditioned medium of hemopoietic colony formation by human bone marrow cells. Blood 49:573, 1977.
3. Schlunk, T, Ruber, E, and Schleyer, M: Survival of human bone marrow progenitor cells after freezing: Improved detection in the colony-formation assay. Cryobiology 18:111, 1981.

QUANTITATION OF THAWED PERIPHERAL BLOOD STEM CELLS

DESCRIPTION	Quantitation of CFU-GM assesses the suitability of a blood stem cell storage specimen for hematopoietic rescue following cytotoxic therapy. However, CFU-GM cultures need to be carried out on cryopreserved samples to indicate cell survival following freezing and storage. These cultures also provide a means of double-checking the results of the initial CFU-GM cultures. The culture system differs from that used on the initial sample only in the nature of stimulus used. Cryopreserved cells require the additional stimulus of leukocyte feeder layers for optimal colony growth.
TIME FOR PROCEDURE	Approximately 2.5 hours, including 2 hours for preparation of feeder layers
SUMMARY OF PROCEDURE	1. Feeder layers are prepared from a leukocyte-enriched fraction of peripheral blood cells from a normal donor.
	2. Cultures are prepared as described in steps 1 through 4 in summary of preceding procedure, "Quantitation of Peripheral Blood Stem Cells Prior to Cryopreservation."
EQUIPMENT	1. Contherm M190 CO_2 controlled incubator (Contherm Scientific, New Zealand, or equivalent)
	2. Class II biologic safety cabinet (BH series, Gelman Sciences, MI, or equivalent)
	3. Olympus dissecting microscope (Model SZH, Olympus, Tokyo, or equivalent)
SUPPLIES AND REAGENTS	1. Iscove's modified Dulbecco's medium (IMDM) with L-glutamine, without bicarbonate, supplied as powder (Gibco Laboratories, New York)
	2. DEAE-Dextran (Pharmacia No. 170350-01, Sweden)
	3. L-asparagine (Sigma, USA)
	4. 2-mercaptoethanol (Sigma, USA)
	5. Bacto-agar (Difco, Detroit)
	6. Fetal calf serum (FCS) (CSL, Australia)
	7. 35- × 10-mm sterile tissue culture dishes (Corning, Ontario)
	8. Human placental conditioned medium (HPCM)
	9. Hydroxyethyl starch (HES), 6 percent solution in 0.9 percent saline (Hespan, American Critical Care, IL)
	10. Hank's balanced salt solution (HBSS) supplied as powder (Flow Laboratories, Australia)
	11. Feeder layers (see Notes)
	12. Sterile individually wrapped 1-mL transfer pipettes (Samco, USA)
PROCEDURE	1. All CFU-GM cultures of thawed cells should be prepared aseptically in a biologic safety cabinet.
	2. Thaw cells by direct transfer of cryotube from $-196°C$ to a $37°C$ waterbath. When thawed, mix sample gently by inversion.

3. As soon as cells are thawed, dilute 1:10 in HBSS and perform a white cell count. Culture cells as soon as possible after thawing and dilution.

4. Thawed cells are usually cultured at the cell concentration that was optimal for cultures on the sample before freezing. In practice this is usually 0.5×10^5 per mL. Generally nine culture dishes are used:
   - two dishes with HPCM added
   - six dishes containing feeder layers (three from each source) with HPCM added
   - one dish with no added stimulus

5. Label culture dishes according to sample and stimulus.

6. Add HPCM to dishes.

7. Prepare culture suspensions in 0.33 percent agar as described in previous procedure, steps 6 through 9.

8. After 14 days colonies are scored as described previously (step 11 of preceding procedure).

9. Colonies are expressed as CFU-GM per 10^6 and optimal results are used.

10. Results are expressed as percentage of CFU-GM numbers (CFU-GM/10^6) in the sample prior to cryopreservation.

ANTICIPATED RESULTS	This culture should yield CFU-GM numbers that are greater than 80 percent of those obtained in the cultures before cryopreservation.
NOTES	1. Feeder layers are prepared from peripheral blood from two normal donors.

      A. A leukocyte-enriched cell suspension is prepared from 20 mL peripheral blood from each donor.

      B. HBSS is added to 20 mL peripheral blood in a sterile 50-mL centrifuge tube to reach a final volume of 45 mL. HES (5 mL) is added and the suspension mixed by inverting the tube several times.

      C. The suspension is incubated at 37°C for approximately 30 minutes or until a clearly defined interface between red cells and plasma can be detected.

      D. The leukocyte-rich plasma is removed to within 1 to 2 mm of the interface using a sterile 1-mL transfer pipette and placed in a 50-mL centrifuge tube.

      E. Wash cells twice with HBSS. Resuspend cells and perform a white cell count.

      F. Prepare suspension of cells in 0.5 percent agar in IMDM with 25 percent FCS and dispense in 1-mL aliquots into 35-mm tissue culture dishes.

      G. Incubate feeder layers at 37°C in 5 percent CO_2 in a humid environment for 3 to 5 days before use.

2. 1 percent agar is prepared by adding 1 g agar to 100 mL distilled water and proceeding as in Note 4 of the preceding procedure. Mixing of equal volumes of 1 percent agar with double-strength IMDM results in 0.5 percent agar.

3. Values less than 80 percent of the value before cryopreservation may indicate that cells have been damaged during cryopreservation. Values greater than 100 percent indicate that the initial assays were suboptimal. Any cultures that show such great variation from the original should be repeated.

If repeated cultures show viability less than 50 percent the suitability of the storage specimen for transplant would be questioned.

4. The effectiveness of feeder layers to stimulate colony formation is very variable, so two sources must be used. When a culture needs to be repeated it is essential that completely different sources of feeder layers be used.

5. Sources of supplies and reagents are suggested. Comparable equivalents may be substituted.

AUTHORS

Pamela G. Dyson, B.Sc.(Hons)
Leukaemia Research Unit
Institute of Medical and Veterinary
  Science
Adelaide, South Australia 5000

David N. Haylock, B.App.Sc.
Leukaemia Research Unit
Department of Haematology
Institute of Medical and Veterinary
  Science
Adelaide, South Australia 5000

Luen Bik To M.D., M.B.B.S.
Leukaemia Research Unit
Division Haematology
Institute of Medical and Veterinary
  Science
Adelaide, South Australia 5000

and

Royal Adelaide Hospital
Adelaide, South Australia 5000

REFERENCE

1. Schlunk, T, Ruber, E, and Schleyer, M: Survival of human bone marrow progenitor cells after freezing: Improved detection in the colony forming assay. Cryobiology 18:111, 1981.

EVALUATION OF T-CELL DEPLETION

Limiting Dilution Analysis for Clonable T Cells— Microtechnique

DESCRIPTION	The low number of residual T cells left after T-cell depletion by soybean lectin agglutination and rosetting with AET-treated sheep red blood cells (see Chapter 7, "T-Cell Depletion of Bone Marrow by Treatment with Soybean Agglutinin and Sheep Red Blood Cell Rosetting"), adherence on the AIS Cellector–T cell (see Chapter 7 "T-Cell Depletion of SBA– Cells by Adherence on the AIS-Cellector–T Cell"), or other T-cell depletion techniques may be detected by a limiting dilution assay (LDA) in which T cells grow in the presence of phytohemagglutinin (PHA), an interleukin-2 (IL-2)–containing supernatant of the MLA gibbon cell line, and irradiated normal allogeneic peripheral blood mononuclear cells. In this miniaturized assay, which uses only 1×10^6 cells per sample, T cells are incubated in 20 μL in Terasaki trays for 11 days, and then examined microscopically for outgrowth. T-cell frequency is determined by the minimum chi^2 method from the Poisson distribution relationship between the cell number seeded per well and the logarithm of the percent of negative wells. Total log_{10} T-cell depletion is the log_{10} of the quotient of the total number of clonable T cells in the unseparated marrow divided by the total number of clonable T cells in the depleted marrow.
TIME FOR PROCEDURE	3 hours sample and feeder preparation and plating; 1 hour examination and analysis
SUMMARY OF PROCEDURE	1. Allogeneic feeder cells are obtained from Ficoll-Hypaque separation of peripheral blood from a normal donor. Following 3000-rad irradiation, feeders are resuspended to 5×10^5 per mL in RPMI-1640 supplemented with 15 percent normal human serum, 4 percent PHA-16, and 5 percent screened MLA supernatant.
	2. Cells from cell populations to be assayed are washed with RPMI, counted, and 1×10^6 cells are resuspended in the feeder cell–MLA medium at 5×10^5 per mL. The cell sample is serially diluted with feeder cell–MLA medium and 20 μL plated into 120 Terasaki wells for each dilution.
	3. Plates are incubated under conditions of high humidity and 5 percent carbon dioxide (CO_2) for 11 days. Plates are examined by inverted microscopy and wells scored for outgrowth.
	4. T-cell frequency is determined from the linear regression analysis of the number of cells seeded per well plotted against the log_{10} of the percent of negative wells at each dilution.
EQUIPMENT	1. 60-well Terasaki plates (Nunc)
	2. Hamilton syringe modified to hold disposable 1-mL tuberculin syringe
	3. Disposable 1-mL tuberculin syringe
	4. 21-gauge, 1⅛-inch needle
SUPPLIES AND REAGENTS	1. RPMI-1640 with 1 mM HEPES, 1 percent glutamine, penicillin (100 U per mL), streptomycin (100 μg per mL)

2. Phytohemagglutinin (PHA-16, Wellcome Diagnostics), reconstituted to 100 μg per mL with RPMI, stored at $-20°$C

3. Normal, pooled human serum, heat inactivated

4. MLA supernatant, conditioned medium from culture of the MLA gibbon cell line (see Notes)

5. Ficoll-Hypaque

PROCEDURE

1. FEEDER CELL PREPARATION

    A. Obtain blood from a normal donor, and separate low-density cells by Ficoll-Hypaque centrifugation at $600g$ for 25 minutes. The peripheral blood mononuclear cells are washed twice with RPMI, with a final centrifugation at $400g$ for 10 minutes for platelet depletion.

    B. Irradiate 25×10^6 feeder cells at 3000 rad and resuspend at 5×10^5 per mL in 50 mL of RPMI supplemented with 15 percent heat-inactivated normal human serum, 4 percent PHA-16, and 5 percent MLA supernatant. Sterile aliquots of PHA-16 and MLA supernatant are stored at $-20°$C and thawed immediately before use. The complete medium is resterilized immediately before feeder cell addition by passage through a 0.2-μm filter.

2. SAMPLE PREPARATION AND PLATING

    A. Wash small aliquots (5×10^6) of marrow at successive steps in T-cell depletion twice with RPMI and count from two independent samples. Suspend 1×10^6 cells in 2.0 mL of irradiated feeders in complete medium.

    B. Serially dilute samples with irradiated feeders in complete medium to yield 1000, 40, 30, 20, and 10 cells per well for unseparated and SBA$^-$ samples; and 800, 600, 400, and 200 cells per well for SBA-E$^-$ and SBA-(CD5/CD8)$^-$ samples. (Dilutions for other T-cell–depletion techniques may vary.) Each dilution is plated into two 60-well Terasaki plates, 20 μL per well, using a Hamilton syringe. The use of 120 wells per dilution allow for narrow 95 percent confidence intervals. A single Terasaki plate is seeded with feeder cells alone as a negative control. The 1000 cell per well dilution of unseparated cells serves as a positive control.

    C. Add 40 μL of RPMI to the corners of the Terasaki plate for additional humidity, and incubate plates in a well-humidified incubator with 5 percent CO_2 for 11 days.

3. ANALYSIS

    A. After 11 days of incubation, examine plates by inverted microscopy and score the wells individually for outgrowth of T cells. T cells appear as clear, healthy round clusters of cells against a background of dark, dead, disintegrating feeder cells.

    B. The relationship between the cell number seeded per well and the logarithm of the percentage of negative wells generates a line whose slope represents the frequency of clonable T cells in cell population. Calculate the total number of T cells for each cell population by multiplying the total number of nucleated cells by the T-cell frequency. Total $\log_{10}$ T-cell depletion is the logarithm of the quotient of the total number of T cells in the unseparated population multiplied by the total number of T cells in the depleted population.

ANTICIPATED
RESULTS

The following are the results of limiting dilution assays performed on all cell populations in 13 T-cell depletions by SBA agglutination and E-AET rosetting.

Cell Population		T-Cell Frequency	Log$_{10}$ T-Cell Depletion
Unseparated	Mean ± SD*	1/44.7 ± 1/37.8	
	(range)	(1/126–1/10)	
	Median	1/25.4	
SBA−	Mean ± SD	1/100.0 ± 1/105.4	1.03 ± 0.30
	(range)	(1/371–1/9)	(0.3–1.35)
	Median	1/55.7	1.15
SBA-E−	Mean ± SD	1/825.6 ± 1/684.1	2.4 ± 0.5
	(range)	(1/2794–1/220)	(1.0–3.0)
	Median	1/703.4	2.6

*SD = Standard deviation.

NOTES

1. MLA supernatant may be replaced or supplemented with 20 U per mL of recombinant IL-2, which will support good outgrowth of T cells.

2. MLA supernatant is generated by culture of the gibbon lymphoma cell line MLA 144 (American Type Culture Collection No. TIB 201) in RPMI with 10 percent fetal calf serum at 3×10^5 per mL until 0.3×10^9 cells are obtained. The cells are concentrated to 2.5×10^6 per mL in RPMI with 1 percent normal human serum and stimulated with 5 ng per mL of phorbol ester myristate acetate (PMA) for 2 hours. After washing and resuspension in fresh RPMI with 1 percent normal human serum, the supernatant is collected and frozen before testing. The supernatant is screened for the support of growth of the IL-2–dependent normal T cells by the incorporation of tritiated thymidine, and for support of T-cell outgrowth in the LDA in comparison to a previously screened batch. The MLA is screened at 5 percent, 10 percent, 15 percent, and 20 percent concentrations. In practice, most supernatants are used at 5 percent of the final assay medium.

3. In a series of 43 HLA-matched T-cell depleted transplants for leukemia, there was a 50 percent incidence of graft-versus-host (GVH) disease when 1×10^5 per kg body weight clonable T cells were present in the graft.

AUTHORS

Nancy A. Kernan, M.D.
Memorial Sloan-Kettering Cancer
  Center
1275 York Ave.
New York, NY 10021

Nancy H. Collins, Ph.D.
Memorial Sloan-Kettering Cancer
  Center
1275 York Ave.
New York, NY 10021

Sharon A. Bleau, M.S.
Memorial Sloan-Kettering Cancer
  Center
1275 York Ave.
New York, NY 10021

Richard J. O'Reilly, M.D.
Memorial Sloan-Kettering Cancer
  Center
1275 York Ave.
New York, NY 10021

REFERENCES

1. Kernan, NA, et al: Limiting dilution microculture assay for quantitation of T lymphocytes in bone marrow. Transplant Proc 27:437, 1985.
2. Kernan, NA, et al: Quantitation of T lymphocytes in human bone marrow by a limiting dilution assay. Transplantation 40:317, 1985.
3. Kernan, NA, et al: Clonable T lymphocytes in T cell depleted bone marrow transplants correlate with development of graft versus host disease. Blood 68:770, 1986.
4. Taswell, C: Limiting dilution assays for the determination of immunocompetent cell frequencies. I. Data analysis. J Immunol 126:1614, 1981.

Limiting Dilution Analysis for Detecting T Cells

DESCRIPTION	Every method used for selective depletion of T lymphocytes from donor bone marrow requires assessment of its efficacy. Limiting dilution analysis (LDA) based on expansion of T cells in medium containing phytohemagglutinin (PHA) and interleukin-2 (IL-2) has higher sensitivity for detecting low numbers of residual T cells than phenotypic analysis. In addition, the method can be used to determine the extent of depletion in bone marrow treated with immunotoxins in which irreversibly damaged T lymphocytes continue to express their surface antigens.
TIME FOR PROCEDURE	Time necessary to set the assay is about 2 hours; each of two refeeding procedures and labeling takes 45 minutes; 2 hours are required for cell harvesting and preparation for counting of incorporated radioactivity
SUMMARY OF PROCEDURE	The method is designed for estimation of the frequency of functional T cells within mononuclear cell population based on a microculture technique with dose-response data analysis. Samples from untreated and depleted bone marrow are cultured at various cell doses in replicate wells of microtiter plates in the presence of PHA and IL-2. The presence or absence of growing T cells in individual wells is assessed by the ability to incorporate [^{3}H]-thymidine. The frequency of T cells in the original fraction is calculated on the basis of Poisson distribution according to which a cell dose that yields a fraction of 0.368 negative wells contains on the average one viable T cell.
EQUIPMENT	1. Laminar flow hood
	2. Incubator
	3. Multiple automated sample harvester (MASH)
	4. Scintillation counter
SUPPLIES AND REAGENTS	1. Culture medium: Iscove's modified Dulbecco's medium supplemented with 10 percent human serum, 20 U per mL of IL-2, 20 μg per mL of PHA, 100 U per mL penicillin, and 100 μg per mL streptomycin.
	2. Human serum
	3. PHA-P (Sigma): prepare 1 mg per mL solution in culture medium and store in adequate portions at $-30°$C.
	4. IL-2 (recombinant, from Cellular Products): make a 300 U per mL dilution in culture medium, aliquot, and store at $-70°$C.
	5. [^{3}H]-thymidine
	6. 96-well round-bottomed microculture plates
	7. Multichannel pipetter and sterile tips
PROCEDURE	Feeder cells and culture medium must be prepared immediately before setting of the assay.
	1. PREPARATION OF FEEDER CELLS: Isolate mononuclear cell fraction from normal peripheral blood by Ficoll-Hypaque density centrifugation. Irradiate washed cells with 50 Gy and suspend them at a concentration of 10^6 cells per mL in culture medium.

2. SETTING THE CULTURE ASSAY
   A. Using culture medium prepare six to eight serial twofold dilutions of untreated (control) and T-cell depleted (treated) mononuclear cells, according to expected T-cell concentration. We usually start with a concentration of 4000 control cells per mL and 800,000 treated cells per mL.
   B. Seed 50 μL of each cell dilution in 24 wells together with 100 μL of feeder cell suspension.
   C. For negative control, seed 48 wells with 100 μL of feeder cell suspension plus 50 μL of medium alone.
   D. Incubate plates at 37°C in 5 percent carbon dioxide (CO_2).
   E. On days 7 and 10 of culture, feed cells in each well by adding 50 μL of freshly prepared culture medium.
   F. On day 14, pulse each well with 1 μCi [^{3}H]-thymidine in 50 μL culture medium for 16 to 18 hours. After pulsing, plates may be stored frozen for further processing.
   G. Harvest cells and evaluate incorporation of radioactivity in each well by scintillation counting.

3. CALCULATION OF T-CELL FREQUENCY
   A. Calculate mean counts per minute (CPM) and standard deviations (SD) for the 48 control wells containing feeders and medium alone.
   B. Score wells from the assayed material as positive or negative, based on whether or not the counts exceed the mean CPM by more than 3 SD.
   C. Calculate the fraction of negative wells for each dose of cells seeded.
   D. Calculate the frequency of T cells on the basis of Poisson distribution by one of the following methods:
      (1) Method of least squares fitting with values derived from logarithmic transformation of the zero term of Poisson equation. Simply do linear regression of log fraction negative cultures (wells) versus cells per culture. The slope expresses the frequency (f) of reactive cells in the assayed population.
      (2) Average frequencies obtained by the single-fit Poisson equation for individual cell doses according to the formula:

$$f = -1 \ np/x$$

where: p = Fraction of negatively responding cultures for a given cell dose
        x = Number of cells per culture

      (3) The best estimation of the T-cell frequency is by the method of chi^2 minimization of Taswell.[1] For details see the publication.
   E. Calculate the extent of T-cell depletion by dividing T-cell frequency found in the control sample by that found in the treated cell population.

ANTICIPATED RESULTS

The frequency of T cells evaluated by LDA in the mononuclear fraction of untreated bone marrow harvested for transplantation ranges from 1 in 7 to 1 in 40 cells (mean 1 in 14 cells). T-cell frequency in depleted bone marrow depends on the method used for depletion.

NOTES	The frequency of proliferating cells estimated by LDA is usually lower than that estimated by phenotypic T-cell analysis. The difference may vary, depending on the efficiency of LDA as a culture assay. Thus, LDA is not an exact method for enumeration of T lymphocytes. However, the frequency ratio of cells scored positive by LDA in untreated and depleted bone marrow does express the extent of T-cell depletion most accurately.

AUTHORS	Ewa Marciniak, M.D. Dept. of Medicine University of Kentucky Medical Center Lexington, KY 40536	P. Jean Henslee-Downey, M.D. Dept. of Medicine University of Kentucky Medical Center Lexington, KY 40536

REFERENCE	1. Taswell, C: Limiting dilution assay for the determination of immunocompetent cell frequencies. J Immunol 126:1614, 1981.

Evaluation of Efficiency of T-Cell Depletion

DESCRIPTION   Several methods are used to evaluate the efficacy of ST1-immunotoxin–mediated T-cell depletion (see "Ex Vivo Immunotoxin-Mediated T-Cell Depletion," Chapter 7). Because ricin-based immunotoxins inhibit protein synthesis, they generally require cell division for cytotoxicity. Fluorescent activated cell sorter (FACS) analysis or other evaluation immediately following the procedure is not appropriate. Therefore, cultures that are dependent on cell proliferation are established and subsequently evaluated. Sensitive and quantitative in vitro analysis of efficacy of mature T-cell removal is critical for the evaluation of the treatment protocol. Typically, three assays are performed on each marrow depletion: (1) cytofluorometric or FACS analysis of residual T cells following phytohemagglutinin (PHA) plus interleukin-2 (IL-2) stimulation (see section A, which follows); (2) proliferative potential of residual T cells contaminating bone marrow cells following stimulation with PHA (see section B); (3) hematopoietic progenitor cell assay to ensure that immunotoxin treatment was not toxic to the marrow. The first two procedures are described in detail subsequently; colony-forming assays are described in detail under "Bone Marrow Cell Culture" earlier in this chapter. In addition, limiting dilution analysis (LDA) is a sensitive assay for residual T cells. It is, however, technically difficult and may not be used by all centers. It is described in detail in "Limiting Dilution Assay for Clonable T Cells—Microtechnique" and "Limiting Dilution Analysis for Detecting T Cells," both also earlier in this chapter.

TIME FOR PROCEDURE   Establishing the cultures for FACS analysis requires approximately 20 to 30 minutes, staining the samples on day 5 requires 2 to 2.5 hours, and cytofluorographic analysis requires an additional 45 minutes. Establishing cultures to evaluate proliferative potential requires approximately 20 minutes and harvesting the cultures on day 5 is accomplished in 20 to 30 minutes.

A. CYTOFLUOROGRAPHIC ANALYSIS OF MATURE T LYMPHOCYTES FOLLOWING CULTURE IN PHA PLUS IL-2

SUMMARY OF PROCEDURE   Following delivery of the ricin A chain into the cytoplasm of the cell and protein synthesis arrest, a great number of cells, unable to divide, continue to have intact cell membranes for some time. Therefore, all methods of evaluation based on the counting of residual T cells directly after treatment are not applicable to the immunotoxin model of T-cell depletion. The method described here is based on the ability of lymphocytes to be stimulated by phytohemagglutinin P (PHA) and interleukin-2 (IL-2). After several days in culture, T-lymphocyte viability is evaluated by indirect immunofluorescence using cytofluorometric analysis and compared with a control culture.

EQUIPMENT
1. Laminar air flow hood
2. 37°C tissue culture incubator, 5 percent carbon dioxide (CO_2)–in–air
3. Flow cytometry capability (FACScan, Becton-Dickinson, Mountain View, CA, or equivalent)

SUPPLIES AND REAGENTS

1. 12-well and 24-well culture plates (Costar or equivalent)

2. Heat-inactivated fetal calf serum (FCS). Heat-inactivate FCS at 56°C for 45 minutes

3. RPMI-1640 (Gibco, Grand Island, NY) supplemented with 15 percent FCS

4. Phosphate-buffered saline (PBS), supplemented with 0.1 percent bovine serum albumin (BSA) and 0.1 percent NaN_3

5. IL-2 (Amgen Biologicals, Thousand Oaks, CA), 20 U per mL final, 400 U per mL initial concentration

6. PHA (Difco Laboratories, Detroit) at 1 percent final, 20 percent initial concentration

7. Tracer beads: nonfluorescent 10-μm beads (Coultronics); wash thoroughly and store in 0.1 percent PBS-BSA with 0.1 percent NaN_3 and 10 percent heat-inactivated FCS

8. Monoclonal antibody (MAb) cocktail: pool of anti-CD5, anti-CD3, anti-CD4, and anti-CD8, at 2 μg per mL final concentration for each antibody; for phenotyping use 100 μL per cell pellet

9. FITC-labeled goat F(ab′)$_2$ antimouse IgG (NEN or Boehringer Mannheim) diluted 1:40 for use

10. Propidium iodide (PI) (Sigma) at 20 μg per mL

11. Particle size standards: traceable polymer microspheres (19.58 μm $\pm$ 0.1 μm Duke Scientific) 4×10^5 beads total in 1-mL sample

PROCEDURE

1. BONE MARROW CELL CULTURE
   A. Wash an aliquot of control bone marrow cells separated by Ficoll-Hypaque, identical to the treated bone marrow except for the absence of immunotoxin, and an aliquot of the immunotoxin treated bone marrow cells, three times in RPMI–15 percent FCS. Resuspend cells in RPMI–15 percent FCS at 2×10^6 nucleated cells per mL.
   B. To each well of 12-well tissue culture plate, add 2×10^6 bone marrow cells in 2 mL RPMI–15 percent FCS. To the cells add:
      (1) 0.05 mL PHA 20 percent initial concentration (1 percent final)
      (2) 0.05 mL IL-2 at 400 U per mL initial concentration (20 U per mL final)
   C. Culture control and treated bone marrow cells in triplicate at 37°C in 5 percent CO_2-in-air for 4 or 5 days.

2. PREPARATION OF CELLS FOR FACS ANALYSIS
   A. On day 4 or 5 after establishing proliferative culture, add to each well 4×10^5 nonfluorescent beads.
   B. Transfer the contents of the wells into 5-mL small plastic tubes.
   C. Wash once in PBS plus 2 percent FCS plus 0.1 percent NaN_3. Spin at 4°C and 1000 rpm ($300g$).
   D. Add to the cell pellet 100 μL of the anti-CD3, -CD4, -CD5, and -CD8 MAb cocktail, each MAb at 2 μg per mL. Incubate at 4°C for 60 minutes with intermittent gentle shaking.
   E. Wash once again in PBS plus 2 percent FCS plus 0.1 percent NaN_3.
   F. Add to the cell pellet 100 μL of FITC-labeled goat antimouse immu-

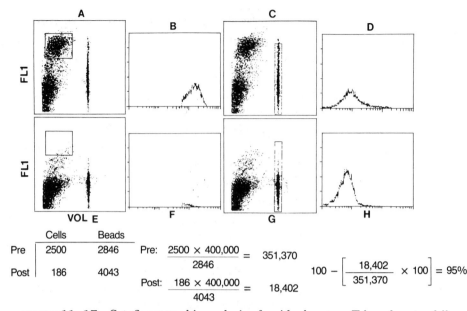

	Cells	Beads
Pre	2500	2846
Post	186	4043

Pre: $\dfrac{2500 \times 400{,}000}{2846} = 351{,}370$

Post: $\dfrac{186 \times 400{,}000}{4043} = 18{,}402$

$$100 - \left[\dfrac{18{,}402}{351{,}370} \times 100 \right] = 95\%$$

FIGURE 11–17 Cytofluorographic analysis of residual mature T lymphocytes following ST1-IT depletion. Untreated (panels A–D) and ST1-IT–treated (panels E–H) bone marrow cells were cultured in PHA in addition to interleukin-2 for 4 to 5 days. Cells were then stained with a combination of anti-CD3, anti-CD4, anti-CD8, and anti-CD5 MAb followed by fluoresceinated goat-anti-mouse Ab. Viable cells, able to exclude propidium iodide, were analyzed by volume versus fluorescence (panels A, C, E, G). Gates were defined to include all stained cells (panels A, E) or nonfluorescent tracer beads (panels C, G). Without changing the defined gates (panels A, E), the number of cells (panels B, F) or beads (panels D, H) were collected by single histogram analysis of cell number versus fluorescence. Percent depletion was calculated as shown above.

noglobin G (IgG), diluted appropriately before use. Incubate 60 minutes at 4°C with intermittent gentle shaking.

   G. Wash again and resuspend the cell pellet with 1 mL of PBS plus 2 percent FCS plus 0.1 percent NaN$_3$. Final volume should be 1 mL (cells with 4×10^5 beads).

3. FACS ANALYSIS OF THE SAMPLE
   A. Add 50 μL of the 20 μg per mL PI solution to the tube to be analyzed.
   B. Resuspend the cells with aid of a syringe or pipette. Analyze (FACScan, Becton Dickinson, Mountain View, CA) according to the following parameters:
     • P_1: Forward light scatter (FLS)
     • P_2: Logarithmic amplification of light diffused at 90 degrees (log PLS)
     • P_3: Logarithmic amplification of fluorescence due to FITC (log FITC)
     • P_4: Fluorescence due to PI
   C. Analyze according to P_1–P_4, setup of a barrier for living cells (PI negative).
   D. Analyze according to P_2–P_3, setup of window (GI) for the T-lymphocyte population, and a window (G2) for the bead population.

E. The number of lymphocytes (N) in the well is calculated as follows:

$$N = \frac{x}{y} \times 400{,}000$$

where: x = Number of T cells in G1
y = Number of beads in G2

F. The ratio of number of T cells counted in the immunotoxin (IT)–treated culture and in the control culture gives the percentage of residual T lymphocytes after treatment with IT.

G. Collect 10,000 events. Volume gate 50 to 250. Volume gate should be kept constant, and SCC should be tuned. Collect control (pre) and treated (post) data, and save data (Fig. 11–17).

H. Draw box around pre cells and print out single histogram of F1 1 or vol. Collect number of events—that is, number of CD3-, CD4-, CD8-, or CD5-positive T cells. Using same box, read post sample. Print out single histograms collecting number of events (Fig. 11–17).

I. Draw box around pre beads and collect number of events using single histogram to be number of beads. Collect number of events in box of post beads using same box.

Example:

	T Cells	Beads
Pre	4087	902
Post	891	1798

pre   *beads*   *T cells*
$(4087 \div 902) \times 4 \times 10^5 = 1{,}812{,}416.851$
post
$(891 \div 1798) \times 4 \times 10^5 =\ 198{,}220.2447$

10.9 expansion or 89.1 percent T-cell depletion

ANTICIPATED
RESULTS

By cytofluorometric analysis, an average of approximately 95 percent of T cells are depleted from the bone marrow inocula using ST1-IT.

B. PROLIFERATIVE POTENTIAL OF RESIDUAL T CELLS

SUMMARY OF
PROCEDURE

Because ricin A chain causes protein synthesis arrest, cells will be unable to undergo cell division. This assay is based on the ability of T lymphocytes to proliferate upon stimulation with phytohemagglutinin (PHA). Control and treated bone marrow cultures are incubated in the presence of PHA for 3 days. Cultures are pulsed with [^{3}H]-thymidine and harvested to determine the incorporation of [^{3}H]-thymidine into dividing cells.

EQUIPMENT

1. Laminar air flow hood
2. 37°C tissue culture incubator, 5 percent carbon dioxide (CO_2)–in–air

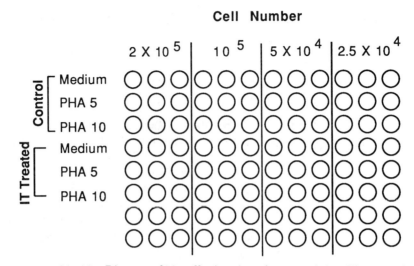

FIGURE 11–18 Diagram of 96-well microtiter plate containing dilutions of control and immunotoxin-treated bone marrow cells for analysis of proliferative potential.

SUPPLIES AND REAGENTS		
	1.	RPMI-1640 (Gibco, Grand Island, NY), supplemented with 20 percent heat-inactivated (56°C for 45 minutes) fetal calf serum (FCS)
	2.	PHA (Difco), 5 μg per mL and 10 μg per mL final concentration
	3.	96-well flat bottom plates (Falcon or Costar)
	4.	[^{3}H]-thymidine (New England Nuclear, Boston, or equivalent)
	5.	Cell harvester (multiple automatic sample harvester [MASH] II, Microbiological Association, Bethesda, MD; or equivalent)

PROCEDURE		
	1.	Count pre and post bone marrow samples and resuspend at 4×10^6 cells per mL. Make three serial twofold dilutions to 2×10^6 cells per mL, 10^6 cells per mL, and 5×10^5 cells per mL. Approximately 500 μL of each sample at each dilution is needed.
	2.	Plate 50 μL of each sample in triplicate on each of three lines in 96-well microtiter plates (Falcon and Costar) (Fig. 11–18).
	3.	Incubate cells in triplicate without (control) or with PHA 10 μg per mL and 5 μg per mL final concentration.
	4.	Final culture volume is 200 μL per well in RPMI–20 percent FCS.
	5.	Incubate at 37°C in tissue culture incubator, 5 percent CO_2–in–air, for 3 days.
	6.	Pulse with 1 μCi per well [^{3}H]-thymidine for final 18 hours.
	7.	Harvest on cell harvester to determine incorporated beta activity.
	8.	Calculate percent inhibition to PHA stimulation for each concentration of PHA.

$$\% \text{ Inhibition} = 100 - \left[\frac{x - y}{x' - y'} \right] \times 100$$

where: x = cpm of stimulated IT-treated cells
        y = cpm of unstimulated IT-treated cells

x' = cpm of stimulated control cells
y' = cpm of unstimulated control cells

ANTICIPATED RESULTS	Approximately 95 percent depletion of residual T lymphocytes is achieved when evaluated by determination of proliferative potential.
NOTES	1. There is often high background proliferation of bone marrow cultures.
	2. Choose a cell concentration (usually 2.5×10^5 cells per well or 10^5 cells per well) on the linear portion of the response curve.

AUTHOR

Barbara E. Bierer, M.D.
Hematology-Oncology Division
Brigham and Women's Hospital
Division of Pediatric Oncology
Dana-Farber Cancer Inst.
Room 1610B
44 Binney St.
Boston, MA 02115

IMMUNOFLUORESCENCE

IMMUNOFLUORESCENCE TEST: COMPLEMENT PURGING

DESCRIPTION	Used as a quality assurance procedure for monoclonal antibody (MAb) and complement marrow purging, the indirect immunofluoresence test detects the presence of MAb after the MAb incubation. A positive result indicates saturating MAb in the supernatant, and that antibodies coat the surface receptors of tumor cells. These cells will pick up fluorescent goat-antimouse conjugate under darkfield.
TIME FOR PROCEDURE	Approximately 90 minutes, including reading 10 slides.
SUMMARY OF PROCEDURE	1. Tumor cells and specimens are incubated (with MAb).
	2. Slides are washed.
	3. Same cells are incubated with goat-antimouse conjugate.
	4. Slides are washed again.
	5. Slides are mounted and read.
EQUIPMENT	Fluorescence microscope
SUPPLIES AND REAGENTS	1. Phosphate-buffered saline (PBS)
	2. Sodium azide
	3. Fetal calf serum
	4. MAb such as IF-5 as positive control
	5. Fluorescein isothiocyanate (FITC) goat-antimouse conjugate
	6. Glycerol
	7. Clear nail polish
	8. Tumor cell lines
PROCEDURE	1. PREPARE SLIDES ON CARDBOARD
	A. Tape both sides of the slides with glossy cellophane tape so that the coverslip will ride on elevated ridges.
	B. Use nail polish to seal two ends of the coverslip, leaving the other ends open for loading cells.
	C. For each slide, prepare a corresponding 15-mL tube. Add 1×10^6 LAM 53 tumor cells in each tube, centrifuge, and aspirate to leave dry pellets.
	D. Add 50 μL of specimen (supernatant from purging procedure) and resuspend cells.
	E. Use IF-5 (1:100) as positive control and use PBS plus 5 percent FCS as negative control.
	F. Incubate on ice for 20 minutes.
	G. Wash once with 10 mL cold PBS plus 0.02 percent azide, centrifuge at 1600 rpm for 5 minutes, and remove supernatant.

    H. Add 50 μL FITC goat-antimouse conjugate (1:10 dilution with PBS plus azide before use) and resuspend pellet.

    I. Incubate on ice for 20 minutes.

    J. Wash once with 10 mL cold PBS plus azide.

    K. Resuspend each pellet with 50 μL 50 percent glycerol in PBS plus azide.

    L. Discharge cells with a pipette tip under the coverslip.

    M. Seal other ends of the coverslips. Cut cellophane tape along the edges of the slides with a blade.

    N. Slide is ready for viewing with fluorescence microscopy.

ANTICIPATED RESULTS	1. The positive control should have fluorescence speckles of dye on the periphery of cells. 2. The negative control should demonstrate evenly stained dark yellow–green cells.

NOTE   The sealed slides can be read later, as long as the slides are refrigerated in the dark.

AUTHOR   Jean T. Yao, M.S., S.B.B.(ASCP)
Research and Development
   Associate
Blood Bank
Methodist Medical Center
221 N.E. Glen Oak Ave.
Peoria, IL 61636

FLUORESCENCE (VISUAL) ASSAY FOR CD34-POSITIVE HEMATOPOIETIC PROGENITORS

DESCRIPTION	Monoclonal antibodies directed against the CD34 differentiation antigen are used, along with fluoresceinated secondary antibodies, to identify hematopoietic progenitor cells in samples of bone marrow or peripheral blood nucleated cells.
TIME FOR PROCEDURE	Total time: 4 hours, 20 minutes
	1. 1 hour, 15 minutes for cell preparation
	2. 30 minutes for first antibody incubation
	3. 40 minutes for first washing
	4. 30 minutes for second antibody incubation
	5. 40 minutes for second washing
	6. 45 minutes for reading
SUMMARY OF PROCEDURE	1. Cells are prepared for antibody labeling by separation of mononuclear cells on Ficoll-Hypaque density gradient and washing in Dulbecco's phosphate-buffered saline (DPBS).
	2. Cells are incubated with CD34 monoclonal antibody.
	3. Excess antibody is removed by washing.
	4. Cells are incubated with fluoresceinated second antibody.
	5. Excess antibody is removed by washing.
	6. The percent of fluorescent cells is determined by epifluorescent microscopic examination.
EQUIPMENT	1. Air-displacement small-volume pipettor, with adjustable volume
	2. Refrigerated centrifuge
	3. Microscope with ultraviolet epifluorescent illumination
SUPPLIES AND REAGENTS	1. Negative control cell line (NALM-6 CALL$^+$ leukemia line recommended)
	2. Positive control cell line (KG-1 or KG-1a acute myelogenous leukemia [AML] line recommended)
	3. CD34 monoclonal antibody (HPCA-1, Becton-Dickinson, Mountain View, CA)
	4. Fluorescein isothiocyanate (FITC)–labeled goat antimurine immunoglobulin (Ig) antiserum (Fisher Scientific)
	5. Conical centrifuge tubes, 15- and 50-mL
	6. Borosilicate glass tubes, 12 mm × 75 mm
	7. Transfer pipettes
	8. Trypan blue dye
	9. Hemacytometer, Neubauer ruled
	10. Slides and *glass* coverslips
	11. Tips for air-displacement small-volume pipettor

12. DPBS with 5 percent serum (DPBSS)

13. Crushed ice in bucket or tray

14. Ficoll-Hypaque 1.077 g per mL density gradient medium (Ficoll-Hypaque, Pharmacia)

PROCEDURES

1. CELL SEPARATION

    A. Layer cell sample on Ficoll-Hypaque density gradient medium (volume of Ficoll-Hypaque should be approximately one-third cell suspension volume)

    B. Centrifuge at *room temperature* as follows: slowly accelerate to 450 to 500g (1500 rpm in standard swinging bucket rotor); maintain speed for 40 minutes; allow centrifuge to stop *without braking.*

    C. Using transfer pipette, remove cells from medium (plasma)/Ficoll-Hypaque interface and transfer to fresh tube.

    D. Harvest positive and negative control cell lines and place in fresh tubes.

    E. Centrifuge all cells (700g for 5 minutes), resuspend pellets with DPBSS. Repeat twice.

    F. Treat cells with trypan blue and count (count only viable, dye-excluding cells: nonviable cells may leak antibodies). Adjust to 10^6 cells per mL.

    G. Transfer 1 mL of cells (10^6 cells total) into borosilicate 12 mm $\times$ 75 mm tubes.

    ALL STEPS FROM THIS POINT TO BE PERFORMED AT 0 TO 5°C

2. LABELING OF CELLS

    A. Centrifuge cell suspensions (700g for 5 minutes at 5°C). Decant excess medium from tubes. Break up pellets by pulling tube across top of test tube rack.

    B. Add 20 μL of CD34 monoclonal antibody plus 20 μL DPBSS to cells. Incubate 30 minutes on ice.

    C. Following incubation: Add 1 to 2 mL *cold* DPBSS to each tube. Centrifuge (700g for 5 minutes at 5°C). Break up pellet by pulling tube over top of test tube rack. Repeat twice.

    D. Add appropriately diluted* secondary (FITC labeled) antibody to tubes in 20 μL, plus 20 μL DPBSS. Incubate 30 minutes on ice and in darkness.

    E. Following incubation: Add 1 to 2 mL *cold* DPBSS to each tube. Centrifuge (700g for 5 minutes at 5°C). Break up pellet by pulling tube over top of test tube rack. Repeat twice.

    F. Centrifuge one more time. Remove as much excess medium from each tube as possible (the last drop may be removed by blotting rim of tube with a tissue). Break up pellet by pulling tube across top of test tube rack.

---

*Secondary antibodies may be sold in a concentration that is greater than that needed for labeling. Each laboratory should determine the ideal dilution for the vendor and lot number of antibody used.

3. ASSAY EVALUATION
   A. Transfer 20 to 30 μL of cell suspension to *clean* microscope slide. Gently place coverslip over drop so as not to form air bubbles.
   B. Keep slides out of light while not viewing.
   C. Check positive and negative controls for proper staining (quality assurance for technique).
   D. Estimate percentage of CD34-positive cells as follows:
      (1) With ultraviolet light source turned OFF, count total nucleated cells in five fields (each corner and center under coverslip).
      (2) Compute average number of cells per field.
      (3) Turn ultraviolet light source ON. Examine at least 20 to 30 fields under coverslip, counting number of fields examined and number of fluorescing cells observed.
      (4) Compute percent CD34-positive cells as follows:

$$\text{\% CD34-positive} = \frac{\Sigma(\text{CD34-positive cells observed})}{(\text{Number fields examined}) \times (\text{Avg. cells per field})}$$

ANTICIPATED RESULTS

We have observed the following levels of CD34-positive cells:

Source of Cells	% CD34-positive
Bone marrow	1.00–5.00
Blood, normal individuals	0.01–0.05
Blood, patients recovering from cyclophosphamide chemotherapy	0.10–0.90

NOTES

1. Erythrocytes that are inadvertently collected from the Ficoll-Hypaque separation may cause the final counting to be inaccurate (use of phase contrast microscopy helps with this problem). We have been examining red cell lytic agents, looking for one that does not interfere with antibody labeling. As of this writing, we have not identified a best agent.

2. A directly conjugated anti-CD34 antibody (HPCA-2, Becton-Dickinson) has recently been introduced. If this antibody is used, the secondary (FITC-labeled) antibody is unnecessary, as are steps 2D and 2E in previous section.

QUALITY CONTROL

1. Positive and negative controls (KG-1a and NALM-6 cell lines) are run with every assay.

2. Assay results from identical samples are plotted on a CUMSUM type of graph, and upward or downward trends watched for.

3. KG-1a, positive control cell line cells that have been labeled with CD34 antibody and secondary FITC labeled antibody, are examined by flow cytometry every time a new lot of CD34 antibodies or FITC secondary antibodies are opened to ensure that the fluorescence per cell is not varying.

AUTHORS

Mary Jane Farmelo, B.A.
  C.L.Sp.(CG)
Bone Marrow Processing and
  Evaluation Laboratory
H. Lee Moffitt Cancer Center and
  Research Institute
University of South Florida
12902 Magnolia Dr.
Tampa, FL 33612-9497

William E. Janssen, Ph.D.
Bone Marrow Processing and
  Evaluation Laboratory
Bone Marrow Transplant Program
H. Lee Moffitt Cancer Center and
  Research Institute
University of South Florida
12902 Magnolia Dr.
Tampa, FL 33612-9497

REFERENCES

1. Siena, S, et al: Flow cytometry for clinical estimation of circulating hematopoietic progenitors for autologous transplantation in cancer patients. Blood 77:400, 1991.
2. Berenson, RJ, et al: Antigen CD34+ marrow cells engraft lethally irradiated baboons. J Clin Invest 81:951, 1988.
3. Civin, IC, et al: Antigenic analysis of hematopoiesis. IV. Flow cytometry characterization of My-10 positive progenitor cells in normal human bone marrow. Exp Hematol 5:10, 1987.

CHROMIUM-51 RELEASE ASSAY

DESCRIPTION	To ensure the effectiveness of the monoclonal antibody (MAb) and complement purging material and procedure, this assay is carried out in parallel with the actual bone marrow purging. A small fraction (5 percent) of tumor cells are mixed with marrow cells. These tumor cells are labeled with chromium-51 (^{51}Cr). After the purging procedure, should have all the tumor cells lysed and all the ^{51}Cr should be in the supernatant instead of in the cell pellet.
TIME FOR PROCEDURE	Approximately 4 hours
SUMMARY OF PROCEDURE	1. Tumor cells are labeled with ^{51}Cr.
	2. Tumor cells are mixed with bone marrow mononuclear cells at 1:20 ratio.
	3. MAb(s) are added and incubated on ice for 30 minutes.
	4. Complement is added and the preparation incubated at 37°C for 1 hour.
	5. Supernatant is centrifuged and saved.
	6. Cells are resuspended; MAb and complement incubation is repeated.
	7. Supernatant is centrifuged and saved.
	8. Cell pellet is saved and gamma scintillation counter is used to determine percentage of killing.
EQUIPMENT	1. Incubator
	2. Centrifuge
	3. Gamma scintillation counter
SUPPLIES AND REAGENTS	1. ^{51}Cr radioisotope
	2. Culture medium RPMI plus 10 percent fetal calf serum (FCS)
	3. Phosphate-buffered saline (PBS)
	4. MAbs and newborn rabbit complement
PROCEDURE	1. Prepare tumor cell line culture (e.g., LAM 53).
	2. Make up the volume of 1×10^6 tumor cells to 1 mL with RPMI plus 10 percent FCS.
	3. Incubate tumor cells and 400 μCi of ^{51}Cr at 37°C for 1 hour. Wash twice with PBS. Pellet cells.
	4. Add 1 mL of a concentration of 2×10^7 per mL bone marrow mononuclear cells that have been treated with MAb(s).
	5. Incubate on ice for 30 minutes.
	6. Add 125 μl (0.125 mL) newborn rabbit complement. Incubate at 37°C for 1 hour.
	7. Centrifuge. Save 100 μL supernatant, and label this S1. Discard the remaining supernatant in a radiation waste container.
	8. Resuspend pellet in 1 mL PBS, repeat MAb(s), and complement incubations.
	9. Centrifuge. Save 100 μL supernatant, and label S2. Discard the remaining supernatant.

10. Wash once with PBS; discard supernatant.

11. Save pellet, and label P1.

12. Calculate percentage of killing:

$$\% \text{ Killing} = \frac{S1 + S2}{S1 + S2 + P1} \times 100$$

ANTICIPATED RESULTS   Percentage of killing should be at least 90 percent.

AUTHORS   Jean T. Yao, M.S., S.B.B.(ASCP)
Research and Development
  Associate
Blood Bank
Methodist Medical Center
221 N.E. Glen Oak Ave.
Peoria, IL 61636

Robert Negrin, M.D.
Hematology Department
Stanford University Hospital
300 Pasteur Dr.
Stanford, CA 94305

12 | OTHER TECHNIQUES

444

SHIPPING OF BONE MARROW

SHIPPING OF FRESHLY HARVESTED BONE MARROW

DESCRIPTION	Bone marrow may be harvested at one institution and transported for processing or for transplantation at another institution (e.g., unrelated donor transplant). Freshly harvested bone marrow must be transported in a timely and *safe* manner between the two centers. Transportation arrangements must be made that will (1) protect the marrow from rough handling and extremes of temperature and pressure; (2) ensure against loss in transit; (3) protect personnel and equipment in case of leakage of marrow in transit.
TIME FOR PROCEDURE	From 1 to 3 hours technician time to make arrangements for transport and to pack marrow for shipment. Transit time must be arranged to require fewer than 12 hours.
SUMMARY OF PROCEDURE	1. Arrangements for marrow transportation are made at least 24 hours in advance of actual shipment. 2. Freshly harvested bone marrow is packaged for shipment. Packing includes double bagging, ice packs (optional), sterile towels (for padding, absorbency, and insulation), and final packaging in a thermally insulated, water-tight container. 3. Package is appropriately labeled and turned over to shipping company or courier.
SPECIMEN	Freshly harvested bone marrow should be contained in a hermetically sealed blood product transfer pack. All lines should be either tightly clamped or heat-sealed.
EQUIPMENT	1. Tube heat sealer 2. Plastic bag heat sealer

SUPPLIES AND REAGENTS	1. 600-mL or 1-L blood product transfer packs
	
	2. Y transfer adaptor with two female spike fittings and one male spike fitting
	
	3. Heavy-duty plastic bag of sufficient size to hold two 1-L blood bags of bone marrow. Ziplock-type bags are adequate, but heat-sealed bags are superior for water tightness.
	
	4. Sterile (or very clean) towels or disposable underpads
	
	5. Picnic cooler "gel-ice" packs (optional)
	
	6. Sturdy insulated shipping container (blood bank shipping containers are recommended)
	
	7. Label, containing the following essential information (Fig. 12–1)
	   A. Contents of shipment: human bone marrow for transplantation
	   B. Name and address of recipient institution
	   C. Name and phone number of responsible individual who can be contacted in case of an emergency with the shipment
	   D. Brief statement describing the packaging, and emphasizing requirement that it be leakproof

URGENT SHIPMENT

HUMAN BONE MARROW
FOR
TRANSPLANTATION

This vessel contains human bone marrow for a life-saving transplant. *BONE MARROW IS NOT REPLACEABLE!* Please treat this shipment accordingly.

IN CASE OF EMERGENCY OR DELAY WITH THIS SHIPMENT PLEASE CALL IMMEDIATELY:

NAME: PHONE:

CONTENTS: CLINICAL SPECIMEN
PACKAGED ACCORDING TO CFR 49-172

FIGURE 12-1   Shipment label for freshly harvested bone marrow.

E. The radiation emitted by security equipment is probably insufficient to be detrimental to the bone marrow stem cells. Nevertheless, it is prudent to carry documentation requesting hand inspection by security personnel and warning that the contents are not to be subjected to x-ray examination owing to the sensitivity of stem cells to radiation damage.

PROCEDURE

1. Contact shipping company at least 24 hours in advance to arrange for shipment. Shipping company (commercial airline is recommended) should be informed of nature of shipment. Obtain assurances of the following:

    A. Cabin or cockpit transit. If all airlines at sending institution's local airport refuse cabin or cockpit transit, temperature-controlled baggage compartment (sometimes referred to as the pet baggage compartment) transit is marginally acceptable.

    NOTE: *Regular baggage compartment transit is unacceptable. The temperatures in these compartments drop precipitously, and the marrow will freeze. Transit in view of the flight crew also provides protection against misrouting.*

    B. Minimal plane changes (not more than one). Direct flights are preferred but are not usually available. If plane changes are expected, cabin or cockpit transit is essential, and the flight crew on each flight should be told to expect the shipment.

    C. Special consideration. Airline personnel need to be aware that a human life is dependent on their performance, and they need to provide assurance of full cooperation.

D. Optional perk: Federal Aviation Administration (FAA) regulations provide for special consideration (e.g., going to the front of the line in the takeoff and landing queues) of "LifeGuard flights." Any aircraft carrying perishable human tissue for transplantation may be so designated, but the airlines frequently need to be reminded of this fact.

2. If these assurances cannot be met, then the marrow must be transported with a human escort—that is, a round-trip ticket must be purchased for an individual, and that person must carry the marrow as carry-on baggage. (In any event, this is the best way to transport marrow and is strongly recommended.)

3. Draw a sample of the bone marrow and perform cell counts. Counts should be recorded, and a copy of record included with the marrow shipment.

4. If the collected bone marrow volume exceeds 1 L, it must be split into two volumes of less than 1 L each (in accordance with United States Government shipping regulations for specimens that potentially may contain pathologic agents).

5. Seal bags with heat sealer.

6. Place transfer bags into outer plastic bag and seal.

7. Wrap in towels or other clean padding and place into shipping container.

8. Seal shipping container, place labeling on outside, and turn package over to airline (or send escort to board the plane).

9. *Upon receipt,* open package immediately, remove marrow bags, and place a thermometer between the two transfer bags. Temperature of the marrow should be neither higher than 37°C nor lower than 2°C. As soon as possible after receipt, draw up a sample and examine it for hemolysis. Cell counts should be performed and checked against those reported by the sending institution.

10. Marrow should be infused as soon as possible after arrival at the recipient institution.

ANTICIPATED RESULTS

Bone marrow should be delivered to recipient institution within 12 hours of completion of harvest, although this may not be possible for centers that are distant from large urban airports. Bone marrow should arrive with minimal hemolysis and with cell counts within 10 percent of those reported by the sending institution.

NOTES

1. Whether it is better to ship bone marrow at room temperature or on ice has not yet been determined. Although it is known that hematopoietic stem cells survive storage at room temperature for 24 hours, observation of small marrow samples in tubes sent on ice or at ambient temperature have shown that the cold shipments have less clumping on receipt. Additionally, it has been shown that marrow stored at 3 to 4°C can be successfully reinfused for up to 3 days.

2. It is advisable to set up hematopoietic colony assays both before and after shipment. However, without standardization of these assays between the sending and the receiving institutions, this measure may be of limited usefulness.

AUTHORS

William E. Janssen, Ph.D.
Bone Marrow Processing and
   Evaluation Laboratory
Bone Marrow Transplant Program
H. Lee Moffitt Cancer Center and
   Research Institute
University of South Florida
12902 Magnolia Dr.
Tampa, FL 33612-9497

Carlos E. Lee, M.T.
Bone Marrow Processing and
   Evaluation Laboratory
Bone Marrow Transplant Program
H. Lee Moffitt Cancer Center and
   Research Institute
University of South Florida
12902 Magnolia Dr.
Tampa, FL 33612-9497

REFERENCE

1. Hoppe, PA, et al (eds): Technical Manual of the American Association of Blood Banks, ed 10. American Association of Blood Banks, Arlington, VA, 1990.

SHIPPING OF LIQUID NITROGEN CRYOPRESERVED (FROZEN) BONE MARROW

DESCRIPTION

Bone marrow that has been cryopreserved at one facility, and is to be infused at another, must be transported in such a manner that the temperature of the marrow does not exceed −150°C. Accordingly, shipment must be carried out in a container that will accommodate the bone marrow and sufficient liquid nitrogen for the duration of the transport. The minimum permissable amount of liquid nitrogen for overnight transport is 25 L. Liquid nitrogen evaporation is hastened by reduced pressures experienced in air transport, as well as by exposure to high temperatures such as might be encountered on airport tarmacs in the summertime and in tropical and subtropical latitudes.

Liquid nitrogen has been determined by the United States Department of Transportation to be a hazardous material. Shipments containing this material must be so labeled (Fig. 12–2) and accompanied by appropriate "hazardous goods" declaration documents.

When available, the CryoMed "Dry" Shipper facilitates shipment of bone marrow at liquid nitrogen temperatures without associated risks of liquid nitrogen spillage in transit. This is accomplished by a solid "sponge," located in the bottom of the tank, that soaks up and retains sufficient liquid nitrogen to maintain a temperature of −193°C for 7 days. Use of this type of shipment container is recommended.

TIME FOR PROCEDURE

Approximately 1 to 2 hours technician preparation time. Shipment may take anywhere from 12 to 36 hours, depending on choice of carrier

SUMMARY OF PROCEDURE

1. An appropriate container for shipment of bone marrow packed with liquid nitrogen is selected.

2. The container is prepared for shipment, with appropriate documentation including *hazardous goods declaration* and *invoice/package inventory*.

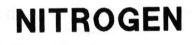

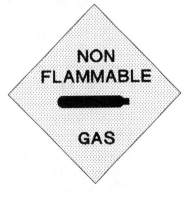

FIGURE 12–2   Label for liquid nitrogen cryopreserved bone marrow.

3. Bone marrow, which has been previously frozen, is placed into container and shipped.

SUPPLIES AND REAGENTS

1. Liquid nitrogen in low-pressure supply cylinder, with phase separator nozzle

2. Hazardous goods declaration forms

3. Airway bill forms for shipping company

4. Label containing essential information regarding contents and recipient institution (see Fig. 12–1)

5. Liquid nitrogen label (Fig. 12–2)

EQUIPMENT

1. Insulated container of heavy construction, with capacity for at least 40 L of liquid

2. *(Recommended)* "Dry" shipping container (CryoMed, New Baltimore, MI)

PROCEDURE

1. Prepare the container 24 hours before shipment by filling at least halfway with liquid nitrogen. Replace the cover on the container and allow it to stand, while both of the following occur:
   A. The while liquid nitrogen will completely chill the inside of the tank
   B. In the dry shipper, the liquid nitrogen will soak into the sponge material in the bottom of the tank.

2. Make arrangements with shipping company for transport. Overnight courier services such as Airborne, Emory, Federal Express, or United Parcel Service Overnight Delivery* have the advantage of door-to-door service. However, the shipment must pass through many sets of hands and has a concomitantly greater risk of being incorrectly routed. (Such events are, however, exceedingly rare.) The commercial airlines have cargo services that offer very reliable delivery to destination. These services generally require that someone from the sending institution deliver the marrow to the airport and that someone from the receiving institution pick it up at the airport on the other end.

3. NECESSARY FORMS TO COMPLETE
   A. Airway bill
   B. Hazardous goods declaration (if using container with free liquid nitrogen)
   C. Customs declaration and invoice (if shipment is to cross an international border)

4. IMMEDIATELY PRIOR TO SHIPMENT
   A. *If using a container with free liquid nitrogen,* add additional liquid nitrogen so that the container is two-thirds full.
   B. *If using a dry shipper,* pour off any remaining free liquid nitrogen.

5. Place the marrow inside. Replace the cover on the tank and secure.

   NOTE: *Do not seal the cover airtight. Evaporating liquid nitrogen requires ventilation to prevent pressure buildup, which could blow the cover off the container.*

6. Turn shipper over to transportation company.

---

*These are in alphabetical order; no recommendation is to be inferred.

7. Upon receipt, receiving institution should remove frozen marrow from shipper and place in local low temperature freezing apparatus (liquid nitrogen storage banks, or ultralow freezers). Presence of liquid nitrogen still in freezer, or the temperature of the dry shipper should be verified.

8. The receiving center should notify the sender that the marrow has been received.

ANTICIPATED RESULTS	Bone marrow should arrive at recipient institution with liquid nitrogen still present in shipping containers. Dry shipper internal temperature should not exceed $-190°C$ at time of receipt.

NOTES

1. EXTREME CARE SHOULD BE EXERCISED WHEN HANDLING LIQUID NITROGEN. IF SPILLED ON SKIN OR SPLASHED IN EYES, LIQUID NITROGEN CAN CAUSE SEVERE BURNS. Properly insulated gloves and eye protection should always be worn whenever liquid nitrogen is present in the work area.

2. Following use, the shipping containers should be left open to allow them to dry out. Otherwise, water condensation will collect and eventually cause corrosion.

AUTHORS

Carlos E. Lee, M.T.
Bone Marrow Processing and
   Evaluation Laboratory
Bone Marrow Transplant Program
H. Lee Moffitt Cancer Center and
   Research Institute
University of South Florida
12902 Magnolia Dr.
Tampa, FL 33612-9497

William E. Janssen, Ph.D.
Bone Marrow Processing and
   Evaluation Laboratory
Bone Marrow Transplant Program
H. Lee Moffitt Cancer Center and
   Research Institute
University of South Florida
12902 Magnolia Dr.
Tampa, FL 33612-9497

REFERENCE

1. Janssen, WE, Gee, AP, and Graham-Pole, Jr: Transporting bone marrow for *in vitro* purging before autologous reinfusion. Prog Clin Biol Res 333:541, 1990.

RECOVERED RED BLOOD CELLS

REINFUSION OF BONE MARROW RED BLOOD CELLS TO THE PEDIATRIC MARROW DONOR

DESCRIPTION	The transfusion of homologous blood to bone marrow donors should be avoided whenever possible. Depending on the age of a pediatric bone marrow donor, it may not be feasible to obtain an autologous blood donation before the bone marrow harvest. To avoid the transfusion of banked blood, red blood cells can be recovered from the bone marrow and reinfused to the donor. This procedure involves centrifuging the bone marrow in an inverted position and withdrawing the red blood cells into a syringe. The red blood cells are then diluted with sterile saline and reinfused into the donor. The remaining marrow may be further processed before infusion.
TIME FOR PROCEDURE	Approximately 40 minutes, to remove red blood cells from 500 mL of bone marrow
SUMMARY OF PROCEDURE	1. Harvested bone marrow is delivered as soon as possible to the processing laboratory.
	2. The marrow is centrifuged in an inverted position for 10 minutes at $600g$ at $22°C$.
	3. The red blood cells are removed by syringe, placed in a transfer pack, and diluted with sterile saline to achieve a hematocrit (Hct) of 65 percent.
	4. The remaining marrow may be further processed if and as required, before infusion.
EQUIPMENT	1. Plasma extractor
	2. Laminar flow hood
	3. Centrifuge
SUPPLIES AND REAGENTS	1. 3 transfer packs (300-mL or 600-mL, depending on volume of bone marrow)
	2. 2 sampling site couplers
	3. Two 16-gauge $\times$ ¾-inch hypodermic needles
	4. Two 30-mL or 60-mL syringes
PROCEDURE	1. CENTRIFUGATION OF MARROW A. If necessary, transfer the marrow to an appropriately sized transfer pack to allow good separation of the red blood cells and plasma. B. Centrifuge the marrow in an inverted position for 10 minutes at $600g$ at $22°C$. 2. PREPARATION OF RED BLOOD CELLS FOR REINFUSION TO DONOR A. After centrifugation hang the marrow bag in an inverted position inside a laminar flow hood. B. Insert a sampling site coupler into one port of the transfer pack. C. Withdraw into a syringe 65 to 70 percent of the red cells in the bone marrow.

D. Insert a sampling site coupler into one port of a new transfer pack.

E. Transfer the marrow red cells from the syringe to the transfer pack. Determine the Hct of the red cells. Calculate the volume of sterile saline required to achieve a final Hct of 65 percent.

F. Remove an aliquot of marrow for a nucleated cell count. Calculate the total nucleated cells in the red cell preparation for donor reinfusion.

ANTICIPATED RESULTS	This procedure should yield 65 to 70 percent of the harvested marrow red blood cells for reinfusion to the donor. The original marrow volume should be decreased by 70 percent. The loss of nucleated cells should be less than 5 percent.
NOTES	1. Sampling for nucleated cell counts, cell cultures, or sterility will vary with each processing laboratory.
	2. In this procedure it is important to calculate the total nucleated cells contained in both the original marrow and in the red blood cells prior to reinfusion to the donor. This will ensure that there is no significant loss of nucleated cells.

AUTHORS

Carol Stanley, A.R.T.
British Columbia Children's
    Hospital
Vancouver, British Columbia
Canada

Sharon Herd, A.R.T.
British Columbia Children's
    Hospital
Vancouver, British Columbia
Canada

L.D. Wadsworth, MB, FRCP(C),
    FRCPath
British Columbia Children's
    Hospital
Vancouver, British Columbia
Canada

REFERENCE

1. Chan, KW, Stanley, CE, and Wadsworth, LD: Bone marrow collection from a 9.4 kg donor avoiding allogeneic blood transfusion (letter to editor). Transfusion 27:441, 1987.

WASHED RECOVERED AUTOLOGOUS RED BLOOD CELLS FROM BONE MARROW

DESCRIPTION	Red blood cells that are recovered from bone marrow for transplantation can be washed and returned to the bone marrow donor postoperatively. This may be of benefit to the donor when autologous units are not available. It also minimizes exposure to transfusion-transmitted infectious diseases in homologous blood products. Blood or blood components that are removed from a donor and stored for subsequent reinfusion are autologous units. Indications for washed recovered autologous red cell transfusions include the following: 1. Allogeneic bone marrow transplant donors with no previously donated autologous blood; donating to patients receiving ABO-incompatible transplants in which the red blood cells will not be used 2. Autologous bone marrow transplant patients unable to predeposit autologous blood
TIME FOR PROCEDURE	1 hour to wash, process, and crossmatch the recovered red blood cell unit.
SUMMARY OF PROCEDURE	1. Harvested bone marrow for transplantation is brought to the processing laboratory in one or two 1-L transfer packs. 2. The bone marrow is centrifuged and the buffy coat harvested. The remaining red blood cells are then washed three times with 0.9 percent normal saline. 3. The COBE 2991 is programmed according to the cell washing program (see step 2 under procedure). 4. The washed red blood cells are labeled, ABO/Rh confirmed, and the unit crossmatched with the recipient's serum before dispensing.
EQUIPMENT	COBE 2991 blood cell processor (COBE Laboratories, Lakewood, CO 80215)
SUPPLIES AND REAGENTS	1. COBE 2991 blood cell processor processing set (No. 912-64-819) 2. Two 1-L bags of 0.9 percent sodium chloride for intravenous (IV) infusion 3. COBE 2991 sampling site and access coupler 4. Tuberculin syringes with 16-gauge needles 5. Alcohol wipes 6. Blood culture bottles 7. Autologous washed red cell labels 8. Sealing clips or heat sealer 9. Hemostats
PROCEDURE	1. INSTALLATION OF COBE 2991 BLOOD PROCESSING SET AND PRIME A. Check hydraulic system prime on 2991 cell processor by the following steps:

(1) Turn the cell washer on.

(2) Press START/SPIN, and allow centrifuge to come to speed.

(3) Press SUPER-OUT. The excess pressure should light up and the alarm sound. Press STOP/RESET.

(4) Repeat steps 1A(1) through 1A(3). The instrument is now primed.

B. Install the set and prime.

(1) Take the set out of the bag and orient it according to the color-coded pinch valves on the front panel. Inspect the set for broken tamperproof caps. If any seal is broken, do not use the set.

(2) Lift the seal weight off the sliding cover's plastic blocks. Open the sliding covers on the machine.

(3) Remove the centrifuge cover by twisting it counterclockwise, while lifting up the circular locking plunger. When the cover tabs are free, lift the cover off.

(4) Slide the centrifuge cover in the holder at the base of the console. Roll the processing bag around the hexagonal seal and pass it through the center hole in the centrifuge cover.

(5) Install the blood processing bag in the centrifuge bowl by positioning the four holes in the bag over the four studs on the centrifuge. Make sure that the bag lies flat over the top of the centrifuge. Position the two white alignment blocks around the inlet stem of the blood processing bag.

(6) Place the bowl cover back on and rotate clockwise until the locking plunger falls. Close the sliding cover, and lower the seal weight. Snap the latex on top of the hexagonal seal into the circular slot at the top of the weight. The ready light should be on.

(7) Press TUBE LOAD.

(8) Push the clear tube into the slot of the red cell detector assembly. The tube must be inserted fully to the back of the slot.

(9) By moving the knobs from V1 through V3, insert the color-coded lines through the pinch valves. Press STOP/RESET.

(10) Place hemostats on the CLEAR line leading to the centrifuge bowl. Hang wash solutions from the GREEN and YELLOW lines.

(11) Clamp off blood line with hemostats and hang waste bag on the three studs on the left side of the machine.

2. MACHINE SETTINGS

Centrifuge Speed	Super-Out Rate	Minimum Agitate Time	Super-Out Volume	Valve Selector
3000	450	60 sec	600	N/A

Spin timer 1: 2½ minutes
Spin timer 2: 1½ minutes
Pump restore rate to 450 mL per minute*
Red cell override to 3.5*
AUTO/MANUAL: AUTO

*Controls found on circuit breaker panel—lower right side of machine.

CONTROL PANEL SETTINGS

	Timer Stop			Valve Stop			RCO STO*
	1	2	PC	1	2	3	RC
1	X	0	0	0	X	0	N/A
2	0	X	0	0	X	0	
3	0	X	0	0	0	X	
4	0	X	X				
5							
6							
7							

*RCO = Red cell override.

3. TO PREDILUTE RED BLOOD CELLS, DO THE FOLLOWING IN ORDER:
   A. Hook up the red blood cells to the red cell line on V1.
   B. Press PRE-DILUTE. Valves 1 and 2 will open and allow the wash solution to flow into the blood bag. Agitate the bag until approximately 100 to 200 mL have entered.

   NOTE: *The volume of wash solution needed to predilute will depend on the volume of red blood cells to be washed. Processing of cell volumes greater than 325 mL per wash precludes adequate washing.*

   C. Press STOP/RESET. This will close all valves.
   D. Hang the red blood cell bag on the left hanger bar.
   E. Remove the hemostat from the clear tube between the red blood cell detector and the rotating seal.

4. WASHING PROCEDURE
   A. Press BLOOD IN. This opens valve 1 and permits the red blood cells to flow into the centrifuge bowl.
   B. Press AIR OUT. This causes the centrifuge to spin and forces air out of the blood processing bag up into the blood container.
   C. When it appears that all the air is out, press BLOOD IN again. Any cells left in the bag or tube will then flow into the processing bag, filling the space formerly occupied by the air.

   CAUTION: *Do not press STOP/RESET while still in the AIR OUT operation. Press BLOOD IN first and allow the centrifuge to stop.*

   D. Press STOP/RESET.
   E. Press START/SPIN. The 2991 will now wash the unit automatically.
   F. When the audible alarm sounds after the final SUPER-OUT, press STOP/RESET. Place hemostats on the CLEAR line.
   G. To obtain red blood cells for compatibility testing (not quality assurance testing), seal along the clear tubing in several places to make segments. Label each one with the unit number assigned to the red blood cells.
   H. Cut the CLEAR line along the sealed end, and remove the processing set as follows:
      (1) Press TUBE LOAD and remove all tubing from each of the valves by using the valve selector switch.

  (2) Open the sliding clear cover and remove the bag with the washed red blood cells.

  (3) The washing process is now complete.

5. PRE-TRANSFUSION TESTING

 A. Specimen: A signed, dated, and timed clotted specimen from the recipient plus an integral segment from the autologous unit of red blood cells

 B. Reagents

  (1) Anti-A

  (2) Anti-B

  (3) Anti-D

 C. In accordance with American Association of Blood Banks (AABB) Standards, ABO/Rh type and antibody screen should have been performed on the patient's specimen in the blood bank. (This is usually performed the day before the bone marrow harvest.)

 D. Perform an ABO/Rh type on the segment made from the washed unit of red blood cells to reconfirm the unit's blood group.

 E. Perform compatibility testing with recipient's serum and donor red blood cells as required.

 F. After completing all the pre-transfusion testing, tag the unit as ready for transfusion. Place a washed red blood cell label on the unit of red cells, indicating the volume of red blood cells contained in the bag, the hematocrit of the recovered red blood cells, and the type of anticoagulant used. The label must also have a green "For Autologous Use Only" sticker placed in a prominent position on the unit (without covering any other labels) (Fig. 12–3).

 G. The transfusion tag should contain information concerning compatibility of the unit crossmatched, ABO/Rh types of the recipient and donor unit, date, time, and signature of the person performing the testing.

 H. The expiration date of the product should be 6 hours from the time of harvest (completed collection).

 I. The label used must also indicate:

  (1) Storage temperature of the product (1 to 6°C)

  (2) Infusion set must have a filter.

  (3) Federal law prohibits dispensing without a prescription.

  (4) Properly identified intended recipient.

  (5) See circular of information for the use of human blood and blood components.

   WARNING: *The risk of transmitting bloodborne diseases is present. No warranties are made or created. Warranties of fitness or merchantability are excluded.*

  (6) ABO retested and confirmed

  (7) Institution's name and address, and Food and Drug Administration (FDA) registration number

6. QUALITY CONTROL

 A. Measure the patient's pre- and post-transfusion Hgb and Hct levels to determine possible increase in Hgb of at least 10 g per L (1 g per dL) and in Hct of 0.3 (3 percent).

RED BLOOD CELLS, WASHED

ABO RETESTED
AND CONFIRMED

Contains_____ ml, collected as_____ ml of Bone
Marrow in_____ ml of Heparin in RPMI 1640
Wash with 0.9% Sodium Choride, Injection, U.S.P.
Expiration Date_____Hour_____

_____
Tech

CAUTIONS:
1. Store between 1 and 6C.
2. Infusion set must have a filter.
3. Federal law prohibits dispensing without a prescription.
4. **Properly identify intended recipient.**
5. See Circular of Information for the Use of Human Blood and Blood Components.
6. WARNING: THE RISK OF TRANSMITTING BLOOD BORNE DISEASES IS PRESENT. NO WARRANTIES OF FITNESS OR MERCHANTABILITY ARE EXCLUDED.
7. **Volunteer Donor.**

_____
Date

_____
Donor Number

Group/Rh

PREPARED BY
BONE MARROW LABORATORY
TRANSFUSION MEDICINE
MUSC MEDICAL CENTER
CHARLESTON, SOUTH CAROLINA 29425-0701
Registration # 1077157

A

EXPIRES

_____

FOR AUTOLOGOUS
USE ONLY
Reserved for

NAME _____
PATIENT ID# _____
HOSPITAL _____
ABO/Rh _ _____
COLLECTION ON _____
REMARKS _____

_____

B

FIGURE 12–3   Labels for red blood cells recovered from bone marrow.

     B. Measure Hct level of the washed unit to ensure Hct does not exceed 80 percent.
     C. Draw blood cultures to ascertain that sterility has been maintained.
     D. An optional quality control test is that of osmotic fragility of the red cells transfused.

7. RECORDS
   A. Date and time of collection
   B. Records of unique numbers assigned to all units.
   C. A record of components prepared from each bone marrow received for processing.
   D. All results of donor and recipient testing must be kept available for a minimum of 5 years.

AUTHORS

Ruth E. Ross, M.H.S., M.T.(ASCP), S.B.B.
Medical University of South Carolina
Charleston, SC 29425

Robert K. Stuart, M.D.
Medical University of South Carolina
Charleston, SC 29425

Elaine K. Jeter, M.D.
Medical University of South Carolina
Charleston, SC 29425

REFERENCES

1. COBE 2991 Model 1, Blood Cell Processor, Operations Manual, Lakewood, CO, 1983.
2. AABB Standards for Blood Banks and Transfusion Services, ed 13, Arlington, VA, 1991.
3. FDA Code of Federal Regulations, ed 21., Washington, DC, April 1990.

4-Hydroperoxycyclophosphamide (4-HC): A cytotoxic derivative of cyclophosphamide that does not require metabolic activation; it is effective in in vitro systems

Agar: Organic material used widely for in vitro cultures of hematopoietic cells

Agglutination: Formation of conglomerates of cells owing to the binding of multivalent antibodies

Allogeneic: Originating from a donor of the same species but genotypically nonidentical with the recipient

Allograft: A graft or transplant from an allogeneic donor

Apheresis: Generally the removal of a blood component, either cellular or noncellular in composition, from the circulation

Aplastic anemia: Severe bone marrow failure usually involving cells of all lineages

Aseptic technique: A technique involving sterile conditions

Autologous (also Authochtonous): Originating from the same individual

Autograft: A graft or transplant from the same individual; that is, the patient serving as his or her own donor (by definition, not a transplant but rather a reimplantation or reinfusion)

Backup marrow: A certain number of marrow cells, preserved, usually in frozen state, to infuse into the patient in case the initially infused marrow does not function satisfactorily

Blast-forming unit—erythroid (BFU-E): Description of a precursor cell of the red blood cell lineage which in vitro forms daughter cells arranged in form of a burst

Buffy coat: The white blood cell layer obtained when centrifuging whole blood

Cell washer: A machine used to remove soluble material—in particular, antibodies from a cell suspension or blood cell preparation

Chemoseparation: Separation or generally elimination of a subpopulation of cells from a cell suspension (usually marrow) by means of incubation with a chemical (for example, glucocorticoids or 4-hydroperoxycyclophosphamide)

Clonogenic: The capacity of cells—often malignant cells—to form daughter cells (i.e., not a terminally differentiated cell)

Cluster of differentiation 34 (CD34): An antigen expressed preferentially on very early multipotent hematopoietic precursor cells, possibly the true stem cells

Colony-forming unit—erythroid (CFU-E): A more differentiated precursor than BFU-E, forming only erythroid elements in culture

Colony-forming unit—granulocyte, erythroid, megakaryocyte, macro-

phage (CFU-GEMM): Hematopoietic precursor cells that in vitro form colonies containing cells of the four lineages indicated

Colony-forming unit—granulocyte, macrophage (CFU-GM): A precursor cell that in vitro forms cells of both granulocytic and macrophage morphology

Colony-stimulating factor: Any one of a number of peptides able to stimulate the growth of hematopoietic colonies in vitro

Complement: A multicomponent enzyme system involved in the lysis of cells

Controlled-rate freezing: Freezing of biologic material at a predetermined rate; that is, a decrease in temperature usually of 1° per minute

Corrected marrow nucleated cell count: Used after bone marrow harvest to describe the number of cells that remain in the aspirate after subtracting the number of cells that would be contained in an identical volume of peripheral blood

Counterflow centrifugation: A centrifuge separation method by which cells are being separated owing to centrifugal forces, as well as size and density in a physiologic environment

Cryopreservation: The preservation of material in a frozen state

Cytokine: A soluble substance mediating signals between different or the same cell populations (e.g., interleukin-1, interleukin-2)

Cytopenia: Literally the lack of cells; abnormally low blood cell counts

Density gradient: A gradient formed by materials of different density either in a discontinuous or in a continuous fashion

Differential: A jargon word usually used to describe a white blood cell count with the relative proportion of cells of different morphology in the total cell number

Differentiation: The development of cells according to different lineages with different morphology and different functions

Dimethyl sulfoxide (DMSO): A cryoprotectant; a chemical used together with tissue culture media to suspend cells in order to protect them against injury that otherwise would be sustained during the cryopreservation process

DNAse: An enzyme that digests DNA

Elutriation: See **Counterflow centrifugation.**

Engraftment: A term describing the fact that donor-derived cells have succeeded in establishing themselves in the recipient to produce daughter cells

Etoposide (VP16): A cytotoxic agent (a topoisomerase inhibitor), a component of numerous chemotherapeutic regimens including those used in preparation for bone marrow transplantation; also used for chemoseparation of bone marrow cells

Ex vivo: Describing material obtained from a patient or an experimental animal for work in vitro; some investigators use the term interchangeably with in vitro; others more correctly differentiate between in vitro (i.e., work with normal cells in an in vitro setting) and ex vivo (i.e., work with cells obtained from individuals who are undergoing a certain treatment, the effect of which cannot be determined in vivo but rather after removal of appropriate material from the subject for testing in vitro)

Ficoll-Hypaque: A material used for density gradients

Flow cytometry (cytofluorometry): Broadly used for the analysis of cells by automated machines determining size, composition of cells, phenotype, and other features

Fluorescein: One agent used to stain cells (usually after attachment to an antibody) so that they can be recognized with a fluorescence microscope or so that they can be used for fluorescence activated cell sorting

Fluorescence-activated cell sorter (FACS): A computerized machine capable of analyzing and separating cells on the basis of fluorescent signals emitted by the cells themselves or by antibodies attached to the cells

Graft-versus-host (GVH) disease: Manifestations of the reaction of grafted donor cells against host tissue; clinical picture classically involving the skin, liver, and intestinal tract, with other organs possibly affected

Graft-versus-leukemia (GVL) effect: The effect of donor-derived cells against leukemic cells in the recipient that cannot be accounted for by radiochemotherapy effects

Granulocyte macrophage—colony-stimulating factor (GM-CSF): A peptide capable of stimulating bone marrow or blood cells to form CFU-GM

Granulocyte—colony-stimulating factor (G-CSF): A peptide or growth factor stimulating the formation of granulocytic colonies

Harvest: In the setting of bone marrow transplantation, usually used to describe the collection of bone marrow cells or peripheral blood stem cells to be used for transplantation

Hematopoietic: Pertaining to the production of blood

Hemacytometer: A counting chamber used in the laboratory to determine the number of leukocytes or red blood cells in a blood sample

Hemopoietic: See **Hematopoietic**

Histocompatibility: Referring to the similarity of tissues between different individuals, the best-known histocompatibility antigens being those of the major histocompatibility complex, termed HLA in humans (other systems less well defined)

Hydroxyethyl starch: A chemical used for mobilization and separation of leukocytes, as well as in some cryopreservation techniques

Immunocompetent: Referring to the ability of an individual to mount normal responses to foreign antigens

Immunophenotype: The type of a cell determined by immunologic methods—usually the use of monoclonal antibodies recognizing cell surface structures

Immunotoxin: Used to describe hybrid molecules usually consisting of a monoclonal antibody and a toxin conjugated to it that is capable of killing cells

Incompatibility, major: ABO incompatibily such that the recipient of a graft may have antibodies against donor cells

Incompatibility, minor: ABO incompatibility such that the donor of a graft (or transfusion) may have antibodies against recipient cells

Interleukin-2 (IL-2): A cytokine released by a subpopulation of T-lymphocytes capable of stimulating itself or other T cells

Inverted microscope: A microscope with relatively limited magnification used to count colonies of cells in suspension or semisolid media

In vitro: Referring to the work on tissue or cells outside the individual from which they were obtained

In vivo: Pertaining to a living patient or experimental animal

Isohemagglutinin: A term used to describe antibodies reactive with major blood group antigens (AB)

Lectin: A plant extract (occasionally also chemical obtained from lower animals) that has been found to bind the mammalian cells and either stimulates them into proliferation or allows to separate them on the basis of binding characteristics

Leukapheresis: The removal of leukocytes (see also **Apheresis**)

Liquid nitrogen: Nitrogen in the liquid state because of extremely low temperatures

Limiting dilution analysis (LDA): A laboratory assay in which the examination of progressively lower concentrations of cells allows for the determination of the frequency of certain precursor cells (for example, cytotoxic T cells) of interest

Mafosfamide (Asta Z): A cyclophosphamide derivative similar to 4-hydroperoxycyclophosphamide, which is active in vitro

Methylcellulose: An organic chemical used to grow hematopoietic cells in vitro

Microsphere: Referring to microscopically small particles of organic material that may have magnetic properties (magnetic microspheres)

Monoclonal antibody (MAb): An antibody generated usually by a hybridoma obtained by fusion of a mouse, rat, or occasional human myeloma cell line and specifically sensitized lymphocytes usually from the same species

Mononuclear cell: Usually referring to blood and marrow cells other than granulocytes and erythrocytes

Nucleated cell: All cells other than red blood cells (and platelets)

Pancytopenia: Abnormally low counts in all cell lineages (see also **Cytopenia**)

Peripheral blood stem cell (PBSC): A hematopoietic cell with multilineage potential obtained from peripheral blood rather than from bone marrow

PHA-LCM: A lymphocyte-conditioned medium obtained by stimulating lymphocytes with PHA

Phytohemagglutinin (PHA): A lectin used to stimulate lymphocytes

Pluripotent: Capable of producing daughter cells of different lineages

Precursor: An early ancestor of a given cell

Progenitor: See **Precursor**

Proliferation: The production of new cells from a given precursor

Purge: Describing the removal of one or several cell populations from a cell suspension

Rebound phase: Usually referring to a period following chemotherapy, during which certain precursor cells are present in an increased frequency in peripheral blood (and possibly bone marrow)

Recovery: In the context of bone marrow transplant, often referring to the gradual increase of lymphohematopoietic cells after transplantation

Ricin (composed of A and B chain): One of the toxins used to prepare immunotoxins

Rosette: Generally referring to the phenomenon of the attachment of one cell population (e.g., sheep red blood cells) to another population (e.g., human T lymphocytes)

Sedimentation: The gradual settling down of cells by gravity

Steady state: A state in vitro or in vivo at which given concentrations or numbers do not change significantly

Stem cell: The cell thought to be capable of producing all necessary components in a given tissue

Stem cell culture: Culture system aimed at discovering the earliest possible precursor cell

Supernatant: Fluid components in culture systems produced in part by the cells in suspension

Syngeneic: Referring to genetically identical individuals (i.e., identical twins); also called monozygotic.

T cell: A lymphocyte subpopulation that requires a functional thymus for normal development

T lymphocyte: See **T cell**

Tissue culture: Broadly referring to the assay and propagation of cells and tissues in an artificial laboratory environment

Tissue culture media: Suspension fluids containing all necessary ingredients to allow the survival of tissue or cells

Tritiated thymidine: A DNA precursor to which ^{3}H is attached that is used to label proliferating cells in vitro

Trypan blue: A dye that is usually taken up only by nonviable cells and excluded by viable cells

Vascular access: Referring to means of easily obtaining blood or transfusing blood components or medications into the circulation

AMERICAN TYPE CULTURE
COLLECTION (ATCC)
12301 Parklawn Dr.
Rockville, MD 20852
800-638-6597

AMERSHAM CORPORATION
2636 S. Clearbrook Dr.
Arlington Heights, IL 60005
800-323-0668

AMGEN BIOLOGICALS
Amgen Center
Thousand Oaks, CA 91320-1789
800-343-7475

APPLIED IMMUNE SCIENCES,
INC.
200 Constitution Dr.
Menlo Park, CA 94025-1109
415-326-7302

BARNANT COMPANY
28W092 Commercial Ave.
Barrington, IL 60010
312-381-7050

BAXTER HEALTHCARE
CORPORATION
Fenwal Div.
1425 Lake Cook Rd.
Deerfield, IL 60015
312-940-5000

BECKMAN INSTRUMENTS, INC.
200 S. Kraemer Blvd.
Brea, CA 92621
800-526-3821

BECTON DICKINSON
IMMUNOCYTOMETRY
SYSTEMS
2350 Qume Dr.
San Jose, CA 95131-1893
800-223-8226

BIO-RAD
Chemical Div.
1414 Harbour Way S.
Richmond, CA 94804
415-232-7000

BOEHRINGER MANNHEIM
BIOCHEMICALS
P.O. Box 50816
Indianapolis, IN 46250-0414
800-428-5433

CHARTERMED, INC.
120 Albany St.
P.O. Box 2623
New Brunswick, NJ 08903
201-249-9393

CISUS, INC.
1983 Marcus Ave.
Lake Success, NY 11042
516-326-8008

COBE LABORATORIES, INC.
1185 Oak St.
Lakewood, CO 80215
302-232-6800

CORNING GLASS WORKS
Corning, NY 14831
607-737-1640

COULTER ELECTRONICS, INC.
P.O. Box 2145
Hialeah, FL 33012-0145
800-327-6531

CRYOMED
51529 Birch St.
New Baltimore, MI 48047
313-725-4614

465

CUTTER BIOLOGICAL
4th and Parker Sts.
P.O. Box 1986
Berkeley, CA 94701
800-227-1762

DIFCO LABORATORIES
P.O. Box 331058
Detroit, MI 48232-7058
800-521-0851

DRUMMOND SCIENTIFIC
COMPANY
Broomall, PA 19008
800-523-7480

DUPONT COMPANY
BIOTECHNOLOGY SYSTEMS
P.O. Box 80024
Wilmington, DE 19880-0024
800-551-2121

DUPONT CRITICAL CARE, INC.
1600 Waukegan Rd.
Waukegan, IL 60085
800-323-4980

FALCON LABWARE
Becton Dickinson Labware
2 Bridgewater La.
Lincoln Park, NJ 07035
800-235-5953

FORMA SCIENTIFIC, INC.
P.O. Box 649
Millcreek Rd.
Marietta, OH 45750
800-848-3080

TERRY FOX LABORATORY
British Columbia Cancer Research
Centre
601 West 10th Ave.
Vancouver, BC V5Z IL3
Canada
604-877-6070

GAMBRO, INC.
600 Knightsbridge Pky.
Lincolnshire, IL 60069
312-634-0004

GIBCO LABORATORIES
Life Technology, Inc.
Grand Island, NY 14072
800-828-6686

HAEMONETICS CORPORATION
400 Wood Rd.
Braintree, MA 02184
617-848-7100

HYCLONE LABORATORIES, INC.
1725 South State Hwy. 89–91
Logan, UT 84321
800-492-5663

ICN BIOMEDICALS, INC.
Research Products Division
P.O. Box 5023
Costa Mesa, CA 92626
800-854-0530

LABCONCO CORPORATION
8811 Prospect
Kansas City, MO 64132
816-333-8811

LAB-LINE INSTRUMENTS, INC.
15th and Bloomingdale Aves.
Melrose Park, IL 60160
800-323-0257

LEE MEDICAL, LTD.
P.O. Box 24288
Minneapolis, MN 55424
612-931-9600

MILLIPORE PRODUCTS
Millipore Corp.
Bedford, ME 01730
800-225-1380

MVE CRYOGENICS
407 7th St. N.E.
New Prague, MN 56071
612-758-8252

METTLER INSTRUMENT
CORPORATION
Box 71
Hightstown, NJ 08520
609-448-3000

NALGE COMPANY
P.O. Box 20365
Rochester, NY 14602-0365
716-586-8800

NORDION INTERNATIONAL,
  INC.
447 March Rd.
P.O. Box 13500
Kanata, Ontario
Canada K2K 1X8
613-592-2790

NOVA PHARMACEUTICAL
  CORPORATION
6200 Freeport Centre
Baltimore MD 21224-2788
301-522-7000

OLYMPUS CORPORATION
Precision Instrument Div.
4 Nevada Dr.
Lake Success, NY 11042-1179
516-488-3880

ORGANON TEKNIKA
  CORPORATION
100 Akzo Ave.
Durham, NC 27704
800-682-2666

PHARMACIA ENI
  DIAGNOSTICS, INC.
8310 Guilford Road
Columbia, MD 21046
800-346-4364

PRECISION SCIENTIFIC, INC.
337 W. Cortland St.
Chicago, IL 60647
312-227-2660

RESEARCH INDUSTRIES
  CORPORATION
Pharmaceutical Div.
Salt Lake City, UT 84119

ROBBINS SCIENTIFIC
1280 Space Park Way
Mountain View, CA 94043
800-752-8585

SEBRA ENGINEERING AND
  RESEARCH ASSOCIATES, INC.
Era Plaza
500 North Tucson Blvd.
Tucson, AZ 85716
602-881-6555

SIGMA CHEMICALS
P.O. Box 14508
St. Louis, MO 63178
800-325-3010

SQUIBB-MARSAM, INC.
34 Olney Ave., Bldg. 31
Cherry Hill, NJ 08034
609-424-8282

STERICON, INC.
2315 Gardner Rd.
Broadview, IL 60153
708-865-8790

STRECO
P.O. Box 636
New Baltimore, MI 48057
313-949-2060

TAYLOR-WHARTON
  CRYOGENICS
P.O. Box 568
Theodore, AL 36509
800-428-3304

TEMPSHIELD, INC.
232 Main St.
Wakefield, MA 01880
617-245-0790

UNIVERSITY OF WASHINGTON
Scientific Instrument Div.
T 283 Health Science Bldg SB-73
Seattle, WA 98195
206-543-5580

WHITTAKER M.A.
  BIOPRODUCTS, INC.
P.O. Box 127
Biggs Ford Rd.
Walkersville, MD 21793-0127
301-898-7025

CARL ZEISS, INC.
One Zeiss Dr.
Thornwood, NY 10594
914-747-1800

INDEX

A "T" following a page number indicates a table; an "F" indicates a figure.

BRITISH COLUMBIA CANCER AGENCY
LIBRARY
600 WEST 10th AVE.
VANCOUVER, B.C.   CANADA
V5Z 4E6

BRITISH COLUMBIA CANCER AGENCY
LIBRARY
600 WEST 10th AVE.
VANCOUVER, B.C. CANADA
V5Z 4E6